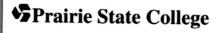
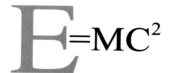

D1087178

# HANDBOOK OF AFRICAN AMERICAN HEALTH

# Handbook of African American Health

*Edited by*
ROBERT L. HAMPTON
THOMAS P. GULLOTTA
RAYMOND L. CROWEL

*Research Assistant*
JESSICA M. RAMOS

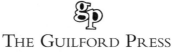

THE GUILFORD PRESS
New York          London

© 2010 The Guilford Press
A Division of Guilford Publications, Inc.
72 Spring Street, New York, NY 10012
www.guilford.com

Printed in the United States of America

This book is printed on acid-free paper.

Last digit is print number:   9   8   7   6   5   4   3   2   1

The authors have checked with sources believed to be reliable in their efforts to provide information
that is complete and generally in accord with the standards of practice that are accepted at the time
of publication. However, in view of the possibility of human error or changes in medical sciences,
neither the authors, nor the editors and publisher, nor any other party who has been involved in
the preparation or publication of this work warrants that the information contained herein is in
every respect accurate or complete, and they are not responsible for any errors or omissions or the
results obtained from the use of such information. Readers are encouraged to confirm the information
contained in this book with other sources.

**Library of Congress Cataloging-in-Publication Data**

Handbook of African American health / edited by Robert L. Hampton, Thomas P. Gullotta,
Raymond L. Crowel.
    p. ; cm.
  Includes bibliographical references and index.
  ISBN 978-1-60623-716-8 (hardcover : alk. paper)
  1. African Americans—Health and hygiene.  2. African Americans—Medical care.  I. Hampton,
Robert L.   II. Gullotta, Thomas P., 1948–   III. Crowel, Raymond L.
  [DNLM: 1. African Americans—United States.  2. Health Status—United States.  3. African
Americans—psychology—United States.   4. Health Services Accessibility—United States.
WA 300 AA1 H236 2010]
  RA448.5.N4H3634 2010
  362.1089′96073—dc22
                                                                                    2009053381

# Preface

This is a book about African Americans: their physical health, their emotional health, and their living environment. The interplay among these three entwined conditions is responsible for the overall health status of this population, and that health status is wanting in many areas. We should note right up front that this volume is intended less to be read by African Americans who live its story every day than by those who would seek to change the reality found within its pages. What is that reality? One story lays bare the challenge that faces health care providers.

That story relates to an episode in American public health history that for African Americans is known simply as "Tuskegee." It began in 1932, when the U.S. Public Health Service funded a study on African American males infected with syphilis. At that time, treatments for syphilis included inducement of fevers and the administration of derivatives of mercury as well as arsenic to destroy the bacteria responsible for the disease. None of these treatments were particularly effective, and each had serious health-harming side effects. Thus, the Tuskegee health study sought to answer the question, Is it less harmful to leave syphilis untreated? Toward this end, the research team recruited 399 poor black sharecroppers infected with syphilis and observed the course of their disease, but did not treat it, for the next 40 years. During that time, these individuals unknowingly infected their wives and partners and fathered children born with congenital syphilis. To add insult to injury, by 1947, 25 years before this study was closed, penicillin was the recognized drug of choice for treating syphilis, and it worked! Thus, not for a quarter of a century, until a white Public Health Service employee, Peter Buxtum, went public, did this travesty end. The outcome of this experiment can be summed up in a single word: mistrust.

For African Americans, Tuskegee became instantaneously synonymous with and representative of a multitude of hurtful practices directed against them and others in our society. Tuskegee equated to harm, harm committed against a group of people by those who should be helping them (medical professionals, counselors) and harm against African Americans by their government. That harm could be unmistakable, as in the sterilization of thousands of women without their consent or knowledge (Roberts, 1997), or, we hope, unintentional, with government welfare practices that sought to assist families in need but established entitlement rules that discouraged black males from "manning up" to their familial responsibilities. Those who did man up did so secretly. Thus, a huge game born in the days of slavery was given new life, one in which deception of authority was necessary for many to survive. Government had become the new overseer. The plantation, without the scenery, was the housing project, and child protective services, with its authority to divide and reunite biological kin, became the new "master." As readers will soon discover, these and other experiences set the stage for the interaction that many African Americans have with helping professionals and the institutions from which they emerge.

To share this story and discuss what can be done to begin to correct these practices, we have divided this volume into two sections to enable the reader to gain an understanding of (1) the barriers that exist between the health care system and African Americans' access to appropriate physical and mental health services and (2) specific issues and general issues of concern. The talented writing teams of scholars who tackled these chapters do not represent a single academic discipline. Thus, the examination of issues and the discussion that follows represent broad and diverse points of view. Even so, readers, if they don the hat of a qualitative investigator, will discern several recurring themes across chapters and disciplines: a fundamental distrust of the establishment and its behavioral and physical health care system; a unity emerging from that distrust that places a high value on the family or, more appropriately, the extended family; and a spiritual but not necessarily a religious underpinning to the worldview that African Americans possess.

Given that this book is intended for graduate students and professionals working in research and practice settings with African American populations, the first chapter, by Briscoe and his associates, examines the strengths of African Americans and an approach to enlisting their support of community research. Chapter 2, by Williams-Washington, begins to place in historical context the barriers that African Americans have needed to overcome and the cost of these impediments to their health. In the chapter that follows, Millet and his associates describe one of the defining moments in African Americans' relationship with health care professions and the American government. The infamous Tuskegee experiment on a group of African American men and, by default, their partners is as sick and perverted an action against a group of people as the prewar German extermination of individuals, "justified" as "the destruction of lives devoid of value" (Chorover, 1979, p. 6).

Chapter 4, by Cook, offers an outstanding examination of the strength and benefit that spirituality offers to African Americans. The role of church as teacher, organizer, and spiritual force is discussed. This is followed by Chao's discussion of how African Americans have prospered under the most trying of circumstances.

The next three chapters examine health-altering interventions. Harvey and his colleagues compare behavioral health models with the scant evidence that exists on their effectiveness among African Americans. The authors offer readers suggestions for where the field and practitioners might go to be more helpful. The next chapter, by Henderson, looks at the growing use of medication in the treatment of behavioral health concerns and the issues this creates for African Americans. In the last chapter in Part I, Simmons and Vaughn focus not on the constructive engagement and enlistment of groups, as does the first chapter, but rather on engaging the individual in a therapeutic, helpful relationship.

The second part of this volume moves away from this more global perspective to focus instead on specific problematic medical concerns. Chapters 9, by Figaro and colleagues; 10, by Cloutier; 11, by Figaro and her associates; 12, by Hennekens and colleagues; and 13, by Beech, examine obesity, asthma, diabetes, cardiovascular disease, and cancer, respectively. Individual, familial, and community factors underlying each disease are examined and best-practice recommendations offered. This is followed by Gilreath and her colleagues' discussion of tobacco use and its contribution to the poorer health outcomes of individuals with the aforementioned and other health issues.

The next chapters focus on behavioral disorders, beginning with anxiety. In the chapter by Neal-Barnett and her colleagues, the authors review the ways in which this behavior can manifest itself and present approaches to successful management. In Chapter 16, Duval-Harvey and Rogers examine attention-deficit/hyperactivity disorder and its occurrence among African American school-age youth. The authors provide readers with several recommendations for best practice in treating this disorder.

Beginning with Chapter 17, on major depressive disorder, by Bailey and his associates, and extending to Chapter 18, on schizophrenia, by Lawson and Gage, and Chapter 19, on suicide, by Barnes, the emphasis moves from a diagnostic perspective to a wider social environmental view. In each of these chapters, the authors describe the African American community's perception of the disorder and the perception of the predominantly non-African American treatment community's view of their clientele. The issues of stigma, mistrust, misdiagnosis, and lack of access to appropriate care are recurrent themes.

This volume concludes with three chapters examining different aspects of violence. In Chapter 20, Harden and White focus on violence against children, while La Taillade and her colleagues, in Chapter 21, devote their attention to violence against domestic partners. In each chapter, the authors cast a broad net investigating the multitude of factors that contribute to these behaviors before offering readers best-practice advice. The final chapter, by Burris-Kitchen, also deals with the subject of violence and imprisonment. It is the incarceration of

African Americans in numbers that defy reason that fuels continued mistrust and suspicion, causing the blindfold over the eyes of justice as she holds her balance to slip a wee bit when people of color stand before her.

In Hampton and Gullotta's epilogue, the editors find hope that the issues examined in this volume will heighten awareness and concern, but also sobering evidence that the recommendations put forward as best practices will not be easily implemented. The journey begun in 1776 toward a unique society, one in which all men and later women are created equal, continues with examples of both progress and failure but with continued hope ever present.

African American scholars will not find much that is either surprising or new in this volume, but this book is not intended for them. Rather, this work is meant for those not of color who in their practices will need to forge that elusive partnership that results in the therapeutic relationship leading to improved health. To achieve this outcome, practitioners cannot ignore the past nor can African Americans remain fixated on what has been and, in too many instances, continues to be. Instead, as this book illustrates, a new beginning founded on promising although tentative findings in many areas of research and practice can mean a better, healthier life for African Americans.

## REFERENCES

Chorover, S. L. (1979). *From genesis to genocide: The meaning of human nature and the power of behavior control.* Cambridge, MA: MIT Press.

Roberts, D. (1997). *Killing the black body.* New York: Random House.

# Contents

# PART I

# Foundations of African American Health

# 1

# The Strengths and Challenges Facing African Americans

*Building Culturally Competent Practices with Communities and Families*

RICHARD BRISCOE
GWEN McCLAIN
TERESA NESMAN
JESSICA MAZZA
MAXINE WOODSIDE

## BACKGROUND

Many of the strengths in the African American community have enabled families and communities to overcome the various challenges present in today's society (Hill, 1999, 2003). These strengths include high achievement orientation, strong kinship bonds, strong religious orientation, and a strong work orientation (Hill, 1972, 1999, 2003). Strengthening African American families requires empowering and mobilizing community residents to increase their knowledge of their own strengths, natural supports, and resources. It also requires increasing their capacity to promote, develop, and implement their own approaches in collaboration with community partners (Briscoe, Keller, McClain, Best, & Mazza, 2009). Those seeking to improve the well-being of African American families need to play an active role in improving research and interventions by increasing their understanding of African American family strengths, culturally competent community based practices, and communitywide interventions.

3

As we look at the African American family in the new millennium, we can observe the economic, social, and political challenges that continue to prevent the healthy development of children and families (McAdoo, 1998; Morial, 2005; Tucker, 1999). Disparities are ever present for African American communities in the areas of health, mental health, and educational practices (U.S. Census Bureau, 2007). Challenges faced by African American families include a declining rate of marriage, a high prevalence of children being raised in single-parent homes, and high levels of adolescent pregnancy (Black, Dubowitz, & Starr, 1999). Disparities in poverty rates and levels of unemployment and overrepresentation of African Americans in the correctional system further compound these challenges (National Association for the Advancement of Colored People [NAACP], 2006; Toldson & Scott, 2006).

## PURPOSE OF THIS CHAPTER

There is a growing body of literature promoting best practices for community-based efforts to improve a range of health behaviors and outcomes for African Americans (Baker, Homan, & Keuter, 1999; Eisinger & Senturia, 2001; Fawcett, Paine-Andrews, & Schultz, 2000). These efforts can improve service delivery for African American children and their families by incorporating specific culturally competent approaches. Although there are multiple perspectives on how to be responsive to the cultural background of African American families and communities, strategies must ensure that all dimensions of research and service delivery are culturally competent. Culturally competent service systems are those that have a high degree of compatibility between the cultural and linguistic characteristics of a community's population and the organization's policies, structures, and processes so that disparities in access, availability, and utilization of services are reduced (Hernandez, Nesman, Isaacs, Callejas, & Mowery, 2006).

This chapter presents four critical components and offers 10 guidelines for the development of a culturally competent approach when partnering with African American families and communities. These components and guidelines can be implemented to enhance the development, refinement, and effectiveness of meaningful relationships with African American community members, human service agencies, planning bodies, foundations, universities and colleges, and community organizations. A key emphasis of the framework is the need to mobilize the African American community to improve service delivery and achieve successful outcomes. The framework also demonstrates the importance of having knowledge about African American cultures in order to inform best practices. This knowledge should include identifying strengths within the African American population, discovering resiliency and protective factors, and identifying natural supports. This chapter offers a guide for developing a culturally competent approach through the implementation of multidimensional strategies, beginning with an understanding of and mobilization of the African American community.

## STRENGTHS OF AFRICAN AMERICANS

African Americans have faced the challenges of slavery, segregation, racism, and discrimination, all of which culminate in specific economic, cultural, psychological, and social stressors (Hines & Boyd-Franklin, 1982; Tucker, 1999). African American families have developed natural supports, resources, and institutions to buffer these challenges and cope with multiple stressors (Bagley & Carroll, 1998; Coner-Edwards & Spurlock, 1988; McAdoo, 1988). Kinship patterns and religious orientations are cultural strengths based in the African culture that have been handed down through the generations. In addition, strengths such as adaptable family roles have been developed through reactive responses to racial or economic oppression associated with the institution of slavery and its aftermath (McDaniel, 1990; Slaughter & McWorter, 1985).

Hill (1972, 1999, 2003) focused on African American family strengths, defining these as traits that facilitate a family's ability to meet the needs of its members and the demands placed upon it by systems outside the family unit. Five important strengths in African American families identified by Hill (2003) include:

1. High achievement orientation

2. Strong work orientation

3. Adaptability of family roles

4. Strong kinship bonds

5. Strong religious orientations

Family strengths are identified as critical resources for the multisystemic needs of the African American community and fundamental supports for educational, health, political, civic, and economic survival (Hill, 1972, 1999, 2003). Hill (2003) further suggests the need for concerted efforts by policymakers and program planners to identify and promote solutions and strategies for African American families that build on and reinforce their strengths.

## EXAMINING CURRENT CHALLENGES
## OF AFRICAN AMERICAN FAMILIES AND COMMUNITIES

Current trends indicate disparities between African Americans and other racial/ethnic groups in terms of income, employment, physical and mental health, and education (NAACP, 2006). Other social issues such as welfare reform, racism, immigration, and urban renewal also contribute to these disparities (Hill, 2003). The current challenges faced by African American families and communities can be a complex set of interrelated factors that make addressing the disparities difficult. Disparities in socioeconomic status for African American families, for example, are strongly related to other challenges in these communities (Brooks-Gunn & Duncan, 1997).

## Socioeconomic Challenges

Poverty is a risk factor for many African Americans, leading to poor physical and mental health outcomes, drug use/abuse, childhood abuse/neglect, and inequities in education (Brooks-Gunn & Duncan, 1997; NAACP, 2006). Approximately 40% of African American families and 30% of African American children live below the poverty line (Toldson & Scott, 2006). A high unemployment rate (> 11%), nearly double that of other racial groups, contributes to the economic disparity (NAACP, 2006; Toldson & Scott, 2006). Furthermore, data show that African Americans earn, on average, $13,000 less than other ethnic/racial groups (NAACP, 2006). These factors, along with a low percentage of homeownership and financial assets, place African American individuals and families at a significantly increased risk of poverty-related challenges. Poverty and the growing challenges of welfare practice continue to have a deleterious effect on the individual, family, and community values of African Americans. The marriage rate is declining, single parenthood is on the rise (Black et al., 1999), and the rate of adolescent pregnancy is higher among the African American community than any other population (Moore & Chase-Lansdale, 2001).

## Health Challenges

Children and families in poverty are at a higher risk of morbidity and mortality (Klevens & Luman, 2001). As of 2000, the mortality rates for African American infants and adults was double that for Whites (NAACP, 2006). Furthermore, there are low rates of vaccinations among children in ethnic neighborhoods, increasing the potential for childhood illnesses that contribute to overall poor health (Klevens & Luman, 2001). Additionally, half of all HIV/AIDS patients in the country are African American, another discouraging statistic (NAACP, 2006). African Americans are less likely to receive effective treatments (such as HIV retroviral therapy) and are more likely to die of cancer and diabetes than White Americans (NAACP, 2006). Moreover, African Americans are approximately 15% less likely than White Americans to have access to health insurance (NAACP, 2006).

Disparities in mental health services for African American community are prevalent. For example, African Americans have a lower rate of receiving community-based, outpatient mental health care (Snowden, 1999). Although there have been calls for creating parity for mental health care (President's New Freedom Commission on Mental Health, 2003), differences in access to and availability of effective mental health treatments continue. African Americans are also less likely than White Americans to seek treatment for mental health problems (Snowden,

1999). Treatment disparities have been linked to the lack of availability of health insurance for people of color (Danish, Forneris, & Schaaf, 2007). Other reasons for mental health disparities include discrimination by providers, lack of availability of African American therapists, lack of information about mental health and treatment, and fear of stigma (Hernandez et al., 2006).

## Educational Challenges

African Americans are less likely to receive a high school diploma than the general population, a statistic that is associated with reduced employment opportunities and economic instability (Davis, Saunders, Williams, & Williams, 2004). Graduation rates for African Americans have been calculated to be as low as 50% (Heckman & LaFontaine, 2007). Furthermore, there are also gender differences in these educational disparities, indicating lower graduation rates for males than females: 43% and 56%, respectively. For males in particular, there are higher rates of suspension and other forms of behavioral discipline (Saunders, Davis, Williams, & Williams, 2004). Only 16% of females and 12% of males pursue college or graduate school (Saunders et al., 2004). In addition, parents of African American students are less likely to be involved with their children's education, also a risk factor for low academic achievement (Overstreet, Devine, Bevans, & Efreom, 2005). Furthermore, gaps in funding for lower income schools are increasing (Arroyo, 2008). A majority of states have large funding disparities between low- and high-income schools, amounting to approximately $1,000 per student (Arroyo, 2008). Between 1999 and 2005, this funding gap increased in 16 states (Arroyo, 2008). Such funding issues decrease the educational resources available to African American children and their families, thereby limiting opportunities for academic achievement.

## Finding Solutions

For African Americans to experience improved health outcomes, changes are essential across all aspects of the economic, social, and political systems. Federal funding agencies, local funders, and researchers must recognize the importance of social, economic, and political systems in addressing the determinants of health and in promoting health behaviors and outcomes (Seifer, Shore, & Holmes, 2003). In the past two decades, numerous programs have been established in both research and practice that have successfully linked communities with efforts to improve health and human services (Suarez-Balcazar, Harper, & Lewis, 2005; Wandersman, 2003). The next step in improving service delivery for African American children, families, and communities is to demonstrate a positive link between cultural adaptations in service delivery and the desired behavioral health outcomes that have been defined through community-based research.

## CREATING A CULTURALLY COMPETENT APPROACH WITH FAMILIES AND COMMUNITIES

Researchers have repeatedly called for culturally competent approaches to improving service delivery and research for ethnically diverse families (Benjamin, 1993; Cross, Bazron, Dennis, & Isaacs, 1989). In order to ensure success, culturally competent approaches must capture the complexity and unique nature of ethnic minority families as well as follow specific principles and guidelines (Benjamin & Isaacs-Shockley, 1996).

The proposed approach emerged as a result of the collaborative efforts of interdisciplinary partnerships of African American social and behavioral science researchers from the University of South Florida (USF) and community- and faith-based organizations (see Briscoe & McClain, 2000; Briscoe, Nixon, Smith, & Favorite, 2004; Briscoe, Smith, & McClain, 2003; Joseph, Briscoe, Smith, Sengova, & McClain, 2001; Oullette, Briscoe, Jones, & Tyson, 2001). These teams conducted several projects using a strengths-based approach with African American families. The culturally competent approach evolved over time as each project was conducted, with a focus on the practical application of findings to refine the approach further. Throughout this iterative process, community stakeholders and university members learned from their experiences, and all the partners engaged in dialogue based on trust in order to promote a strengths-based, effective collaborative effort. The shared philosophy and values of the partnership included a commitment to culturally competent research protocols and acknowledgment of the historical, cultural, socioeconomic, and political circumstances and experiences of African Americans (e.g., physical, mental, and psychological well-being and survival). The approach that emerged from this work blends strengths-based principles and practices, a system-of-care framework, an emphasis on collaboration, and community-based participatory research methods to create culturally competent guidelines for service providers and researchers (see Tables 1.1 and 1.2).

A strengths-based approach was identified as an effective way to serve African American families because it emphasizes creating linkages with existing informal resources, church networks, community centers, organizations, and extended family members (Alston & Turner, 1994; Bagley & Carroll, 1998). The strengths-based approach was seen as reflecting the natural supports and experiences of African American families in coping with challenges to survival and advancement presented by slavery, racism, and oppression (Martin & Martin, 1985). The partners found that, because of the complexity and uniqueness of factors that contribute to problems experienced by African American children and their families, intensive and sustained solutions are required that take into account strengths identified in well-functioning African American communities (Hines & Boyd-Franklin, 1982; Lewis & Looney, 1983; McAdoo & McAdoo, 1985; Rosnow & Marianthi, 1986).

In contrast, a system-of-care framework was adopted as a way to develop effective services for children with mental health challenges because of its empha-

**TABLE 1.1. Critical Components of the Research Approach**

| Critical components | Activities |
| --- | --- |
| Community–university partnership | Mutually beneficial and equal partnership that guides the structure for all aspects of research activities |
| Cultural competence | Preserves and enhances the historical, cultural, socioeconomic, and political circumstances and experiences of participants |
| Community based | Identification of the target population as a group of people who form a functionally cohesive group within their perceived boundaries |
| Community driven | Active participation of community members in central decision making at all levels |
| Strengths based | Emphasizes identifying and enhancing natural supports, networks, and assets |
| Capacity building | Resources are made available to the group that can be sustained after the completion of the research |
| Comprehensive services | Recognize that children, youth, and families have multisystem needs and require supports, resources, and services to become self-sustaining |
| Multifaceted research | Emphasizes mixed methods; data emerge that will promote relevant solutions |

sis on addressing numerous needs involving a range of conditions through interventions and services delivered by multiple agencies (Stroul & Friedman, 1986). Similar to the strengths-based approach, the system-of-care framework includes the integration of formal and informal resources in delivering effective and quality services and supports (Stroul & Friedman, 1986). This framework was identified as particularly relevant to African American families because it requires the support of a broad network of family, church, friends, and other resources available in the community (Friesen & Koroloff, 1990).

Collaboration was found to be an essential feature of all components of the culturally competent approach. Collaboration requires specific practices for building effective partnerships in order to design and deliver services that match the needs and resources of all stakeholders, including children and families (Anderson, McIntyre, Rotto, & Robertson, 2002). Collaboration is also identified as an important component of a community-based participatory research approach, which was a priority for the partners. By definition, community-based participatory research involves community stakeholders in designing and implementing research to effectively solve problems, thereby benefiting the community (Turnbull, Friesen, & Ramirez, 1998). Collaborative practices were found to be essential across all aspects of planning, implementation, and evaluation of the partnership projects.

Collaboration and all other components of the cultural competence approach overlap and contribute in additive ways, making each theoretical perspective

**TABLE 1.2. Critical Components of the Culturally Competent Approach**

| Components | Activities |
| --- | --- |
| Cultural competence | A conceptual model to operationalize the definition of cultural competence<br>• Community context to understand the population being served.<br>• Compatibility of organizational structures and process.<br>• Knowledge of the population.<br>• Domains of the organizational structure and processes.<br>  • Infrastructure<br>  • Direct service<br>  • Compatibility between the organizational infrastructure and direct service<br>• Outcomes (Hernandez et al., 2006). |
| Strengths based | • Importance of recognizing and enhancing strengths, protective factors, assets, family supports, and community networks (Hill, 1972, 1998; Tucker & Herman, 2002; Yokshikawa & Seidman, 2000).<br>• Incorporates the building of resiliency and protective factors for at-risk children and families (Furstenberg, Cook, Eccles, Elder, & Sameroff, 1999; Li, Nussbaum, & Richards, 2007). |
| System of care | • Children and families have multiple needs to address.<br>• Child and family centered.<br>• Emphasizes multiagency involvement, community-based nonresidential services.<br>• Strong partnership between parents and professionals.<br>• Meets the needs of ethnically and racially diverse populations.<br>• Supports the advancement of community-based programs to meet the needs of this varied population of children.<br>• Emphasis on family and culturally sensitive approaches (Stroul & Friedman, 1994). |
| Collaboration | • A collaboration of needs, agencies, and systems for children and families.<br>• Mutually responsible and equal partnerships that guide the structure for all aspects of services and supports.<br>• Collaboration is maintained through shared values and communication (Anderson et al., 2002). |
| Community-based participatory research | • An applied social process that involves a partnership between trained evaluation personnel and practice-based decision makers, organization members with program responsibility, and people with a vital interest in the program, the primary users of the program (Cousins & Earl, 1992; McKernan, 1988).<br>• Characterized by direct involvement and influence in the real-world experience of participants.<br>• Frames community issues, determines possible solutions to address these concerns, places solutions into practice, studies outcomes.<br>• Local practitioners play central roles in simultaneous action and enlightenment through the process of problem framing, planning, action, observation, and reflection.<br>• Participatory action research helps the community build resiliency in solving problems and utilize research findings to promote the community's well-being.<br>• Participatory action research also gives an equal share of control to the community engaged in the research (Israel et al., 1998; Turnbull et al., 1998). |

essential to the whole conceptual model. Omitting any one perspective would potentially create a gap in culturally competent guidelines. The partnership proposed that the creation of a culturally competent approach can help direct the attention of service providers, practitioners, researchers, and other stakeholders to begin the process of using African American strengths along with other strategies in a manner that will improve overall service delivery. This approach may be applied to specific neighborhood efforts, broader community collaborations, or research projects that can be generalized to other communities. By including community-driven approaches, understanding unique and complex needs and strengths, and sustaining collaboration among families, communities, and service providers, our USF research team is working to develop successful culturally competent approaches to further inform the implementation of programs, interventions, and changes in social policy.

## Description of Critical Components of the Approach

The critical components of this approach are designed to make research with African American families and neighborhoods culturally competent. Cultural competence is a set of beliefs, behaviors, and processes that allow professionals to work with other staff and clients across cultures (Cross et al., 1989). It should be recognized that culture, race, and ethnicity shape the ways in which individuals perceive and experience events, and all of these viewpoints should be considered when trying to increase the effectiveness of any type of intervention with African American families (Cauce et al., 2002). Although the need for services and interventions is great the availability of services specifically targeting diverse racial/ethnic groups is significantly lacking (Padgett, Patrick, Burns, & Schlesinger, 1994).

Cultural competence requires that individuals striving to serve diverse families appropriately must (1) hold diversity as a value, (2) be willing to conduct a self-assessment of beliefs and attitudes, (3) understand and balance those dynamics that arise from cultural differences, (4) continually learn about other cultures, and (5) apply these principles to the unique racial, ethnic, and other cultural contexts within the communities they are serving (Cross et al., 1989).

Cultural competence is critical for maximizing the impact of research and treatment with African American families and communities (Nagayama Hall, 2001). Cultural competence can be integrated into both practice and research by using specific strategies to engage community members in developing and studying the effectiveness of programs for individuals in their diverse neighborhoods (Hernandez et al., 2006).

The following components of the approach and action steps are intended to make working with African American families and communities both culturally competent and optimally effective. All of these critical components are built on the foundation of culturally competent practice and research.

### Strengths–Based Principles and Practices

Interdisciplinary social scientists have recognized that traditional approaches were ineffective when working with African American families because of the social, economic, educational, cultural, and historical conditions unique to their communities. Early studies provided major insights into understanding the causes of and solutions to African American family crises (Billingsley, 1968; Du Bois, 1899/1967; Frazier, 1939). However, there was a need to go beyond the narrow, critical views of African American families held by policymakers and service providers, whose decisions had direct repercussions for African American families (McAdoo, 1988). A shift to a strengths-based approach was considered ideal. This approach can increase cultural competence by promoting the natural supports for African American families that are relevant and sustainable.

### System–of–Care Philosophy

The holistic nature of a system of care can contribute to improving the quality and effectiveness of services for African American families. A system-of-care approach emphasizes multiagency involvement, child-centered and family-focused services, coordinated community-based service systems, a strong partnership between parents and professionals, accountability, and culturally competent practices that meet the needs of ethnically and racially diverse populations (Stroul & Friedman, 1986, 1994). It supports the advancement of community-based programs so that children with serious mental health issues are able to remain in their home communities, where appropriate networks of informal and formal supports can best be maintained. In a community-based system of care, the focus is broadened to include not only the children but their network of family, churches, friends, and other supports available in the community (Friesen & Koroloff, 1990; Slaughter, 1988) (see Figure 1.1). Service delivery is expanded to incorporate culturally appropriate resources using a systematic approach to support children and families in their community, thereby increasing culture competence.

### Collaborative Practices

Collaboration is required to develop services that address the multiple risk factors faced by African American children and families, including low SES, low-quality education, low occupational status, single-parent homes, large families, and challenging neighborhood characteristics (Carnegie Council on Adolescent Development, 1995; Ford, 1993; Masten & Coatsworth, 1998; McLoyd, 1990; Sameroff, Seifer, Baldwin, & Baldwin, 1993). A single-target program is insufficient to address these risk factors. Because of the complex needs of African American families, a collaborative effort is needed to identify the risk factors that are pertinent to a particular community or neighborhood and to marshal the resources required to address them.

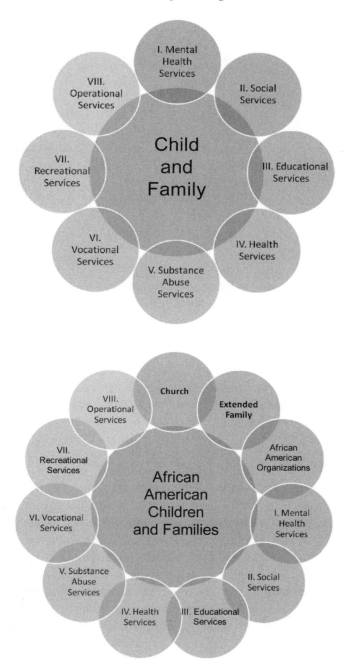

**FIGURE 1.1.** Eight major dimensions of service of a system of care (top) and 11 major dimensions of services for African Americans (bottom). From Stroul and Friedman (1986), with permission of the National Technical Assistance Center for Children's Mental Health, Center for Child and Human Development, Georgetown University.

A critical component in creating a culturally competent community-based program is the commitment to building a mutually beneficial collaboration (Vey, 2005). Collaboration can meet the needs of children and their families by facilitating the development of a comprehensive and coordinated network of services across both formal and informal sectors of the community (Ross-Gordon, Martin, & Briscoe, 1990). In addition, collaboration has been identified as essential to the work of community–researcher partnerships in a wide range of fields such as public health (Greenberg, Howard, & Desmond, 2003; Roussos & Fawcett, 2000; Sullivan & Kelly, 2001), community psychology (Nelson, Prilleltensky, & MacGillivary, 2001), sociology (Park & Lee, 1999), community development (Panet-Raymond, 1992), urban planning (Gills, Butler, Rose, & Bivens, 2001), and medicine (Hatch, Moss, Saran, Presley-Cantrell, & Mallory, 1993). The goal of many such collaborative efforts is to have both professionals and community members serve as equal partners in decision making.

Collaboration can also build cultural competence by joining different community efforts so they can work in conjunction with one another rather than separately (Axelsson & Axelsson, 2006). Collaborating individuals can share the responsibility of partnership development and commit to common goals for improving the community (Anderson et al., 2002). Open and frequent communication, funding transparency, and a focus on shared values and leadership facilitate such collaboration (Anderson et al., 2002). Strong collaboration and communication are highlighted as fundamental components of successful partnerships between African American communities and professionals (Hatch et al., 1993; Lefley & Bestman, 1991; Reed & Collins, 1994).

### Community-Based Participatory Research

Participatory research is an applied social process that involves a partnership among trained researchers, decision makers, program implementers, primary users of a program, and other community stakeholders (Cousins & Earl, 1992; McKernan, 1988). The term community-based participatory research (CBPR) encompasses a field of research that includes various approaches such as participatory research, action research, participatory action research, constituency-oriented research, emancipatory research, empowerment research, and discovery research (Turnbull et al., 1998). In general, participatory research includes direct involvement of community members in all aspects of research. This comprehensive approach occurs in the natural community context, where community members and researchers can generate practical knowledge and interventions (Israel, Schulz, Parker, & Becker, 1998). The real-world experience of community members contributes to framing community issues, developing possible solutions to address community concerns, incorporating solutions into practice, and analyzing the outcomes (King & Lonnquist, 1992; Lonnquist & King, 1993; Turnbull et al., 1998). Community partners represent diverse ethnic, economic, social, and professional backgrounds with a range of experiences and, therefore, contribute to comprehensive, culturally competent solutions (Eisinger & Senturia, 2001).

In a community-based approach, the role of community members is central to the simultaneous action and enlightenment that occurs during problem framing, planning, action, observation, and reflection (King & Lonnquist, 1992; McKernan, 1988). This type of research is based on information gathered within the community (e.g., in the form of surveys, community meetings), which is then used to generate interventions designed to solve community challenges (Israel, Schulz, Parker, & Becker, 1998). The research process also helps communities identify social justice issues and create workable solutions that are effective in addressing local priorities (Hall, 1981). Participatory research ideally gives an equal share of control to the community engaged in the research, which can build resiliency in solving problems and increase the use of research findings to promote the community's well-being (Hughes, 2003). These approaches contribute to cultural competence by developing greater understanding of community strengths, resources, and challenges and identifying the most appropriate service system reforms.

## Guidelines for Establishing and Maintaining Cultural Competence

The following 10 guidelines are provided as a resource for researchers and service providers who are entering a community for the first time to ensure culturally competent and collaborative research, service planning, and community involvement.

1. *Identifying strengths and natural supports.* Before entering the community, it is important for service providers and researchers to learn the strengths and positive qualities of African American families in general and the community or neighborhood in particular. It is suggested that the process begin with contacting and working with African American researchers who are familiar with the professional research literature. Other African American professionals and community leaders may serve as direct sources of information about local community strengths and resources. To further enhance understanding of local strengths and resources and build trust, several actions can be taken. The first step requires formal and informal interactions with community members to learn firsthand their values, attitudes, historical experiences, and specific local knowledge. Professionals can attend community meetings and activities, assist with and participate in local organizations, and communicate with community members face to face or by phone and e-mail. The information gathered can be used to inform the research and develop the mutual goals that will ensure long-term sustainability of the collaboration. This first step allows professionals to work in collaboration with African American families and communities to discover skills or resources that have been successful in the past and promote a strengths-based perspective. Through careful, targeted research, professionals and community members can

identify specific African American family and community strengths and abilities that have enabled them to overcome obstacles. Professionals can also work with members of specific neighborhoods or broader community groups to identify natural supports and networks within their locale or membership. This approach allows professionals to work together with families and communities to discover and enhance strategies to reach mutually defined goals, such as raising healthy and successful children and families.

In another step to ensure a successful collaborative partnership, one's understanding of the African American community must be thorough in several areas: the population's functioning at the individual, family, and community levels (Suarez-Balcazar et al., 2005); the historical context of the community, which can include family, political, and religious histories; and the current issues encountered by community members (Higgins & Metzler, 2001).

In a third step, professionals who are initiating a community partnership can develop joint task forces with existing agencies or collaboratives that are addressing issues important to the community. To help initiatives share resources efficiently and maximize their impact, partners must thoroughly process and assess what is occurring within, and across, various collaborative groups and the effect of these interactions on the community and other stakeholders. Professionals seeking to develop a new partnership also need to learn about the history of research within this community, including the level of understanding about research methods, experiences with discriminatory or culturally incompetent research approaches, and other barriers to developing trust (Callejas, Nesman, Mowery, & Hernandez, 2008; Slaughter, 1988). The team must identify potential community issues and concerns, resources, and strengths that might impact the research process (Jordan, Bogat, & Smith, 2001).

These collaborative processes can contribute to improved neighborhood life through the development of common goals and increased commitment to work together; however, there are also dangers of fragmenting the community and polarizing groups. Discovering existing community efforts and the issues that are already being addressed can reduce the potential for conflict and enhance the potential for sustainability of the partnership. It is important for professionals and community residents to develop an appreciation for each others' skills, knowledge, and potential contributions to the partnership. In addition, desired benefits for both community members and professionals should be identified and celebrated. Benefits might include increased awareness of and involvement in activities and events in the community, increased personal growth, increased appreciation for individual and community strengths, and improved ability to identify specific actions to enhance quality of life in the community.

2. *Community-driven solutions and community ownership of sustainable solutions.* Community-driven research places the work within a unique community rather than in a clinical setting that does not reflect the complexities of the families and neighborhood interactions (Schensul et al., 2006). Once community sup-

ports and resources are identified, those strengths can be tapped to improve the community. Partners will then know that the community will drive action and take the leader in planning change. This entails active participation of community members in driving the central decision making at all levels of research. Active participation of neighborhood members is crucial for a project because it brings their practical knowledge and experiences into the process and elicits real interests and concerns and identifies needs (Eisinger & Senturia, 2001). When community participation is emphasized in this way, community buy-in to the project typically increases, and more realistic and practical goals and strategies are adopted because residents are directly involved in its planning and implementation (Stith et al., 2006).

When considering community participation, it is important to distinguish between active involvement of community members in research or service development and passive roles such as community outreach or information gathering. Community members should be active partners who have a substantial role in all aspects of research and program development.

3. *Building trust by using established channels of communication and trust building.* Trust building is initiated by acknowledging community strengths, supports, resources, and skills, which can be called on for developing solutions. Once this strengths-based approach is established, discussions can move to a focus on how the partnership will further contribute to change. A trusting partnership is fundamental to a culturally competent approach (Suarez-Balcazar et al., 2005; Tucker et al., 2007). Developing this trust requires time, especially when individuals in the community adopt a wait-and-see attitude, and, therefore, needs to be strategically addressed in the initial stages of the partnership (Killon, 2007; Slaughter, 1988). Each community and cultural context for community-based practice has unique characteristics and must be examined to determine what strategies may or may not be effective (Greenbaum, 1998). Opportunities for open dialogue must be made available throughout the project to clarify issues, nurture relationships, and attain and celebrate the project's objectives (Slaughter, 1988; Suarez-Balcazar et al., 2005). For example, the partnership can maintain ongoing progress notes, hold more frequent meetings at the outset, set up listserves, and promote individualized discussions among members to increase mutual understanding and shared goals. Promotion and coordination of two-way communication can facilitate partnership development by reducing the potential for individuals to violate the trust that is being built across the partnership (Lefley & Bestman, 1991; Reed & Collins, 1994). Communication between professionals and community partners should be included as aspects of the project to monitor, manage, and evaluate, and this should include analysis of power differentials. The partnership can also measure outcomes of communication and trust building such as the degree to which all participants are involved in carrying out partnership activities.

4. *Timely feedback to community.* The partnership must provide ongoing information in a written report to community members and obtain feedback reg-

ularly. Communities and family members should be kept informed of research and practice findings (via, e.g., multimedia presentations, roundtable discussions, community forums). This process can promote community ownership of information, which can result in greater utilization of planned activities and services. It is important for professional and community partners to report information together and in a variety of venues, including community, professional, and academic meetings, workshops, and conferences.

5. *Neighborhood based.* A neighborhood-based approach includes the identification of the target population as a group of people who form a functionally cohesive neighborhood within their perceived boundaries. The term *neighborhood* implies an emphasis on the locality and history of a group of people. A "neighborhood-based" approach develops micro-level strategies for a specific geographical area and involves residents in the design and operation of a targeted project. It is essential to work at the neighborhood level in order to plan, implement, and evaluate projects that are truly accountable and responsive to the needs of the residents. Often planners initiate programs that have a macro-level focus targeting several different neighborhoods and addressing a wide range of community issues that are predetermined and possibly irrelevant to specific neighborhoods. When such broad-based programs are implemented in many different neighborhoods without having roots in any of them, low utilization and poor outcomes likely result. A neighborhood-based approach is initiated by identifying local residents who are willing to commit to the project and participate in a core group. This micro-level neighborhood group can serve as a key mechanism through which effective dialogue, resource mobilization, skill training, needs assessment, strategic planning, and action occur within the neighborhood (Jordan et al., 2001).

6. *Comprehensive approach.* The multiplicity and complexity of the needs of children/youth and their families underscore the necessity for intervention efforts to be multilayered and integrative (see Tables 1.3 and 1.4). A community-based partnership should acknowledge that children, youth, and families have numerous and varying needs (i.e., health, social, educational, vocational, and recreational) that require local supports, resources, and services to be relevant and sustainable (Stroul & Friedman, 1986). Community-based efforts that target African American families must include holistic conceptualizations of children within their families and communities. Also, comprehensive frameworks for interventions must be considered. Such interventions should include both formal services and informal (natural) supports, such as extended family and faith-based and community-based organizations (Briscoe & McClain, 2000; Briscoe et al., 2003, 2004).

7. *Multidisciplinary partnerships.* The complexity of African American communities requires the involvement of interdisciplinary professionals in community-based partnerships (Reich & Reich, 2006). The multiple needs of children, families, and communities lie in a complex web of risk and resiliency factors that cannot easily be addressed by any single discipline or practice (Reich & Reich,

**TABLE 1.3. Action Steps of a Culturally Competent Approach**

| Principles | Actions |
|---|---|
| 1. Gaining an understanding of strengths, natural supports, resources, and community context | • Begin by establishing a history and maintain active involvement with community members.<br>• Researchers and practitioners should have a thorough understanding of African American functioning at the individual, family, and community levels (Suarez-Balcazar et al., 2005).<br>• The team must quickly develop an understanding of the specific community issues, concerns, resources, and strengths (Jordan et al., 2001). |
| 2. Community driven for community ownership of sustainable solutions | • Communities implement their own strategies/solutions and maintain proactive decision making at all levels.<br>• Communities must be involved with research and intervention to promote sustainability when reducing disparities (Schensul et al., 2006). |
| 3. Building trust by established channels of communication | Continuous verbal/written communication with residents. |
| 4. Timely feedback to the community | Information reported to community throughout the project for feedback, input, and utilization. |
| 5. Neighborhood based | • Identification of the target population as a group of people who form a functionally cohesive neighborhood within their perceived boundaries.<br>• Micro-level strategies for a specifically identified geographical area; involves residents in the design and operation of a project targeted to that neighborhood. |
| 6. Comprehensive approach | Practitioners should recognize that children, youth, and families have multisystemic needs (i.e., health, social, educational, vocational, recreational) and require supports, resources, and services to become self-sustaining (Stroul & Friedman, 1986). |
| 7. Multidisciplinary partnerships | Engaging various partners and community members of varied educational, professional, and practical expertise. |
| 8. Community capacity building | Resources must be available to assist community organizations by providing technical assistance in the areas of leadership, development, program planning, advocacy, implementation, and evaluation (Seifer et al., 2003). |
| 9. Expanding financial resources | Professionals should help community partners to obtain increased funding through joint presentations, fund-raising efforts, and strategic planning (Children's Defense Fund, 2006; Jones & Wells, 2007). |
| 10. Multifaceted accountability, evaluation, and research | • Collecting information on the outcomes or *impact* of services is critical when trying to implement culturally competent interventions (Scott & Usher, 1996; Tebes, 2005).<br>• Multiple perspectives are required to fully document change; researchers must utilize qualitative techniques (interviews, focus groups, observation) and quantitative methodologies (surveys, statistical data collection, asset maps) in order for findings to be generalized (Knapp, 1995). |

2006). Interdisciplinary collaboration brings a variety of perspectives together to create new questions, new solutions, and a broader view of community problems and solutions (Pickett, Burch, & Grove, 1999; Snowden, 2005). Community-based partnerships must develop an understanding of specific factors impacting African American communities and formulate unique conceptualizations of the issues and challenges in order to develop and implement culturally competent community-based interventions.

**TABLE 1.4. Examples of Each Strategy from Briscoe and McClain (2000)**

1. *Gaining an understanding of strengths, natural supports, resources, and community context*

This study focused on the African American community developing a comprehensive analysis of family and community resources and strengths in order to be able to use these strengths to support educational achievement, social development, and neighborhood development.

2. *Community driven for community ownership of sustainable solutions*

A core team of partners, stakeholders, family members, and other involved participants joined forces with policymakers, administrators, and practitioners to plan, design, and coordinate this consumer-driven research project.

3. *Building trust through "open" and honest communication*

The process itself was very gradual and developmental in nature. Open communication was established and maintained among core group members and target communities. These groups did not lose sight of their overall goal and mission; they remained committed and focused, with any obstacles serving as learning experiences.

4. *Timely feedback to the community*

Core team members, including residents from all four communities, participated in biweekly meetings over a period of 9 months, produced a newsletter, held meetings in the community, and sponsored a community summit.

5. *Neighborhood based*

The aim of this project was to collect information that could be used by human service providers to more effectively support families in four predominantly African American neighborhoods in the county.

6. *Comprehensive approach*

The core team consisted of a wide range of conscientious social service providers and agencies, among them the Department of Children and Families, the housing authority, the school district, the Development of African American Men support group, the Department of Juvenile Justice, the university, the community college, and the African American church.

7. *Multidisciplinary partnerships*

This was a collaborative project involving several university departments and 31 agencies, programs, churches, and community organizations.

8. *Community capacity building*

This project resulted in recommendations for use by school personnel and human service providers that built on identified strengths. These neighborhood stakeholders developed specific action steps and conducted work sessions to mobilize local communities to use strengths-based approaches to enhance service delivery and quality of life by building on the natural system of support and family strengths within the African American community.

9. *Expanding financial resources*

It was decided by the core team that an African American church would be the financial agent for the project because religious institutions are still considered cornerstones for the African American community, and it was a key player in the project. A community coordinator and an administrative aide, both part time, were hired from within the target communities.

10. *Multifaceted accountability, evaluation, and research*

The approach used in this study included several different research methods: an in-depth census analysis to help identify demographic factors; an examination of local data (articles, reports, surveys, newspaper articles) provided by African American organizations and individuals, governmental agencies, and universities; a review of the research literature; asset mapping; summit meetings where providers, residents, and other professionals identified perceptions, strengths, and resources within the four target communities; and focus groups with successful children, parents of successful children, senior citizens, at-large residents, educators, and service providers in the target neighborhoods.

8. *Community capacity building.* Community-based partnerships should seek change in both individual beliefs and broader social policy (Albino & Tedesco, 1983; Weissberg, Caplan, & Harwood, 1991) through strategic planning, capacity building, and information sharing. For example, the partnership can seek technical assistance in the areas of leadership development, program planning, advocacy, implementation, and evaluation (Seifer et al., 2003). Information and education can also be provided to children and families in the community to build the capacity for meeting partnership goals (Spoth & Greenberg, 2005). The partnership can assist existing community programs and providers with fundraising, obtaining grants for new projects, and implementing and evaluating novel interventions (Flick, Reese, Rogers, Fletcher, & Sonn, 1994).

9. *Expanding financial resources.* Historically, African American organizations, including faith-based initiatives, have had limited financial resources (Mincy, 1994; Wiener, 1994). Funding that is sought for projects must include an allocation of resources for the community and its residents. Community members should not be expected to participate and serve in voluntary roles alone; they should also be included as paid staff. For example, community members can be hired initially as coordinators or program assistants and later promoted to more responsible positions as capacity increases and credentials are gained. Open communication about expectations for funding and resources that are brought to the community should be an explicit goal of the partnership. Community-based partnerships working with African American communities need to balance their approach between a recognition of and respect for the boundaries of local resources (Jones & Wells, 2007) and a commitment to bringing in new funding and resources to benefit the community. Professionals and community partners can work together to increase financial resources through joint presentations to funding sources, collaborative fund-raising efforts, and strategic planning to gain the maximum benefit from existing resources (Children's Defense Fund, 2006; Jones & Wells, 2007).

10. *Multifaceted accountability, evaluation, and research.* In examining the outcomes of any community-based intervention, it is important to measure the effectiveness of programs or services implemented (Massey, 1996). Collecting information on the outcomes, or impact, of services is critical when implementing culturally competent interventions (Scott & Usher, 1996; Tebes, 2005). Monitoring programs and services for positive outcomes creates accountability, which ensures that community resources and efforts are not wasted on ineffective programs.

Significant advances have been made in social research methodologies that apply to complex community interventions (Rossi, Freeman, & Lipsey, 1999). CBPR is one such tool, which also emphasizes community ownership of the research and problem-solving process (Lantz, Viruell-Fuentes, Israel, Softley, & Guzman, 2001; Randall, Swenson, & Henggeler, 1999). To fully document change brought about by community-based partnerships, researchers must utilize a variety of qualitative (e.g., interviews, focus groups, observation) and quantitative (e.g., surveys, statistical data collection, asset maps) methods (Knapp, 1995). Using mixed methods can also broaden the application of data to provide both locally relevant and more generalized findings that can be applied to other communities or used in theory development (Cronbach, 1986).

## DISCUSSION

This chapter explores some of the ways in which culturally competent approaches can be used to carry out community-based research and develop effective interventions for African American communities, families, and children. The first recommendation is designing a strengths-based approach to understanding and promoting positive strategies and outcomes. For African Americans, this inspires a healthy personal and interpersonal approach for building on life successes. This approach highlights positive factors that will help African American families become more proactive participants in the long-term sustainability of their communities and culture as well as help change perceptions held by professionals. In turn, the professionals engaged in the process benefit from the knowledge and commitment gained from working within the community. Every step of the process is designed to improve the skills and techniques of partnership members so that meaningful relationships can be built among academic researchers, other professionals, and community members. This process can result in increased ownership and empowerment of families and the community as well as increased commitment of professionals. Successful partnerships share responsibility, create a relationship of mutual learning, and increase the skill level of both community members and professionals in carrying out research and program implementation. Such collaborative work can foster the development of iterative cycles of quality improvement as well as strategies for sustainability beyond initial funding sources. It is important that researchers who are entering communities for the first time carefully focus on and develop the skills necessary to build and sustain relationships with its members. The learning process that comes with building and sustaining community- and neighborhood-based partnerships can be of immense value for both professional partners and residents who engage in the process.

Critical elements of a culturally competent approach have been described as overlapping components that include a focus on strengths in families and communities, a holistic and comprehensive view of children and service systems, multidisciplinary and multiperspective collaboration, and CBPR, program implementation, and evaluation. By orienting themselves to these components, professionals and residents can design strategies that are uniquely adapted to fit their specific community and can be documented for greater generalizability. This approach recognizes the importance of integrated interventions at the individual, family, and neighborhood/community levels that take into account existing community structures, issues, and relationships. It fosters local ownership of problems, development of long-term working partnerships, and commitment to creating viable community solutions. The approach has both unique elements that stand alone (e.g., focusing on African American strengths) and overlapping qualities (e.g., collaboration, community participation), which together can contribute to the development of interventions that are culturally acceptable and relevant. The application of each component independently of the others can result in the development of strategies and interventions that do not address the critical factors affecting African American communities. A single approach comprising all the components can more effectively guide the development of culturally competent research and interventions and provide maximum benefits for African American communities and the professionals who work with them.

## REFERENCES

Albino, J., & Tedesco, L. A. (1983). Women's health issues. *Issues in Mental Health Nursing, 5*, 157–172.

Alston, R., & Turner, W. (1994). A family-strengths model of adjustment to disability for African-American clients. *Journal of Counseling and Development, 72*(4), 378–383.

Anderson, J. A., McIntyre, J. S., Rotto, K. I., & Robertson, D. C. (2002). Developing and maintaining collaboration in systems of care for children and youths with emotional and behavioral disabilities and their families. *American Journal of Orthopsychiatry, 72*(40), 514–524.

Arroyo, C. G. (2008). *The funding gap 2007*. Washington, DC: Education Trust.

Axelsson, R., & Axelsson, B. (2006). Integration and collaboration in public health: A conceptual framework. *International Journal of Health Planning and Management, 21*, 75–88.

Bagley C. A., & Carroll, J. (1998). Healing forces in African-American families. In H. I. McCubbin, E. A. Thompson, A. I. Thompson, & J. A. Futrell (Eds.), *Resiliency in African-American families* (Vol. 2, pp. 117–142). Thousand Oaks, CA: Sage.

Baker, E. A., Homan, S., & Keuter, M. (1999). Principles of practice for academic/practice/community research partnership. *American Journal of Preventive Medicine, 16*, 86–93.

Benjamin, M. (1993). *Child and adolescent service system program minority initiative research monograph*. Washington, DC: CASSP Technical Assistance Center, Georgetown University Child Development Center.

Benjamin, M. P., & Isaacs-Shockley, M. (1996). Culturally competent services approaches. In B. Stroul (Ed.), *Children's mental health: Creating systems of care in a changing society* (pp. 475–491). Baltimore: Brookes.

Billingsley, A. (1968). *Black families in White America*. Englewood Cliffs, NJ: Prentice Hall.

Black, M. M., Dubowitz, H., & Starr, H. R. (1999). African-American fathers in low income, urban families: Development, behavior, and home environment of their three-year-old children. *Child Development, 70*(4), 967–978.

Briscoe, R., & McClain, G. (2000). *African-American family support analysis: Strengths of African-American families*. Tampa, FL: Children's Board of Hillsborough County.

Briscoe, R., Nixon, R., Smith, A., & Favorite, J. (2004). *Spiritual Educational Network Directory (SEND): A resource directory of educational and social service programs for children and families provided by African-American faith-based institutions.* Tampa, FL: University of South Florida, Louis de la Parte Florida Mental Health Institute, Child and Family Studies.

Briscoe, R., Smith, A., & McClain, G. (2003). Implementing culturally competent research practice: Identifying strengths of African-American communities, families, and children. *Focal Point, 17*(1), 10–16.

Briscoe, R. V., Keller, H. R., McClain, G., Best, E., & Mazza, J. (2009). A culturally competent community-based research approach with African American neighborhoods: Critical components and examples. In S. Y. Evans, C. M. Taylor, M. R. Dunlap, & D. S. Miller (Eds.), *African Americans and community engagement in higher education: Perspectives of race in community service, service-learning, and community-based research* (pp. 205–224). New York: State University of New York Press.

Brooks-Gunn, J., & Duncan, G. (1997). The effects of poverty on children. *Children and Poverty, 7*(2), 55–71.

Callejas, L. M., Nesman, T., Mowery, D., & Hernandez, M. (2008). *Creating a front porch: Strategies for improving access to mental health services* (Making Children's Mental Health Services Successful Series, FMHI Publication No. 240-3). Tampa, FL: University of South Florida, Louis de la Parte Florida Mental Health Institute, Research and Training Center for Children's Mental Health.

Carnegie Council on Adolescent Development. (1995). *Great transitions: Preparing adolescents for a new century.* New York: Author.

Cauce, A. M., Domenech-Rodriguez, M., Paradise, M., Cochran, B. N., Shea, J. M., Srebnick, D., et al. (2002). Cultural and contextual influences in mental health help seeking: A focus on ethnic minority youth. *Journal of Counseling and Clinical Psychology, 70,* 44–55.

Children's Defense Fund. (2006). *Improving children's health: Understanding children's health disparities and promising approaches to address them.* Washington, DC: Author.

Coner-Edwards, A. F., & Spurlock, J. (1988). *Black families in crisis: The middle class.* New York: Brunner/Mazel.

Cousins, J. B., & Earl, L. M. (1992). The case for participatory evaluation. *Educational Evaluation and Policy Analysis, 14,* 397–418.

Cronbach, L. J. (1986). *Social inquiry by and for earthlings.* In D. W. Fiske & R. A. Shweder (Eds.), *Metatheory in social science: Pluralisms and subjectivities* (pp. 83–107). Chicago: University of Chicago Press.

Cross, T. L., Bazron, B. J., Dennis, K. W., & Isaacs, M. R. (1989). *Towards a culturally competent system of care: Volume I.* Washington, DC: CASSP Technical Assistance Center, Georgetown University Child Development Center.

Danish, S., Forneris, T., & Schaaf, K. (2007). Counseling psychology and culturally competent health care: Limitations and challenges. *The Counseling Psychologist, 35*(5), 716–725.

Davis, L., Saunders, J., Williams, H. J., & Williams, T. (2004). Gender differences in self-perceptions and academic outcomes: A study of African-American high school students. *Journal of Youth and Adolescence, 33*(1), 81–90.

Du Bois, W. B. (1967). *The Philadelphia Negro.* New York: Shocken Books. (Original work published 1899)

Eisinger, A., & Senturia, K. (2001). Doing community-driven research: A description of Seattle partners for health communities. *Journal of Urban Health, 78*(3), 519–534.

Fawcett, F., Paine-Andrews, A., & Schultz, J. (2000). A model memorandum of collaboration: A proposal. *Public Health Reports, 115,* 174–179.

Flick, L. H., Reese, C. G., Rogers, G., Fletcher, P., & Sonn, J. (1994). Building community for health: Lessons from a seven-year old neighborhood/university partnership. *Health Education Behavior, 21,* 369–380.

Ford, D. (1993). Black students' achievement orientation as a function of perceived family achievement orientation and demographic variables. *Journal of Negro Education, 14*(3), 130–136.

Frazier, E. F. (1939). The present status of the Negro family in the United States. *Journal of Negro Education, 8*(3), 376–382.

Friesen, B. J., & Koroloff, N. M. (1990). Family-centered services: Implications for mental health administration and research. *Journal of Mental Health Administration, 17*(1), 13–25.

Furstenberg, F. F., Jr., Cook, T. D., Eccles, J., Elder, G. H., Jr., & Sameroff, A. (1999). *Managing to make it: Urban families and adolescent success.* Chicago: University of Chicago Press.

Gills, D. C., Butler, M., Rose, A., & Bivens, S. (2001). Collaborative research and action in communities: Partnership building in the Chicago empowerment zone. In M. Sullivan & J. G. Kelly (Eds.), *Collaborative research: University and community partnership* (pp. 25–44). Washington, DC: American Public Health Association.

Greenbaum, S. D. (1998). The role of ethnography in creating linkages with communities: Identifying and assessing neighborhoods' needs and strengths. In M. Hernandez & M. R. Isaacs (Eds.), *Promoting cultural competence in children's mental health services* (pp. 119–132). Baltimore: Brookes.

Greenberg, J. S., Howard, D. E., & Desmond, S. (2003). A community-campus partnership for health: The Seat Pleasant/University of Maryland Health Partnership. *Health Promotion Practice, 4,* 393–401.

Hall, B. L. (1981). Participatory research: An approach to change. *Convergence, 14*(3), 6–17.

Hatch, J., Moss, N., Saran, A., Presley-Cantrell, L., & Mallory, C. (1993). Community research: Partnership in black communities. *American Journal of Preventive Medicine, 9,* 27–31.

Heckman, J. J., & LaFontaine, A. P. (2007). *The American high school graduation rate: Trends and levels* (NBER Working Paper 13670). Cambridge, MA: National Bureau of Economic Research.

Hernandez, M., Nesman, T., Isaacs, M., Callejas, L. M., & Mowery, D. (Eds.). (2006). *Examining the research base supporting culturally competent children's mental health services* (Making Children's Mental Health Services Successful Series, FMHI Publication No. 240-1). Tampa, FL: University of South Florida, Louis de la Parte Florida Mental Health Institute, Research and Training Center for Children's Mental Health.

Higgins, D. L., & Metzler, M. (2001). Implementing community-based participatory research centers in diverse urban settings. *Journal of Health, 78,* 488–494.

Hill, R. (1972). *The strengths of Black families.* New York: Emerson Hall Press.

Hill, R. (1998). Enhancing the resilience of African-American families. *Journal of Human Behavior in the Social Environment, 1,* 49–61.

Hill, R. (1999). *The strengths of Black families: Twenty-five years later.* Lanham, MD: University Press of America.

Hill, R. (2003). The strengths of Black families revisited. In L. A. Adams (Ed.), *The state of Black America* (pp. 107–146). New York: National Urban League.

Hines, P. M., & Boyd-Franklin, N. (1982). Black families. In M. McGoldrick, J. K. Pearce, & J. Giordano (Eds.), *Ethnicity and family therapy* (pp. 87–107). New York: Guilford Press.

Hughes, J. N. (2003). Commentary: Participatory action research leads to sustainable school and community improvement. *School Psychology Review, 32*(1), 38.

Israel, B. A., Schulz, A. J. Parker, E. A., & Becker, A. B. (1998). Review of community-based research: Assessing partnership approaches to improve public health. *Annual Review of Public Health, 19,* 173–202.

Jones, L., & Wells, K. (2007). Strategies for academic and clinician engagement in community-participatory partnered research. *Journal of the American Medical Association, 297,* 407–410.

Jordan, L. C., Bogat, G. A., & Smith, G. (2001). Collaborating for social change: The Black psychologist and the Black community. *American Journal of Community Psychology, 29,* 599–620.

Joseph, R., Briscoe, R., Smith, A., Sengova, J., & McClain, G. (2001). *Strengths of African-American families: A cross-site analysis of families in Baltimore, Detroit, Plant City, San Diego and Savannah.* Tampa, FL: Louis dela Parte Florida Mental Health Institute, University of South Florida, Child and Family Studies.

Killon, C. M. (2007). Patient-centered culturally sensitive health care: Trend or major thrust in health care delivery? *The Counseling Psychologist, 35,* 726–734.

King, J. A., & Lonnquist, M. P. (1992). *A review of writing on action research.* Minneapolis: Center for Applied Research and Educational Improvement, University of Minnesota.

Klevens, R. M., & Luman, E. T. (2001). U.S. children living in and near poverty: Risk of vaccine-preventable diseases. *American Journal of Preventive Medicine, 20*(4), 41–46.

Knapp, M. S. (1995). How shall we study comprehensive, collaborative services for children and families? *Educational Researcher, 24*(4), 5–16.

Lantz, P. M., Viruell-Fuentes, E., Israel, B. A., Softley, D., & Guzman, R. (2001). Can communities and academia work together on public health research?: Evaluation results from a community-based participatory research partnership in Detroit. *Journal of Urban Health, 78,* 495–507.

Lefley, H., & Bestman, E. (1991). Public-academic linkages for culturally sensitive community mental health. *Community Mental Health Journal, 27,* 473–491.

Lewis, J. M., & Looney, J. G. (1983). *The long struggle: Well functioning working-class Black families.* New York: Brunner/Mazel.

Li, S., Nussbaum, K., & Richards, M. (2007). Risk and protective factors for urban African-American youth. *American Journal of Community Psychology, 39,* 21–35.

Lonnquist, M. P., & King, J. A. (1993, April). *Changing the tire on a moving bus: Barriers to the development of professional community in a new teacher-led school.* Paper presented at the annual meeting of the American Educational Research Association, Atlanta.

Martin, J. M., & Martin, E. P. (1985). *The helping tradition in the Black family and community.* Silver Spring, MD: National Association of Social Workers.

Massey, O. T. (1996). *Evaluating human resource development programs. A practical guide for public agencies.* Boston: Allyn & Bacon.

Masten, A. S., & Coatsworth, J. D. (1998). The development of competence in favorable and unfavorable environments: Lessons from research on successful children. *American Psychologist, 53*(2), 205–220.

McAdoo, H. P. (1988). The study of ethnic minority families: Implications for practitioners and policymakers. *Family Relations, 37,* 265–267.

McAdoo, H. P. (1998). African-American families: Strength and realities. In H. I. McCubbin, E. A. Thompson, A. I. Thompson, & J. A. Futrell (Eds.), *Resiliency in African-American families* (pp. 17–30). Thousand Oaks, CA: Sage.

McAdoo, H. P., & McAdoo, J. L. (Eds.). (1985). *Black children: Social, educational and parental environments.* Beverly Hills, CA: Sage.

McDaniel, A. (1990). The power of culture: A review of the idea of Africa's influence on family structure in antebellum America. *Journal of Family History, 15,* 225–238.

McKernan, J. (1988). The countenance of curriculum action research: Traditional, collaborative and critical-emancipatory conceptions. *Journal of Curriculum and Supervision, 3,* 173–200.

McLoyd, V. (1990). The impact of economic hardships on Black families and children: Psychological distress, parenting, and socioeconomic development. *Child Development, 61,* 311–346.

Mincy, R.B. (1994). Conclusions and implications. In R. B. Mincy (Ed.), *Nurturing young Black males: Challenges to agencies, programs, and social policy* (pp. 187–204). Washington, DC: Urban Institute Press.

Moore, R. M., & Chase-Lansdale, L. P. (2001). Sexual intercourse and pregnancy among African-American girls in high poverty neighborhoods: The role of family and perceived community environment. *Journal of Marriage and Family, 63*(4), 1146–1157.

Morial, M. H. (2005). The state of Black America: Prescription for change. In L. A. Daniels, R. Jefferson-Frazier, & S. Jones (Eds.), *The state of Black America 2005* (pp. 11–14). Washington, DC: National Urban League.

Nagayama Hall, G. C. (2001). Psychotherapy research with ethnic minorities: Empirical, ethical, and conceptual issues. *Journal of Consulting and Clinical Psychology, 62,* 502–510.

National Association for the Advancement of Colored People. (2006). *The state of the disparity.* Baltimore, MD: Author.

Nelson, G., Prilleltensky, I., & MacGillivary, H. (2001). Building value-based partnerships: Toward solidarity with oppressed groups. *American Journal of Community Psychology, 29,* 649–677.

Oullette, P., Briscoe, R., Jones, A., & Tyson, C. (2001). *West Tampa TeleNetworking Initiative: Towards the development of a technology-supported school and community networking strategy.* Tampa, FL: Children's Board of Hillsborough County.

Overstreet, S., Devine, J., Bevans, K., & Efreom, Y. (2005). Predicting parental involvement in children's schooling within an economically disadvantaged African-American sample. *Psychology in the Schools, 42*(1), 101–111.

Padgett, D. K., Patrick, C., Burns, B. J., & Schlesinger, H. J. (1994). Ethnicity and the use of outpatient mental health services in a national insured population. *American Journal of Public Health, 84,* 222–226.

Panet-Raymond, J. (1992). Partnership: Myth or reality? *Community Development Journal*, *27*, 156–165.

Park, P., & Lee, W. L. (1999). A theoretical framework for participatory evaluation research. *Sociological Practice*, *1*(2), 89–100.

Pickett, S. T., Burch, W. R., & Grove, J. M. (1999). Interdisciplinary research: Maintaining the constructive impulse in a culture of criticism. *Ecosystems*, *2*, 302–307.

President's New Freedom Commission on Mental Health. (2003). *Achieving the promise: Transforming mental health care in America. Final Report* (DHHS Publication SMA-03-3831). Rockville, MD: U.S. Department of Health and Human Services.

Randall, J., Swenson, C. C., & Henggeler, S. W. (1999). Neighborhood solutions for neighborhood problems: An empirically based violence prevention collaboration. *Health Education and Behavior*, *26*, 806–820.

Reed, G. M., & Collins, B. E. (1994). Mental health research and service delivery: A three communities model. *Psychological Rehabilitation Journal*, *17*, 71–81.

Reich, S., & Reich, J. (2006). Cultural competence in interdisciplinary collaborations: A method for respecting diversity in research partnerships. *American Journal of Community Psychology*, *38*, 51–62.

Rosnow, R. L., & Marianthi, G. (1986). *Contextualism and understanding in behavioral science: Implications for research and theory.* New York: Praeger.

Ross-Gordon, J. M., Martin, L. G., & Briscoe, D. B. (1990). *Serving culturally diverse populations.* San Francisco: Jossey-Bass.

Rossi, P. H., Freeman, H. E., & Lipsey, M. W. (1999). *Evaluation: A systematic approach.* Thousand Oaks, CA: Sage.

Roussos, S. T., & Fawcett, S. B. (2000). A review of collaborative partnerships as a strategy for improving community health. *Annual Review of Public Health*, *21*, 369–402.

Sameroff, A. J., Seifer, R., Baldwin, A., & Baldwin, C. (1993). Stability of intelligence from preschool to adolescence: The influence of social and family risk factors. *Child Development*, *64*, 80–97.

Saunders, J., Davis, L., Williams, T., & Williams, J. H. (2004). Gender differences in self-perceptions and academic outcomes: A study of African-American high school students. *Journal of Youth and Adolescence*, *33*, 81–90.

Schensul, J., Robison, J., Reyes, C., Radda, K., Gaztambide, S., & Disch, W. (2006). Building interdisciplinary/intersectoral research partnerships for community-based mental health research with older minority adults. *American Journal of Community Psychology*, *38*, 79–93.

Scott, D., & Usher, R. (1996). *Understanding educational research.* New York: Routledge.

Seifer, S., Shore, N., & Holmes, S. (2003). *Developing and sustaining-community university partnership for health research: Infrastructure requirement.* Seattle, WA: Community-Campus Partnerships for Health.

Slaughter, D. (1988). Programs for racially and ethnically diverse American families: Some critical issues. In H. B. Weiss & J. F. Helene (Eds.), *Evaluating family programs* (pp. 461–476). New York: Aldine de Gruyter.

Slaughter, D. T., & McWorter, G. A. (1985). Social origins and early features of the scientific study of Black Americans and children. In M. B. Spencer, G. K. Brookins, & W. R. Allen (Eds.), *The social and affective development of Black children* (pp. 5–18). Hillsdale, NJ: Erlbaum.

Snowden, L. (1999). African American service use for mental health problems. *Journal of Community Psychology, 27,* 303–313.

Snowden, L. (2005). Racial, cultural and ethnic disparities in health and mental health: Toward theory and research at community levels. *American Journal of Community Psychology, 35,* 1–8.

Spoth, R., & Greenberg, M. (2005). Toward a comprehensive strategy for effective practitioner-scientist partnerships and larger-scale community health and well-being. *American Journal of Community Psychology, 35,* 107–126.

Stith, S., Pruitt, I., Dees, J., Fronce, M., Green, N., Som, A., et al. (2006). Implementing community-based prevention programming: A review of the literature. *Journal of Primary Prevention, 27,* 599–617.

Stroul, B. A., & Friedman, R. (1986). *A system of care for severely emotionally disturbed children and youth.* Washington, DC: CASSP Technical Assistance Center, Georgetown University Child Development Center.

Stroul, B. A., & Friedman, R. (1994). *A system of care for children and youth with severe emotional disturbances* (rev. ed.). Washington, DC: Georgetown University Child Development Center, Georgetown University Child Development Center.

Suarez-Balcazar, Y., Harper, G. W., & Lewis, R. (2005). An interactive and contextual model of community-university collaborations for research and action. *Health Education and Behavior, 32*(1), 84–101.

Sullivan, M., & Kelly, J. G. (2001). *Collaborative research: University and community partnership.* Washington, DC: American Public Health Association.

Tebes, J. (2005). Community science, philosophy of science, and the practice of research. *American Journal of Community Psychology, 35,* 213–230.

Toldson, I. L., & Scott, E. L. (2006). *Poverty, race and policy: Strategic advancement of a poverty reduction agenda.* Washington, DC: Congress Black Caucus Foundation.

Tucker, C. (1999). *African-American children: A self-empowerment approach to modifying behavior problems and preventing academic failure.* Needham Heights, MA: Allyn & Bacon.

Tucker, C. M., & Herman, K. C. (2002). Using culturally sensitive theories and research to meet the academic needs of low-income African-American children. *American Psychologist, 57,* 762–773.

Tucker, C. M., Herman, K. C., Ferdinand, L. A., Bailey, T. R., Lopez, M. T., Beato, C., et al. (2007). Providing patient-centered culturally sensitive health care: A formative model. *Counseling Psychologist, 35,* 679–705.

Turnbull, A. P., Friesen, B. J., & Ramirez, C. (1998). Participatory action research as a model for conducting family research. *Research and Practice for Persons with Disabilities, 23,* 178–188.

U.S. Census Bureau. (2007). *The American community—Blacks: 2004: American community survey reports.* Washington, DC: U.S. Department of Commerce, Economics and Statistics Administration, U.S. Census Bureau.

Vey, J. S. (2005). *Higher education in Pennsylvania: A comprehensive asset for communities.* Washington, DC: Brookings Institution.

Wandersman, A. (2003). Community science: Bridging the gap between science and practice with community-centered models. *American Journal of Community Psychology, 31,* 227–242.

Weissberg, R., Caplan, M., & Harwood, R. (1991). Promoting competent young people in competence-enhancing environments: A systems-based perspective on primary prevention. *Journal of Consulting and Clinical Psychology, 59,* 830–841.

Wiener, S. J. (1994). Funding youth development programs for young Black males: The little we know. In R. B. Mincy (Ed.), *Nurturing young Black males: Challenges to agencies, programs and social policy* (pp. 205–229). Washington, DC: The Urban Institute.

Yokshikawa, H., & Seidman, E. (2000). Competence among urban adolescents in poverty: Multiple forms, context, and developmental processes. In R. Montemayor, G. R. Adams, & T. P. Gullotta (Eds.), *Adolescent diversity in ethnic, economic and cultural contexts* (pp. 9–42). Thousand Oaks, CA: Sage.

# 2

# Historical Trauma

Kristin N. Williams-Washington

**B**y definition, trauma is the result of exposure to a stressful event that overwhelms a person's ability to effectively cope with a stressor (van der Kolk, 1997). Race-based discrimination is an undeniable stressor. The severity and specific circumstances of the trauma endured can have psychological consequences. Research has indicated that African Americans have suffered from multiple traumas—cultural, historical, and intergenerational—as a result of slavery, racism, and discrimination. Studies have documented the negative impact of widespread racial discrimination against African Americans (Franklin-Jackson & Carter, 2007; Landrine & Klonoff, 1996).

Because of the incongruent nature of the different criteria that must be met to acquire a diagnosis of posttraumatic stress disorder (PTSD), the concept of historical trauma was created to embody the specific symptoms that African Americans may experience. Furthermore, many trauma researchers have criticized the text revision of the fourth edition of the *Diagnostic and Statistical Manual of Mental Disorders* (DSM-IV-TR; American Psychiatric Association, 2000) definition and criteria for their lack of inclusiveness (Brown, 2008). Daniel (2000) indicated that it is erroneous to refer to the distress suffered by individuals of color as *post*traumatic because racism is not a specific, time-limited event; it is perpetual.

PTSD is a relatively new diagnostic category, first making its appearance in the third edition of the DSM (American Psychiatric Association, 1980). According to the fourth edition of the DSM (American Psychiatric Association, 1994), three specific types of events can lead to PTSD: (1) incidents that are, or are perceived as, threatening to one's own life or bodily integrity; (2) being a witness to acts

31

of violence to others; and (3) hearing of violence to or the unexpected or violent death of close associates. All of these categories differ from historical trauma.

Category 1 can encompass historical trauma but only if, in this case, African Americans believe they are currently in physical danger because of slavery, racism, and discrimination. Category 2 is probably the closest match to historical trauma in that African Americans have read and heard stories or watched movies that depict violence against slaves. Category 3 can be loosely interpreted to include historical trauma in that African Americans often hear of the violence endured by slaves, but these individuals from generations ago may not be considered close associates.

Because of this incongruence between PTSD and historical trauma, different terms are needed. Additionally, PTSD implies a pathology in which inflicted individuals are unable to cope with daily life. In contrast, historical trauma typically is not so overwhelming or debilitating that individuals cannot function in their daily activities. Similar to intergenerational trauma, some theories of trauma transmission identify a response to the trauma endured by previous generations as second-generation psychological trauma rather than psychopathology (Baranowsky, Young, Johnson-Douglas, Williams-Keeler, & McCarrey, 1998).

Historical trauma has been defined as "cumulative emotional and psychological wounding over the life span and across generations, emanating from massive group trauma experiences" (Yellow Horse Brave Heart, 2003, p. 7). Brown (2008, p. 167) confirms "the likelihood that a person whose culture of origin has a history of oppression or genocide may be living with effects of trauma exposure that occurred not to the individual but to their forebearers." The use of the term *historical trauma* typically has been limited to the experiences of American Indians and recently has been expanded to include the trauma endured by Holocaust survivors.

A more specific working definition of historical trauma was framed during a focus group held in Washington, DC, and should be considered when exploring the African American experience: the collective spiritual, psychological, emotional, and cognitive distress perpetuated intergenerationally deriving from multiple denigrating experiences originating with slavery and continuing with pattern forms of racism and discrimination to the present day.

A validating observation that historical trauma can be expanded to include the African American experience comes from Maria Yellow Horse Brave Heart, who, in a news interview with Edna Steinman of *Spero News*, indicated that "historical or intergenerational trauma is similar to that suffered by the Jewish people as a result of the Holocaust, the Japanese Americans interned in California at the beginning of World War II and African Americans suffering the aftermath of slavery" (Steinman, 2005; Whitbeck, Adams, Hoyt, & Chen, 2004). Furthermore, many have argued that racism is indeed a form of trauma (Brown, 2008; Sue, 2003). Given the context of racism and subjugation, the concept of historical trauma can be applied to the case in which specific groups of individuals have been subdued to denigrating or disenfranchising standards such that individuals representative of those specific groups generations later may still be adversely impacted.

Similar to the impetus set forth by American Indians, there is a necessity to foster an understanding of the potential impact on African Americans of more than 300 years of captivity in America, ethnic cleansing under the guise of eugenics, and forced acculturation. This understanding is threefold. First, it is necessary to determine whether the grief and trauma currently endured are due to historical issues or to current racism and discrimination practices. Next, to comprehend historical trauma fully, an understanding of how trauma is transmitted from one generation to the next (i.e., intergenerational trauma) is imperative. Last, an understanding of the symptoms of historical trauma is essential in order to interpret accurately the prevalence of this newly acknowledged phenomenon among African Americans (Whitbeck et al., 2004).

Intergenerational (or multigenerational or transgenerational) trauma refers to the transmission of traumatic experiences across generations. Yellow Horse Brave Heart (1999) defines it as "the collective emotional and psychological injury both over the life span and across generations, resulting from a cataclysmic history of genocide" (p. 7). Additionally, a new term has been coined: *posttraumatic slave syndrome*, a derivative of PTSD that includes the notion that the legacy of slavery goes beyond single generations, creating residual psychological effects (Blitz, 2006).

Akbar (1996) believes that, despite being currently five to six generations removed from slavery, the trauma at the time was so severe as to implant a psychological and social shock in the minds of African Americans, and the current generations still carry the scars mentally and socially. In support of this position, Clark (as cited in Akbar, 1996, p. 3) points out that slavery has shaped the mentality of present-day African Americans more than any other single event.

Research on the detriment of perceived racism and discrimination is sparse. The general consensus has been to call for further research in order to achieve a better understanding of the effects of racism on the mental well-being of those afflicted (Rollins & Valdez, 2006). Specifically, additional research should be conducted on the historical aspects of the African American experience to foster an understanding of how they may still resound within the psyche of African Americans today.

## BIOLOGICAL/GENETIC FACTORS
## AND HISTORICAL TRAUMA

> Our brains are sculpted by our early experiences. Maltreatment is a chisel that shapes a brain to contend with strife, but at the cost of deep, enduring wounds.
>
> —TEICHER (2000, p. 67)

Historical trauma may manifest itself in terms of numerous biological responses. Symptoms may resemble those of PTSD in that the stress endured impacts both the endocrine and the immune systems. Furthermore, perceptions, feelings, and behaviors serve to alter the functioning of the brain and the central nervous system. However, the main factor is race: Being African American is the main criterion that increases one's risk for African American historical trauma.

Research has found that stress is a major cause of disease and illness, and long-term exposure can pose significant health complications as a result of maladaptive response. The body's natural goal is to maintain a state of homeostasis or balance. However, chronic stress upsets this balance, potentially resulting in an allostatic load. *Allostatic load* refers to the physiological toll of consistent or long-term exposure to the neuroendocrine stress response (McEwan, 2000). There are four conditions under which an individual can acquire allostatic load:

1. Repeated frequency of stress responses to multiple novel stressors.
2. Failure to habituate to repeated stressors of the same kind.
3. Inadequate response, leading to compensatory hyperactivity of other mediators.
4. Failure to turn off each stress response.

Each condition contributes to the stress response indicative of historical trauma.

The first two conditions deal with the frequency and manner of coping with both novel and habitual stressors. In historical trauma, the individual will treat each stressor, whether novel or habitual, as though it is the first time it has ever been encountered. This is indicative of the failure to habituate or to learn to accommodate the stressor. It is detrimental to the psyche in that the psychological wounding recurs every time the stress is experienced. The latter two conditions reflect the prolonged and persistent state of hyperarousal or hypervigilance that the individual may manifest as a result of stressors and lack of appropriate response. Thus, an individual's fight-or-flight response is constantly ready to react should he or she be faced with a subversive or denigrating experience. The dysfunctional response to allostasis causes allostatic load, which may be either a single or a contributing factor in the long-term effects associated with acquiring a disease or illness.

Similar to PTSD, individuals suffering from historical trauma may experience a biphasic state of arousal, which causes them to cycle between hypo- and hyperarousal. Hypoarousal involves psychological numbing; individuals refuse to acknowledge or feel anything in response to a stressor. The hyperarousal response is similar to the aforementioned hypervigilance, which causes a constant state of fight or flight. This biphasic state fails to include a state of homeostasis, so the body is never at rest. Lack of homeostasis may lead to increased heart rate, elevated blood pressure, hyperalertness, and amplified muscle tension and blood sugar levels. Many of these conditions are already disproportionately found within the African American population and often the risk of acquiring these conditions is increased through genetics.

The main system within the brain that is impacted by historical trauma is the limbic system. The limbic system, which is housed in the temporal lobe and regulates emotions, is composed of the amygdala, the hippocampus, and the hypothalamus. Disruption of any structure within the limbic system affects mood and behavior. The hypothalamus makes CRH (corticotropin-releasing hormone), which stimulates the pituitary gland to release adrenocorticotropic hormone (ACTH). ACTH then makes the adrenal glands secrete the hormone cortisol into the blood. The hypothalamus monitors cortisol levels. However, in a person suffering from either hypo- or hyperarousal, the hypothalamus may continuously influence the pituitary gland to over- or underproduce CRH regardless of the level of cortisol currently in the brain, causing imbalance. Structurally, research has indicated that the amygdala, which controls functions for arousal, is enlarged in individuals facing chronic stress.

In addition to specific biological and genetic factors, there are historical contexts that can precipitate historical trauma. This biological phenotype consists of race, culture, and trauma; the intermingling of these concepts serves to foster the notion of historical trauma and even make it more fathomable. According to the external locus of control theory, it is plausible that the prolonged circumstances under which African Americans lived since their arrival in America, as well as their personal experiences of loss of autonomy and persecution (e.g., being torn from their homeland, witnessing the deaths of friends and family during the middle passage, being sold as property, being forced to denounce their name and heritage), bred the collective notion among this population that control of their lives lies in the hands of others. This same external locus of control today operates in the form of institutional racism (e.g., inferiority stereotyping, derogatory appellations such as "nigger"). There are numerous situations and memories that may foster African Americans' mistrust of Whites, a constant sense of hyperarousal, and even lessened feelings of self-worth.

In May 1851, Louisiana physician Dr. Samuel A. Cartwright published his "Report on the Diseases and Physical Peculiarities of the Negro Race." In this article, Cartwright (as cited in Bynum, 2000, p. 1615) introduced two psychological disorders that he believed were specific to African Americans: drapetomania and dysaesthesia aethiopis. Drapetomania was defined as a disease of the mind that caused Black slaves to run away from White slave owners. This was technically referred to as "absconding from service." The psychological aspect of this "disorder" comes from the fact that slaves were thought to be crazy for running away (Bynum, 2000). Dysaesthesia aethiopica was a disorder that caused Black slaves to have a lack of work ethic. Symptoms included a refusal to work, disobedience, and insolence in addition to physical lesions (as cited in Bynum, 2000, p. 1615). The treatment for both disorders was the whip.

# INDIVIDUAL FACTORS INFLUENCING
# RISK AND RESILIENCY

One ever feels his twoness—an American, a Negro; two souls, two thoughts, two
unreconciled strivings; two warring ideals in one dark body, whose dogged strength
alone keeps it from being torn asunder.

—W. E. B. Du Bois (1989, p. 299)

The means and extent to which an individual is susceptible to historical trauma
are impacted by three factors: level of identity development, exposure to racism,
and knowledge of subjugation and denigrating experiences by previous generations. The most widely used model of identity development for African Americans
is Cross's (1994) model of nigrescence. This model discusses the four psychological stages that lead to true Black identity and self-acceptance (see Table 2.1).

In Stage 1, preencounter, individuals are fully cognizant of the negative
implications associated with being Black and deliberate whether their hue is light
enough to pass for White to avoid the subjugation and racism to be endured if they
live a "Black life." Thus, they fall victim to deracination in an effort to deny their
Blackness. To ensure complete acceptance, they tend to possess very pro-White
and anti-Black views. In Stage 2, encounter, Blacks view their race as an irrelevant
factor and wish to be viewed and accepted as simply a human being. Once they
realize that society tends to categorize people and fails to view everyone as just
human beings, the Black individuals defiantly accept their Black identity.

Stage 3 is immersion–emersion, which entails the possession of a pro-Black
and anti-White attitude. In this stage, Black individuals delve deep within the
Black culture, perhaps even embracing stereotypes by wearing "Black" clothes
and "Black" hairstyles and listening to "Black" music. In the final stage, internalization, anti-White feelings die out and give way to indifference. Emotional energy
gives way to psychological flexibility and Black individuals become comfortable
with their Blackness.

The natural progression through these stages can trigger a sense of historical
trauma. This is due to the fact that having a pro-White and anti-Black attitude
(Stage 1) implies a knowledge of Black denigration and a wish to escape the denigration by idealizing all that is White. Believing that race is irrelevant (Stage 2) is
indicative of the same wish to escape denigration: One longs to believe that everything endured by African Americans can be avoided if one is seen as a member
of the universal human race, not of a particular race. The possession of the pro-
Black and anti-White attitude (Stage 3) demonstrates assertiveness and resiliency
in spite of the persecution and a willingness to persevere through ownership of
one's race. Psychological flexibility (Stage 4) is achieved when both the good and
bad are accepted in both African American and White people and individuals are
comfortable in their own skin. As previously stated, having knowledge of denigrating experiences was one of the key points associated with African American
historical trauma, and each of the aforementioned stages involves knowledge.

**TABLE 2.1. Cross's (1994) Model of Nigrescence**

| | |
|---|---|
| • Stage 1: Pre-encounter | Pro-White/anti-Black attitude |
| • Stage 2: Encounter | Race is irrelevant; want to be seen as a human being |
| • Stage 3: Immersion–emersion | Pro-Black/anti-White attitude |
| • Stage 4: Internalization | Psychological flexibility; no hatred toward White people |

Thus, just being African American implies knowledge of the discriminatory, racist, and denigrating experiences endured by this population.

In a position statement titled *Resolution against Racism and Racial Discrimination and Their Adverse Impacts on Mental Health*, the American Psychiatric Association (2006, p. 1) acknowledged the following:

- Racism and racial discrimination adversely affect mental health by diminishing the victim's self-image, confidence, and optimal mental functioning.
- Attempts should be made to eliminate racism and racial discrimination by fostering a respectful appreciation of multiculturalism and diversity.
- Racism and racial discrimination are two of the factors leading to mental health disparities.
- Further research should be conducted on the impact of racism and racial discrimination as an important public mental health issue.

The fact that the American Psychiatric Association wrote and approved this document indicates that its membership believes that the detriments imposed by racism should not be taken lightly, especially in a society with a rapidly changing racial and ethnic composition.

Racial and ethnic minorities currently comprise approximately one-third of the U.S. population and, according to the U.S. Census Bureau (2008), by the year 2042 will become the majority. As the minority population increases, it logically follows that a positive correlation will occur among the individuals subjected to racism, racial discrimination, acculturation, and various other forms of denigration and marginalization.

Disparities between ethnic and racial minorities and Caucasians in the United States are well documented (U.S. Department of Health and Human Services, 1999). For example, in his 2001 report *Mental Health: Culture, Race and Ethnicity, A Supplement to Mental Health—A Report of the Surgeon General* (U.S. Department of Health and Human Services, 2001), U.S. Surgeon General Satcher noted numerous disparities in mental health services for racial- and ethnic-minority populations. Report data show that these populations are:

- Less likely to have access to available mental health services.
- Less likely to receive needed mental health care.

- Significantly underrepresented in mental health research.
- Likely to receive poorer quality of care.

These data indicate that the needs of African Americans are still failing to be adequately met.

Thorton (1997) believes that racism is harmful to health and, therefore, it is imperative that African Americans develop coping strategies to combat its effects. Evidence has been presented regarding the negative consequences of racism on both physical and mental health at all levels: personal, family, and community (Dole et al., 2004; Feagin & McKinney, 2003). Sellers and Shelton (2003) found that perceived discrimination is a predictor of future psychological distress among African Americans. Additionally, Clark, Anderson, Clark, and Williams (1999) indicate that the impact of racism on the historical legacy of African Americans should not be discounted, and that the negative stereotypes and rejecting attitudes toward African Americans do have measurable and adverse consequences on their mental health.

In addition to slavery, African Americans have been forced to endure a plethora of detrimental experiences, including iatrogenic treatments and experiments in eugenics. In *Bad Blood: The Tuskegee Syphilis Experiment,* Jones (1993) states, "No scientific experiment inflicted more damage on the collective psyche of Black Americans than the Tuskegee study" (p. 38). The Tuskegee study was a government-sponsored experiment conducted between 1932 and 1972. Throughout the course of this 40-year experiment, 399 African American males from Macon County, Alabama, were denied effective treatment for syphilis for the specific purpose of documenting the natural course of the disease. This study constitutes the longest nontherapeutic experiment on human beings in medical history (Thomas & Quinn, 1991).

The crippling legacy of the Tuskegee experiment is not an isolated incident of scientific or psychological abuse of African Americans. Some experts have long debated and studied whether Blacks are inherently and innately inferior to Whites (Dove, 1998; Franklin & Collier-Thomas, 1996), including in terms of mental capacity, even postulating that light-skinned Blacks are more intelligent than dark-skinned Blacks, although still inferior to Whites because of the Black blood running through their veins. Still today, human racial classification is a focus of scientific investigation by evolutionary biologists whose goal is to categorize individuals on the basis of presumed biological difference (Bonam, Warshauer-Baker, & Collins, 2005).

Some research suggests that females may be equipped with more protective or proactive racial socialization characteristics than males (Stevenson, 1994). However, other investigations report that perceived discrimination among African American women was related to a decrease in psychological well-being (Schmitt, Branscombe, Kobrynowicz, & Owen, 2002).

The knowledge of and exposure to racist, denigrating, and subjugating experiences are risk factors for historical trauma. The ability to avoid or mentally and physiologically tolerate racist experiences and evade the knowledge of denigration by previous generations may prove to be protective factors against historical trauma. Attempting to reduce the risk for historical trauma poses a dilemma, however: While being knowledgeable of African American history, and by extension African American historical figures, may increase the likelihood of historical trauma, avoidance behaviors could allow the history of African Americans to once again be subjugated or, worse, forgotten.

## FAMILY FACTORS INFLUENCING RISK AND RESILIENCY

At the heart of the deterioration of the fabric of Negro society is the deterioration of the Negro family.

—DANIEL PATRICK MOYNIHAN (1965)

In addition to the historical trauma endured psychologically, the detriments have transcended to impact African Americans socially, as reflected in the breakdown of the traditional family structure. The collapse in family structure can increase the risk for and decrease the resiliency to historical trauma. Socioeconomic status plays a formative role in the current construction of many African American families.

As a result of economic stagnation caused by unemployment, disenfranchisement, the welfare cycle, and other factors, African American families are more likely to have several generations living under one roof. Thus, the typical nuclear family is extended to include not only parents and children but grandparents, aunts, uncles, and cousins as well. Additionally, because many African Americans make use of the collective "we," friends are often included within the family structure. Brown (2008) indicates that in communities of color individuals are identified as family based on their role in people's lives, not merely on their shared genetics.

Often, African American families may have as many as three generations cohabitating. Many believe that this multigeneration system is beneficial for childrearing and for socioemotional support (Taylor, Chatters, & Jackson, 1993). Although this family structure seems all-encompassing, a key component is often missing: the father. The lack of African American men within the family dynamic is becoming more apparent. In his book *Come On People*, Bill Cosby indicates that approximately 70% of African American children are born to single mothers. African American women have thus had to assume the responsibility of not only being the backbone of the family system but also of being the sole provider. The reason for this phenomenon is unclear, but social theorists have postulated that the instability, disorganization, and stagnation in Black families can be attributed to the effects of slavery (Ruggles, 1994).

The deterioration/demise of Black families began with slavery, when many individuals were taken from their families and sold to masters in different areas. The Black man was not in control of his family, this being the master's privilege, and grew to lack the pride and entitlement associated with having a family and being the head of a household. It is believed that African American men still lack this sense of pride and entitlement, and for myriad reasons, among them a disproportionate number of available women because of high incarceration rates for men, do not feel compelled to "settle down."

However, although currently many African American families lack a father figure, which is a point of ridicule, this model of African American family structure is being used by divorced European American families in their struggles to protect the general welfare of dependent children, resolve confusion about family roles, and redefine the family (Crosbie-Burnett & Lewis, 1993). That this model is being mirrored by other populations is a testament to the resiliency and strength of African American women for attempting to maintain family structure.

African American parents raise their children to deal with racism, and the family structure operates accordingly. African American children are taught that they must work twice as hard to achieve the same as their Caucasian counterparts. This is a significant burden to bear as a child, and having this knowledge increases both the risk for and resiliency to historical trauma. Knowing at a young age that the world is an unfair place and that you are the individual who will be treated unfairly increases the risk, but this knowledge also increases resiliency and strength: A child will not be completely thrown off guard when he or she encounters racism.

Additionally, the African American parent–child dyad may be tested because of the absolute necessity for the parent to work, which often forces children to grow up faster. For example, the eldest child becomes the parent figure to younger siblings and is thus held to higher standards than same-age counterparts. In their study of parents' experience with racism and its effects on children, Caughy, O'Campo, and Muntaner (2004) found greater problem behaviors among children whose parents were in denial about racist encounters. Additionally, a study involving parents of African American 3-year-olds found that children's well-being was positively influenced by the presence of the father in the home (Black, Dubowitz, & Starr, 1999). Thus, the absence of Black fathers creates a cycle that will only further cripple the African American family.

Ultimately, a two-parent family structure is the most protective factor against historical trauma and results in increased resiliency. Although African American women possess qualities of resilience to adequately maintain a family in the absence of African American men, they are more likely to suffer from stress caused by racism, inadequate resources, and relationship conflicts (McCallum, Arnold, & Bolland, 2002). This stress often trickles down to the children, causing them to experience an inordinate amount of stress at an early age.

The combination of adolescent stress and lack of a paternal figure often produces a cycle either negative or positive: Boys who grow up without a father figure can decide to become better fathers themselves or to repeat their father's behavior, believing that, just as they experienced, fatherhood is optional. Likewise, girls who grow up without a father can be determined that their own children will not be fatherless or can, not uncommonly, repeat their mother's single-parent experience.

## SOCIAL AND COMMUNITY FACTORS INFLUENCING RISK AND RESILIENCY

Trauma tends to be a central issue for individuals with mental health problems, and there are both social and community liabilities associated with ignoring trauma. This concept is better explained by examining the condition of African Americans in the United States. The great majority of African Americans live within an urban center of concentric circles, or ghettos. Not uncommonly, the middle class, looking for affordable city housing, will come in and rebuild the ghettos for their own benefit, thereby displacing—and revictimizing—impoverished African Americans, in this process of gentrification.

According to one census interpretation, the African American population seems to be holding steady rather than increasing, possibly because of Black on Black crime, increased abortion rates, or mortality from diseases such as diabetes and hypertension. Following slavery, a group mentality was established among African Americans that partially persists to this day: a "collective Black psychology" (Covington, 1999), defined as the bonding among African Americans as a result of segregation throughout American history. It was once believed that it "takes a village to raise a child" and African Americans used to subscribe to this notion. Not only has this principle been forgotten, but it seems like "the streets" are plagued with the promotion of "I" at the expense of the collective "we," best described using the analogy of crabs in a barrel: Not one crab can get out because another will pull it down.

It appears that the lack of 40 acres and a mule increased the risk for historical trauma, when the provision of these items could have altered life courses and enhanced resiliency. Instead, because of spatial and institutional racism, many African Americans are running a losing race. *Spatial racism* refers to the trend in which the affluent displacing the poor in city homes leave the impoverished in deteriorating portions of cities or dilapidated suburbs while maintaining racial and economic segregation. In *institutional racism*, White privilege is maintained at the expense of people of color.

A contributing factor to the current state of African American economic stagnation is the lack of business, finance, and economic classes in the curricula of predominantly African American high schools. In predominantly White high schools, students have access to courses that teach the basics of finance management—the pros and cons of credit cards and the importance of remaining debt free, for example—and they have the opportunity to learn how to create business and marketing plans, thus preparing them for success. Predominantly African American schools do not have the same access to funding to ensure a complete, wide-ranging curriculum, limiting students' options in school and, in turn, their opportunities for success later. Many African American students do not have career or education counseling advocates who steer them on a path to success. African American students need champions who will give them tools for success: the knowledge that it is important to plan ahead, that they need to capitalize on their skills if they enter trade in order to be self-sufficient, and that higher education is a viable option. Whereas White students are encouraged to take college preparatory classes, attend evening SAT preparation courses, and consider their college options during their sophomore year in high school, predominantly African American schools fail to ask students if they are even interested in college until the end of their junior year.

The problem does not lie solely within the educational system, however; many African Americans do not even graduate high school because they are incarcerated instead. Upon release, their police record renders their employability difficult at best. Unemployment postincarceration is a huge factor for recidivism. For those who choose to "stay clean," welfare is often the last and only resort.

The socioeconomic status of Black people in America has long been a huge factor in the social issues affecting their community (e.g., crime, teenage pregnancy, high school dropout, single-parent families, and premature death among young Black men). The lack of opportunities and self-help tools for Blacks will only mire them deeper in poverty. This long-standing relationship with poverty has become a psychological barrier thwarting the ascension of the African American race as a whole. Many Blacks feel stagnant in their surroundings but have no hope that there is a better alternative within reach, because the ghetto has been the way of life for them for generations.

## THEORIES TO EXPLAIN
## AND UNDERSTAND HISTORICAL TRAUMA

Specific treatments for historical trauma do not yet exist. Theories for treatment, however, are those that serve as the foundation of treatment for PTSD. The majority of treatments and interventions for PTSD are based on cognitive theory, on the belief that improvements are fostered by changing the way a traumatized individual thinks about that experience. The goal is the reduction or removal of the negative feedback loop that has been created around the traumatic experience. This feedback loop is reactivated whenever the traumatized individual encounters something perceived as a threat. This threat is typically rather mild in comparison to the initial traumatic experience. This mild threat activates the threat-response structures, which cause the individual to interpret mild threats as extremely threatening, resulting in more arousal and activating the feedback loop to an even greater extent.

Cognitive action theory (Chemtob, Roitblat, Hamada, Carlson, & Twenty-man, 1988) views PTSD from an information-processing perspective. The information-processing network consists of several interrelated nodes, and information can be processed in one or more nodes at any given time. In an individual with PTSD, only one node is processing the information regarding threat arousal. This node, however, was weakened by the initial traumatic experience and thus interprets subsequent ambiguous or mild threats as catastrophic. The activation of this node arouses an expectancy that a threat will occur, causing the fight-or-flight response to be in a constant state of activation. It is believed that the greater the node activation for threat arousal, the more likely that intrusive memories will occur (Chemtob et al., 1988).

Psychological stress and coping theory uses cognitive appraisal and coping to interpret stressful encounters between individual and environment. Cognitive appraisal is a process in which an individual thinks about whether his or her well-being can be jeopardized by the environment. If a threat is perceived, the individual attempts to figure out in what ways the environment poses a threat. The individual makes use of both primary and secondary appraisal processes to determine whether the environment is primarily threatening (capable of inflicting harm or loss) or challenging (warranting a competition) (Folkman, Lazarus, Dunkel-Schetter, DeLongis, & Gruen, 1986). Coping is the process of consistently altering both thoughts and behaviors to achieve the most desirable outcome. Stress and coping theory incorporates balanced cognitive appraisal and coping for the benefit of the individual in dealing with stressful encounters.

Other theories relevant to the topic are based on the learning theory, model of stress response syndromes, and dual-representation theory. The learning theory approach to PTSD has its origins in Mowrer's (1956) two-factor learning theory. The theory postulates that cues during a traumatic episode can be considered conditional stimuli and the traumatic event serves as an unconditional stimulus. The cues elicit conditional responses. These conditional responses can be considered comparable to the unconditional responses of fear and anxiety elicited by the traumatic episode (Chemtob et al., 1988). The responses are strengthened/reinforced by the reduction in fear and anxiety.

Stress response syndromes in relation to PTSD are expressed in two phases: intrusive state and denial state. The intrusive state consists of thoughts, ideas, beliefs, and feelings, along with compulsive actions, while the denial state encompasses emotional numbing. The progression between these two states is linear.

The dual-representation theory of PTSD views traumatic memories as being processed in two systems and creating two representations. The two systems are the verbally accessible memory (VAM) system and the situationally accessible memory (SAM) system. All memories are encoded in either the VAM or SAM system. The VAM system is the basis of verbal accounts of a traumatic experience, and the SAM system stores sensory information and is accessed when a new exposure to a perceived threat is encountered. The dual-representation theory of PTSD is a way of looking at the systems underlying intrusive images characteristic of PTSD (Holmes, Brewin, & Hennessy, 2004).

Additional means of understanding historical trauma by proxy of PTSD and its effects can be interpreted through neuroimaging techniques and eye movement desensitization and reprocessing (EMDR). Research has shown that neuroimaging studies of individuals with PTSD have identified brain structural and functional changes. The brain may, in fact, be damaged by psychological trauma (Hull, 2002). The particular structures of interest include the hippocampus and amygdala. Studies of brain function in people with PTSD have utilized positron emission tomography (PET) or single-photon emission computed tomography (SPECT) and functional magnetic resonance imaging (fMRI). PET and SPECT detect radiation-emitting radioisotopes to measure blood flow. Other researchers have chosen fMRI over PET or SPECT because fMRI detects changes in blood oxygenation levels and offers better spatial resolution. Hull (2002) found hippocampal volume reduction and increased activation in the amygdala following symptom provocation and reduction of activity of the Broca's area. These results have implications for the emotional memory related to PTSD in the amygdala and the difficulty in labeling a traumatic experience in the Broca's area.

EMDR is a derivation of information-processing therapy that attempts to resolve symptoms caused by stressful or traumatic life experiences. EMDR makes use of cognitive restructuring to address past traumatic experiences. Some clinical trials suggest that EMDR may be useful in the treatment of PTSD (Alto, 2001). These theories are specified for the treatment of PTSD, but may have implications for the treatment of historical trauma among African Americans because of the general congruency of symptoms.

## Psychopharmacology

Historical trauma is not a diagnosable disorder by DSM-IV-TR standards. However, it may be a contributing factor to persistent depression and anxiety.

There are several neurotransmitters within the brain. Neurotransmitters are messengers that deliver neurological information from one cell to another. Mental illnesses that have a biological basis often originate from an inconsistency in the manner in which the neurotransmitter is either released from the presynaptic neuron or taken up into the postsynaptic neuron. The neurotransmitters of interest include serotonin, norepinephrine, dopamine, and gamma-aminobutyric acid. Three of these neurotransmitters have been found to be associated with clinical depression: serotonin, norepinephrine, and dopamine. The specific role of these neurotransmitters in depression is unclear, but there is a connection between the function of neurotransmitters and the successful use of antidepressant medication.

## RECOMMENDED BEST PRACTICES

That which must be achieved from a psychological viewpoint is the inclusion of African American historical trauma as a culture-bound syndrome within the DSM. The addition of this phenomenon will enlighten clinicians to the fact that slavery, racism, and denigrating experiences may be a contributing factor to an African American client's presenting problem in a therapeutic setting. It is pertinent to recognize and acknowledge the link between historical trauma and a patient's current life stressors. However, it should be noted that further harm may be caused by discussing these issues if it does not appear to be a relevant part of a client's presenting problem. Brown (2008) suggests that clinicians should engage in therapeutic work "with an enhanced awareness of the possibility of the impact of historical trauma on functioning" (p. 167).

Currently, only a few clinicians are well versed in providing therapy to clients with diverse racial and cultural backgrounds. However, in order to meet the growing demands of a changing population, it is imperative that all clinicians be equipped with the skills necessary to possess cultural competence:

1. Actively working to become aware of their own assumptions about human behavior, values, biases, preconceived notions, personal limitations, and so forth.
2. Actively attempting to understand the worldview of culturally different clients without negative judgments.
3. Actively developing and practicing appropriate, relevant, and sensitive intervention strategies and skills in working with culturally different clients (Sue, Arredondo, & McDavis, 1992, p. 481).

Bentacourt, Green, Carillo, and Ananeh-Firempong (2003) define a culturally competent health care system as "one that acknowledges and incorporates—at all levels—the importance of culture, assessment of cross-cultural relations, vigilance toward the dynamics that result from cultural differences, expansion of cultural knowledge, and adaptation of services to meet culturally unique needs" (p. 294).

Clinicians should be cognizant of how pivotal a thorough understanding of their clients' experience is to the psychotherapy process. Not only are there a limited number of clinicians who possess cultural competence, but there are also a limited number of researchers who include ethnic minority populations in their samples (U.S. Department of Health and Human Services, 2001). Hall (2001) stresses the need for psychotherapies for ethnic minority populations that are evidence based and that are culturally competent. This can only be achieved with further research on the detriments of race-related stress on African Americans.

Clinicians providing psychotherapy from a monocultural perspective do their clients a disservice. There are many differences between races and cultures that need to be addressed to form a healthy therapeutic alliance. The lack of empirically supported and culturally sensitive psychotherapies has two important consequences. First, minorities may refrain from seeking psychotherapy services because of their awareness of previous iatrogenic treatments. Second, empirical research that excludes ethnic minorities lacks external validity because minorities were not included in the norm sample, and thus the treatments may not have the same results when applied to ethnic minority groups.

For years, it has been suggested that merely matching/pairing a client with a racially ethnically similar clinician solves the issue of cultural competence (Schoenwald, Halliday-Boykins, & Henggeler, 2003; Snowden, Hu, & Jerrell, 1995). Although it is true that dissimilarity between clinicians and clients can cause misunderstandings, miscommunication, and cultural biases within counseling services, it has also been found that ethnic similarity between clinician and client is not a significant predictor of premature termination or of retention in overall treatment. Thus, the seemingly contradictory nature of current findings necessitates further research on the motivating factors of ethnic minority clients to abstain from seeking mental health services. Empirical research to date indicates that racial-ethnic matching does not increase the success rate of therapy and that it is more important for clinicians to be culturally competent (Maxie & La Roche, 2003; Shin et al., 2005).

The premise behind cultural competence is that clinicians should "not only appreciate and recognize other cultural groups, but also be able to effectively work with people from different cultural backgrounds" (Sue, 1998, p. 445). At a minimum, clinicians should initiate conversations regarding ethnic and racial differences in psychotherapy in order to foster the therapeutic alliance. Discussions of this nature enable clinicians to gain more insight into their clients. Once the concern of race and ethnicity is uncovered, clinicians may be able to provide a more holistic means of psychotherapy. By being more open to clients' experience, clinicians may be better prepared to empathize with them, thus making it easier to provide ethical treatment to actually get to the root of the clients' needs. Ethnic minority clients in one study reported that they preferred sensitive remarks regarding their concerns about racial issues rather than having clinicians ignore or avoid their concerns (Maxie, Arnold, & Stephenson, 2006).

Ultimately, clinicians should strive to be culturally competent as a means of maintaining ethical behavior toward their clients, as declared in Principle A: Beneficence and Nonmaleficence of the American Psychological Association's Ethical Principles of Psychologists and Code of Conduct. Principle A states that psychologists should benefit their clients and seek to do no harm. However, clinicians who lack cultural competence may be prone to treating all clients in the same manner without considering their cultural, racial, gender, or ethnic backgrounds. This may prove to be a hindrance or even a disservice to clients' psychological well-being.

# REFERENCES

Akbar, N. (1996). *Breaking the chains of psychological slavery*. Tallahassee, FL: Mind Productions.

Alto, C. (2001). *Meta-analysis of eye movement desensitization and reprocessing efficacy studies in the treatment of PTSD*. Retrieved August 28, 2008, from Digital Dissertations database (UMI No. 3015591).

American Psychiatric Association. (1980). *Diagnostic and statistical manual of mental disorders* (3rd ed.). Washington, DC: Author.

American Psychiatric Association. (1994). *Diagnostic and statistical manual of mental disorders* (4th ed.). Washington, DC: Author.

American Psychiatric Association. (2000). *Diagnostic and statistical manual of mental disorders* (4th ed., text rev.). Washington, DC: Author.

American Psychiatric Association. (2006). *Resolution against racism and racial discrimination and their adverse impacts on mental health*. Retrieved November 16, 2009, from *www.psych.org/Departments/EDU/Library/APAOfficialDocumentsandRelated/Position Statements/200603.a.SDX*.

American Psychological Association. (2006). *APA resolution on prejudice, stereotypes, and discrimination*. Retrieved February 25, 2007, from *www.apa.org/pi/prejudice_discrimination_resolution.pdf*.

Baranowsky, A. B., Young, M., Johnson-Douglas, S., Williams-Keeler, L., & McCarrey, M. (1998). PTSD transmission: A review of secondary traumatization in Holocaust survivor families. *Canadian Psychology, 39*(4), 247–256.

Bentacourt, J. R., Green, A. R., Carillo, J. E., & Ananeh-Firempong, O. (2003). Defining cultural competence: A practical framework for addressing racial/ethnic disparities in health and health care. *Public Health Reports, 118*, 293–302.

Black, M. M., Dubowitz, H., & Starr, R. H., Jr. (1999). African American fathers in low income, urban families: Development, behavior, and home environment of their three-year-old children. *Child Development, 70*(4), 967–978.

Blitz, L. V. (2006). *Racism and racial identity: Reflections on urban practice in mental health and social services*. Philadelphia: Hawthorne Press.

Bonam, V., Warshauer-Baker, E., & Collins, F. (2005). Race and ethnicity in the genome era: The complexity of the constructs. *American Psychologist, 60*(1), 9–15.

Brown, L. S. (2008). *Cultural competence in trauma therapy: Beyond the flashback*. Washington, DC: American Psychological Association.

Bynum, B. (2000). Discarded diagnosis. *Lancet, 356*, 1615.

Caughy, M. O., O'Campo, P. J., & Muntaner, C. (2004). Experiences of racism among African American parents and the mental health of their preschool-aged children. *American Journal of Public Health, 94*(12), 2118–2124.

Chemtob, C., Roitblat, H. L., Hamada, R. S., Carlson, J. G., & Twentyman, C. T. (1988). A cognitive action theory of post-traumatic stress disorder. *Journal of Anxiety Disorders, 2*, 253–275.

Clark, R., Anderson, N. B., Clark, V. R., & Williams, D. R. (1999). Racism as a stressor for African Americans: A biopsychosocial model. *The American Psychologist, 54*(10), 805–816.

Covington, J. (1999). African-American communities and violent crime: The construction of race differences. *Sociological Focus, 32,* 7–24.

Crosbie-Burnett, M., & Lewis, E. A. (1993). Use of African-American family structures and functioning to address the challenges of European-American postdivorce families. *Family Relations, 42*(3), 243–248.

Cross, W. E. (1994). Nigrescence theory: Historical and explanatory notes. *Journal of Vocational Behavior, 44,* 119–123.

Daniel, J. H. (2000). The courage to hear: African American women's memories of racial trauma. In L. C. Jackson & B. Greene (Eds.), *Psychotherapy with African American women: Innovations in psychodynamic perspective and practice* (pp. 126–144). New York: Guilford Press.

Dole, N., Savitz, D. A., Siega-Riz, A. M., Hertz-Picciotto, I., McMahon, M. J., & Buekens, P. (2004). Psychosocial factors and preterm birth among African American and White women in central North Carolina. *American Journal of Public Health, 94,* 1358–1365.

Dove, N. (1998). African womanism: An Afrocentric theory. *Journal of Black Studies, 28*(5), 515–539.

Du Bois, W. E. B. (1989). *Souls of Black folk.* New York: Penguin Books.

Feagin, J. R., & McKinney, K. D. (2003). *The many costs of racism.* Lanham, MD: Rowman & Littlefield.

Folkman, S., Lazarus, R. S., Dunkel-Schetter, C., DeLongis, A., & Gruen, R. J. (1986). Dynamics of a stressful encounter: Cognitive appraisal, coping, and encounter outcomes. *Journal of Personality and Social Psychology, 50*(5), 992–1003.

Franklin, V. P., & Collier-Thomas, B. (1996). Biography, race vindication, and African-American intellectuals: An introductory essay. *Journal of Negro History, 81*(1/4), 1–16.

Franklin-Jackson, D., & Carter, R. T. (2007). The relationship between race-related stress, racial identity, and mental health for Black Americans. *Journal of Black Psychology, 33*(1), 5–26.

Hall, G. C. (2001). Psychotherapy research with ethnic minorities empirical, ethical, and conceptual issues. *Journal of Consulting and Clinical Psychology, 69*(3), 502–510.

Holmes, E. A., Brewin, C. R., & Hennessy, R. G. (2004). Trauma films, information processing, and intrusive memory development. *Journal of Experimental Psychology: General, 133*(1), 3–22.

Hull, A. M. (2002). Neuroimaging findings in post-traumatic stress disorder: Systematic review. *British Journal of Psychiatry, 181,* 102–110.

Jones, J. H. (1993). *Bad blood: The Tuskegee syphilis experiment.* New York: Free Press.

Landrine, H., & Klonoff, E. A. (1996). The schedule of racist events: A measure of racial discrimination and a study of its negative physical and mental health consequences. *Journal of Black Psychology, 22*(2), 144–168.

Maxie, A. C., Arnold, D. H., & Stephenson, M. (2006). Do therapists address ethnic and racial differences in cross-cultural psychotherapy? *Psychotherapy: Theory, Research, Practice, Training, 43*(1), 85–98.

Maxie, A. C., & La Roche, M. J. (2003). Ten considerations in addressing cultural differences in psychotherapy. *Professional Psychology: Research and Practice, 34*(2), 180–186.

McCallum, D. M., Arnold, S. E., & Bolland, J. M. (2002). Low-income African-American women talk about stress. *Journal of Social Distress and the Homeless, 11*(3), 249–263.

McEwan, B. S. (2000). Allostasis and allostatic load: Implications for neuropsychology. *Neuropsychopharmacology*, 22(2), 108–124.

Mowrer, O. H. (1956). Two-factor learning theory reconsidered, with special reference to secondary reinforcement and the concept of habit. *Psychological Review*, 63(2), 114–128.

Moynihan, D. P. (1965). The Negro family: The case for national action. Office of Planning and Research, United States Department of Labor. Retrieved November 16, 2008, from *www.dol.gov/oasam/programs/history/webid-meynihan.htm*.

Rollins, V. B., & Valdez, J. N. (2006). Perceived racism and career self-efficacy in African American adolescents. *Journal of Black Psychology*, 32(2), 176–198.

Ruggles, S. (1994). The origins of African-American family structure. *American Sociological Review*, 59(1), 136–151.

Schmitt, M. T., Branscombe, N. R., Kobrynowicz, D., & Owen, S. (2002). Perceiving discrimination against one's gender group has different implications for well-being in women and men. *Personality and Social Psychology Bulletin*, 28, 197–210.

Schoenwald, S. K., Halliday-Boykins, C. A., & Henggeler, S. W. (2003). Client-level predictors of adherence to MST in community service settings. *Family Process*, 42(3), 345–359.

Sellers, R. M., & Shelton, J. N. (2003). The role of racial identity in perceived racial discrimination. *Journal of Personality and Social Psychology*, 84, 1079–1092.

Shin, S., Chow, C., Camacho-Gonsalves, T., Levy, R. J., Allen, I. E., & Leff, H. S. (2005). A meta-analytic review of racial-ethnic matching for African American and Caucasian American clients and clinicians. *Journal of Counseling Psychology*, 52(1), 45–56.

Snowden, L. R., Hu, T., & Jerrell, J. M. (1995). Emergency care avoidance: Ethnic-matching and participation in minority serving programs. *Community Mental Health Journal*, 31(5), 463–473.

Stevenson, H. C., Jr. (1994). Validation of the Scale of Racial Socialization for African American adolescents: Steps toward multidimensionality. *Journal of Black Psychology*, 20, 445–468.

Sue, D. W. (2003). *Overcoming our racism: The journey to liberation*. San Francisco: Wiley.

Sue, D. W., Arredondo, P., & McDavis, R. J. (1992). Multicultural counseling competencies and standards: A call to the profession. *Journal of Counseling and Development*, 70, 477–486.

Sue, S. (1998). In search of cultural competency in psychotherapy and counseling. *American Psychologist*, 53(4), 440–448.

Taylor, R. J., Chatters, L. M., & Jackson, J. S. (1993). A profile of familial relations among three-generation Black families. *Family Relations*, 42(3), 332–341.

Teicher, M. D. (2000). Wounds that time won't heal: The neurobiology of child abuse. *Cerebrum: The Dana Forum on Brain Science*, 2(4), 50–67.

Thomas, S. B., & Quinn, S. C. (1991). The Tuskegee syphilis study, 1932–1972: Implications for HIV education and AIDS risk education programs in the Black community. *American Journal of Public Health*, 18(11), 1498–1505.

Thorton, M. C. (1997). Strategies of racial socialization among Black parents: Mainstream, minority, and cultural messages. In R. J. Taylor, J. S. Jackson, & L. M. Chatters (Eds.), *Family life in Black America* (pp. 201–215). Thousand Oaks, CA: Sage.

U.S. Census Bureau. (2008, August 14). *An older and more diverse nation by midcentury*.

Retrieved November 16, 2008, from *www.census.gov/Press-Release/www/releases/archives/population/012496.html.*

U.S. Department of Health and Human Services. (1999). *Mental health: A report of the surgeon general.* Rockville, MD: Author.

U.S. Department of Health and Human Services. (2001). *Mental health: Culture, race, and ethnicity–A supplement to mental health: A report of the surgeon general.* Rockville, MD: Author.

van der Kolk, B. (1997, March 1). Posttraumatic stress disorder and memory. *Psychiatric Times, 14*(3). Retrieved July 19, 2008, from *www.psychiatrictimes.com/p970354.html.*

Whitbeck, L. B., Adams, G. W., Hoyt, D. R., & Chen, X. (2004). Conceptualizing and measuring historical trauma among American Indian people. *American Journal of Community Psychology, 33*(3/4), 119–129.

Yellow Horse Brave Heart, M. (1999). Gender differences in the historical trauma response among the Lakota. *Journal of Health and Social Policy, 10*(4), 1–21.

Yellow Horse Brave Heart, M. (2003). The historical trauma response among natives and its relationship to substance abuse: A Lakota illustration. *Journal of Psychoactive Drugs, 35*(1), 7–14.

# 3

## Beyond Tuskegee

### *Why African Americans Do Not Participate in Research*

Peter Edmund Millet
Stacey Kevin Close
Christon George Arthur

**A** review of the clinical literature provides evidence that African Americans are often underrepresented in clinical trials and other forms of research compared with Whites in both medical (Freimuth et al., 2001; Gamble, 1997; Lichtenberg, Brown, Jackson, & Washington, 2004) and behavioral (Graham, 1992; Hamilton et al., 2006) settings. The most frequently cited reason for this dearth of participation by African Americans is the infamous Tuskegee Study of Untreated Syphilis in the Negro Male.

In this project, 600 African American men, 399 of whom had syphilis, were unknowingly included as subjects in a longitudinal research project. These men were never given the opportunity to consent and did not even know they were part of an ongoing research project. They were misled to believe that their medical conditions, among them "bad blood," were being appropriately addressed by doctors, even though these medical researchers had no intention of providing treatment. Furthermore, these men were not given appropriate medical treatment even after penicillin was proven successful and was identified as the treatment of choice for syphilis in 1945. Although this study was initially scheduled to last for only 6 months, it continued for 40 years, from 1932 and 1972 (Centers for

Disease Control and Prevention, 2008). Many believe that this project caused irreparable damage to the trust between African Americans and both researchers and the medical community (Corbie-Smith, Thomas, Williams, & Moody-Ayers, 1999; Freimuth et al., 2001). This incident, however, although certainly a factor in the low research participation rates among African Americans, is only partially responsible for the current state of affairs.

In this chapter, we examine this phenomenon by discussing the experiences of African Americans in the United States from a historical perspective and the possible link between this history and current levels of African American research participation. Next, we examine apparent health disparities between African Americans and White Americans and their consequences for both researchers and African Americans. Finally, we examine some of the reasons why African Americans do and do not participate in research and make recommendations for researchers on how they can increase the participation of African Americans in both behavioral and medical research.

## HISTORICAL CONTEXT

A number of factors contribute to the paucity of African American participation in research. In order to understand these low levels of research involvement, it is necessary to examine the historical context within which African Americans found themselves upon their introduction to this country. According to John Hope Franklin, as the Pilgrims voyaged to North America to establish a Christian utopia in 1619, a Dutch merchant vessel stopped at Jamestown to sell/trade "19 odd negroes" to English settlers in Virginia (Franklin, 1972, p. 3). The European trade in Africans eventually brought millions of Africans to the Western Hemisphere. For people of African ancestry, the early founding of the English colonies and the United States came with terror, violence, and death. For much of their lives in North America, the majority of people of African ancestry lived in chattel slavery and state-sanctioned neo-slavery. The records of the horror of the slave trade and slavery can be found in the writings of John Hope Franklin, Hugh Thomas, and Eric Williams. From New England to the South, slaveholders maintained the system through the lash, terror, and the courts. The cases of abuse of slave men, women, children, and older adults are well documented by historians such as Wilma King (1995) and Eugene Genovese (1976). Along with the dreadful treatment of people of African ancestry, White leaders justified their actions through their biased interpretations of Christian teachings and scientific racism. Given such a history, scores of African Americans were, and remain, skeptical about the use and misuse of research by White scholars.

Historically, in the United States, African Americans have been described as intellectually (Jefferson, 1955), physically (Baker, 1998–1999), and spiritually (Johnson & Bond, 1934) inferior to Whites. Founding fathers such as Thomas Jefferson regarded enslaved Africans as inferior to Whites, even in the "secretion of bodily fluids." Jefferson believed that people of African ancestry lost most of their bodily fluids through sweating, which gave them a foul odor (Jefferson, 1954). He also argued in his *Notes on the State of Virginia* that people of African ancestry lacked the intelligence necessary to understand Euclidian geometry. Even when confronted with the work of Benjamin Banneker, Jefferson and most of his contemporaries continued to believe in the inherent inferiority of Africans (Jefferson, 1954, pp. 139–143).

Similarly, although noted fugitives such as Frederick Douglass and Harriet Tubman and thousands of others disproved these research claims with their intellectual and physical prowess, efforts to establish the inferiority of people of African ancestry continued. In the decades before the Civil War, noted anthropologist Samuel Morton "linked cranial capacity with moral and intellectual endowments and assembled a cultural ranking scheme that placed the large brained Caucasoid at the pinnacle." By 1854 George Glidden and Josiah Nott, a Morton protégé, published *Types of Mankind*. According to Lee D. Baker, their work bolstered "proslavery arguments by scholars and lay people" (Baker, 1998–1999, pp. 88–89).

The ideas of leading scholars such as Daniel G. Britton, John Wesley Powell, Frederic Ward Putnam, and Nathaniel Southgate Shaler further sanctioned the mindset for the denigration of people of African descent. Britton's *Races and People* proved to be one of the most influential publications of the period. Britton argued that based on scientific evidence the "European or White race stands at the head of the list, the African or negro at the foot" (Baker, 1998–1999, p. 91). His assumptions rested on "cranial capacity, color, muscular structure, vital powers, and sexual preference." Such research served to support segregation and its pain. These arguments also bolstered the thirst and actions of lynch mobs (Baker, 1998–1999, p. 91).

More recently, Carl Campbell Brigham, the developer of the Scholastic Aptitude Test (SAT), used the IQ tests taken by soldiers during World War I to argue that African Americans were the "least intelligent" people who took the test. As reported in the *Journal of Blacks in Higher Education* ("Carl Campbell Brigham," 1997, pp. 72–73), Brigham believed that a goal of the nation should be to develop a method to counter damage done to the "pool of American intelligence" by African Americans. Given this history, mistrust of standardized tests such as the SAT and research sponsored by White researchers remains in the African American community.

On September 4, 1969, the *Hartford Courant* published an Associated Press article on the work of Dr. William Shockley ("Study asked again," 1969). Shockley, who received a Nobel Prize in Physics and worked as a professor of engineering science at Stanford University, began to release the results of studies he conducted on the "loss of ground for Negro genetic potential for intelligence." The Nobel Prize winner believed that the intelligence of African Americans would continue to fall given their high birth rates. His research led him to believe that even changing the living conditions would not improve the hereditary intelligence of African Americans. Shockley also refuted the commonly held belief that African

Americans were inferior to Whites. In fact, the results of his statistical studies on African American and White athletes in the Olympic Games led him to believe that many African Americans were actually superior to Whites. Shockley ("Study asked again," 1969, p. 59) noted that African American athletes were "50 per cent more successful per capita in winning gold medals."

The physicist's arguments were well aligned with those of University of California–Berkeley's Arthur Jensen, whose findings were published in the *Harvard Educational Review*. Jensen and Shockley considered it useless to pump money into antipoverty, welfare, and busing programs. The two announced loudly and clearly to the American public that African Americans would never duplicate the educational achievements of Whites ("Study asked again," 1969).

Whites have used the Bible to justify the enslavement of African people (Johnson & Bond, 1934, p. 328). According to Genesis 5:5, in the words of Noah, "And he said, Cursed be Canaan: a servant of servants shall he be unto his brethren" Foster, 1974, p. 176). Herbert J. Foster argued:

> It is in the Babylonian Talmud, a collection of oral traditions of the Jews, that appeared in the sixth century A.D., that the sons of Ham are cursed by being Black. Throughout the Middle Ages and to the end of the eighteenth century, the Negro was seen by Europeans as a descendant of Ham, bearing the stigma of Noah's curse to be, forever, the White man's drawer of water and hewer of wood. (1974, p. 177)

For years racists in the United States have used this verse to justify and sanction the enslavement and inferiority of people of African ancestry. In addition, enslaved Africans often became pawns in cruel and callous experiments.

During times of slavery, research and experimentation were conducted on both the living and the dead. Historian Todd Savitt wrote that the Medical College of the State of South Carolina "continued to use Black patients for surgical demonstrations throughout the antebellum years" (Savitt, 1982, p. 335). He noted that White physicians "found it more convenient to obtain Black specimens than White" (Savitt, 1982, p. 337). Whites even purchased or hired slaves to rob graves for research purposes. One owner bought Grandison Harris, an enslaved African American, and ordered him to buy dead bodies for research. Harris even removed bodies from graves for his owner's use. On another occasion, a White physician in South Carolina paid a young boy "two dollars" for the body of a deceased slave child of 1 or 2. The youngster dug the body from the ground and brought it to the physician to be studied (Savitt, 1982, p. 340).

White physicians conducting research using live African Americans had little concern about the well-being of the subjects. When one Georgia physician/planter desired to test his theories on "heat stroke," he borrowed Fed, an enslaved man, wrapped him in wet blankets, and buried him up to his neck in a heating pit (Savitt, 1982, p. 344). To make sure that Fed had a greater propensity to faint in the pit, the physician made sure that he first completed the workday (Savitt, 1982).

In another instance of research on a slave, Dr. James Marion Sims, a physician, sought to find a cure for vesicovaginal fistula. This was a "break in the wall separating the bladder from the vagina, which allows urine to pass involuntarily to the outside from the vagina rather than from the urethra" (Savitt, 1982, p. 344). The severity of suffering associated with vesicovaginal fistula—its odor, pain, and infections—was well known. Although Sims eventually found a cure, he was quite open in reporting that his work on slave women was experimental (Savitt, 1982).

Some slaves found the strength and courage to flee slavery. For those bold enough to run, sometimes escaping to freedom via the Underground Railroad, some Whites attributed their actions to disease. For example, Dr. Samuel Cartwright, a Virginia-born physician, was summoned to a plantation in Mississippi to investigate why slaves continued to try and escape. He concluded that slaves have a physiological disorder, which he called "drapetomania" (literal translation: "running away mania"), that caused them to run away. Once slaves contracted this disease, they could not prevent themselves from running away, even if it was against their will (Duffy, 1968, p. 270).

Cartwright also believed that "rascality," a problem that overseers found among enslaved people, was a disease. He referred to the disease as "dysaesthesia." People stricken by this disease became lethargic or lazy. The prescribed treatment for both drapetomania and dysaesthesia included whippings with cat o' nine tails and bullwhips in an attempt to beat the illness out of the slaves (Johnson & Bond, 1934, p. 336).

Although the northern victory in the Civil War and Reconstruction Era amendments eventually brought legal freedom to more than 4 million slaves, most African Americans in the South continued to be shackled by a system of legalized segregation. It controlled their economic, political, and social lives. Both the judicial system and the American Association for the Advancement of Science supported legalized segregation in the South. The justices in the 1896 *Plessy v. Ferguson* decision argued that "the [Fourteenth] Amendment was intended to enforce equality between the two races before the law." They further concluded that the "amendment was not intended to impose an unnatural or impossible social equality" (Baker, 1998–1999, p. 91). Their decision gave legal sanction to terrorist lynch mobs that swept down on African American communities, often with the support of southern state leaders and the silence of national leaders. Some years earlier, writing in the *Atlantic Monthly* in the 1880s, Nathaniel Southgate Shaler, once a dean at Harvard University, considered African Americans unworthy of the vote. He proposed that a "scientific rationale" existed that supported this point (Baker, 1998–1999, p. 92).

One of the greatest changes in the lives of African Americans came with the development of an educational system for this population in the South. In the 19th century North, African Americans attended public and private educational institutions at all levels. The key to educating the masses of African Americans was the development of institutions in the South. Howard University in Washington, DC, eventually included both a law school and medical school, and Atlanta University became a well-known graduate school. African American education in the South emerged from a strong yearning for advancement, deliberate African American sacrifice, and northern support.

However, no name remains linked to this development more significantly than that of Booker T. Washington. Because of his strong hand and tireless work, Washington turned Tuskegee Institute into a school of world renown. Washington argued for the education of the masses through vocational and industrial training. His accommodating manner allowed him to easily move among the super rich and powerful like Andrew Carnegie, Theodore Roosevelt, and John Rockefeller. As World War I in Europe entered its second year in 1915, Booker T. Washington passed away. His death left a huge void in African American leadership (Harlan, 1983).

During World War II, Tuskegee Institute served as the home for the legendary Tuskegee Airmen. Despite the fact that many White military personnel circulated rumors that African Americans were innately prone to violence and rape (Franklin & Moss, 1988), the record of service and sacrifice of the airmen was well documented. The U.S. Public Health Service's Tuskegee syphilis study, discussed earlier, remains a sensitive and tragic issue, however. Few events or tragedies invoke such anger, fear, and skepticism about America's disregard for African American life as this study. Reverby (2001) argued that the U.S. Public Health Services 40-year study of "untreated syphilis in the male negro" continues to be mired in "historical fog and fact." She wrote that many African Americans believed that the U.S. Public Health Services deliberately infected some of the 399 men in the study who had syphilis and that, even after being informed otherwise, the idea remained firmly planted. Reverby says that the idea of deliberate infection even made its way onto "an NBC evening broadcast, an Eddie Murphy cartoon series, a scholarly scientific paper, talk radio call-in show, and community rumors." Other African Americans thought that the government's true targets were the Tuskegee Airmen (Reverby, 2001, p. 24). Incidents like this are clearly at the root of the mistrust many African Americans have for medicine and research (Gamble, 1997).

## THE TUSKEGEE LEGACY

Freimuth and colleagues (2001) found that African Americans' feelings about medical research in general and the Tuskegee study in particular were not predicted by socioeconomic status, gender, or geographical region. These same researchers found that African Americans were significantly more likely to be familiar with the Tuskegee study than White persons. Shavers, Lynch, and Burmeister (2001) found that 81% of surveyed African Americans had knowledge of the Tuskegee experiment, and that 51% of these reported they were less likely to take part in medical research because of it. Hamilton and colleagues (2006) corroborated these findings but found that the Tuskegee experiment was more of a deterrent for older than for younger participants. For younger participants, a general distrust of society and social institutions contributed more strongly to a reluctance to participate in research. Findings such as these are prevalent in the clinical literature (Corbie-Smith, Thomas, Williams, & Moody-Ayers, 1999) and suggest that the Tuskegee legacy continues to have a negative effect on the participation of African Americans in clinical trials.

However, Tuskegee is just one of many factors that contribute to the minimal levels of research participation by African Americans. Other barriers involve characteristics of both potential participants and researchers and recruiters. Barriers for potential participants include characteristic beliefs of African Americans about research, structural barriers, and conceptual barriers. Structural barriers involve real-world obstacles that make research participation difficult if not impossible (e.g., transportation, child care, time from work). These challenges, however, are often amenable to expedient resolution if appropriate resources are available (Chandra & Paul, 2003). Conceptual barriers involve attitudes, perceptions, beliefs, and particular theoretical orientations held by or imposed upon research participants. Typically, these are more subjectively experienced and are not easily modified. They may require greater time and effort to adequately address (Freimuth et al., 2001). A review of the literature suggests that there may be significantly more conceptual barriers than structural barriers.

Researcher and recruiter attitudes and actions may also play a part in the underinvolvement of African Americans in the research process. It has been shown that there is a correlation between researchers' and recruiters' attitudes toward African Americans and the amount of effort expended to recruit them (Chandra & Paul, 2003).

## CONSEQUENCES OF SUBOPTIMAL LEVELS OF PARTICIPATION BY AFRICAN AMERICANS IN CLINICAL RESEARCH

"Numerous reports have argued that the Tuskegee Syphilis Study is the most important reason why many African Americans distrust the institutions of medicine and public health. Such an interpretation neglects a critical historical point: the mistrust predates public revelations and the Tuskegee study" (Gamble, 1997, p. 1773). Gamble argues that the Tuskegee study is simply a metaphor that symbolizes the racism, misconduct, arrogance, and abuse that has been meted out to African Americans. Although one may acknowledge and understand the historical origins of this mistrust, African Americans' reluctance to participate in research studies and their mistrust of the institutions of medicine and public health persist, often with adverse consequences.

Kennedy and Burnett (2007) report that one of the consequences of abusive clinical research trials is that African Americans continue to refrain from participating in research trials because of lingering doubt, fear, resentment, and mistrust of researchers. Even if current research trials are monitored correctly, the effects of previous government-sponsored racism remain (Shavers, Lynch, & Burmeister, 2000; Thomas, Pinto, Roach, & Vaughn, 1994). However, as was documented earlier, this prolonged nonparticipation of African Americans in clinical research trials has significant adverse effects. For example, African Americans and other minorities are disproportionately affected by high blood pressure, high cholesterol, heart disease, cancer, Type II diabetes, and obesity (Singh, Kochanek, & MacDorman, 1996; Smedley, Stith, Nelson, & the Committee for Understanding and Eliminating Racial and Ethnic Disparities in Health Care, 2003). The nonparticipation of American Americans in clinical trials "jeopardizes generalizability of findings, limits ability to conduct subgroup analysis, denies patients access to state-of-the-art treatment for disease, and raises issues about equity in health" (Kennedy & Burnett, 2007, p. 141).

This lack of generalizability is not limited to the medical sciences. Research in the social sciences is also affected. According to Goss, Julion, and Fogg (2001), participation bias and high dropout rates among African Americans in a study on parenting made it difficult to conclude that the parent training models identified as effective were also successful among African Americans.

## CONSEQUENCES OF A LACK OF TRUST IN THE HEALTH CARE SYSTEM

Undoubtedly, the consequences that result from African Americans' mistrust and nonparticipation in clinical trials research are multifaceted (Simmonds, 2008). In addition to limited generalizability of research findings, another consequence is mistrust of medical providers and thus underuse of health care programs. According to Taxis (2006), African Americans underutilize the care provided by hospice programs. In 2003, of the 885,000 persons served, 82% were Caucasians and only 8% were African Americans. As stated by Cort (2004), "Cultural mistrust is an unfortunate dynamic of the relationship between African Americans and the healthcare system in America" (p. 67). Fears of mistreatment, the withholding of life-saving treatment, and the dominance of Whites in health care professions might have led to underutilization of services (Taxis, 2006). This cultural mistrust of the health care system is somewhat unique to African Americans because the death of African Americans has "often been associated with social injustice" (Cort, 2004, p. 64).

Another possible reason for this cultural mistrust is the fact that White professionals dominate the health care industry (Kennedy, Mathis, & Woods, 2007; Randall, 1996). Because of the ethnic disparity between the health care provider and the African American patient, there is no cultural connection between them.

Providers are ignorant of culturally relevant medical issues, and friction arises. These differences between patient and provider create barriers that threaten meaningful partnerships and effective communication, traits that are necessary for successful treatment (Kennedy et al., 2007). When a trusting patient–provider relationship exists, patients tend to be more participatory in their health care decision making (Mechanic, 1998; Mechanic & Schlesinger, 1996).

The fact that a significant level of mistrust remains among African Americans is alarming. This mistrust affects not only their involvement in research but also their compliance with medication and health care. The irony is that some African Americans cite the Tuskegee study, a study that denied them access to health care, as the basis for their rejection of needed health care. The consequence of Tuskegee's medical disenfranchisement of African Americans is self-disenfranchisement of the said group.

This self-denial of access to needed health care has contributed to the fact that African Americans, who comprise 12% of the U.S. population, account for 50% of AIDS cases (Centers for Disease Control, 2002; Hagan, 2005). Although it is understandable that African Americans might have just cause for mistrusting health care professionals, their self-denial of access is a major concern. The disenfranchisement that was orchestrated during the Tuskegee study is now realized when African Americans fail to participate in clinical trials. Abstinence of African Americans from clinical trials prevents drug companies from ascertaining which medications have the maximum health benefits for them. Hagan (2005) argues that it is unethical to dispense medications to a group of persons for whom there is little or no preexisting dose and safety information.

To document the mistrust that African Americans feel toward health care professionals, Hagan (2005) recounted a conversation overheard between two HIV/AIDS clients in an outpatient clinic:

> "'What did they give you?'
>
> "A prescription for that new drug AZT, an appointment for a breathing treatment to keep me from getting the AIDS pneumonia, and some vitamins."
>
> "OK, here's what you do. Go down the street and fill the vitamin and AZT prescriptions, because they'll know if you don't—the doctors can look on their computer and see if you went to a pharmacy and filled your prescriptions or not—but don't take the AZT. Take the vitamins, and you definitely want to do the breathing treatment because you don't want to get the pneumonia, but don't take the AZT. None of us are taking it. If your doctor asks you, 'Are you taking your AZT?', tell him you are, but throw it away instead. It's poison and it doesn't work in Black people anyway. It's just like Tuskegee all over again. They are just using it to experiment on Black people." (Hagan, 2005, p. 31)

For example, LaViest, Nickerson, and Bowie (2000) conducted a study to examine the attitudes about racism, medical mistrust, and satisfaction with care among African American and Caucasian cardiac patients. They found "a consistent racial disparity in reports of racism" (LaViest et al., 2000, p. 151). African

Americans consistently reported evidence of racism being meted out to them. They also consistently registered higher indices of medical mistrust and were consistently less satisfied with hospital care. Real or perceived, feelings of racial discrimination, mistrust of medical providers, and dissatisfaction with hospital care permeate the psyche of African Americans.

Similarly, a study by Oliver (2007) revealed several themes regarding African American males' lack of participation in prostate cancer screening: (1) their feelings of "disparity when accessing health care"; (2) a general "lack of knowledge" about what is involved in prostate cancer screening; (3) "past family practices" (i.e., the vicious cycle of nonparticipation is passed from generation to generation); (4) "mistrust of health care providers and the health care system"; (5) fear; and (6) the rectal exam being seen as "a threat to manhood" (i.e., during the exam, the men expressed feelings of being violated). Although many themes emerged from this study, mistrust of health care providers and the health care system is a prevailing reason for not participating in clinical trials, avoiding medical examinations, and not taking prescribed medications.

Like African American males, African American females do not have full access to medical care. In a study conducted by Cronan and colleagues (2008), only 64.4% of African American women reported undergoing a mammography screening within the past 2 years compared with 74% of Caucasian women. Similarly, Caucasian women reported lower medical mistrust than African American women. This finding is consistent with other scientific findings (Bolden & Wicks, 2005; Chow, Jaffee, & Snowden, 2003; Diala et al., 2001; Minsky, William, Miskimen, Gara, & Escobar, 2003; U. S. Department of Health and Human Services, 1999) that African Americans tend to delay seeking medical care and are thus more severely ill when they do present. Consequently, their hospitalizations are significantly longer (Bolden & Wicks, 2005) and their "symptoms precipitate behaviors that lead to a crisis, forcing individual and family to seek treatment in an emergency room" (p. 11). Compounding this, according to Bolden and Wicks (2005), emergency room care is "crisis-oriented, episodic, and less likely to enhance long term recovery" (p. 11), possibly impairing quality of life. Additionally, in an emergency room setting, patients are more likely to be treated by clinicians who are pressured for time, increasing the possibility of misdiagnosis (Bolden & Wicks, 2005; Institute of Medicine, 2003; Neighbors, Trierweiler, Ford, & Muroff, 2003; Rollock & Gordon, 2000).

## CLINICAL TRIALS: THE GOLD STANDARD

For the majority of medical and behavioral researchers, the randomized (single or double-blind) controlled clinical trial is the most widely utilized design for the evaluation of clinical interventions (Killien et al., 2000) and is commonly referred to as the gold standard of research (Israel, Schulz, Parker, & Becker, 1998). Historically, however, for a number of reasons, African Americans and members of other minority groups have been excluded from most clinical trials (Corbie-Smith et al., 1999; Shavers-Hornaday & Lynch, 1997). Recognizing the deleterious effects of this practice, since 1993, the National Institutes of Health (NIH) have required that in order for research projects to qualify for federal funding, women and minorities must be included in all clinical research or clinical trials:

> It is the policy of NIH that women and members of minority groups and their subpopulations must be included in all NIH-funded clinical research, unless a clear and compelling rationale and justification establishes to the satisfaction of the relevant Institute/Center Director that inclusion is inappropriate with respect to the health of the subjects or the purpose of the research. Exclusion under other circumstances may be made by the Director, NIH, upon the recommendation of an Institute/Center Director based on a compelling rationale and justification. Cost is not an acceptable reason for exclusion except when the study would duplicate data from other sources. Women of childbearing potential should not be routinely excluded from participation in clinical research. This policy applies to research subjects of all ages in all NIH-supported clinical research studies. (U.S. Department of Health and Human Services, 1993)

Similarly, research by Hamilton and colleagues (2006) stresses the importance of clinical trials including participants from all available demographic groups in both medical and psychological research. This is necessary "to ensure that any benefits associated with participation are equitably shared" (Hamilton et al., 2006, p. 18). Mason (2005) adds that since the 1980s there has been documented evidence that certain drugs, for both medical and psychiatric symptoms, have differing effects on African American, Hispanic, and White patients. Despite these finding, African Americans continue to be underrepresented in most types of empirical research.

## PARTICIPANT CHARACTERISTICS

Any discussion of barriers to the participation of African Americans in research should recognize what is perhaps the most core obstacle: the beliefs held by African Americans regarding research and researchers' motives. One common theme is that African Americans will be mistreated or harmed in some way if they participate in a research program. Although this perception is not universal among African Americans, it is common in certain segments of this population. Corbie-Smith and colleagues (1999) found that this belief may remain rooted even when evidence to the contrary is provided. This study, in which participants were questioned about their knowledge of the Tuskegee study, revealed much misinformation. The majority of participants refused to accept historically accurate information that was subsequently provided by the researchers. They appeared unwilling to accept information they could not personally verify.

Freimuth and colleagues (2001) found that some African Americans espoused the belief that research participants in general were mistreated and that African Americans were even more likely to be the recipients of this mistreatment. In addition, some of their respondents believed that White researchers thought of African Americans as animals and would probably treat them as such. Findings by a number of researchers (Ammerman et al., 2003; Shavers et al., 2001) indicate a common belief that, although all research may carry some risk, these risks are not distributed equally. African Americans saw themselves as the group most likely to be exposed to unnecessary risk and least likely to receive a complete and thorough explanation of the research. Furthermore, some research participants believed that medical researchers sometimes intentionally inflicted harm on African Americans (Corbie-Smith et al., 1999; Shavers-Hornaday & Lynch, 1997). For example, AIDS and Agent Orange exposure were seen as afflictions deliberately inflicted upon the African American community.

Other beliefs held by African Americans that are reported in the literature have nothing to do with a perceived fear of harm by researchers. According to Freimuth and colleagues (2001), some African Americans believe that researchers who come into their communities with the expressed intention of wanting to help are not completely altruistic: Although participants may receive help during the study, the researchers' ultimate goal is profit. Finally, Shavers-Hornaday and Lynch (1997) suggests that low levels of participation in medical research are a function of beliefs about the causes and treatment of physical or mental illnesses. Millet (2001) found that African Americans were significantly more likely than White Americans to believe in the effectiveness of spiritual treatments for certain illnesses, perhaps suggesting a diminished necessity for involvement in research or clinical interventions. In sum, although it is critical to look at various barriers that contribute to the low participation rates of African Americans, it is also important to first explore the belief systems of their communities.

## STRUCTURAL BARRIERS TO RESEARCH PARTICIPATION

To some degree, structural barriers to research participation may be construed as inconveniences that disrupt the daily functioning of potential participants, making it difficult for them to become engaged in the research process. Common structural barriers involve child care issues; time commitment (Shavers et al., 2001); study schedule; follow-up visits; concern about treatment side effects (Chandra & Paul, 2003); transportation issues, including traveling in unknown areas; and financial compensation (Chandra & Paul, 2003). However, most of these issues can be readily addressed with planning and forethought when developing the project methodology.

## CONCEPTUAL BARRIERS TO RESEARCH PARTICIPATION

The more challenging obstacles to address are conceptual in nature. These barriers may be divided into three broad categories: trust, education, and culture. Trust involves issues that are related to distrust of researchers based on personal or historical experiences of discrimination or prejudice, including concerns about researchers taking advantage of African American participants. Education refers to the amount of accurate information potential research participants have regarding the research process itself, the value of research participation, and perceptions of data and how they are used. Culture refers to beliefs about the stigma associated with some illnesses and the treatment of illness in the African American community.

The clinical literature is replete with instances of African American research participants reporting a lack of trust in both researchers and the medical community at large (Chandra & Paul, 2003; Corbie-Smith et al., 1999; Freimuth et al., 2001; Hamilton et al., 2006). This lack of trust often results in potential participants being less willing to engage in the research enterprise (Shavers-Hornaday & Lynch, 1997), specifically that they will be treated like guinea pigs (Corbie-Smith et al., 1999) or subject to experimentation. According to Shavers-Hornaday and Lynch (1997), some African American research participants feared they might be exposed to riskier research conditions and unnecessary or subpar treatments or might be seen by less experienced staff in poorer work environments using suboptimal technology. Finally, a number of researchers reported participant concerns regarding ethics and ethical misconduct and whether researchers' good is to truly help them or to just make a profit.

Many potential research participants expressed concerns regarding informed consent. The purpose of informed consent is to enable persons to voluntarily decide whether or not to participate as a research subject and to protect them from any potential risks (U.S. Department of Health and Human Services, 2005). A review of the literature provides data suggesting that some members of the African American community may not be aware of this purpose. Interviews conducted by Corbie-Smith and colleagues (1999) revealed that some participants believed the purpose of informed consent was to protect the researcher. Indeed, some of the physicians interviewed appeared to view informed consent as more of an inconvenient legal requirement than an opportunity to inform and engage patients. Similarly, Freimuth and colleagues (2001, p. 801) reported participants' beliefs that the purpose of informed consent was to protect doctors and that to sign it was equivalent to "signing away your rights." Additionally, they reported a common belief that all of the potential risks of a particular trial were not included on the informed consent form so as to minimize participation dropout.

The second type of conceptual barrier, education, involves participants' level of knowledge regarding various components of the research process. Freimuth and colleagues (2001) reported that some African American research participants demonstrated a lack of understanding of the research process, and Hamilton and colleagues (2006) found lack of knowledge of the structure or function of clinical trials to be one reason for the low participation among African Americans. Freimuth and colleagues' participants reported concerns about the maintenance of privacy and the perception that research might not be beneficial to African Americans but would ultimately benefit the researchers (Corbie-Smith et al., 1999).

Cultural barriers are beliefs or attitudes prevalent within a particular community that may have an impact on research participation. Hamilton and colleagues (2006) note that mental health research can be particularly difficult to conduct because of the stigma often associated with mental illness. Furthermore, Gary (2005) notes that African Americans are less likely than Whites to utilize the mental health system partially because of the stigma associated with such services. Similarly, research by Alvarez, Vasquez, Mayorga, Feaster, and Mitrani (2006) suggests that some physical conditions such as HIV and AIDS have a social stigma that may deter potential participants from taking part in research studies. Shavers-Hornaday and Lynch (1997) add that other cultural factors such as language and nonverbal communication patterns, as well as beliefs in alternate disease models, may contribute to the reluctance of African Americans to engage in medical research.

## RESEARCHER CHARACTERISTICS

Although the low level of research participation by African Americans may be partially the result of participant characteristics, some of the responsibility for this phenomenon may also lie with the researchers and recruiters who develop and implement the processes. Chandra and Paul (2003) identify a number of researcher-related factors. First, recruiters who are paid based on the number of participants they successfully engage may be more motivated to make money than to select individuals who fully meet the study requirements and thus may recruit candidates who are not appropriate for a particular study. Second, recruiters may believe that African American participants are too difficult to recruit and as a result may fail to actively seek them out for study inclusion. Third, some researchers may offer too much money as an incentive for research participation. This may have a coercive effect on financially challenged individuals, encouraging them to supply false data in order to meet the inclusion requirements. Shavers and colleagues (2001) note that:

1. Researchers sometimes have a tendency to exclude from research people with various diseases. They might be well advised to note that the world is not disease free and challenged to include people with various physical or mental conditions as appropriate.
2. Researchers should be mindful of their own cognitive processes. There is sometimes a propensity for researchers to exclude African Americans

because of a belief that they have a high attrition rate. This concern may, however, be addressed with proper planning and rapport building.

3. Researchers must sometimes choose between recruiting a sample that is truly reflective of the population of interest and selecting a group that may not accurately reflect the population of interest but that have a higher retention rate. There are costs and benefits associated with both of these options, which the researcher should carefully consider before starting an active recruitment campaign.

4. Often recruitment of participants for clinical trials is assisted by referring physicians or other professionals. It has been noted that on occasion some African American physicians may have the same lack of trust and level of skepticism as the patients whom they refer. This may lead to a reduction in the number of potential referrals.

In sum, a number of barriers lead to suboptimal levels of research participation by African Americans. Some are primarily caused by the thoughts and experiences of the potential research participants, others by the practices and beliefs of recruiters and researchers, and still others by the interaction of the two. In order to increase research participation by African Americans, it is crucial that all of these factors be taken into account in the planning stages of the research project. In the next section, we present some recommendations for addressing these issues both proximally and distally.

## ADDRESSING PARTICIPANT CHARACTERISTICS

The characteristics of participants who choose not to participate in research are closely aligned with many of the conceptual barriers to research involvement that have been discussed thus far. For this reason they are not addressed separately in this section. The following discussion of ways to respond to these barriers also applies to the issue of participant characteristics and beliefs.

## ADDRESSING STRUCTURAL BARRIERS

As stated previously, structural barriers are those that involve real-world obstacles that make research participation difficult if not impossible. Killien and colleagues (2000) suggest that a primary concern of researchers who are attempting to increase participation among minority persons should be making the process as convenient as possible for research participants. This may include planning for issues such as transportation, scheduling, and study location site.

Killien and colleagues (2000) recommend scheduling at least part of the research hours in the evenings or on weekends to make participation more convenient for persons who work a traditional schedule. Others suggest the use of van pools or free transportation to the research site to minimize the burden on potential participants (Alvarez et al., 2006; Freimuth et al., 2001). Taking this concept one step further, Killien and colleagues recommend taking the research to the participants in their own communities.

Similarly, Weinrich, Boyd, Bradford, Mossa, and Weinrich (1998) suggest performing the research in multiple locations; this not only can increase participation but can increase the likelihood of getting a representative sample of the group of interest. Additionally, they recommend scheduling the research activity so that it is part of an already established community activity. For example, participation may be greater if data collection takes places immediately after a church service where the participants are already in attendance and will not have to make a return trip to the research location.

Other researchers have identified simple tasks that, if implemented, may also have a positive effect on research participation. Alvarez and colleagues (2006) suggest contacting potential participants with a simple reminder of the time, place, and location of the research project. This may prevent a number of willing participants from missing sessions simply because they have forgotten the location or the correct date. Ammerman and colleagues (2003) suggest minimizing the paperwork required of community partners or organizations: These groups were more likely to sponsor and advocate for research that did not involve excessive paperwork or administrative processes.

Financial compensation is often a powerful inducement for participation in research studies (Ammerman et al., 2003; Freimuth et al., 2001). However, Chandra and Paul (2003) caution that excessive compensation may be coercive, and that some potential participants may falsify requisite information to make themselves appear eligible for inclusion in the study. They recommend setting an appropriate amount that is sufficient to serve as an incentive but not so extravagant as to be coercive. Additionally, care should also be taken in situations where recruiters are financially compensated based on the number of participants they engage. A tendency toward rapacity may lead some recruiters to exercise poor judgment when identifying persons who truly meet the criteria for inclusion in the study.

Finally, Chandra and Paul (2003) found that African Americans may be more likely to participate in research that is noninvasive. In their study, persons were more likely to take part in research that did not involve potentially painful or risky treatments (e.g., shots, ingestion) and that involved low-risk behavior (e.g., excretion monitoring).

## ADDRESSING CONCEPTUAL BARRIERS

Earlier conceptual barriers were described as involving attitudes, perceptions, beliefs, and particular theoretical orientations held by or imposed upon research participants. Typically, these are more subjectively experienced than structural barriers and are not easily modified. Conceptual barriers involve issues of trust, education, and culture. Trust issues may be addressed by establishing credibility, thoroughly exploring and explaining informed consent, and actively engaging the community; education issues by accurately and completely informing participants of what happens in the research process, dispelling commonly held myths, and exploring issues of data utilization and privacy; and culture issues by utilizing culturally sensitive methods to recruit and retain research participants, addressing the stigma associated with research held by many members of the African American community, and acknowledging the history of race-related abuse in this community.

## Trust Building

One of the first tasks to be addressed in trust building involves establishing credibility. Without this, it will not be possible to involve the community or get to the point where issues of informed consent can be discussed. Mason (2005) found that some research participants were positively influenced by the belief that they would be associated with a well-respected group of researchers. Distributing biographies of the research team was suggested as a way to familiarize participants with the researchers. Similarly, distributing reprints or summaries of past research (written in understandable layperson's language) was recommended as a way of letting participants know they are working with an experienced team. Mason also indicated that introducing participants to research team members during a community meeting or forum might be useful in establishing the credibility of and rapport with the research team. Finally, credibility might also be built by practicing professional behaviors, such as starting and ending on time. Actions such as these convey respect for the participants.

Wilson and colleagues (2006) suggest having previous research participants provide testimonials, where they describe their experiences as part of the project. This might be done via radio or television or in a live group presentation.

Trust-building efforts must also involve instructing participants regarding exactly what they will be asked to do (Freimuth et al., 2001) and informing them of any associated risks (Earl & Penney, 2001). Stated differently, it is critical that informed consent is thoroughly discussed and explored with project participants. In addition, they must also be informed of any alternative treatments that are available and clearly instructed that their participation in the study is completely voluntary and can be discontinued at any time (U.S. Department of Health and Human Services, 2005). Conversely, Corbie-Smith and colleagues (1999) and Earl and Penney (2001) note the importance of emphasizing the mutual benefits of research participation for both the researchers and the participants. People are more likely to participate in research if they can plainly see the benefit for themselves or their families. Killien and colleagues (2000) add that researchers should also point out how the research will benefit participants' communities. Earl and

Penney stress that honest, clear, and complete communication is a prerequisite to African American involvement in research.

Part of this progression toward complete transparency in the research process involves ensuring that informed consent documents are readily understandable to participants (Chandra & Paul, 2003). More specifically, documents must be of appropriate length and complexity and at a reading level suitable for the sample of interest (Chandra & Paul, 2003; Earl & Penney, 2001). They suggest emphasizing the fact that questions are always welcome and encourage researchers to include complete contact information, including more traditional methods of communication because many participants may not have e-mail. Mason (2005) found a relationship between literacy and distrust, which suggests that the inability of some research participants to read and understand informed consent documents diminished their trust of research situations.

One strategy that may be used to increase the likelihood that an informed consent form is appropriate for a particular sample would be to have community partners such as churches and schools help with the development of understandable documents (Earl & Penney, 2001). Additionally, once created, it may be beneficial to pilot test the consent forms with community partners to ensure appropriate length, content, and readability.

A third area to be addressed involves maximizing community involvement. A mutually beneficial, ongoing relationship between researchers and community members should be cultivated (Alvarez et al., 2006) in which participants are treated as true partners in the research, not just as subjects of clinical trials (Ammerman et al., 2003).

One of the most effective ways to actively and genuinely involve communities in research is through community-based participatory research (CBPR). CBPR differs from more traditional community research in that it involves having community partners more intimately involved in the research project. Killien and colleagues (2000) state that with CBPR community members should be involved in all phases of research: from design to implementation and from recruitment of participants to dissemination of the final results. In more traditional research, the research takes place in participants' home communities where they are typically viewed as subjects in the research project or experiment rather than active partners.

Savage and colleagues (2006) have identified four key components of CBPR: trust, collaboration, excellence, and ethics. Trust, in this context, means that researchers actively work to build a trusting environment by having appropriate community members serve as equal partners in creating a research project that is both meaningful to and appropriate for a particular community. Killien and colleagues (2000) and Mason (2005) note that this might initially be approached by the creation of advisory councils, which include community partners. These partnerships could assist in the conceptualization, design, and implementation of community-based research projects. Similarly, a number of researchers suggest that the inclusion of pastors or other community leaders might be useful in strengthening the relationships between the researchers and the community and may give the community members a sense of ownership in the project (Hatchett, Holmes, Duran, & Davis, 2000; Killien et al., 2000).

Collaboration infers that both community partners and researchers share in the decision-making process. Killien and colleagues (2000) and Mason (2005) recommend allowing community partners to assist not only in determining project goals but also in planning and implementing the project. Complete collaboration would involve incorporating community members' input during the entire process: from project conceptualization to development of the methodology, vetting of the informed consent, recruitment of project participants, carrying out of the study, and dissemination of results to project stakeholders.

Excellence requires that the project adhere to the most rigorous scientific methods possible. Savage and colleagues (2006) recommend providing community members with basic information on research methods and the scientific method. This will enable them to render more informed judgments about the project.

Ethics requires that all persons involved with the research project receive training in ethics and appropriate forms of behavior. Savage and colleagues (2006) suggest providing community members with basic information on ethics and the informed consent process. This will help them to better understand the safeguards that need to be implemented to protect research participants.

## Education

When working with African American research participants, it will be necessary to inform them accurately and completely regarding what happens in the research process, dispel commonly held myths about the research process, and explore issues of data utilization and privacy.

Hamilton and colleagues (2006) found that one reason for low participation among African Americans was a lack of knowledge of the structure or function of clinical trials. Research participants need to be given a clear and complete understanding of how the research process works. A number of researchers suggest that this should start with a complete and honest description of the study (Ammerman et al., 2003; Freimuth et al., 2001). Hamilton and colleagues add that providing research participants with accurate and comprehensive information from trusted community sources may serve to "dispel myths and correct faulty assumptions" (p. 18). The transparency of the research study may be heightened if participants are given information both verbally and in written form in language that is easy to understand. Mason (2005) recommends then having participants repeat the instructions in their own words to ensure complete comprehension. Additionally, involving participants' families in the decision-making process and possibly introducing them to research team members as appropriate may increase confidence in the research process (Mason, 2005).

It will be important for researchers to share with participants the importance of participation in research studies (Corbie-Smith et al., 1999), that is, how their participation may be able to help them personally and also be beneficial to others in their racial group. Participants should also be informed, in a noncoercive manner, regarding the negative consequences of nonparticipation for their particular group. It might be helpful at this point to state clearly why some research projects appear to target only African American or other minority groups as opposed to White participants (Chandra & Paul, 2003).

Corbie-Smith and colleagues (1999) remind us of the importance of addressing myths and correcting any identified misconceptions related to research. Common myths include beliefs that (1) the primary purpose of informed consent is to protect the researchers; (2) once individuals commence participation in a research study, they cannot discontinue it; (3) the only people who take part in research studies are either physically or mentally ill; (4) once they sign the consent form, participants can be made to do things against their will. These issues can be largely addressed by giving participants a clear and complete description of the current research project and information about what typically happens in research studies. Freimuth and colleagues (2001) stress the importance of informing potential research participants of their rights and add that they must be informed of any options or alternatives to the treatment prescribed by a particular clinical trial.

Finally, it is critical that researchers address any concerns held by participants about data utilization and issues of privacy. Participants must be informed honestly and completely about how the data will be used and reported. If their results will be combined with the results of others, the process of data aggregations should be explained. However, in situations where the design of the study is such that it is possible for participants to be individually identified, it is critical that they be told (1) why such identification is necessary and (2) what safeguards are in place for their protection.

Many potential participants decline involvement because they are fearful that their privacy will be threatened and the results used against them. Shavers-Hornaday and Lynch (1997) gave the example of a company that tested employees for sickle cell trait. These same results were later used to stigmatize the affected employees and deny them employment and health insurance benefits. In light of these situations, it is not surprising that many African Americans are wary of researchers. The more researchers are able to educate participants about how they will be protected, the more likely they are to garner participation.

## Culture

Addressing culture-related barriers involves utilizing culturally sensitive methods to recruit and retain research participants, addressing the stigma associated with research held by many members of the African American community, and acknowledging the history of race-related abuse in the lives of many members of the African American community.

When recruiting African American research participants, Freimuth and colleagues (2001) recommend using publicity and recruitment campaigns that are geared specifically toward the African American community. This might include advertising in newspapers and periodicals frequently read by African Americans, making presentations to community groups, or hosting radio or TV ads (Hatchett et al., 2000; Killien et al., 2000). Additionally, researchers can post advertisements in venues frequented by African Americans, for example in college dormitories, barber shops, hair salons, religious institutions, and community centers and at sporting or musical events.

Hatchett and colleagues (2000) note that, consistent with the oral tradition of many African Americans, word of mouth can be a very effective form of communication when recruiting research participants. Alvarez and colleagues (2006) recommend the "snowballing technique": having a small group of people initially notified of a particular project, who, in turn, contact others, ultimately forming an exponentially expanding network of social contacts.

A number of researchers (Mason, 2005; Shavers-Hornaday & Lynch, 1997) stress the importance of addressing the stigma associated with research participation. Although negative connotations abound (Mason, 2005), the stigma is especially strong when research addresses culturally sensitive issues such as mental illness (Hamilton et al., 2006) or certain medical conditions such as HIV/AIDS (Alvarez et al., 2006; Shavers-Hornaday & Lynch, 1997). Research by Millet (2001) found that African Americans were significantly more likely than White Americans to view the cause of mental illness as moral weakness; the condition was perceived as being largely attributable to the person him- or herself.

Researchers will be more successful in recruiting African Americans if these stigmas are addressed. Researchers can approach this challenge by presenting participants with factual information that refutes the validity of certain stigmas or other erroneous beliefs regarding research participation. However, because of the highly subjective nature of stigmas, many of which are not factual in origin, the mere presentation of facts and statistics may have only marginal success. Researchers may have more success by acknowledging the stigmas but countering them with arguments demonstrating how the potential benefit to the individual and his or her community may outweigh the negative beliefs. An alternative strategy might involve having past research participants provide testimonials about their experience having emerged none the worse for the wear. Finally, it might also be prudent to seek advice from collaborative community partners. These individuals might be in the best position to offer suggestions on how to address research-related stigmas in their particular community.

One final culture-related issue that has been shown to negatively influence research participation by African Americans is the race-related abuse that has been experienced, either personally or vicariously, by many members of this population (Corbie-Smith et al., 1999). Hamilton and colleagues (2006) found that the historical and current mistreatment of African Americans was a significant deterrent to their present-day research participation. Older African Americans were reluctant to participate in research because of knowledge of the Tuskegee syphilis study. Younger African Americans were dissuaded from participation by their current levels of social distrust, particularly in terms of involvement in physically intrusive types of research. Earl and Penney (2001) and Mason (2005) suggest that researchers need to acknowledge past incidences of abuse and be willing to engage in honest and open communication where they address any concerns presented by participants. Corbie-Smith and colleagues (1999) suggest that engaging in such a dialogue may serve to repair the trust that was damaged as a result of the Tuskegee study.

## ADDRESSING RESEARCHER-RELATED BARRIERS

Although any attempt to increase the level of research participation by African Americans must certainly start by looking at relevant characteristics of that particular group, it is also necessary to consider potential barriers stemming from the beliefs and actions of researchers and recruiters. Addressing this issue will most likely involve building a competent and culturally sensitive team and exploring researchers' beliefs about and behaviors toward African Americans.

Earl and Penney (2001) suggest that researchers must strive to create a trusting research environment, one in which participants feel safe and valued. This starts with listening, which conveys respect and is the basis for trust. The research staff must also acknowledge and be sensitive to the mistreatment and prejudice experienced by many members of the African American community (Killien et al., 2000). A history of negative societal experiences may cause some potential research participants to be wary of involvement in research activities. Shavers and colleagues (2001) state that, in addition to listening to and validating the concerns of the research participants, at the outset of the study, the researchers must clearly state their commitment to ethical principles and to the protection of research participants. Doing so communicates to the participants that their concerns have been heard and affirms the researchers' commitment to appropriate professional behavior.

Freimuth and colleagues (2001) note that African Americans may be reluctant to participate in research because of a concern of being viewed as personally responsible for any adverse conditions they may be experiencing. In all types of research, particularly medical, it is critical that the focus be steered away from behaviors or conditions that may be construed as the participant's fault. The same may be said about certain mental conditions, the cause of which is often attributed to personal characteristics. Researchers are advised to remain as objective and nonjudgmental as possible when dealing with sensitive issues, especially those that engender particular stigmas.

A number of researchers suggest that having diverse research teams may positively influence African Americans' participation (Chandra & Paul, 2003; Freimuth et al., 2001). According to Killien and colleagues (2000), not only should there be diversity, but the researchers should resemble the community to the greatest extent possible. Researchers would be well advised to work with community partners to accurately assess the relevant demographic characteristics of the community of interest. Utilizing researchers and field staff who match the community will likely put the participants at greater ease and facilitate data collection and community involvement.

One often overlooked reason why many African Americans do not take part in research is simply that they are not asked (Hatchett et al., 2000), this despite the fact that many would be willing to participate. In Shavers and colleagues' (2001) survey, 56% of African Americans indicated a willingness to take part in a research study if they were approached. Common reasons that researchers give for not actively recruiting African Americans include concerns about a perceived high attrition rate, methodological problems attributable to a small sample size, and the additional costs that might be incurred when attempting to recruit members of this group (Shavers-Hornaday & Lynch, 1997). There are ways to address all of these concerns. For example, when working with small sample sizes, researchers could make statistical corrections or adjustments, which may necessitate the use of nonparametric or other appropriate types of analyses. These issues should be addressed when planning the study's method. Additionally, the National Institutes of Health requires research projects to include women and minorities in order to qualify for federal funding (U.S. Department of Health and Human Services, 1993). As another example, Shavers-Hornaday and Lynch (1997) suggest that a significant factor in attrition is the quality of the researcher–participant relationship. They suggest that researchers pay careful attention to both conceptual and structural issues to strengthen the bond.

These barriers constitute the primary reasons behind African Americans' less-than-optimal levels of research participation. Zealously working with community partners to overcome these obstacles may significantly increase participation and may start to narrow the health disparity gap between African Americans and White Americans.

## SUMMARY

Currently, African Americans participate in clinical trials and other forms of research at levels significantly lower than those of White Americans. These suboptimal levels of participation may be largely attributed to the history of abusive and prejudicial treatment experienced by many African Americans. Starting with the introduction of slavery in the early 1600s, African Americans have been subjected to physical and mental atrocities and death at the hands of White Americans. Despite the abolition of slavery in the late 1800s, African Americans continued to be mistreated and to be thought of as subhuman. Using everything from theories of genetic inferiority to pronouncements that Blacks were cursed by God, Whites in America created a very oppressive environment for African Americans.

A classic example of the horrific mistreatment of African Americans is the infamous Tuskegee Study of Untreated Syphilis in the Negro Male, in which African American men were unknowingly included as subjects in a longitudinal research project, were misled to believe that they were receiving medical treatment, and were denied effective treatment in the form of penicillin. Having experienced these types of negative interactions with researchers and with American society in general, it is understandable that there would remain a significant lack of trust for research and researchers.

The unfortunate consequence of this low level of research participation is a significant health disparity between African Americans and White Americans. African Americans are affected by a number of physical conditions such as hypertension, diabetes and some types of cancer at higher proportions than White Americans. Suboptimal levels of research participation result in fewer data gathered on issues that impact the health of African Americans, and thwart the advancement of new or experimental treatments for certain health conditions. This is problematic because research suggests that certain drugs have differing effects on African Americans and White Americans for both medical and psychiatric symptoms.

Four primary factors contribute to the low levels of research participation among African Americans: (1) participant characteristics, (2) structural barriers, (3) conceptual barriers, and (4) researcher characteristics.

A commonly held belief among African Americans is that they will be harmed in some way if they participate in research. Although research is seen as having the potential for harming all participants regardless of race, African Americans believe their race may be disproportionately mistreated. Not all beliefs, however, are related to threats of harm. Other commonly held beliefs are that (1) researchers' main interest is profit, not participants' well-being and (2) there may not be a significant need for the research. Additionally, for many African Americans, spirituality or other nontraditional methods of healing may be seen as effective in treating both mental and physical maladies, thereby lessening the importance of or need for research.

Other hindrances to African American participation in research include both structural and conceptual barriers. Structural barriers impede African Americans willingness to participate because of the inconvenience. These include difficulties such as child care issues, transportation problems, and financial issues. Addressing structural barriers basically means finding ways to make the research experience convenient and worthwhile for the participant. These challenges can typically be overcome with careful planning and forethought. Solutions that may be easily implemented include providing child care and transportation, scheduling convenient times and locations, sending reminders, and providing financial compensation. Conceptual barriers are more challenging to address. They deal with the way participants think about and view their world and are more resistant to change than are structural barriers. They comprise three broad but interrelated categories: trust, education, and culture. Each of these areas includes thoughts, beliefs, attitudes, and subjective emotions that have been well ingrained into the psyche of African Americans. These beliefs may be thought of as lenses through which potential participants view the research world, often with the result of invoking feelings of fear, mistrust, and skepticism. Conceptual barriers can often be addressed satisfactorily if the researcher is willing to empathize with research participants and focus on their trust, education, and culture. Toward this end, in terms of trust building, researchers should (1) establish their credibility as professionals; (2) thoroughly explore the informed consent process; and (3) become actively involved in the community of interest, most effectively through CBPR, which views the community members as true partners rather than just subjects of a research project. In terms of education, research should (1) inform participants of exactly what happens in a research study; (2) dispel commonly held myths; (3) explore issues of data utilization and privacy; and (4) discuss the benefits of participation in research and the consequences of nonparticipation. In terms of culture, researchers should (1) use culturally sensitive methods of recruitment; (2) address the stigma so often associated with research; (3) acknowledge the many negative experiences that African Americans have historically endured in this country; and (4) be willing to recognize the source of mistrust among many African Americans and to engage in open, honest dialogue.

Finally, it is possible that certain researcher characteristics and attitudes may be correlated with suboptimal levels of African American research participation. For instance, researchers may not assiduously seek out African Americans because they believe that (1) this population will have a poor retention rate, (2) African Americans are difficult to recruit, and (3) recruitment will be too costly. Researchers and recruiters are advised to monitor their own cognitive process and potential biases and assess the effects of their beliefs on their recruitment efforts. It is critical that researchers establish creating a trusting environment, demonstrate sensitivity to the negative social situations many African Americans have experienced in the United States, and demonstrate their commitment to ethical principles and the well-being of research participants.

Future research should use this information as a starting point for an even more thorough examination of the complexities related to suboptimal levels of participation in research by African Americans. This might include differentially analyzing data based on participant sex, age, and level of education.

## REFERENCES

Alvarez, R., Vasquez, E., Mayorga, C., Feaster, D., & Mitrani, V. (2006). Increasing minority research participation through community organization outreach. *Western Journal of Nursing Research, 28*(5), 541–560.

Ammerman, A., Corbie-Smith, G., St. George, D., Washington, C., Weathers, B., & Jackson-Christian, B. (2003). Research expectations among African-American leaders in the PRAISE! Project: A randomized trial guided by community based participatory research. *American Journal of Public Health, 93*(10), 1720–1727.

Baker, L. D. (1998–1999, Winter). Columbia's Franz Boas: He led the undoing of scientific racism. *Journal of Blacks in Higher Education, 22*, 89–99.

Bolden, L., & Wicks, M. N. (2005). Length of stay, admission types, psychiatric diagnosis, and the implications of stigma in African-Americans in the nationwide impatient sample. *Issues in Mental Health Nursing, 26*, 1043–1059.

Carl Campbell Brigham: The man who devised the SAT. (1997). *Journal of Blacks in Higher Education, 17*, 72–73.

Centers for Disease Control. (2002). *HIV/AIDS Surveillance Report.* Atlanta, GA: Author. Retrieved January 18, 2009, from *www.cdc.gov/hiv/topics/surveillance/resources/reports/2002report/pdf/2002SurveillanceReport.pdf.*

Centers for Disease Control and Prevention. (2008). *U.S. public health service syphilis study at Tuskegee.* Atlanta, GA: Author. Retrieved February 27, 2008, from *www.cdc.gov/tuskegee/timeline.htm.*

Chandra, A., & Paul, D. (2003). African-American participation in clinical trials: Recruitment difficulties and potential remedies. *Hospital Topics: Research and Perspectives on Healthcare, 81*(2), 33–38.

Chow, J., Jaffee, K., & Snowden, L. (2003). Racial/ethnic disparities in the use of mental health services in poverty areas. *American Journal of Public Health, 93*(5), 792–797.

Corbie-Smith, G., Thomas, S., Williams, M., & Moody-Ayers, S. (1999). Attitudes and beliefs of African-Americans toward participation in medical research. *Journal of General Internal Medicine, 14*, 537–546.

Cort, M. A. (2004). Cultural mistrust and use of hospice care: Challenges and remedies. *Journal of Palliative Medicine, 7*(1), 63–71.

Cronan, T. A., Villalta, I., Gottfried, E., Vaden, Y., Ribas, M., & Cornway, T. L. (2008). Predictors of mammography screening among ethnically diverse low-income women. *Journal of Women's Health, 1*(4), 527–537.

Diala, C., Muntaner, C., Walrath, C., Nickerson, K., LaViest, T., & Leaf, P. (2001). Racial/ethnic differences in attitudes toward seeking professional mental health services. *American Journal of Public Health, 91*(5), 805–807.

Duffy, J. (1968). A note on ante-bellum southern nationalism and medical practice. *The Journal of Southern History, 34*(2), 266–276.

Earl, C., & Penney, P. (2001). The significance of trust in the research consent process with African-Americans. *Western Journal of Nursing Research, 23*(7), 753–762.

Foster, H. (1974, December). Ethnicity of ancient Egyptians. *Journal of Black Studies, 5*(2), 175–191.

Franklin, J. (1972). The great confrontation: The south and the problem of change. *Journal of Southern History, 38*(2), 3–20.

Franklin, J., & Moss, A. (1988). *From slavery to freedom: The history of Negro Americans* (6th ed.). New York: Knopf.

Freimuth, V., Quinn, S., Thomas, S., Cole, G., Zook, E., & Duncan, T. (2001). African-Americans' views on research and the Tuskegee syphilis study. *Social Science and Medicine, 52*(5), 797–808.

Gamble, V. (1997). Under the shadow of Tuskegee: African-Americans and health care. *American Journal of Public Health, 87*(11), 1773–1778.

Gary, F. (2005). Stigma: Barrier to mental health care among ethnic minorities. *Issues in Mental Health Nursing, 26*, 979–999.

Genovese, E. (1976). *Roll, Jordan, roll: The world the slaves made.* New York: Vintage Books.

Goss, D., Julion, W., & Fogg, L. (2001). What motivates participation and dropout among low-income urban families of color in a prevention intervention? *Family Relations, 50,* 246–254.

Graham, S. (1992). Most of the subjects were White and middle class: Trends in published research on African-Americans in selected APA journals, 1970–1989. *American Psychologist, 47,* 629–939.

Hagan, K. S. (2005). *Bad blood: The Tuskegee syphilis study and legacy recruitment for experimental AIDS vaccines* (New Directions for Adult and Continuing Education, No. 105). Wilmington, DE: Wiley.

Hamilton, L., Aliyu, M., Lyons, P., May, R., Swanson, C., Savage, R., et al. (2006). African-American community attitudes and perceptions toward schizophrenia and medical research: An exploratory study. *Journal of the National Medical Association, 98*(1), 18–27.

Harlan, L. (1983). *Booker T. Washington: The wizard of Tuskegee, 1901–1915.* New York: Oxford University Press.

Hatchett, B., Holmes, K., Duran, D., & Davis, C. (2000). African-Americans and research participation: The recruitment process. *Journal of Black Studies, 30*(5), 664–675.

Institute of Medicine. (2003). *Unequal treatment: Confronting racial and ethnic disparities in healthcare.* Washington, DC: National Academy of Science.

Israel, B., Schulz, A., Parker, E., & Becker, A. (1998). Review of community-based research: Assessing partnership approaches to improve public health. *Annual Review of Public Health, 19,* 173–202.

Jefferson, T. (1954). *Notes on the state of Virginia.* Chapel Hill: University of North Carolina Press.

Jefferson, T. (1955). *Notes on the state of Virginia.* Chapel Hill: University of North Carolina Press.

Johnson, C., & Bond, H. (1934). The investigation of racial differences prior to 1910. *Journal of Negro Education, 3*(3), 328–339.

Kennedy, B. M., & Burnett, M. F. (2007). Clinical research trials: Factors that influence and hinder participation. *Journal of Cultural Diversity, 14*(3), 141–147.

Kennedy, B. R., Mathis, C. C., & Woods, A. K. (2007). African Americans and their distrust of the health care system: Healthcare for diverse populations. *Journal of Cultural Diversity, 14*(2), 56–60.

Killien, M., Bigby, J., Champion, V., Fernandez-Repollet, E., Jackson, R., Kagawa-Singer, M., et al. (2000). Involving minority and underrepresented women in clinical trials: The National Centers of Excellence in Women's Health. *Journal of Women's Health and Gender-Based Medicine, 9*(10), 1061–1070.

King, W. (1995). *Stolen childhood: Slave youth in the nineteenth-century America.* Bloomington: Indiana University Press.

LaViest, T. A., Nickerson, K. J., & Bowie, J. V. (2000). Attitudes about racism, medical mistrust, and satisfaction with care among African American and White cardiac patients. *Medical Care Research and Review, 57*(1), 146–161.

Lichtenberg, P., Brown, D., Jackson, J., & Washington, O. (2004). Normative health research experiences among African-American elders. *Journal of Aging and Health, 16*(78), 78S–92S.

Mason, S. (2005, November). Offering African-Americans opportunities to participate in clinical trials research: How social workers can help. *Health and Social Work, 30*(4), 296–304.

Mechanic, D. (1998). The functions and limitations of trust in the provision of medical care. *Journal of Health Politics, Policy and Law, 23,* 661.

Mechanic, D., & Schlesinger, M. (1996). The impact of managed care on patients' trust in medical care and their physicians. *Journal of the American Medical Association, 275,* 1693–1697.

Millet, P. (2001, August). *Conceptualizations of mental illness: A racial comparison.* Paper presented at the 109th Annual Convention of the American Psychological Association, San Francisco.

Minsky, S., William, V., Miskimen, T., Gara, M., & Escobar, J. (2003). Diagnostic patterns in Latino, African-American and European American psychiatric patients. *Archives of General Psychiatry, 60,* 637–644.

Neighbors, H., Trierweiler, S., Ford, B., & Muroff, J. (2003). Racial differences in DSM diagnosis using a semi-structured instrument: The importance of clinical judgment in the diagnosis of African-Americans. *Journal of Health and Social Behavior, 43,* 237–256.

Oliver, J. S. (2007). Attitudes and beliefs about prostate cancer and screening among rural African American men. *Journal of Cultural Diversity, 14*(2), 74–80.

Randall, V. (1996). *Slavery, segregation and racism: Trusting the health care system ain't always easy. An African American perspective on bioethics.* Retrieved December 22, 2008, from *academic.udayton.edu/health/05bioethics/slavery.htm.*

Reverby, S. (2001). More than fiction: Cultural memory and the Tuskegee syphilis study. *Hastings Center Report, 31*(5), 22–28.

Rollock, D., & Gordon, E. (2000). Racism and mental health into the 21st century: Perspectives and parameters. *American Journal of Orthopsychiatry, 70*(1), 5–13.

Savage, C., Xu, Y., Lee, R., Rose, B., Kappesser, M., & Anthony, J. (2006). A case study in the use of community-based participatory research in public health nursing. *Public Health Nursing, 23*(5), 472–478.

Savitt, T. (1982). The use of Blacks for medical experimentation and demonstration in the old south. *Journal of Southern History, 48*(3), 331–348.

Shavers, V. L., Lynch, C. F., & Burmeister, L. F. (2000). Knowledge of the Tuskegee study and its impact on the willingness to participate in medical studies. *Journal of the National Medical Association, 266,* 2730–2751.

Shavers, V. L., Lynch, C., & Burmeister, L. (2001). Factors that influence African-Americans' willingness to participate in medical research studies. *Cancer Supplement, 91*(1), 233–236.

Shavers-Hornaday, V., & Lynch, C. (1997). Why are African-Americans under-represented in medical research studies?: Impediments to participation. *Ethnicity and Health, 2*(1–2), 31–45.

Simmonds, G. (2008). African-American participation in public health research. *Association of Black Nursing Faculty Journal, 19*(2), 69–72.

Singh, G. K., Kochanek, D. K., & MacDorman, M. F. (1996). Advanced report of final mortality statistics, 1994. *Mortality Vital Statistics Report, 45*(Suppl.), 23–33.

Smedley, B. D., Stith, A. Y., Nelson, A. R., and the Committee for Understanding and Eliminating Racial and Ethnic Disparities in Health Care. (2003). *Unequal treatment: Confronting racial and ethnic disparities in health care.* Washington, DC: National Academies Press.

Study asked again to find if Negro genetically inferior. (1969, September 4). *Hartford Courant,* p. 59.

Taxis, C. J. (2006). Attitudes, values, and questions of African-Americans regarding participation in hospice programs. *Journal of Hospice and Preventative Nursing, 8*(2), 77–85.

Thomas, C. R., Jr., Pinto, H. A., Roach, M., III, & Vaughn, C. B. (1994). Participation in clinical trials: Is it state-of-the-art treatment for African-American and other people of color? *Journal of National Medical Association, 86,* 177–182.

U.S. Department of Health and Human Services. (1993). *NIH policy and guidelines on the inclusion of women and minorities as subjects in clinical research.* Retrieved April 12, 2008, from *grants.nih.gov/grants/funding/women_min/ guidelines_amended_10_2001. htm.*

U.S. Department of Health and Human Services. (1999). *Mental health: A report of the Surgeon General.* Rockville, MD: Substance Abuse and Mental Health Services Administration.

U.S. Department of Health and Human Services. (2005). *Title 45: Public welfare. Part 46: Protection of human subjects.* Retrieved April 15, 2008, from *www.hhs.gov/ohrp/ humansubjects/guidance/45cfr46.htm#46.116.*

Weinrich, S., Boyd, M., Bradford, D., Mossa, M., & Weinrich, M. (1998, January–February). Recruitment of African-Americans into prostrate cancer screening. *Cancer Practice, 6*(1), 23–30.

Wilson, J., Mick, R., Wei, J., Rustgi, A., Markowitz, S., Hampshire, M., et al. (2006). Clinical trial resources on the Internet must be designed to reach underrepresented minorities. *Cancer Journal, 12*(6), 475–481.

# 4

# Spirituality and the Power
# of Religion

DONELDA A. COOK

**S**pirituality and the power of religion have historically been a lifeline to social, emotional, physical, material, and economic survival and well-being for African Americans (Billingsley, 1999; Boyd-Franklin, 2003; Cook & Wiley, 2000; Lincoln & Mamiya, 1990). African American spirituality derived from the experiences of African peoples making meaning of the presence and activity of the divine (God) in the midst of captivity in their own homeland and their transport, enslavement, oppression, and fight for freedom and justice in America (Floyd-Thomas, Floyd-Thomas, Duncan, Ray, & Westfield, 2007). These historical beginnings set the stage for the power of religion for most African Americans. As Frederick (2003) explains:

> Spirituality is specific to particular groups. ... It is informed first by an individual's relationship with God—nurtured by religious doctrine, holy scriptures, pastors, televangelists, and other mediators of faith. It is further informed by historical traditions—learned understandings of what it means to serve God. Finally, it is informed by social relations—one's positioning in society, which in the United States is inevitably raced, classed, and gendered. These three contributing elements form vast and complicated systems through which [African Americans] navigate their spiritual experiences. (p. 16)

Spirituality and religion continue to serve as a foundation for life satisfaction and well-being for many African Americans and a buffering influence on racial group, gender, class, and personal life stressors (Floyd-Thomas et al., 2007; Jang & Johnson, 2004; Marks, Nesteruk, Swanson, Garrison, & Davis, 2005; Taylor, Chatters, & Levin, 2004). This chapter draws from the disciplines of psychology, theology, and Black Church studies to examine African American religious involvement and health and the dynamics of African American churches that influence the health psychology of African Americans. Particular emphasis is given to ways in which health psychologists might cooperate and collaborate with African American religious practices and institutions.

## DEFINITIONS

Before discussing how African American religious involvement relates to health psychology, it is important to address the conceptual interplay among spirituality, religion, and the Black Church (the scope of this chapter is limited to the Black Christian Church tradition). For research purposes, defining spirituality and religion operationally calls for delineation between the two concepts. However, in discussing spirituality and religion in the context of African Americans, there exists a dynamic interplay between inherited remnants of African spirituality, an adapted Christian religious faith, and the most powerful institution in African American communal life: the Black Church. Spirituality and religious influences are integrated into the personal and collective identities of most African Americans (Dillard & Smith, 2005; Nobles, 1991), and the Black Church serves to aid African Americans in living out their faith in a historically oppressive society (Dillard & Smith, 2005; Lincoln & Mamiya, 1990). It is important to also note that some African Americans have sought the Nation of Islam for similar purposes, but the majority of African Americans adhere to the Christian faith (Cook & Wiley, 2000; Harley, 2005).

Koenig, McCullough, and Larson argue, in their *Handbook of Religion and Health* (2001), the importance of delineating characteristics that distinguish between religion and spirituality; however, such delineations may not be as distinguishable in the African American context. Koenig and colleagues characterize *religion* as (1) community focused; (2) observable, measurable, objective; (3) formal, orthodox, organized; (4) behavior-oriented, outward practices; (5) authoritarian in terms of behaviors; and (6) doctrine separating good and evil. *Spirituality* is characterized as (1) individualistic; (2) less visible and measurable, more subjective; (3) less formal, less orthodox, less systematic; (4) emotionally oriented, inward directed; (5) not authoritarian, little accountability; and (6) unifying, not doctrine oriented (Koenig et al., 2001). African American spirituality, however, is rooted in African spirituality, which is communal rather than individualistic (Nobles, 1991), visible in that God is seen in all things, both inward and outward directed, in communion with all of the created universe (Mitchell & Mitchell, 1989), and accountable to the community (Mbiti, 1969).

Many African Americans who do not subscribe to any particular *community focused, observable, organized, authoritarian, doctrinal religion* participate in the Christian religious beliefs, practices, symbols, and rituals ingrained by their familial religious influence (e.g., swearing on the Bible, wearing crosses, praying, foremost giving thanks to God our Creator) (Boyd-Franklin, 2003; Cook & Wiley, 2000). For instance, Taylor and colleagues (2004) report national survey data revealing that even persons who identified themselves as "religiously uninvolved" indicated that they prayed frequently and characterized themselves as fairly religious (p. 47). They also report survey findings of African American women who never or rarely (once a year) attend church but who identify themselves as "very" or "fairly religious" (Taylor et al., 2004, p. 47).

Most African Americans reverence the religious, social, and political power of the Black Church, honoring the social significance of the Church and its leaders in "functioning as the center of Black life, culture, and heritage for much of the history of the African American experience in North America" (Floyd-Thomas et al., 2007, p. xxxi). The Black Church in many respects is a receptacle for the collective Black experience (Floyd-Thomas et al., 2007; Harley, 2005). The term *Black Church* designates not a monolithic religious institution but rather a religious tradition that preserves sacred aspects of African American culture within the narrative of the relationship between an enslaved and oppressed people and their God (Floyd-Thomas et al., 2007). The Black Church tradition has given generations of African Americans a belief in the power of prayer and the grace of God as the source of their resiliency in surviving as a people. God's grace has been evident through the Middle Passage, slavery, Jim Crow laws, the civil rights movement, integration, and prevailing economic, educational, health, and social inequities. To survive and succeed in all that people of African descent have endured and fought to change in this country, the *power of religion* is recognized as *the power of God's Spirit manifested* in the activity of the Black Church (Floyd-Thomas et al., 2007).

## RELIGIOUS INVOLVEMENT OF AFRICAN AMERICANS

Research has consistently shown high levels of religious involvement among African Americans (Chatters, Taylor, & Lincoln, 1999; Levin, Taylor, & Chatters, 1994; Taylor, Chatters, Jayakody, & Levin, 1996). Taylor and colleagues (2004) posit a three-dimensional conceptualization of religious involvement: *organizational* (e.g., "church attendance, membership, participation in auxiliary groups"), *nonorganizational* (e.g., "private prayer, reading religious materials, watching or listening to religious television and radio programs"), and *subjective* (e.g., "perceived importance of religion, the role of religious beliefs in daily life, individual perceptions of being religious") (p. 32). Health psychology assessments of the role of religion in people's lives can be developed using Taylor and colleagues' model of religious involvement. There is a need to assess both organizational and nonorganizational religious involvements to identify potential benefits to individuals' health. Organizational involvements offer resources external to the individual (i.e., social support), whereas nonorganizational religious involvements offer internal resources (i.e., coping with distress).

Taylor and colleagues (2004) have conducted research on African American religious involvement for more than 20 years. They reported findings of a variety of national surveys revealing that only 10% of African Americans did not participate in organizational religion. Further examination of that 10% revealed that "80% report that they pray nearly every day, 27% report that they read religious books, and 21% watch or listen to religious programming on television or radio almost daily" (p. 33). National survey and qualitative studies have shown religious involvement among African Americans to be related to decreased distress (Jang & Johnson, 2004); increased social support (Marks et al., 2005); positive coping with serious problems (Ellison & Taylor, 1996); and positive therapeutic outcomes in affect, cognition, and behavior (Thompson & McRae, 2001). Most African Americans are very loyal to their faith and church traditions, as they have witnessed powerful spiritual experiences and practical benefits that have sustained them throughout their lives.

## MECHANISMS OF INFLUENCE IN AFRICAN AMERICAN CHURCHES

Because of the traditional role of the Black Church in the African American community, it is tempting to perceive the Church as monolithic. Skepticism of the profession of psychology has traditionally been voiced in the Black Church. A schism has existed between the worldviews of religion and psychology. However, clergy have become more open to the professional expertise of health psychologists as (1) more clergy have become seminary educated, (2) ministry has become more of a mainstream profession, and (3) the life circumstances and mental and physical health of church members have become increasingly challenging.

Floyd-Thomas and colleagues (2007) note W. E. B. Du Bois's observation over a century ago that "the Black Church's key role in the local community was to provide a total support system for its members" (p. 43). Support of members remains a unified mission of African American churches; however, today greater diversity in religious experience exists among African American churches. The diversity in African American churches offers varied mechanisms of influence on the health psychology of African Americans. The Church provides both positive and negative influences on the promotion of African American physical and mental health care.

### Diverse Orientations within African American Churches

Lincoln and Mamiya (1990) have characterized the diversity that exists among African American churches in terms of six dialectical tensions or polar opposites of a continuum. Cook and Wiley (2000) proposed that the dialects had implications for attitudes about counseling and psychotherapy that may be helpful to health psychologists in assessing clergy and church congregations' openness to health collaborations. Churches may integrate aspects of both sides of the dialectical tensions in their mission, operating practices, and worship experiences; however, one of the two tensions usually predominates. The following six dialectical tensions have different emphases:

1. *Priestly* functions (i.e., worship and spiritual life of members) *and prophetic* functions (i.e., community service and political concerns)
2. *Otherworldly* orientation (i.e., heaven and eternal life) *and this-worldly* orientation (i.e., affairs of the world in the here and now)
3. *Universalism* (i.e., universalism of the Christian gospel, one family in Christ) *and particularism* (i.e., confrontation of racial history of oppression and racism of White Christianity)
4. *Communal* (i.e., political, economic, educational, and social concerns of members and the wider community) *and privatistic* (i.e., responding only to the needs of the church congregation)
5. *Charismatic* (i.e., charismatic personality and divine gifts of the pastor, eliciting a strong cathartic response) *and bureaucratic* (i.e., organizational hierarchy and structure, membership and financial record keeping, educational credential of the pastor)
6. *Accommodation* (i.e., influenced by larger society, concerned with expectations of White society) *and resistance* (i.e., autonomously affirms African American cultural perspective and fosters self-determination and self-affirmation) (Lincoln & Mamiya, 1990, pp. 12–15).

Lincoln and Mamiya (1990) argue that African American churches are dynamic institutions that move within dialectical continua in response to social conditions.

Each dialectal tension may have implications for a church's focus on the health of the whole person (e.g., mind, body, spirit) and their receptiveness to referrals and collaborations with external health care providers. Churches emphasizing priestly functions and otherworldliness tend to focus primarily on the spiritual lives and to some degree the physical well-being of members of their congregations. Weekly prayer meetings provide an opportunity for members to bring their physical and emotional cares and "lay them on the altar for the Lord." The names of members who are "sick and shut in" at home or hospitalized for physical illnesses or surgery are often placed on a prayer list and visited by ministers or church leaders. However, mental health concerns are less likely to be acknowledged because of perceived stigma. Priestly churches may be open to health care professionals from the congregation offering preventive health interventions. The otherworldly orientation tends to espouse tolerance for enduring suffering in this life, while encouraging members to focus on the glory of the afterlife. As Harley (2005) proposes:

African Americans have developed a strength to suffer, struggle, survive, and succeed ... it is not acquiescence to victimization but an acknowledgement of perseverance. However, the Christian faith's interpretation and the public's perceptions of the word *strength* among African Americans, along with the stigma attached to appearing weak, are one explanation of African Americans' reluctance to seek mental health treatment. (p. 191)

Prophetic and this-worldly churches tend to focus on the physical and, to a lesser degree, emotional lives of the larger community. As part of their social services mission, counseling services and health education may be offered, particularly for persons of low income. Prophetic churches may be invested in culturally responsive health care interventions that serve to build up the African American community and recognize and combat the negative effects of racism and classism on African Americans' health. Predominantly prophetic churches may be more concerned with social activism and less responsive to individual members. Both prophetic and this-worldly churches tend to have more open attitudes regarding mental and physical health care than priestly and otherworldly churches.

Churches that ascribe to universalism and accommodation may focus more on the whole person, recognizing the links among mind, body, and spirit. They may be very open to health care interventions, as they are more in tune with, and trusting of, dominant-culture influences. Pastors are likely to collaborate with and refer members to local health care agencies and professionals. In contrast, those who ascribe to particularism and resistance would likely be skeptical of traditional medical and mental health care agencies and providers, noting the historical negligible treatment of African Americans through national health care policies and practices. However, similar to the prophetic church, pastors may trust health care professionals with Africentric orientations, and they may prefer to establish their own health care services.

Both the communal and privatistic churches may also be more likely to embrace the mind, body, and spirit approach of health psychology. The communal church tends to be more interested in providing large-scale services to the surrounding community, while the privatistic focuses on the congregation. Communal churches ascribe to the historical role of the Black Church of providing for all aspects of African Americans' lives. They might seek faith-based grant funding to provide health care services to the community.

Finally, the charismatic and bureaucratic churches may operate very differently in terms of mental and medical health care for their congregations. Charismatic churches may rely heavily on spiritual healing, under "the divine anointing" of the pastor, to provide physical and emotional healing. Pastors periodically offer healing services in which persons come before the pastor for laying-on of hands and healing prayer. The congregation may be most receptive to professional health care providers who have been endorsed by the pastor as having faith in the healing power of God and inviting the presence of God in their health practices. If a health care professional is perceived as doubting God's healing power, there may be concern that he or she may hinder God's healing blessings in response to the perceived lack of faith. Charismatic churches take to heart the gospel scriptures of Jesus saying, "Your faith has made you whole" (Matthew 9:22; Mark 5:34; Luke 7:50; 8:48), after healing someone. Bureaucratic churches are likely to be open to referring members for external health care services because they often interface with external agencies.

There is division among the Black Church community, both religious scholars and clergy, over the tensions between the prophetic and priestly dialects in today's African American churches. The arguments center on some African American churches' apparent deemphasis on the historical prophetic function of the Black Church, that is, social justice and activism (e.g., fighting against oppression, injustice, poverty). Rather, some churches are focusing primarily on priestly functions, personal salvation from sin, "winning souls for Christ," charismatic spiritual experiences, and "name-it-and-claim-it" prosperity preaching (Frederick, 2003, p. 150; Harris, 1991, p. 4). As Barnes (2004) explains:

> In its priestly role, the Church provides religious symbols, worship, and events to enable members to strengthen their relationship with the Deity ... enables congregants to survive in a society that is often unwelcoming and motivates them to look forward to a more promising afterlife ... tends to focus on use of scripture, songs, and church gatherings to strengthen the religious character of congregants to live lives that are set apart from secular society rather than challenging social problems in society. (p. 204)

Although the prophetic and priestly dialectical tensions are at the forefront of Black Church debates, additional dialectical tensions contribute to the concern that individual churches are doing more to promote their own institutional welfare over that of the African American community (privatistic vs. communal).

Some churches have accommodated to the success of White evangelical church growth movements, which have resulted in mega-churches and major television ministries (Harris, 1991). Mega-churches are defined by "a sustained average attendance of tens of thousands of church goers attending weekly worship services as well as the church's overall membership" (Floyd-Thomas et al., 2007, p. 42). Evangelical pastor Rick Warren's book, *The Purpose-Driven Church* (1995), was very influential in encouraging many African American churches to make a feel-good, spirit-filled worship experience a major focus of the church's agenda and to be consumer oriented in catering to the unchurched as an avenue for church growth. Harris (1991) argues, "The Black minister cannot morally or politically afford to be oblivious to the reality of the urban condition and preach as if the goal of Black people is to be mesmerized into an otherworldly frenzy without a real concern for eradicating the dehumanizing force of the present" (p. 49). However, Barnes (2004) posits, "The Church must address diverse sub-groups whose religious needs are not met using traditional methods ... and competition due to expanded religious social options. ... These challenges explain possible tensions associated with the Church's priestly and prophetic roles" (p. 203). (Discussion of the influences of mega-churches and television ministries on African American health psychology follows shortly). Finally, the influence of universalism over particularism has promoted an emphasis on multiculturalism, which seeks racial integration of traditionally African American churches, yet often fails to address and confront issues of racial discrimination and injustices, which impact the daily lives of most African Americans (Frederick, 2003).

The aforementioned debate over churches veering from the traditional Black Church prophetic tradition has implications for their influence on the health psychology of African Americans. The prophetic function has been responsible for the Black Church providing a host of social services to members of the African American community, particularly those of low income. Billingsley (1999) reports the results of a national Black Church survey designed to investigate the contemporary Black Church's participation in Lincoln and Mamiya's (1990) communal orientation. The study surveyed more than 1,000 African American churches, examining their provision of community outreach programs. More than two-thirds of the churches offered one or more community outreach programs "of nonreligious character and extended to members of the community including those not members of the particular church or any church" (Billingsley, 1999, p. 199). Nonreligous outreach programs include those that provide basic needs (e.g., food, clothing, housing), financial services, family counseling, teen parenting/sexuality seminars, prevention program for youth, and support programs for ex-offenders and their families (Taylor et al., 2004). Education and awareness initiatives are also provided, including health education for HIV/AIDS, diabetes, hypertension, and substance abuse. Seventy-one percent of the churches reported collaborations with social agencies (Billingsley, 1999, p. 201), the most frequent being local police departments and schools, welfare departments, and hospitals (p. 201).

The church survey data (Billingsley, 1999) reveal that the prophetic and communal functions of the Black Church offer opportunities for health psychology collaborations. The number of programs offered by individual churches ranged from none to 25 programs, with a median of three. The more active churches shared several qualities: They (1) were older and more established; (2) had a mixture of middle- and working-class members; (3) had larger congregations; (4) owned their own buildings; (5) had more paid clergy on staff; and (6) had senior pastors with various common characteristics (e.g., younger, married, more educated, seminary trained, active in the community) (Billingsley, 1999). Methodist and Baptist (particularly churches associated with the Progressive National Baptist Convention) denominations were more likely to provide community outreach services than Pentecostal churches. Churches that have strong community outreach programs demonstrate concern for the health of African Americans and tend to be open to collaborations with mental and medical health care providers.

## Contemporary Trends in African American Churches

The prevalence of charismatic worship styles in African American churches also has roots in the African American neo-Pentecostal movement that began in the 1960s and has spawned numerous Black mega-churches (Lincoln & Mamiya, 1990). According to Weems (2005):

> Neo-Pentecostalism, which was once associated only with the smaller, even marginalized Holiness and Pentecostal denominations of the '30s, '40s and '50s can be characterized by a lively, exuberant worship style, expository preaching that applies the scripture toward personal transformation and successful living, and at least a token acceptance in worship of gifts of the spirit as outlined in the New Testament (ecstatic praise, tongue-speaking, gift of prophesy, etc.). . . . Neo-Pentecostalism has contributed to phenomenal church growth in urban areas where many conservative mainstream churches were dying, unable or unwilling to evangelize new, younger members. (p. 122)

The neo-Pentecostal movement sought to integrate the charismatic, deeply spiritual worship experience with community outreach and social action. As Lincoln and Mamiya (1990) posit, "In contrast to most White churches in which the Pentecostal spirit and political conservatism seem to appear in tandem, the majority of the Black pastors and their churches in the neo-Pentecostal movement tend to be politically progressive" (p. 386). The deep charismatic spirituality of the neo-Pentecostal movement draws power from the Holy Spirit. According to Weems (2005), "In order to fight for justice, you have to have a strong spiritual life . . . the Holy Spirit, not human beings, is the one who rights the wrongs, establishes peace, melts cold hearts and ushers in the beloved community characterized by equality among peoples and human dignity for all" (p. 123). The charismatic worship experience consists of spiritual aspects that may influence African American health psychology.

Some researchers have found aspects of charismatic worship experiences to be therapeutic (Frederick, 2003; Griffith, English, & Mayfield, 1980; Griffith, Young, & Smith, 1984). In a handbook for evidenced-based treatment and prevention approaches, it may seem a contradiction to recommend that health psychologists accept individuals' self-reports of church experiences providing general feelings of well-being, physical or emotional healing, or deliverance from addictions. As Queener and Martin (2001) argue, health care providers "may view religion or spirituality as unscientific. Hence . . . interpret talk of God as passivity, dependence, superstition, hyperreligiosity, or magical thinking" (p. 116). However, by inquiring into individuals' responses to aspects of their church's worship, clinicians may discover ways that worship experiences can complement their medical or mental health treatment (Helms & Cook, 1999). Health psychologists who are interested in collaborating with African American clergy and churches must develop a bicultural attitude about religion and psychology, recognizing the strengths of both disciplines and managing the tension between two opposing perspectives on the basis of "evidence." For psychologists, evidence is perceived as outcomes that are operationally measurable. In Christian religion, evidence consists of scripture, church tradition, reason, and personal experiences of faith in the providence and promises of God that are both seen and unseen.

Accompanying the mega-church movement has been an increase in television ministries. There are 24-hour cable networks dedicated to televangelism. African Americans watch not only African American church broadcasts but also many White evangelical mega-church broadcasts, thereby receiving a variety of religious and spiritual perspectives. As Frederick (2003) explains:

> Television ministries . . . contribute information on how "to make things better." From marital relationships and financial problems to health and race issues, these television ministries offer a variety of solutions to individuals' everyday problems. Some scholars suggest this counseling discourse in television ministries is one of the reasons for their significant rise over the last several decades . . . marketed along the lines of providing assistance to the individual looking for motivation to change his or her life circumstances. (p. 134)

The trust that African Americans have had in their pastors for counseling and healing has extended to clergy with whom they have no personal relationship but rather a spiritual connection through television, radio, and Internet transmittals.

Frederick (2003) conducted a qualitative study of African American women's spirituality. Interview data reveal what televangelism offers (1) practical, no-nonsense "Bible-based" solutions to people's questions; (2) direct application of scriptural interpretations to daily life, which brings about change; (3) clear messages that sustain attention; (4) teachings about family and raising children; (5) teachings about financial prosperity in the believer's life; (6) encouragement for radical changes in the individual; (7) response to the emotional and spiritual needs of individual believers; and (8) encouragement to think beyond current circumstances (Frederick, 2003, pp. 131–159). The appeal of the positive, solution-focused message of media ministries may be similar to that of self-help and positive psychology interventions. Health psychologists and other health care professionals can collaborate with media ministries to reach out to African Americans in addressing their physical and emotional needs.

Celebrity preachers and spiritual teachers host national conferences and sell books, CDs, and DVDs. They provide "highly personal messages like 'How you can overcome your fears,' 'Five ways that you can tackle your finances,' or 'Seven steps to a more joy filled you'" (Frederick, 2003, p. 143). African Americans' receptivity to practical messages of hope provided by televangelists, regardless of race, suggests comfort in being able to anonymously access health and psychological information that speaks to their personal life circumstances. Their receptivity is based on their faith in the God of whom the televangelists are speaking and in the scripture-based instruction for living that offers hope in "things not yet seen" in their day-to-day existence.

Some of the preaching and teaching approaches of televangelists, however, may discourage persons from seeking help for personal problems because
this might be perceived as accepting and surrendering to life's difficulties. For
instance, prosperity preaching based on the Word of Faith movement "promises
that Christians should expect to achieve health, wealth, success, happiness, and
personal fulfillment ... during this life" (Frederick, 2003, p. 151). It prescribes a
"name-it-and-claim-it" approach to spirituality (Frederick, 2003, p. 150). Believers in Christ are encouraged to practice "positive confession" (Frederick, 2003, p.
146) in claiming the things that they want, believing that it is God's plan for all
Christians to be financially prosperous and physically healthy (Frederick, 2003).
Persons may go so far as to begin living today as if they have already received their
desired blessings. This exemplifies an "act of 'positive confession,' speaking and
acting according to profession ... [and a] demonstration of faith in God's promise"
(Frederick, 2003, p. 146). Persons may deny medical or mental health treatment
because they do not want to claim the illness; instead, they live and "walk in"
their profession of health and healing.

## Pastoral Leadership Styles

Pastoral leadership is a mechanism of influence in African American churches.
Although survey data reveal that African Americans have historically sought
counseling from their pastors rather than mental health providers and agencies
(Taylor et al., 2004), the changing role of pastors may inhibit their availability for
personal counseling. With the advent of the mega-church, senior pastors hold a
business executive or celebrity status that does not afford them time to respond
to individual congregants. With increased membership and the senior pastor's
visionary and executive function responsibilities, many churches now hire additional clergy to serve as secondary pastors over various ministries (e.g., youth
pastor, congregational life pastor, administrative pastor). The senior pastor may
be engaged in oversight of economic development, multiple building projects,
real estate ventures, development of educational institutions, and investment in
church-run businesses in addition to their focus on "receiving a word from the
Lord." Senior pastors with resources for church-based business ventures tend to
be progressive in providing for the health care of the congregation and the surrounding community, with services ranging from counseling and hospital visits
by ministers assigned to respond to the physical and emotional health of the congregation to the development of professionally staffed counseling services.

Some senior pastors are nationally recognized celebrities whose charismatic
preaching and spiritual healing services attract national followings. They espouse
extravagant lifestyles (e.g., elaborate church edifices, private jets, luxury auto-
mobiles, mansions) as signs of God's favor on their lives and ministries (Frederick, 2003). Television audiences are encouraged to "sow seeds into their ministries" by sending financial donations, with hopes that they will receive God's
favor in return (Frederick, 2003). Some televangelists sell prayer cloths or offer

to pray for persons in return for donations. Although their messages may address the emotional and spiritual needs of tens of thousands church members and a national broadcast audience, they offer limited personal attention. Perceived as God's anointed vessels, their word, prayers, healing touch, and books and taped sermons provide the healing and life application teachings that their followers trust. Rarely do celebrated pastors use their influence to promote secular healing practices; some speak against the necessity for counseling, psychotherapy, psychiatry, or medication.

Frederick's (2003) research led her to attend a national T. D. Jakes "Woman Thou Art Loosed" conference. Women from all over the country filled a sports arena believing that "God had sent this messenger, T. D. Jakes, and had given him a vision to 'loose women' from their social, economic, and spiritual chains" (p. 161). Frederick quoted the famed televangelist's remarks to the audience:

> "Many thousands of women ... are going to be loosed today. Suicide is going to be loosed today; spirits of depression are going to be loosed from you today; hallelujah, homosexuality is going to be loosed from you today; right women in wrong relationships. You're going to be loosed. Addictive behaviors, where somebody's abusing you, you're going to be loosed today. Loosed today from spirits of bondage, manipulation and control." (p. 163)

The authoritative charismatic preaching, accompanied by "signs and wonders" of God's spiritual powers manifested in an arena filled with women being "slain in the spirit," crying, shouting, dancing, and rejoicing as they claim their deliverance from emotional, physical, and spiritual bondage, promotes faith in spiritual healing.

Health psychologists must be open to individuals' personal testimonies of healing from spiritual experiences. Acceptance of their spiritual healing may help in building a trusting therapeutic health care relationship. The challenge is to find ways to collaborate with celebrity pastors. Suggestions include the following:

1. Appeal to their concern for the physical and emotional well-being of their followers.

2. Offer education to clergy on the prevalence of various medical and mental health concerns of African Americans and the ways that the two healing practices can work together.

3. Inform spiritual healers of incidence rates, lethality and mortality statistics, and treatment modalities for major health concerns.

4. Attempt to promote mutual healing strategies, honoring what spiritual and medical healing practices offer.

Both sides have the same intention: the health and well-being of the African American community. Partnerships must be formed in fulfilling that intention.

# HEALING POTENTIAL OF SPIRITUALITY AND RELIGION

## The Power of Faith

The healing potential of African American Christian spirituality and religion stems from a *lived* belief in the core faith doctrine of the Holy Trinity, of God the Father, Jesus the Son, and the Holy Spirit. The Three Persons of the Trinity serve as a living communal spiritual force that is always with and available to Christian believers. African Americans gain solace and strength in their relationship with God, who is omnipotent, known through scriptures and experienced as "the One to whom all power belongs (Psalm 147:5), for whom all things are possible (Luke 1:37; 19:26), and who is able to accomplish far more than humans can ask or imagine (Ephesians 3:20)" (Butler, 1991, p. 1049). The oral tradition of memorized scriptural verses, the preached word, and church hymns keep God's saving power ever present in the hearts and minds of African American Christians.

The scriptures remind African Americans of "who they are and whose they are," in that they are created in the image of the omnipotent God and they belong to God. The Bible provides a narrative of God's relationship with the people of God, which is compatible with the oral tradition of ancestral storytelling in African and African American cultures. The retelling of a story of the past brings the events of the story into the actual life of the present. Thus, the story of God's saving power in the lives of the people of Israel becomes the story of God's saving power in the lives of African Americans today. God's power is revealed

> in God's creating and sustaining the universe (Psalm 65:6; Jeremiah 32:17), in God's deliverance of Israel from Pharoah's forces (Exodus 15:1-18) … in the incarnation [of Christ] (Luke 1:35), in Christ's death on the cross [for humankind] (1 Corinthians 1:17-18, 23-24), and in the ongoing ministry of the church (1 Corinthians 2:5; Ephesians 3:20). (Butler, 1991, p. 1049)

The healing potential rests in believing that one's relationship with God gives one access to the healing power of God, and the scriptures are reminders of the inherited spiritual power. People have faith that God will heal them directly and that God will use health care providers as instruments of God's healing (Taylor et al., 2004).

The prophetic tradition of the church holds to the liberating power of Jesus Christ, which forms the basis of Black liberation theology. Although societal oppression has been an aspect of the legacy of African Americans in this country, Black liberation theology affirms Jesus's liberating power for all. Jesus serves as a model of the One who was oppressed, who brings about the liberation of oppressed people (Floyd-Thomas et al., 2007). Jesus was sent to "proclaim release of the captives … to let the oppressed go free" (Luke 4:18). The gospel message preached in the Black Church has traditionally sought to reveal Jesus's power to transform the oppressive structures of society. Furthermore, through Jesus, "God is free to demonstrate what it means to suffer and be in bondage as well as what it means to be free by sending Jesus into the world so that the world might be saved (cf. Phil. 2:5ff.)" (Harris, 1991, p. 11).

Jesus gives hope through the power of His resurrection. To most African American believers, Jesus is a "very real and present help in times of trouble," a living presence. Many believe that to merely "call on the name of Jesus" invites His resurrection power, the power to overcome, into their life circumstances. Also, the gospel narratives reveal God in Jesus as a loving, compassionate, and caring God who fed, healed, and delivered persons, through personal encounters with individuals and with the masses. As health care providers hear patients speaking the name of Jesus, they should inquire into the healing presence that Jesus provides and collaborate with that presence.

Jesus promised the Holy Spirit would come into believers after His ascension, to assure believers of the indwelling Spirit of Jesus within them (John 16:7–11; 1 John 3:24). The Holy Spirit serves to remind believers of the nature of Christ's Spirit that dwells in them. The "fruit of the Spirit" (Galatians 5:22), love, joy, peace, patience, kindness, goodness, faith, meekness, and self-control builds up the church as a community. The fruit of the Spirit are virtues of healing that the Holy Spirit is able to manifest in believers. God works through the Holy Spirit, disclosing God's personal presence and empowering believers with God's Spirit. The Holy Spirit is most acknowledged in charismatic church traditions, which believe strongly in the use of the miraculous and healing spiritual gifts that God gives through the Holy Spirit.

The Holy Trinity provides believers with a powerful spiritual support system. Through scriptures, church tradition, and ancestral and personal experiences, African American Christians know that they are never alone. They rely on their personal connection and relationship with God, Jesus, and the Holy Spirit for comfort, protection, provision, direction, and healing. Individuals and different church traditions may rely on one Person of the Trinity more than the others.

Relationship with God holds persons accountable in trying to live a life that is pleasing to God, which includes a healthy lifestyle. Similarly, persons who participate in organized religious involvement have the support of their church "family," who also serves as a source of accountability. According to Taylor and colleagues' (2004) review of focus group data, African American men and women reported that participation in church involved them in healthier lifestyles than friends and family members who did not attend church.

## Worship and Prayer

Both organized (e.g., church attendance and membership, participation in worship services, auxiliary group participation) and nonorganized (e.g., prayer, reading scripture, living in relationship with God) religious involvements demonstrate the desire for reciprocal communication with the Godhead through worship and prayer. Aspects of worship and prayer may be particularly helpful to the health psychology of African Americans (Taylor et al., 2004). Worship and prayer may produce positive feeling states (e.g., gratitude, forgiveness, inner peace, ecstasy) that are conducive to positive health and well-being as well as physical and emotional healing (Taylor et al., 2004, p. 204).

Worship acknowledges who God is and the many acts of unconditional love that God provides. Worship is founded on participation in a healthy, loving, personal, and collective relationship with God. As Mitchell and Mitchell (1989) explain, "The mainstream of worship is a communal experience of the divine Presence, or the Holy Spirit, manifested often in involuntary acts of praise" (p. 105). Often leaders of contemporary worship services call the congregation to worship with phrases or call-and-response chants that praise God's presence and invoke God's blessings. Common worship chants include "When praises go up, blessings come down"; "God is good ... all the time ... All the time ... God is good"; "God inhabits the praises of God's people"; "This is the day that the Lord hath made, let us rejoice and be glad in it"; and "For a spirit of heaviness [i.e., emotional heaviness], put on a garment of praise." Such chants indicate that God responds to the praise and worship offered by God's people, and praising God is helpful, especially in troubling life circumstances. These worship techniques often incite enthusiastic corporate singing, clapping, waving of hands, jumping, ecstatic dancing, shouts and tears of joy, and "involvement of the higher emotions and of the senses and limbs" (Mitchell & Mitchell, 1989, p. 380). Anecdotally, many church members report feeling better, physically and mentally, in the aftermath of corporate worship. Physical and psychological benefits of the worship experience might be explained as reactions to spiritual (e.g., divine) or physiological (e.g., relaxation response, neurological, endocrine, and immune systems) interventions (Taylor et al., 2004, p. 205).

Some researchers have found evidence that aspects of African American worship services are psychologically therapeutic (Griffith et al., 1980, 1984). Griffith and colleagues (1984) conducted a qualitative study of a charismatic worship service in which persons were asked to describe their personal reactions (feelings and behaviors) to the service as a whole and to four different aspects of the service: testimony, spirit possession, dancing, and speaking in tongues. Participants reported benefits of the service as a whole, including "receiving help, gaining strength, expressing feelings ... group closeness, and a conviction that they could help other worshipers" (p. 466). Testimony was described as a religious experience. Griffith and colleagues defined spirit possession as a "religion-based altered state of consciousness," which is a "voluntary ... short-term state induced in ritual ceremonies" (p. 465). Reported individual reactions to spirit possession included "notable emphasis on clarification and security; that is, members spoke of enhanced understanding and a sense of direction, of inner peace and security ... few heard voices ... an inner spiritual experience rather than an auditory one. Two members [asserted] that possession was helpful for relationships outside the immediate group" (p. 467). Responses to dancing were of a depersonalized, or "outside of myself," experience (p. 467). The dominant feeling associated with speaking in tongues was "a sense of strength" (Griffith et al., 1984, p. 467).

Griffith and colleagues (1984) likened the worship service experiences to Yalom's curative factors of instillation of hope, group cohesiveness, social learning, universality, existential factors, and catharsis (p. 467). Health psychologists should assess immediate and long-term responses to various aspects of worship in relation to reports of general well-being and presenting health concerns. Positive experiences of worship may be integrated into health care treatment plans (Cook & Wiley, 2000).

As previously mentioned, Taylor and colleagues (2004) found that prayer, even for the unchurched, is a predominant spiritual resource for African Americans. For most African Americans, prayer is a daily, continual spiritual activity for (1) communicating with God, (2) developing and sustaining their relationship with God, (3) listening to God, and (4) petitioning God for help as a coping resource (Taylor et al., 2004). As Cook and Wiley (2000) posit, "Individuals turn their anxieties and worries over to God through prayer and receive psychological, spiritual, and sometimes physical relief from their pain" (p. 389). In their examination of the social and situational predictors of prayer for African Americans, Ellison and Taylor (1996) found that those coping with health problems, bereavement, and feelings of lack of control in their personal lives were most likely to use prayer as a coping strategy (p. 111). Taylor and colleagues (2004) describe three categories of prayer—reflective, protective, and supportive (p. 52)—and report on focus group data revealing that prayer "works to strengthen and sustain one's endurance in order to deal with life issues" (p. 100). Focus group members found prayer to impart strength, reduce stress, and ease their worries (Taylor et al., 2004, p. 109), all of which have health benefits. Health psychologists can assess people's timing, frequency, duration, type of prayer, and circumstances for prayer to determine the role that prayer plays in individuals' lives and assess the appropriateness of utilizing prayer as a health intervention.

## STRATEGIES THAT WORK

Two church-based preventive health programs offer successful strategies for collaboration with African American churches. One program trains volunteers from church congregations to develop and implement substance abuse prevention programs in the community (Brown et al., 2006). The other consists of efforts to change the health behavior of church members (Resnicow et al., 2005).

Brown and colleagues (2006) developed a university-based program that provided training to volunteer church members in the development and implementation of substance use prevention. Volunteers were solicited through letters to churches, recommendations from community leaders, and churches that had previously received substance abuse prevention grants. Volunteers were trained to increase their knowledge, skills, and strategies for providing substance abuse prevention programs for families and communities. The 3-year grant-funded program had volunteers from 16 churches in the first year, 20 in the second year, and 23 churches in the third year of the program.

Quarterly training workshops were conducted to address all aspects of developing substance abuse prevention programs, including content on substance abuse prevention, role-plays, group facilitation, budgeting and fiscal management, and program evaluation (Brown et al., 2006, p. 49). Volunteers were divided into groups that targeted youth, family, or men and women. The trainers provided ongoing technical support for the volunteers once they began developing and implementing their own programs.

Program evaluation methods included surveys for participants and nonparticipants, focus groups, individual interviews, and program data reviews (Brown et al., 2006). Survey data revealed that volunteer participants' knowledge of training topics was increased, and the majority of participants were able to implement substance abuse prevention programs at their church. Interview data revealed key aspects of successful prevention programs:

> Having participants: 1) who have a determination or "passion" to implement a prevention program despite family, work, or school obligations, 2) who can mobilize assistance from relatives or other volunteers to implement program activities, and 3) who can aggressively seek funding (from different sources) for their prevention program either on their own or with assistance with proposal development. (Brown et al., 2006, p. 59)

Barriers to program implementation included:

> 1) Lack of support from minister or key persons at the church ... to implement a program, 2) lack of assistance (e.g., unsuccessful collaborations with other [volunteer] participants) with implementing program activities, and 3) work, school, and family obligations. (Brown et al., p. 59)

Program evaluation data suggest program modifications. Changes included (1) a needs assessment before the program implementation to assess readiness for program development and for shaping training topics, (2) restructure training to provide more individual technical assistance rather than group training sessions, and (3) make quarterly training sessions available on videotape (Brown et al., 2006, p. 62).

Resnicow and colleagues (2005) implemented a comprehensive "Healthy Body Healthy Spirit" intervention to increase fruit and vegetable consumption and physical activity with volunteers from 16 African American churches. Volunteers were divided into three different treatment groups. Group 1 (representing five churches) received standard health education materials on nutrition and physical activity, including a commercial aerobics video and health education brochures from government and health care agencies. Groups 2 (six churches) and 3 (five churches) received culturally targeted self-help materials, including a nutrition and a physical activity videotape, a healthy eating cookbook, an exercise guide, and an audiocassette containing gospel music. All of the interventions for Groups 2 and 3 were developed specifically for African American church populations. The cookbook included recipes from members of the participating churches. The fruits and vegetables videotape used biblical and spiritual themes to motivate healthy eating and was a dramatization comparing two families, one with healthy eating habits and the other with poor eating habits. "Woven into the story line is information about the health benefits of [fruits and vegetables], analysis of costs, recipes, and cooking tips" (Resnicow et al., 2005, p. 340).

The exercise videotape was hosted by local African American celebrities; 10 families were recruited from the churches to document one parent's efforts at increasing or maintaining a desired level of physical activity over a 4-week period. "The goal of this 'documentary' component was to provide real-world role models to whom participants could relate.... The two pastors [who were videotaped participants] were also filmed giving sermons on the importance of exercise and maintaining a healthy body" (Resnicow et al., 2005, p. 341). Biblical scriptures related to health were also spliced throughout the video. The 37-page exercise guide accompanied the videotape and consisted of instruction and skills-building information utilizing biblical themes and scripture. "The guide provides an activity program for three levels: beginner, intermediate, and advanced. It emphasizes walking as a core strategy.... To encourage walking, all participants in Groups 2 and 3 were provided with a pedometer.... The guide also addresses other forms of activity" (Resnicow et al., 2005, p. 341). The gospel music audiocassette was also designed to accompany exercise activities, with biblical quotes and excerpts from the pastor's sermons interspersed with the music. Group 3 differed from Group 2 in that they also received four telephoned motivational interviewing counseling calls over intervals of 4, 12, 26, and 40 weeks.

The average program included 66 participants from each of the 16 churches, with a total of 906 participants. Approximately 45% of participants reported a moderate or large change in either an increase in fruit and vegetable consumption or an increase in physical activity, 17% reported changes in both fruit and vegetable consumption and physical activity, and 39% reported little or no change in either health behavior (Resnicow et al., 2005). Groups 2 and 3 showed a significantly large change in fruit and vegetable consumption and, to a lesser degree, physical activity. Motivational interviewing was somewhat effective for increasing fruits and vegetables but not for physical activity (Resnicow et al., 2005).

Both church-based preventive health programs reveal the receptivity of church congregations to collaborations with health psychologists. The approach that one takes in gaining entry into the church system is critical to the success of preventive health programming. Taking time to assess the relationship of the church to the community and the cultural values and mission, communication patterns, and leadership hierarchy of each church setting is important (Cook, 1993).

## STRATEGIES THAT MIGHT WORK

The primary strategies for intervening in the health psychology of African Americans through spirituality and religion consist of cooperation between and collaboration with the personal and institutional resources provided by their organizational and nonorganizational religious involvements. Best practices in implementing health psychology strategies within the context of African American spirituality and churches consist of assessment and cooperation with the unique spiritual/cultural dynamics of the individual or institution. Health prevention interventions have the most potential for success in collaborations with African American churches.

### Assessment

Assessment takes place at both individual and institutional levels. Richards and Bergin (2004) offer recommendations for religious-spiritual assessment at the individual level. They recommend that the religious-spiritual dimension of individuals' functioning be assessed along with their physical, social, behavioral, intellectual, educational-occupational, and psychological-emotional functioning (p. 22). The religious-spiritual dimension should be included in whatever form typical initial assessments are conducted (e.g., clinical interviews, objective assessment measurements). The goal is to investigate the degree to which individuals' spiritual and religious participation may be a motivating factor in health prevention or may complement health treatment planning. An adaptation of some of Richards and Bergin's assessment questions follow:

- Does the individual have a relationship with God that is a source of comfort or strength? With which Person(s) of the Trinity does the individual most relate?
- Does the individual have a religious-spiritual affiliation? If so, how important is the affiliation?
- Does the individual believe that his or her spiritual beliefs, practices, and lifestyle contribute to his or her health? If so, give specific examples of spiritual practices, frequency of participation, and health-related benefits of spiritual practices.
- Is the individual open to using religious and spiritual resources to assist her or him in efforts to cope, heal, and change health-related behavior? If so, what encouragement or support does he or she need to commit to beneficial spiritual practices? (Richards & Bergin, 2004, pp. 23–24)

Furthermore, it is important to assess an individual's view of God (i.e., loving, punishing, forgiving) (Richards & Bergin, 1997) because this may have ramifications for the degree to which he or she believes that God will intervene on his or her behalf.

Additional spiritual-religious criteria to be considered in developing health psychology strategies include religious orthodoxy and religious problem-solving style (Richards & Bergin, 1997). Religious orthodoxy considers how strongly individuals believe and practice the doctrines and teachings of their religion and the degree to which religious doctrines and practices influence individuals' health care attitudes and behaviors (Richards & Bergin, 1997). Many persons compartmentalize their religious beliefs and practices from other aspects of their lives, whereas others fully integrate their beliefs into every aspect of their lives. Therefore, it is important to assess relevant religious beliefs and practices and assess their compatibility with proposed health psychology strategies to determine the level of cooperation the health psychologist may receive (Richards & Bergin, 1997). For some persons, strong commitment to religious beliefs leads them to practice healthy lifestyles that prohibit smoking, drinking, and substance abuse and encourage healthy diets (Taylor et al., 2004). Strong commitment to religious beliefs may also work against persons' health, if, for instance, their belief in divine healing discourages them from seeking preventive or remedial health care services.

Religious problem-solving style considers how persons use their religious beliefs to solve problems (Pargament et al., 1988). Pargament and colleagues (1988) delineated three religious problem-solving styles. The first, the *self-directing* style, consists of individuals relying on themselves to solve their life's problems: "God is viewed as giving people the freedom and resources to direct their own lives" (p. 91). The second, the *deferring* problem-solving style, consists of waiting on God to solve one's problems. The third, the *collaborative* problem-solving style, consists of persons working together with God to solve their problems. The self-directing problem solver might be most likely to seek immediate help from health care providers when a health concern arises and may be most likely to engage in preventive health behaviors. The deferring problem solver may be most in danger of delaying or ignoring health care issues. Finally, the collaborative problem solver might recognize health care providers as resources that God uses to minister to people's health care needs.

Institutional assessment entails investigating churches to determine their existing resources for promoting congregational and community health psychology as well as their potential for developing such resources. Lincoln and Mamiya's (1990) description of dialectical tensions of Black Churches provides a model for institutional assessment. Investigating church website pages, Sunday bulletins, and advertisements in the religion section of newspapers provides useful information on community outreach programs and church services. Visiting worship services, viewing television broadcasts, and attending religious conferences provide more in-depth information on health psychology attitudes and activities of church congregations.

## Health Prevention and Support Interventions

The continuation of social inequalities for African Americans, including health disparities, makes it imperative that health psychologists join forces with African American churches in providing health prevention interventions for African American church congregations, their surrounding communities, and national church audiences. In January 2008, a coalition of more than 25 national health advocacy and civil rights organizations submitted a report to the United Nations Committee on the Elimination of Racial Discrimination—*Unequal Health Outcomes in the United States*—documenting inequality in health care, health outcomes, and environmental health in the United States related to race, ethnicity, immigration, and socioeconomic status (CERD Working Group on Health and Environmental Health, 2008). Racial health disparities reveal that

> Racial and ethnic gaps exist across a range of health conditions ... African Americans, American Indians, and Pacific Islanders face some of the most persistent and pervasive disparities relative to Whites and Asian Americans. They experience a disproportionate burden of poor health in problems ranging from infant mortality and diabetes to cardiac disease, HIV/AIDS, and other illnesses. (CERD, 2008, p. 9)

Furthermore, the American Cancer Society reports that cancer is the second leading cause of death among African Americans, surpassed only by heart disease (American Cancer Society, 2007, p. 1).

Church-based preventive health programs, such as screening and education programs for hypertension, cardiovascular disease, stroke, diabetes, HIV/AIDs, have been shown to be effective (Collins, Whiters, & Braithwaite, 2007; Frank & Grubbs, 2008). Cancer prevention and support programs are needed, including, for example, education regarding (1) the leading sites in the body of new cancer cases for African Americans, (2) cancer screenings, and (3) cancer prevention lifestyles (e.g., diet, exercise, spirituality). There is also need for support services for persons diagnosed with cancer, such as (1) transportation and escort to doctors' visits, (2) assistance and advocacy in negotiating medical care, (3) assistance with practical needs (e.g., meal preparation, grocery shopping, pharmacy deliveries), and (4) support for family and caregivers.

Developing health-conscious churches goes beyond short-term prevention workshops. Health psychologists must be invested in sustaining relationships with church congregations that raise consciousness, address patterns of denial and unhealthy life choices, motivate toward change, and help organize church resources to effect change. This entails a long-term, collaborative relationship that is built on trust and faith in common religious beliefs and practices. Consciousness raising about major health concerns for African Americans tends to be a welcomed intervention by most African American churches, particularly given the historical prophetic tradition of Black Churches. However, breaking through patterns of denial may require helping churches overcome stereotypical and judgmental thinking (e.g., in terms of developing church-supported HIV/AIDS interventions, many churches still consider these to be gay male diseases and are reluctant to deal openly with sexuality). Regarding unhealthy life choices, some church traditions are hard to break, like the unhealthy food choices frequently offered in fellowship meals. Moving through these barriers takes time, time to develop a trusting relationship that honors the spiritual and cultural traditions of the church while establishing healthy spiritually based lifestyle changes. To be fully integrated into the life of the church, health interventions need to be tailored to the spiritual language, communication styles, attitudes, rituals, and cultural characteristics specific to the congregation.

## SUMMARY OF RECOMMENDATIONS
## FOR CHURCH COLLABORATIONS

The Black Church is a recognized American institution; it has historically responded directly to the interests and needs of African Americans and has impacted the course of human rights for all Americans. Therefore, social scientists, health care providers, and mental health professionals, regardless of race and religious affiliation, should consider partnering with churches in responding to the holistic health care of African Americans. By working with churches, social scientists and health professionals can reach a significant proportion of the African American population, through the large number of African Americans who hold church membership as well as churches' community outreach with the unchurched. Imagine the difference that could be achieved!

Major public health initiatives for African Americans could be developed through church collaborations. It is no coincidence that the civil rights movement came out of the Black Church, because of its extensive human resources, control of their own financial and material resources, and combined spiritual and social action mission. Today, with the national influence of television and other media ministries and the host of stadium-filled ministry conferences, African American health concerns could become part of their agenda, if social scientists and health professionals would initiate church partnerships. From the smallest storefront church to the most extravagant mega-church corporation, at the heart of their ministries is the spiritual and physical health, welfare, prosperity, and social equality of African Americans. Why wouldn't clergy be open to collaborations and partnerships with social scientists, health care providers, and mental health professionals who honor their church's mission?

Perhaps the greatest challenges to overcome in church collaborations are the competing worldviews regarding healing. Traditional religious healing differs from healing in the social and medical sciences in that religion emphasizes "supernatural or spiritual etiologies of emotional [and to some extent, physical] problems and subsequent healing practices" (Helms & Cook, 1999, p. 254). For successful collaborations, social scientists and mental and physical health care practitioners must be open to religious healing worldviews and respect the professional status of religious leaders. In the complex world of African American health, all professionals (e.g., clergy, researchers, physicians, psychologists, social workers, public health professionals) are equipped with the tools of their disciplines to contribute to the amelioration of health disparities of African Americans. Therefore, it is important to communicate respect for spiritual healing and to demonstrate that social and medical research and practice are a complement to religious practices. It would be a mistake to seek collaborations with churches solely for their role as social institutions without recognizing the benefits of their spiritual beliefs and practices.

The easiest method for gaining entry into church systems is for health care providers and social scientists who attend church to offer their knowledge and skills to their own congregation. However, often individuals separate their religious and professional practices, perhaps unconsciously compartmentalizing spirituality from other aspects of their lives or consciously seeking anonymity in their church attendance. For some, church is the one place that they can go to receive help rather than taking care of others or upholding a professional role. Professionals must weigh the costs to themselves versus the potential benefits to the health of African Americans in deciding whether or not to include their professional talents in their church giving. Should they choose to partner with their churches, it will be important to set healthy and ethical professional boundaries in working within their own congregations. Developing a collaborative church partnership must include educating clergy and the congregation on the importance of ethical and procedural boundaries in the social scientific and health care professions because boundaries within the church tend to be less restrictive and procedures less formal (e.g., consent forms, confidentiality, time limits, dual relationships) (Helms & Cook, 1999).

Finding a church with which to partner is as simple as looking to the nearest corner in any city, viewing a television ministry, researching churches on the Internet, or reading the religion section of the local newspaper. Professionals must determine what resources are important to a particular research study or health intervention and consider selecting a church that meets the necessary criteria. Alternatively, they can select a church with limited resources to help "the least of these" in their community outreach efforts. Professionals seeking to collaborate with churches with which they are not affiliated should begin by carefully getting to know the church. They can attend not only Sunday worship services but also some of the midweek activities in order to understand the culture, the church leadership structure, communication patterns, resources, and congregation-community relations.

Professionals should adapt research methodologies and health care language to practices and language that are common to the church (Helms & Cook, 1999). For instance, Helms and Cook (1999) described how a church-based counseling program adapted the language and procedures of traditional counseling interventions to the church culture. The traditional language for components of a counseling services program (e.g., individual and group counseling, paraprofessional counseling training, preventive and developmental outreach interventions) was adapted to form the Ministry of Spiritual Nurturing, consisting of "(1) individual nurturing; (2) group nurturing; (3) reaching out/lending a helping hand; (4) church-community conferences; and (5) networking" (Helms & Cook, 1999, p. 266). It is important to develop interventions that are geared to the educational levels of the congregation and that reflect the church's culture, similar to the Resnicow and colleagues (2005) "Healthy Body Healthy Spirit" intervention. Also, professionals should consider how church rituals might be opportunities for advancing health care initiatives. African American churches tend to hold annual days for the different segments of the congregation (e.g., Women's Day, Men's Day, Children's Day); these are opportune times to promote health care initiatives to the specific populations.

Social scientists and health professionals must recognize that they need pastors as partners in responding to African American health care needs. They can actually learn from pastors' professional knowledge and experience with large and diverse segments of the African American community. When ready for a formal introduction, professionals should reflect on and appeal to pastors' (1) concern for the congregation and community, (2) spiritual and social influence, (3) understanding of African American Christian life, and (4) application of theology to everyday life. Professionals must learn from clergy how to integrate scripture into practical health care instruction in reaching out to the congregation, but also must be realistic that churches have long-standing traditions that will not change. Although African American churches may be idealized institutions, they are not perfect. Multicultural competencies, expertise in group dynamics, and clinical assessment skills are useful collaboration tools.

Finally, for professionals who believe in a Supreme Power, or God, it is helpful to reflect on how one's role as a social scientist or health professional may actually be a "vocational calling," that is, a divine calling into one's profession for the greater good. Professionals should consider the possibility of God instilling within them the passion and aptitude for research and health care practice, the likelihood that God calls and uses some researchers and clinicians just as He calls clergy. Churches alone cannot change the quality of life for African Americans. However, as the social and spiritual home of African American culture, they are the base from which professionals from all disciplines can channel their expertise in answering the call to make a significant difference: through the agency of the trusted church.

## REFERENCES

American Cancer Society. (2007). *Cancer facts & figures for African Americans 2007–2008.* Atlanta, GA: Author.

Barnes, S. L. (2004). Priestly and prophetic influences on Black Church social services. *Social Problems, 51,* 202–221.

Billingsley, A. (1999). *Mighty like a river: The Black Church and social reform.* New York: Oxford University Press.

Boyd-Franklin, N. (2003). *Black families in therapy* (2nd ed.). New York: Guilford Press.

Brown, D. R., Scott, W., Lacey, K., Blount, J., Roman, D., & Brown, D. (2006). Black churches in substance use and prevention efforts. *Journal of Alcohol and Drug Education, 50,* 43–65.

Butler, T. (Ed.). (1991). *Holman Bible dictionary.* Nashville, TN: Broadman & Holman.

CERD Working Group on Health and Environmental Health. (2008). *Unequal health outcomes in the United States: Racial and ethnic disparities in health care treatment and access, the role of social and environmental determinants of health, and the responsibility of the state.* Retrieved January 26, 2009, from *www.prrac.org/pdf/CERDhealthEnvironmentReport.pdf.*

Chatters, L. M., Taylor, R. J., & Lincoln, K. D. (1999). African American religious participation: A multi-sample comparison. *Journal of the Scientific Study of Religion, 38,* 132–145.

Collins, C. E., Whiters, D. L., & Braithwaite, R. (2007). The Saved Sista Project: A faith-based HIV prevention program for Black women in addiction recovery. *American Journal of Health Studies, 22,* 76–82.

Cook, D. A. (1993). Research in African American churches: A mental health counseling imperative. *Journal of Mental Health Counseling, 15,* 320–333.

Cook, D. A., & Wiley, C. Y. (2000). Psychotherapy with members of African American churches and spiritual traditions. In P. S. Richards & A. E. Bergin (Eds.), *Handbook of psychotherapy and religious diversity* (pp. 369–395). Washington, DC: American Psychological Association.

Dillard, J. M., & Smith, B. B. (2005). African Americans' spirituality and religion in counseling and psychotherapy. In D. A. Harley & J. M. Dillard (Eds.), *Contemporary mental health issues among African Americans* (pp. 279–292). Alexandria, VA: American Counseling Association.

Ellison, C. G., & Taylor, R. J. (1996). Turning to prayer: Religious coping among Black Americans. *Review of Religious Research, 38,* 111–131.

Floyd-Thomas, S., Floyd-Thomas, J., Duncan, C. B., Ray, S. G., & Westfield, N. L. (2007). *Black Church studies: An introduction.* Nashville, TN: Abingdon Press.

Frank, D., & Grubbs, L. (2008). A faith-based screening/education program for diabetes, CVD, and stroke in rural African Americans. *Association of Black Nursing Faculty Journal, 19,* 96–101.

Frederick, M. F. (2003). *Between Sundays: Black women and everyday struggles of faith.* Berkeley: University of California Press.

Griffith, E. E. H., English, T., & Mayfield, V. (1980). Possession, prayer, and testimony: Therapeutic aspects of the Wednesday night meeting in a Black church. *Psychiatry, 43,* 120–127.

Griffith, E. E. H., Young, J. L., & Smith, D. L. (1984). An analysis of the therapeutic elements in a Black church service. *Hospital and Community Psychiatry, 35,* 464–469.

Harley, D. (2005). The Black church: A strength-based approach in mental health. In D. A. Harley & J. M. Dillard (Eds.), *Contemporary mental health issues among African Americans* (pp. 191–203). Alexandria, VA: American Counseling Association.

Harris, J. H. (1991). *Pastoral theology: A Black church perspective.* Minneapolis, MN: Fortress Press.

Helms, J. E., & Cook, D. A. (1999). *Using race and culture in counseling and psychotherapy: Theory and process.* Boston: Allyn & Bacon.

Jang, S. J., & Johnson, B. R. (2004). Explaining religious effects on distress among African Americans. *Journal of the Scientific Study of Religion, 43*, 239–260.

Koenig, H. G., McCullough, M. E., & Larson, D. B. (2001). *Handbook of religion and health.* New York: Oxford University Press.

Levin, J. S., Taylor, R. J., & Chatters, L. M. (1994). Race and gender differences in religiosity among older adults: Findings from four national surveys. *Sociological Quarterly, 36*, 157–173.

Lincoln, C. E., & Mamiya, L. H. (1990). *The Black church in the African American experience.* Durham, NC: Duke University Press.

Marks, L., Nesteruk, O., Swanson, M., Garrison, B., & Davis, T. (2005). Religion and health among African Americans: A qualitative examination. *Research on Aging, 27*, 447–474.

Mbiti, J. S. (1969). *African religions and philosophy.* London: Heinemann.

Mitchell, E. P., & Mitchell, H. H. (1989). Black spirituality: The values of the "ol' time religion." *Journal of the Interdenominational Theological Center, 17*, 102–109.

Nobles, W. W. (1991). African philosophy: Foundations of Black psychology. In R. L. Jones (Ed.), *Black psychology* (3rd ed., pp. 47–63). Berkeley, CA: Cobb & Henry.

Pargament, K. I., Kennell, J., Hathaway, W., Grenvengoed, N., Newman, J., & Jones, W. (1988). Religion and the problem-solving process: Three styles of coping. *Journal of the Scientific Study of Religion, 27*, 90–104.

Queener, J. E., & Martin, J. K. (2001). Providing culturally relevant mental health services: Collaboration between psychology and the African American church. *Journal of Black Psychology, 27*, 112–122.

Resnicow, K., Jackson, A., Blissett, D., Wang, T., McCarty, F., Rahotep, S., et al. (2005). Results of the Healthy Body Healthy Spirit trial. *Health Psychology, 24*, 339–348.

Richards, P. S., & Bergin, A. E. (1997). *A spiritual strategy for counseling and psychotherapy.* Washington, DC: American Psychological Association.

Richards, P. S., & Bergin, A. E. (2004). *Casebook for a spiritual strategy in counseling and psychotherapy.* Washington, DC: American Psychological Association.

Taylor, R. J., Chatters, L. M., Jayakody, R., & Levin, J. S. (1996). Black and White differences in religious participation: A multi-sample comparison. *Journal for the Scientific Study of Religion, 35*, 403–410.

Taylor, R. J., Chatters, L. M., & Levin, J. (2004). *Religion in the lives of African Americans: Social, psychological, and health perspectives.* Thousand Oaks, CA: Sage.

Thompson, D. A., & McRae, M. B. (2001). The need to belong: A theory of the therapeutic function of the Black Church tradition. *Counseling and Values, 46*, 40–53.

Warren, R. (1995). *The purpose driven church: Growth without compromising your message and mission.* Grand Rapids, MI: Zondervan.

Weems, R. (2005). Black American and religion. *Ebony, 61*, 122–125.

# 5

# Well-Being and Resilience
## *Another Look at African American Psychology*

RUTH CHU-LIEN CHAO

African Americans have historically lived in a traumatic environment of oppressive discrimination. Their fortitude, communal and personal, has been sorely tested through years of slavery, Jim Crow laws, and slavery-like conditions that persisted even after the civil rights movement. All these circumstances are attended with various stressors of discrimination and stereotypes under which African Americans have suffered.

For several hundred years, African Americans have lived with racism in regard to use of public facilities and transportation, housing, business operations, and other areas of life. These traumatic life experiences are flatly contradictory to the three Civil War amendments to the U.S. Constitution meant to secure personal freedom and political rights for African Americans. The Thirteenth Amendment prohibited slavery. The Fourteenth Amendment defined American citizenship by requiring states to honor the same due-process guarantees in criminal proceedings that are required for the federal government and to not "deny to any person within its jurisdiction the equal protection of the laws." The Fifteenth Amendment guaranteed "the right of the citizens of the United States to vote ... [regardless] of race, color, or previous condition of servitude." These guarantees are as firm as the federal government stands. Unfortunately, throughout history and until quite recently, the majority of African Americans did not totally receive the treatments guaranteed by these amendments. Now, in this, the 21st century, are African Americans finally freed from these past barriers and adversity? Sadly, the answer for many is still a tragic "no."

The U.S. Department of Health and Human Services Surgeon General reported (USDHHS, 1999) that compared with Whites, African Americans were more likely to live in poverty, experience unemployment and homelessness, and reside in high-crime neighborhoods. In addition, as recently as 2002, the National Center for Health Statistics reported that African Americans suffered from fewer resources, financial and otherwise, to support them through their struggles. They had higher mortality rates and a shorter life expectancy; were three times more likely to suffer from diabetes; had a 40% higher incidence of heart disease and prostate cancer; were seven times more likely to become infected with HIV; were at greater risk for breast cancer; and had a higher infant mortality rate. Yet, despite this long list of adverse conditions and centuries of exclusion from the socioeconomic mainstream, African Americans have managed to forge striking contributions to American society. Examples are legion: vibrant Africentric cultural independence; a unique legacy of social activism; unparalleled advances in art, sports, and businesses; and a distinctive creativity of spirit, all of which have enriched our nation historically, continuously, and enormously.

Understandably, as social scientists, we are interested in exploring what protective factors supported and enabled many African Americans to successfully cope with their deleterious circumstances and soar high in their achievements. Empirical evidence links cultural factors to their coping behaviors. Culture has been shown to influence how African Americans define stressors (Parks, 1998), evaluate their coping resources (Daly, Jennings, Beckette, & Leashore, 1995), and provide a context for coping (Constantine, Donnelly, & Myers, 2002). The most prominent of cultural factors are resilience and well-being. These cultural factors do not necessarily remove African Americans from harm, but they do appear to reduce its negative effects. Researchers reported that individuals with greater cultural resources tend toward more positive mental health than those with fewer resources (Potts, 1996; Simoni, Martone, & Kerwin, 2002; Wilson & Miles, 2001). Because many African Americans succeed despite adversity, the traditional linear assumption that their psychological problems are mostly caused by adverse environment appears inadequate. Instead, the research suggests that well-being and resilience are two indispensable factors for coping with adversity and even thriving in spite of it.

## HISTORY OF THE STUDY OF WELL-BEING AND RESILIENCE AMONG AFRICAN AMERICANS

Although well-being and resilience are highly correlated with each other, they are two separate factors in African Americans' ability to manage adversity and even flourish in the face of it.

## Well-Being

Well-being means a state of happy contentment, with low psychological distress, overall physical and mental health, and a positive outlook on life: in other words, good quality of life (VandenBos, 2007). In recent years, many psychologists have shifted their focus from an emphasis on disorder and dysfunction to one on well-being and robust health. Early proponents of the health perspective included Seligman (1991), Ryff (1989a, 1989b), and Diener (1984), who built on the earlier works of investigators like Bradburn (1969) and Argyle (1987). This positive asset perspective has also enriched the Constitution of the World Health Organization (1948), in which even as early as 1948 health was defined as a state of physical and social well-being and not merely the absence of disease.

Historically, most work on African Americans' well-being utilized a deficit model focused on shortcomings like poverty, residency in a high-crime neighborhood, low socioeconomic status, and victimization by racism and discrimination. This asset-less approach spawned two lines of thought: bottom-up theories and adaptation theories.

Bottom-up explanations argue that it is the sum of life events that is important: A happy life is the accumulation of positive events. A person who is asked to judge his or her life satisfaction is imagined to perform a mental calculation weighing good events against bad ones. Headey, Veenhoven, and Wearing (1991) argued that the whole is the sum of all its parts; satisfaction with life domains of, for example, marriage, family, employment, and health, determined life satisfaction.

A second theoretical model infers that subjective well-being arises from discrepancies between objective circumstances and subjective evaluations. It suggests that happiness or satisfaction results from subjective processes in which comparisons are made between one's status and reference points of importance. This theoretical framework has, in turn, produced social comparison theories and adaptation theories.

In social comparison theories, subjective well-being means that other individuals are used as reference points, and that happiness is gauged by comparing how much better one individual is compared with another. Based on this theory, downward comparison with less fortunate Americans was tested as a predictor of change in general life satisfaction. For example, an African American woman may feel satisfied living in her small studio when she compares herself to a homeless person living on street.

Because the adversities African Americans encounter are often cultural, multicultural scholars focus more on the negative cultural consequence (e.g., identity crisis, traumatic experience related to discrimination) than on the strengths of African Americans. This has resulted in neglecting the various adaptation strategies African Americans under adverse conditions have used to succeed.

Adaptation theories propose that individuals use some point in their life as the prior reference point for comparison to determine their current status of happiness. Well-being or life satisfaction results when present status is better than the comparison point. In one study, Adams (1999) reported that African Americans' general life satisfaction, happiness, and family satisfaction were interrelated with one another. In this study, well-being and happiness were strong predictors of each other.

Since the 1970s, racial segregation and integration have been seen as unique experiences for African Americans. In fact, racial segregation was understood to decrease well-being, whereas integration was believed to potentially improve well-being. This second belief is often referred to as the *contact hypothesis*. It is, however, controversial, with both supporters and detractors.

Supporters of the *contact hypothesis* argue that specific and direct interpersonal contact can reduce prejudice and hostility among formerly segregated groups (Pettigrew & Tropp, 2000). It was this argument that Kenneth B. Clark (1974) used in his successful plea to the U.S. Supreme Court to overturn the practice of racial segregation in public schools, resulting in the historical *Brown v. Board of Education of Topeka* (1954) decision. On the other hand, some studies have shown that African Americans could emotionally benefit from segregation in terms of increased self-esteem and well-being (Allport, 1953; Coleman, 1966).

Another line of research on African Americans' well-being follows the assumption that well-being equals the *lack* of psychological disorders. Thus, the fewer psychological disorders one has, the higher level of well-being one enjoys. This line of research has not proven fruitful. Edwards (1999) contends that it does not accommodate African Americans' definition of mental health, which contains three themes: (1) moral worth and ideological and belief references; (2) competence and determination for youth and religion and spirituality for elders; and (3) interpersonal attributes, particularly self-expression, ability to communicate feelings, having a secure relationship, and assertiveness. Fulfilling these themes is not necessarily dependent on one's state of mental health, and psychological issues may not automatically reduce well-being.

## Resilience

Resilience is "the process and outcome of successfully adapting to difficult or challenging life experiences, especially through mental, emotional, and behavioral flexibility and adjustment to external and internal demands. A number of factors contribute to how well people adapt to adversities, predominant among them are (a) the ways in which individuals view and engage with the world, (b) the availability and quality of social resources, and (c) specific coping strategies" (VandenBos, 2007, p. 792).

In the research literature, resilience and invulnerability frequently have been used interchangeably to describe individuals who do not exhibit psychological, behavioral, or mental health problems despite predisposing factors (Bowen-Reid & Rhodes, 2003). Historically, Garmezy (1972) is credited with first using the concept to describe a sample of highly competent, urban-reared Black children who adjusted well despite environmental conditions conducive to various dysfunctions. Unfortunately, recent research seldom uses invulnerability as an empirical operational concept, although resilience as an operational concept continues to stimulate much interest (Masten, 2001).

Thus, resilience has two meanings for African Americans: It describes both Blacks at high risk who have not succumbed to dysfunction-inducing factors and those who have recovered after a dysfunctional episode, whether brief or protracted. Both types of resilience denote the ability to overcome adversities in environments or internal stresses and live a life that functions well.

The concept of resilience in the face of adversity is rooted in antiquity. In myth, children's fables, epic literature, and art, heroes and heroines succeed despite huge obstacles. However, it was not until the 1970s that social science began to pay serious attention to it, in particular to at-risk children who succeeded in life (Masten, 2001). The study of resiliency remains in its infancy, especially in regard to African Americans (Utsey, Bolden, Lanier, & Williams, 2007). For example, more needs to be understood regarding the manner in which many African Americans have emotionally managed the uncertainty of employment and financial stability. The lack of jobs and thus inadequate finances often contribute to emotional unrest, ill health, or both. Yet many African Americans are able to maintain their integrity and life purpose in spite of seemingly overwhelming stress. For their neighbors, these individuals' serene composure provides a beacon of hope. Besides, these resilient heroes are not those one would have expected, such as the educated or the skillful. We cannot help but ask, "What sources of strength are these admirable African American heroes and heroines drawing upon?"

## THE CONTRIBUTION OF AFRICAN AMERICANS TO OUR UNDERSTANDING OF THEIR WELL-BEING AND RESILIENCE

The key to understanding how these African Americans have forged themselves lies in the adaptive capacity of their culture to interpret events for the group. They have not sulked or negatively reacted to institutional abuses or laid down awaiting some inevitable fate. Rather, they have actively made choices to enable the group to continue. Adaptation, culture, and choice are important factors in understanding how many African Americans have creatively responded to oppression and dire conditions.

Understanding the process of successful adaptation under stressful life conditions offers a conceptual base on which treatment and preventive interventions can be framed.

# THEORETICAL MODELS OF WELL–BEING AND RESILIENCE FOR AFRICAN AMERICANS

There are three theoretical models in which studies of well-being and resilience among African Americans are based: (1) well-being and resilience as outcome variables, (2) well-being and resilience as moderator variables, and (3) well-being and resilience in a cultural–ecological framework.

## Model 1: Well–Being and Resilience as Outcome Variables

This theoretical model can be divided into two subsets: a model on well-being and a model on resilience.

### *Well–Being*

Recent studies of positive well-being as an outcome variable are generally conceptualized in three distinct traditions: subjective well-being (SWB), psychological well-being (PWB), and objective well-being (OWB) (Keyes, Shmotkin, & Ryff, 2002). The SWB engages in "more global evaluations of affect and life quality," and the PWB examines "perceived thriving vis-à-vis the existential challenges of life (e.g., pursuing meaningful goals … establishing quality ties to others)" (Keyes et al., 2002, p. 1007).

One of the most widely cited theories of PWB is that by Ryff (1989a, 1989b, 1995), who proposes a multidimensional model derived from three bodies of theoretical literature: (1) life span developmental psychology (e.g., the writings of Erickson, Buhler, and Neugarten); (2) mental health (e.g., the writings of Maslow, Rogers, Jung, and Allport); and (3) personal growth (e.g., the writings of Jahoda). Ryff reviewed the characteristics of well-being described in these writings and found six points of convergence, which she put forth as an integrative model of PWB in adult life: self-acceptance, positive relations with others, autonomy, environmental mastery, purpose in life, and personal growth. To illustrate, higher levels of private religious behaviors correlate positively to more favorable perceptions of one's religiosity and more favorable perceptions of interpersonal relationships and self-acceptance. For many African Americans, private religious behaviors and positive feelings about one's religion seem to be related to increased PWB. Besides, a more favorable perception of one's religiosity and public participation was found to be associated with a favorable perception of mastery over one's environment, personal growth, good relationships with others, purpose in life, and self-acceptance. In other words, a favorable internal perception of one's religiosity, coupled with public behaviors, was associated with several well-being indicators, including self-acceptance and a sense of mastery (Taylor, 1993).

The second tradition of studies, SWB, is based on satisfaction indicators used by social psychologists to assess individuals' quality of life.

The third tradition of studies, OWB, is based on evaluative-descriptive indicators used primarily by economists and sociologists to analyze the quality of life of specific groups or subgroups. Between 1980 and 1992, indicators of OWB for African Americans, such as health, education, and economic status, either remained stagnant or deteriorated. Yet the University of Michigan's National Panel Survey of Black Americans, a subset of the National Survey of Black Americans, showed a marked increase from 1980 to 1992 in the number of respondents reporting "high general life satisfaction," a measure of subjective well-being (Jackson & Adams, 1992). Specifically, in 1992, 39% of African Americans were very satisfied, 48% were somewhat satisfied, and 13% were dissatisfied with general life. These data raise the question of why there was a substantial increase in the proportion of respondents reporting positive life satisfaction during a period of decline in objective standards such as health, education, and income.

"Positive coping" is a possible answer to this seeming contradiction. Rising subjective evaluations of one's well-being may facilitate efforts to remain viable—psychologically, spiritually, and physiologically, individually, and groupwise—in the face of stagnation or decline of objective condition. The key here is that the underlying psychological processes are functioning to adjust respondents' subjective interpretation of environment.

Perhaps this is their adaptive process. Bowman (1990) has noted that extended family systems, strong spiritual beliefs, and ethnic pride (or ethnic identity) serve as sources of personal empowerment. These cultural resources may have facilitated coping schemata and cognitive strategies and motivated adaptive responses that, in turn, increased perception of well-being (Bowman, 1990). An alternative explanation is that another variable mediated the relationship between objective and subjective well-being. For example, social support, spirituality, religion, and family can be mediators to associate objective with subjective well-being.

Numerous studies have used religion or spirituality as an independent variable or predictor to African Americans' well-being. For example, Taylor (1993) documented the salutary impact of Black Churches on their lives, revealing that they perceived their churches as providers of sustenance, strength, assistance, and moral guidelines for conduct and a source of unity, a community gathering place, and a help in attaining social, economic, and educational goals.

Clearly, the Black Church is a powerful force for many African Americans (Coke, 1992). Given this, it is not surprising that strong ties are found between religiosity and indicators of Black healthy well-being. For example, the higher the religiosity, the lower the use of tobacco products (Ahmed, Brown, Gary, & Saadatmand, 1994; Brown & Gary, 1994) and alcohol (or even abstention) (Brown & Gary, 1994; Darrow, Russell, Cooper, Mudar, & Frone, 1992) and the lower the rates of incarceration (Parson & Mikawa, 1991). Religious involvement is a critical component in understanding African American well-being.

In contrast, racial discriminatory experiences have been found to be detrimental to well-being. African Americans with less positive feelings about Blacks have more depressive symptoms and lower well-being than those with positive feelings about Blacks (Caldwell, Guthrie, & Jackson, 2006).

## Resilience

Masten (2001) defines resilience as good outcomes despite serious threats to adaptation or development. Two conditions are necessary to identify resilience: (1) The presence of a significant threat (e.g., poverty, parental history of mental illness) or exposure to severe adversity (e.g., victim of a violent crime, death of a parent) and (2) a determination that positive adaptation has occurred in the face of such adversity (Masten & Coatsworth, 1998). Thus, adversity is a risk factor that correlates with poor social, psychological, and health outcomes (Masten, 2001). Risk factors have an additive effect (loss of job + inability to pay mortgage = ill health) that can increase in the chances for poor outcomes. Balancing risk factors are protective factors or assets that encourage an adaptation (healthier response) in the face of adversity. Protective factors can include individual characteristics such as cognitive ability and disposition, family cohesiveness, and extrafamilial factors such as an adequate societal safety net of unemployment compensation and available affordable health care.

This model offers an explanation of African Americans' resilience. In addition, their culture provides additional protective factors such as extended familial bonds to cope effectively and adapt to adversity (Brosky, 2000; Taylor, Chatters, & Levin, 2004).

To illustrate, Brown (2008), using multiple regression analyses, reported that racial socialization inculcation and receiving social support explained the most variance in African Americans' resilience. Racial socialization is a set of behaviors, communications, and interactions between parents and children that address how they should feel about their cultural heritage and how they should respond to racial hostility in American society (Stevenson, Cameron, Herrero-Taylor, & Davis, 2002).

In another study, spirituality again appeared as a protective factor among 1,013 African American students at two historically Black universities that contributed to resilience (Bowen-Reid & Rhodes, 2003). Furthermore, parents' religious behavior appeared important among their children and adolescents (Christian & Barbarin, 2001), whose higher level of resilience, fewer oppositional behaviors, less expressed depression, and less perceived immaturity were related to parents' regular church attendance.

This relation could be explained in at least in two ways. First, regular church attendance might serve as a coping strategy that reduces parental distresses and makes them more effective parents. Second, religiosity could be passed on to their children, enhancing their capacity for self-regulation.

## Model 2: Well-Being and Resilience as Moderator Variables

### Well-Being

Self-perceived well-being is a critical variable affecting individuals' level of distress. For example, some individuals with apparently strong social support and functional coping experience distress; others do not. This dilemma might be resolved by evaluating their well-being as emotional reactions to and cognitive judgment of events. In this instance, well-being is a mediator between two predictors (social support and coping) and an outcome variable (mental distress).

A variable (e.g., well-being) is said to act as a mediator when it partially or completely accounts for the relationship between a predictor and an outcome variable. Stevens, Hill, Heiner, and Chao (2007) investigated the role of well-being as mediator between social support/coping and mental distress. Their survey of 156 African American college students indicated that before well-being was entered as a mediator, social support and coping significantly contributed to the variance of mental health. When well-being was entered as a mediator, there was no significant relation between social support/coping and mental distress.

The relationship between racial attribution and lower well-being and mental health problems has generated conflicting explanations. For example, some studies report that external racial attribution has served as a protective factor enabling African Americans to avoid self-blame and brush off adversity by attributing it to external racial issues (e.g., African Americans are always the target of discrimination) and thereby maintain their self-esteem and well-being.

On the other hand, Christian and Barbarin (2001) have suggested that external racial attribution was related to lower well-being, resulting in more behavior problems such as social withdrawal. For example, the use of external racial attribution might indicate individuals' inability to take responsibility, mobilize resources to solve problems, and overcome adversity in life. This behavior might lower well-being and increase psychological distress.

### Resilience

Gordon (1995) examined 40 African American high school students from homes with low socioeconomic status and high stress. Resilient students had healthier self-concepts, felt more positive about their cognitive abilities, and stressed extracurricular activities more than their nonresilient peers. Furthermore, resilient students were focused more on future financial security and independence, despite their low socioeconomic background and high stress.

## Model 3: Well-Being and Resilience in a Cultural-Ecological Framework

Bronfenbrenner's (1979) ecological framework suggests that humans live in an environmental context. This human ecology includes four levels: macrosystem, exosystem, mesosystem, and microsystem. The macrosystem consists of institutional patterns and economic, social, educational, and political influences on the individual. The exosystem includes social settings, such as neighborhood, school, and church interactions. The mesosystem is a network of connections among close-knit environments such as home and schools. The microsystem contains the intimate and immediate environments such as family, school, peer group, neighborhood, and child care.

Culture can be understood as an acquired system of beliefs and values that incorporates and represents the worldview held in common by its members; well-being and resilience are recognizable as two Africentric values.

One approach to understanding the resilience and well-being of African Americans is to examine the biographies of successful African Americans. Charles Henry Turner, for example, has the unique distinction of having published a summary of his undergraduate thesis in the prestigious journal *Science* (Turner, 1892). By the time he received his master's degree, he had published three additional papers, one of these in *Science*. Despite this productivity and a PhD from the University of Chicago, Turner could not secure a university appointment. Ultimately, he accepted a teaching position at Sumner High School in St. Louis. Rather than accept his rejection as a researcher, he continued his studies, eventually publishing more than 70 papers; consistently attended conferences; and became, despite those who sought to deny him, a pioneer in comparative psychology. Applying the model of "well-being and resilience in a cultural-ecological framework," Turner suffered from stresses from the macrosystem, exosystem, mesosystem, and microsystem. His macrosystem consisted of nearly every institutional barrier imaginable in the late 19th and early 20th centuries placed before African Americans. After earning a prestigious PhD from the University of Chicago, this exosystem denied him rightful employment. During several undesirable jobs, he had to endure mesosystemic disdain because of his color and the microsystemic loss of his beloved wife while in his late 30s.

How did Turner survive these chronic and acute stressors? How was he able to channel his frustration into an outstanding publication record of more than 70 academic papers? How did he cope with being denied a university career and seemingly adapt to a career as a high school teacher? His biographers offer evidence that Turner demonstrated a high level of resilience and positive perception of life and well-being (Dewsbury, Benjamin, & Wertheimer, 2006). Turner and other historical figures like Malcolm X offer examples of the ability of well-being and resilience to buffer African Americans from deleterious conditions and enable them to succeed.

## Summary of Findings on Well–Being and Resilience

Interest in resilience and well-being in children and adults has grown rapidly in recent years (Masten, 2001). Despite the importance of understanding well-being and resilience (Seligman, 1991), current knowledge remains limited, primarily because most research was not conducted in an African cultural context.

An Africentric worldview places the highest value on interpersonal relations and groups. Resistance to oppression is shaped in a wide *social* environment, involving interactions between how the larger social context affects everyday experiences and, conversely, how day-to-day activities help shape the social context (Bagley & Carroll, 1998).

Research on African Americans' well-being and resilience found that the experience of enslavement required them to draw on their capacity to live above conditions. This experience caused African Americans to develop a unique style of resilience and well-being.

To illustrate, Levine (1977) quotes Aunt Aggy, an enslaved African American woman, who speaks of being *blessed* to see things that the slave captor could not see and reality unknown to the materially powerful captor. The tenacious legacy of that awareness is what underpins optimal well-being and resilience.

Heartfelt knowledge of spiritual connections beyond all manners of abuse and prejudice is reputed to be the source of energy that empowers African Americans to emerge intact from cultural trauma and injustice. Although deficit-focused scholars emphasize cultural traumas and psychological distress, other researchers tell us that well-being and resilience are two major themes in African American life that enable them to thrive in the midst of adversity.

## STRATEGIES TO FOSTER WELL-BEING AND RESILIENCE AMONG AFRICAN AMERICANS

Life experience supported by research (see Duncan, 2003) shows that people can foster well-being and resilience. Seligman, Rashid, and Parks (2006) demonstrated that well-being can be enhanced through planned interventions. What is important is that these interventions be tailored to the African American culture.

African Americans have long held that a virtuous life is the foundation for well-being. For example, in 1926, Sumner, writing on the philosophy of Negro education, encouraged personal cultivation of the following: physical well-being; simplicity in living; belief in God; fondness for literature, art, and music; industry; a contempt for loud and indiscreet laughing and talking; thrift; honesty; courteousness; respect; race pride; and punctuality (p. 43).

Given the importance of the family in every culture, family-based, coping-focused interventions have the potential to promote resilience and break linkages in the pernicious cycle of poverty (Wadsworth & Santiago, 2008). Coping effectively with stressors created and exacerbated by poverty could buffer families from various types of problems.

Wadsworth and Santiago (2008) studied two types of coping, the first to bolster the ability of adults to break the links of economic distress by reducing stress and enhancing problem-solving ability and the second to strengthen children's ability to cope with poverty-related stress that may trigger developmental problems. They found that people's beliefs about a situation could empower them to cope with difficulties.

In other work, African American preadolescent girls benefited from interventions with a relational and Africentric focus (Belgrave, Chase-Vaughn, Gray, Addison, & Cherry, 2000). Belgrave and colleagues (2000) sought to successfully increase bonding and mutually empowering relationships among girls, their peers, and female role models, via relational, gender-focused activities, thereby increasing self-esteem and gender identity. Belgrave and colleagues' study successfully enhanced African American preadolescent girls' self-esteem and gender identity.

Belgrave and colleagues' (2000) program also tried to strengthen Africentric and ethnic beliefs as a foundation for resilience. The Africentric worldview expounds on the core African values and uses the rich traditions for support during adversity and suffering (Akbar, 1996). Its organizing principles include spirituality, harmony, collective responsibility, oral tradition, sensitivity to emotional cues, authenticity, balance, concurrent time orientation to past, present, and future, and interpersonal/communal orientation.

High ethnic identity has been associated with higher achievement and self-esteem among African American youth (Phinney & Chavira, 1992) and with less risky sex and drug activity. Thus, it is necessary to increase resilience by appreciating Africentric values and ethnic identity, particularly values that promote communal responsibility, self-determination, purpose, and faith.

## CONCLUSION

A good deal of previous research has dwelt on differences between Blacks and Whites and described the physical and mental difficulties African Americans experienced to a greater degree than Whites (Williams, Yu, Jackson, & Anderson, 1997). Less attention has been given to intragroup differences discerning why some individuals cope and adapt better than others.

In fact, based on all these minutely researched reports discussed here, there is reason for excitement. We cannot help but conclude that resilience is a modus operandi of well-being itself. Well-being seldom lays passively back on the beach, basking in the ocean breeze, sipping soft drinks. On the contrary, as African Americans show us, well-being is an active process of living, remaining tough in adversity, which strengthens our stamina to resiliently thrive through it. Well-being is "to be well no matter what," to live abundantly in adversity, and to make creative contributions to the world, precisely through thick and thin. To live well, to be well, is to live in resilience.

## REFERENCES

Adams, V. H., III (1999). Predictors of African American well-being. *Journal of Black Psychology, 25,* 78–104.

Ahmed, F., Brown, D. R., Gary, L. E., & Saadatmand, F. (1994). Religious predictors of cigarette smoking: Findings for African-American women of childbearing age. *Behavioral Medicine, 20,* 34–43.

Akbar, N. (1996). African metapsychology of human personality. In D. A. Azibo (Ed.), *African psychology in historical perspective and related commentary* (pp. 29–46). Trenton, NJ: Africa World Press.

Allport, G. W. (1953). The trend in motivational theory. *American Journal of Orthopsychiatry, 23,* 107–119.

Argyle, M. (1987). *The psychology of happiness.* London: Routledge.

Bagley, C. A., & Carroll, J. (1998). Healing forces in African American families. In H. I. McCubbin, E. A. Thompson, A. I. Thompson, & J. A. Thompson (Eds.), *Resiliency in African-American families* (pp. 117–142). Thousand Oaks, CA: Sage.

Belgrave, F. Z., Chase-Vaughn, G., Gray, F., Addison, J. D., & Cherry, V. R. (2000). The effectiveness of a culture- and gender-specific intervention for increasing resiliency among African American preadolescent females. *Journal of Black Psychology, 26,* 133–147.

Bowen-Reid, T. L., & Rhodes, W. A. (2003). Assessment of marijuana use and psychological behaviors at two historically Black universities. *Journal of Black Psychology, 29,* 429–444.

Bowman, P. J. (1990). Coping with provider role strain: Adaptive cultural resources among Black husband-fathers. *Journal of Black Psychology, 16,* 1–21.

Bradburn, N. M. (1969). *The structure of psychological well-being.* Oxford, UK: Oxford University Press.

Bronfenbrenner, U. (1979). *The ecology of human development: Experiments by nature and design.* Cambridge, MA: Harvard University Press.

Brosky, A. E. (2000). The role of religion in the lives of resilient, urban, African American, single mothers. *Journal of Community Psychology, 28,* 199–219.

Brown v. Board of Education of Topeka, 347 U.S. 483 (1954).

Brown, D. L. (2008). African American resiliency: Examining racial socialization and social support as protective factors. *Journal of Black Psychology, 34,* 32–48.

Brown, D. R., & Gary, L. E. (1994). Religious involvement and health status among African American males. *Journal of the National Medical Association, 86,* 825–831.

Caldwell, C. H., Guthrie, B. J., & Jackson, J. S. (2006). Identity development, discrimination, and psychological well-being among African American and Caribbean Black adolescents. In A. J. Schulz & L. Mullings (Eds.), *Gender, race, class, and health: Interpersonal approaches* (pp. 125–136). San Francisco: Jossey-Bass.

Christian, M. D., & Barbarin, O. A. (2001). Cultural resources and psychological adjustment of African American children: Effects of spirituality and racial attribution. *Journal of Black Psychology, 27,* 43–63.

Clark, K. B. (1974). *Pathos of power.* New York: Harper & Row.

Coke, M. M. (1992). Correlates of life satisfaction among elderly African Americans. *Journal of Gerontology: Psychological Sciences, 47,* 316–320.

Coleman, P. (1966). Verbal discrimination reversal as a function of overlearning and percentage of items reversed. *Journal of Experimental Psychology, 72,* 271–275.

Constantine, M. G., Donnelly, P. C., & Myers, L. J. (2002). Collective self-esteem and Africultural coping styles in African American adolescents. *Journal of Black Studies, 32,* 698–710.

Daly, A., Jennings, J., Beckette, J. O., & Leashore, B. R. (1995). Effective coping strategies of African Americans. *Social Work, 40,* 240–248.

Darrow, S. L., Russell, M., Cooper, M. L., Mudar, P., & Frone, M. R. (1992). Sociodemographic correlates of alcohol consumption among African American and White women. *Women and Health, 18,* 35–51.

Dewsbury, D. A., Benjamin, L. T., & Wertheimer, M. (2006). *Portraits of pioneers in psychology* (Vol. VI). Washington, DC: American Psychological Association.

Diener, E. (1984). Subjective well-being. *Psychological Bulletin, 95,* 542–575.

Duncan, M. J. (2003). *African American history.* Indianapolis, IN: Alpha Books.

Edwards, K. L. (1999). African American definitions of self and psychological health. In R. L. Jones (Ed.), *Advances in African American psychology* (pp. 287–312). Hampton, VA: Cobb & Henry.

Garmezy, N. (1972). *Models of etiology for the study of children at risk for schizophrenia.* Minneapolis: University of Minnesota Press.

Gordon, K. E. (1995). Self-concept and motivational patterns of resilient African American high school students. *Journal of Black Psychology, 21,* 239–255.

Headey, B., Veenhoven, R., & Wearing, A. (1991). Top-down versus bottom-up theories of subjective well-being. *Social Indicators Research, 24,* 81–100.

Jackson, J. S., & Adams, V. H. (1992, August). *Changes in reports of subjective well-being among African Americans, 1979 to 1989.* Paper presented at the 100th Annual Convention of the American Psychological Association, Washington, DC.

Keyes, C. L. M., Shmotkin, D., & Ryff, C. D. (2002). Optimizing well-being: The empirical encounter of two traditions. *Journal of Personality and Social Psychology, 82,* 1007–1022.

Levine, L. W. (1977). *Black culture and Black consciousness.* New York: Oxford University Press.

Masten, A. S. (2001). Ordinary magic: Resilience process in development. *American Psychologist, 56,* 227–238.

Masten, A. S., & Coatsworth, J. D. (1998). The development of competence in favorable and unfavorable environments: Lessons from research on successful children. *American Psychologist, 53,* 205–220.

National Center for Health Statistics. (2002). *National vital statistics report* (Vol. 50, No. 16). Hyattsville, MD: Author.

Parks, F. M. (1998). Models of helping and coping: A transgenerational theory of African-American traditional healing. *Revista Interamericana de Psicologia, 32,* 95–110.

Parson, N. M., & Mikawa, J. K. (1991). Incarceration and nonincarceration of African-American men raised in Black Christian churches. *Journal of Psychology, 125,* 163–173.

Pettigrew, T. F., & Tropp, L. R. (2000). Does intergroup contact reduce prejudice?: Recent meta-analytic findings. In S. Oskamp (Ed.), *Reducing prejudice and discrimination* (pp. 93–114). Mahwah, NJ: Erlbaum.

Phinney, J. S., & Chavira, V. (1992). Ethnic identity and self-esteem: An exploratory longitudinal study. *Journal of Adolescence, 15,* 271–281.

Potts, R. (1996). Spirituality and the experience of cancer in an African-American community: Implications for psychosocial oncology. *Journal of Psychosocial Oncology, 14,*
1–19.

Ryff, C. D. (1989a). Beyond Ponce de Leon and life satisfaction: New directions in quest of
successful ageing. *International Journal of Behavioral Development, 12,* 35–55.

Ryff, C. D. (1989b). Happiness is everything, or is it?: Explorations of the meaning of psychological well-being. *Journal of Personality and Social Psychology, 57,* 1069–1081.

Ryff, C. D. (1995). Psychological well-being in adult life. *Current Directions in Psychological Science, 4,* 99–104.

Seligman, M. E. P. (1991). *Learned optimism.* New York: Knopf.

Seligman, M. E. P., Rashid, T., & Parks, A. C. (2006). Positive psychotherapy. *American
Psychologist, 61,* 774–788.

Simoni, J. M., Martone, M. G., & Kerwin, J. F. (2002). Spirituality and psychological adaptation among women with HIV/AIDS: Implication for counseling. *Journal of Counseling Psychology, 49,* 139–147.

Stevens, F. L., Hill, S., Heiner, M., & Chao, R. (2007, August). *Social support, coping, and
mental health: Well-being as a mediator.* Poster presented at the 115th Annual Convention of the American Psychological Association, San Francisco, CA.

Stevenson, H. C., Cameron, R., Herrero-Taylor, T., & Davis, G. Y. (2002). Development
of the Teenager Experience of Racial Socialization Scale: Correlates of race-related
socialization frequency from the perspective of Black youth. *Journal of Black Psychology, 28,* 84–106.

Sumner, F. C. (1926). The philosophy of Negro education. *Educational Review, 71,* 42–45.

Taylor, R. J. (1993). Religion and religious observances. In J. Jackson, L. Chatters, & R.
Taylor (Eds.), *Aging in Black America* (pp. 101–123). Newbury Park, CA: Sage.

Taylor, R. J., Chatters, L. M., & Levin, J. (2004). *Religion in the lives of African Americans:
Social, psychological, and health perspectives.* Thousand Oaks, CA: Sage.

Turner, C. H. (1892). A few characteristics of the avian brain. *Science, 19,* 16–17.

U.S. Department of Health and Human Services. (1999). *Mental health: A report of the
surgeon general.* Retrieved June 15, 2008, from *www.surgeongeneral.gov/library/men-
talhealth/summary.html.*

Utsey, S. O., Bolden, M. A., Lanier, Y., & Williams, O., III. (2007). Examining the role of
culture-specific coping as a predictor of resilient outcomes in African Americans
from high-risk urban communities. *Journal of Black Psychology, 33,* 75–93.

VandenBos, G. R. (Ed.). (2007). *APA dictionary of psychology.* Washington, DC: American
Psychological Association.

Wadsworth, M. E., & Santiago, C. D. (2008). Risk and resiliency process in ethnically
diverse families in poverty. *Journal of Family Psychology, 22,* 399–410.

Williams, D. R., Yu, Y., Jackson, J., & Anderson, N. (1997). Racial differences in physical and mental health: Socioeconomic status, stress, and discrimination. *Journal of
Health Psychology, 2,* 335–351.

Wilson, S., & Miles, M. (2001). Spirituality in African-American mothers coping with a
seriously ill infant. *Journal of Social Pediatric Nursing, 6,* 116–122.

World Health Organization. (1948). *Preamble to the constitution of the World Health Organization.* Geneva, Switzerland: Author.

# 6

# Evidence-Based Practice

Aminifu R. Harvey
Oliver J. Johnson
Annie McCullough-Chavis
Tamara M. Carter

This chapter examines several theoretical schools of thought explaining human behavior and their appropriateness with African Americans.

## PSYCHOANALYTIC THEORY

Psychoanalytic theory was developed by the Austrian physician Sigmund Freud from the late 1800s to the 1930s. Freud viewed personality from six perspectives: topographic, which involves conscious versus the unconscious; dynamic, which entails interaction of psychic forces; genetic, concerned with the origin and development of psychic phenomena through oral, anal, phallic, latency, and genital stages; economic, involving the distribution, transformation, and expenditure of energy; structural, which revolves around the functional units of the id, ego, and superego; and adaptive, which involves the instinctual preparedness to interact with an evolving series of normal and predicable environments (Prochaska & Norcross, 2007). Psychoanalytical theory is the foundation for psychoanalysis and can be defined as a conflict model leading to compromise formation. That is, the mind is in continuous conflict between the conscious and the unconscious, between what the individual immediately desires and the acceptable norms of society.

## Tenets and Principles

The basic dynamics motivating personality from a psychoanalytic perspective are life and sex (Eros) and death and aggression (Thanatos). From this perspective, the person desires immediate gratification of sexual and aggressive impulses; these complementary forces are instincts that possess a somatic basis. The demand for instant gratification (id) leads to conflict with social rules (ego) that demand some control over sex and aggression, if there is to be order in society. In order to manage these conflicting impulses, the person's id is forced to develop defense mechanisms. The defense mechanisms safeguard the individual from the danger of punishment from the ego for breaking the social order and from experiencing guilt and anxiety from the superego while allowing indirect satisfaction of these impulses. Some of the most common defense mechanisms include denial, or the closing off on a cognitive level of threatening aspects of one's life; projection, placing the negative phenomena that occur in one's life onto others; incorporation, making images of others an aspect of one's own life; reaction formation, or expressing the opposite of what one desires; and intellectualization, which is neutralizing affect-laden experiences by talking in intellectual or linear logical terms. Other defense mechanisms include displacement, which involves taking out our frustrations, feelings, and impulses on less threatening people or objects; and compensation, repression, and sublimation, which allows us to act out unacceptable impulses by converting these behaviors into a more acceptable form. When confronted by stressful events, people sometimes abandon coping strategies and revert to patterns of behavior used earlier (developed by Anna Freud, 1966, in her work with children). Repression acts to keep information out of conscious awareness. However, these memories do not just disappear; they continue to influence our behavior. Consciously forcing the unwanted information out of our awareness is known as suppression.

Probably, the most well-known and controversial concept of psychoanalytical theory is the "Oedipal conflict." This involves the sexual desires of the son for the affection of his mother with the expectation that she fulfill these desires. Of course, the son fears that the father will punish him because the father already has these privileges of the mother's affection. The fear is that the punishment will be the father removing his son's penis. This is known as castration anxiety. In order to deal with this anxiety, the son represses his desire for his mother, represses his hostile rivalry toward his father, and identifies with his father's rule so he can avoid castration. Based on this theoretical proposition, Freud concluded that females were subject to penis envy and became hostile toward their mothers for not providing them with a penis.

## General Effectiveness of the Theory

It is important to remember that psychoanalytical theory is the basis and the foundation for the development of insight-oriented psychotherapy and, at the time of its introduction, was a positive, hopeful major contribution to the science of human development and the treatment of mental disorders. The basic premise of the theory was that personality development was completed by roughly age 6 (Rickman, 1957), that dysfunctional behavior was the result of psychic trauma experienced earlier in the individual's life, and that, through free association and the retelling of dreams to an analyst, the origins of this trauma would be revealed. This revelation and the individual's desire to please the analyst (transference) would enable the individual to move beyond this painful experience to lead a more personally fulfilling life. There are major criticisms of the theory. Thematically, the most critical ones are that the theory is patriarchal and Eurocentric. The theory is patriarchal in the sense that the theory places emphasis on the biological superiority of the male while simultaneously oppressing females. The question is, Who says having a penis is superior to having a vagina and why should women be envious of a male's penis? The other question in terms of patriarchy is, Where is the father in the development of the child? In this theoretical orientation, it is the mother who is held responsible for all the misgivings of the child and the father seems to be exonerated. The lead author tends to believe it is this Freudian concept that has led men to believe they play no significant role in the development of the child. Thus, their presence is not essential and they can, therefore, just be "baby makers."

Other criticisms of the theory are that it ignores the self as a part of the family system, and that many mental health problems have their genesis in dysfunctional families or with the social environment. When psychoanalysis does consider relationships, it is sexist in that it engages in mother bashing. In a literature review, Prochaska and Norcross (2007) reported finding reports that classical psychoanalysis was an effective mental health intervention. However, these reports must be treated cautiously because there have been no controlled outcome studies on classical psychoanalysis or relational psychoanalysis.

## Major Theorists

There were a number of people who were part of Freud's inner circle until their deviation from his teachings led to their expulsion (Gay, 1988). Wilhelm Reich (cited in Prochaska & Norcross, 2007) developed character analysis. He worked to pass laws against child abuse and for the equal rights for women. Alfred Adler (cited in Prochaska & Norcross, 2007) advanced his theoretical perspective, individual psychology, that each person was unique and no one theory applied to all; he is known for the development of the concepts of inferiority and superiority complexes. Carl G. Jung (cited in Prochaska & Norcross, 2007) rejected Freud's emphasis on sex and formed his own theoretical orientation: analytical psychology. Jung believed the psyche consisted of the conscious mind, the unconscious mind, and the collective unconscious; he believed the best means for understanding the mind was through dreams, in which the content is loaded with symbols of archetypes. Additionally, there was Anna Freud (cited in Prochaska & Norcross, 2007), Freud's youngest daughter, who is identified with child psychoanalysis.

## Normalization

Not surprisingly, psychoanalytic theory was grounded in a Eurocentric worldview. It was developed by an Austrian atheist Jewish physician in the late 19th and early 20th centuries who was influenced by the secular and spiritual traditions of the Hebrew sojourn.[1] He was particularly interested in Jewish mysticism, especially the Kabbala (Bynum, 1999). The Kabbalalistic approach probably has its roots in African mysticism (see Bynum, 1999).

The theory is focused on the individual and intrapsychic phenomena; from an Africentric perspective, a child chooses his or her family of birth and it is the responsibility of the community to raise the child. This perspective articulates the role of the father in the development of the child. An Africentric theory adheres to the equality of the sexes, as seen in the story of Isis, Osiris, and Horus. In this story, which is a metaphor for the philosophy of African culture just as the story of Oedipus is a metaphor for Eurocentric culture, Osiris is mutilated by his jealous brother, but it is his wife, Isis, who plays the major role in restoring him whole again (Karenga, 1990; Budge, 1994). Africentric theory also holds that many of the mental health issues are not as much due to an individual deficient or intrapsychic instinctual conflict but to the oppression of people of African descent and is manifested in the concept of posttraumatic slave disorder (Leary, 2005).

Another question arises: Is psychoanalysis a functional theory for all ethnic groups or has it totally missed the target? Are there some theoretical propositions and assumptions that are valid, and does this validity rely more on one's philosophical orientation and worldview rather than one's biological, racial, and ethnic makeup? If it relies on the latter, then if one is African in origin but adheres to a European worldview, could not psychoanalysis be the most appropriate theoretical underpinning for psychotherapy?

## Applicability for African Americans

In reviewing the literature, there are a few articles that provide case studies of psychotherapy (Addams, 2002) but none support the application of psychoanalysis to African Americans. If there is a derivative of this theory that might have applicability with people of African descent, then it is the work with the unconscious found in Jungian psychology. Jung revealed to the Western world the concept of the collective unconscious based on his study of African culture. Interestingly,

---

[1]Freud's (1939) last book published shortly before his death in England was devoted to his belief that Moses was an Egyptian, not a Jew, and a believer in unlimited polytheism. Thus, the Hebrew religion is descended from ancient rejected Egyptian beliefs. He further contended that Moses was put to death by the Jews.

Jung obtained many of his ideas from his prolonged stays in Africa, even though he considered Africans primitive in their interactions with the world, especially psychologically (Hill, 1997).

Richard King (2001) developed this concept of the collective unconscious for people of African descent and established its roots in African culture. This form of psychotherapy incorporates the use of archetypes and universal symbols (including numerology and astrology) to express the hidden meanings of the unconscious world in relationship to one's life and has meaning for African Americans. King speculates that it is melanin in its form as neuromelanin in the nervous system that acts as a neurotransmitter to pass on the collective unconscious from one generation to the next.

The applicability of psychoanalysis in all its forms and its effectiveness with African Americans does not have a simple "yes" or "no" answer but dictates further study, with a closer evaluation of which aspects of which theories are applicable and possibly helpful. I suspect Jungian psychology could be useful in clinical work with people of African descent if the therapist incorporated the work of Dr. Richard King (2001). As a means of testing for theory appropriateness, Azibo (1996) has developed a structural framework, an emic theory-derived steady-state approach. This approach contends that in researching people of African descent one must understand the Black personality (Kambon, 1992), a theoretical construct that attempts to explain the psychological functioning of persons of African origin. Pasteur and Toldson (1982) contend that unlike the Eurocentric mind, which is more left brain and compartmentalizes, the Black/African mind is more right brain, mentalizes human awareness holistically, and is spontaneous. Thus, there is a propensity to use song, dance, oratory, and creativity to expel impulses that probably become the material of the unconscious in the Western mind. Pasteur and Toldson said the right brain:

> Characterized by spontaneous, spiritual, and ecstatic, it demands immediate release of energy through action, and expressive discharge experiences in the direction of total freedom in both the feelings and movement domains. (1982, p. 19)

It seems reasonable to assume that those rooted in an African mindset, relying more on the right brain and because of the melanin factor, trigger emotions and feelings that are fundamental to Black expressive behavior (Boykin & Toms, 1985). Boykin and Toms (1985) specified nine related but distinct dimensions of expressions in African Americans: spirituality, harmony, movement, verve, affect, communalism, expressive individualism, orality, and social time perspective (p. 41). Given this discussion, it seems that there needs to be a systematic development of an African-oriented psychological therapeutic intervention that takes into account the total aspects of aforementioned discussion.

## HUMANISTIC PSYCHOLOGY AND THEORY

The humanistic approach to psychology has emphasized the incessant search for a philosophical and ultimately pragmatic comprehension of human existence that supports the quest for highest aspirations uniquely associated with human achievement and human potential. The earliest humanistic psychologists (Jourard, 1961; Maslow, 1967; May, 1965; Sutich, 1949) centered their collective efforts on questions pertaining to the existential search for what it means to be fully, completely, and genuinely human.

They sought to formulate psychological methodologies that would assist humans in arriving at their full potential. These developments were viewed as particularly fruitful from 1954 to 1973, which interestingly enough was a period of significant advancement for African Americans in a wide variety of spheres, including, not insignificantly, an interest in the evidence-based articulation of African American cultural and familial strengths. Connections between these developments are explored later in this section. Indeed, humanistic psychologists issued scholarly critiques aimed principally at conventional psychological schools in the first half of the 20th century for promulgating a narrow-minded view of human potential and human existence (Moustakas, 1962).

Abraham Maslow (cited in Prochaska & Norcross, 2007) is the person largely responsible for the creation of the humanistic psychology movement. Maslow galvanized the growing interest in psychology for alternative paradigms for understanding human behavior into a radically new theory of the self and self-actualization that stands as a blueprint for later generations of humanistic psychologists.

### Tenets and Principles

Maslow (1967) conceptualized key dimensions of humanistic psychology as a new and decidedly distinct viewpoint for exploring the whole person based on a study of emotionally healthy, resilient, and creative persons. He believed that the overwhelming majority of psychologists focused their energies on persistent examinations of human deficits, deviance, abnormalities, and pathology. Maslow elected to launch empirically based explorations into the lives of who he defined as "self-actualizing persons," believing instead that those persons have a great deal to teach us regarding how we may become fully human and fully alive, embracing life's rich complexities and living life to the absolute fullest. Consequently, humanistic perspectives on psychology were conceptualized as the "third force" (i.e., in stark contrast to the views of human nature articulated by behaviorist and psychoanalytic schools) (Winthrop, 1962).

Humanistic psychology primarily concerns itself with the individual person and his or her capacities to strive toward the pinnacle of self-actualized growth and development. Chein (1972, p. 6) observed that the humanistic perspective views the person as "an active responsible agent," not as a person completely at the whim of, for example, environmental influences.

## General Effectiveness of the Theory

It seems that humanistic psychology would have a great deal to offer African American people. However, African American psychologists have raised questions regarding the relevance of tenets integral to humanistic psychology and issues central to the African American experience and attendant worldview. Again, humanistic psychology values and elevates the primacy of selfhood. Its chief focus tends to rest exclusively on methods of accomplishing ever-improving psychological and psychosocial functioning of the *individual* person. Conversely, Nobles (1973) has asserted:

> We have contended that African psychology is rooted in the nature of Black culture which is based on particular forms of African philosophical principles. Consequently, the understanding of the psychology of Black people (more appropriately classified as Americanized Africans) must be African-based. Similarly, if we are to rid the literature of its scientific, colonialistic tone, the proper understanding of Black self-concept must be based on African assumptions and must incorporate African-based analyses and conceptualizations. In this regard, we can clearly see the importance of understanding the African self-concept and its psychological basis for Black self-concept. (p. 23)

The emphasis on the primacy of individuality is uniquely characteristic of Western societies. Sampson (1988) referred to this orientation as "self-contained" individualism, that is, an orientation that is defined by "firm boundaries demarcating the sense of self from non-self other, an emphasis on personal control and independence, and an exclusionary singular sense of the self" (p. 16). Conversely, the principal construction for genuine personhood that seems to be embraced globally appears to be centered on an African worldview (e.g., "I am because we are, and because we are, therefore, I am") (Nobles, 1973, pp. 23–24).

Myers (1988) argues that the individual person is not a separate and distinct entity. She asserts that the individual person is rooted within the very fabric of what she refers to as the "tribe," and that this sense of personhood is not (in sharp contrast to the dominant worldview) linked to external accomplishments, titles, or accoutrements, but that its sense of worth is simply intrinsic "in being." The dominant paradigm elevates and evaluates a person's worth and importance according to largely impermeable standards of separateness, impersonality, a quantitative orientation, and strict objectivism, indeed constructs that are decidedly Eurocentric. Alternatively, an Africentric worldview would not give primacy to conventional attributes, patriarchal perspectives, or paternalistic standards. An Africentric paradigm would evaluate a person's worth and importance according to standards of the inherent worth and dignity of all human beings. This paradigm specifically structures relations with others around recognition of the interconnected and always personal nature of and with the elements of the world around us. Separateness and impersonality (again, key characteristics of the dominant worldview) are seen as obstacles to constructing effective therapeutic relationships. The dominant worldview focuses preeminently and exclusively on the primacy of the "self." Complementary and integrative perspectives constitute essential Africentric characteristics. The dominant worldview espouses principles that represent both ways of knowing and what is considered worth knowing within the confines of the dominant culture. Not surprisingly, these same perspectives have heavily influenced the development of theoretical and practice-related guidelines uniquely associated with humanistic psychology in particular and American psychology in general.

Humanistic treatment modalities that are consistent with an appreciation for the primacy of family and social networks as key therapeutic agents would seem to be more appropriate. These approaches would not elevate individual autonomy and separateness as critical ingredients to wholeness, wellness, and healing.

## Major Theorists

Abraham Maslow (cited in Prochaska & Norcross, 2007) stands as the individual most responsible for the development of humanistic psychology. Maslow articulated the ever-burgeoning quest for a different type of psychological theory and practice into a cohesive and coherent perspective. Carl Rogers (cited in Prochaska & Norcross, 2007) provided the primary clinical framework for humanistic clinicians (i.e., "client-centered" therapy), and Fritz Perls (1973) sharpened humanistic psychology's focus on the self and self-awareness by body-oriented interpretations of what stifles human growth and potential.

## Intended Population

Humanistic psychologists outlined a conceptual framework of theory and practice that was rooted in the decidedly self-centered system of values espoused by the dominant culture. It seems as if the very system of values that served to give birth to the evolution and development of humanistic psychology is diametrically opposed to the family- and community-minded principles that mark Africentric philosophy and, ultimately, practice paradigms.

## Applicability for African Americans

According to Jenkins (2001), there are a number of pivotal sociological dimensions that would necessarily impinge upon these issues. For example, this nation places a premium on individual advancement, success, and unrelenting achievement. These beliefs stand in direct contrast to the life-sustaining principles of Africentricity. There are several psychosocial dimensions as well. As African Americans began to restore and reclaim the Africentric emphasis on community empowerment, dramatic improvements were achieved regarding substantive quality of life measures, as evidenced by gains won during the civil rights movement.

Significantly, the notion of group advancement represents the key strand of thought regarding Africentric worldviews, a notion that appears to be decidedly contrary to the focus on individual growth and self-actualization so intrinsic to humanistic psychology.

## SOCIAL LEARNING THEORY AND BEHAVIOR THERAPY

In the United States, social learning theory and its application was well known in the closing decades of the 19th century. Its use as a mental heath intervention grew in popularity in the late 1950s as interest in insight-oriented approaches waned. Today, behavioral therapy is widely used with many individuals to change specific dysfunctional behaviors. Unlike analytic interventions, behavioral therapies are not concerned with the underlying causes of the behavior but rather with the observable demonstrable behaviors themselves (Prochaska & Norcross, 2007).

### Tenets, Principles, and Assumptions of Behavior Theory

Behaviorists take the position that people's thoughts, feelings, and actions are a result of learning, and that established principles and assumptions determine how the learning process works. Kazdin (1984, as cited in Kazdin, 2001) suggests that the major characteristics of behavioral treatments are the primacy of behavior, the importance of learning, the directive and active nature of the treatments, the importance of assessment and evaluation, and the use of persons in everyday life. Behavior therapy is derived from social learning theory, which posits that:

1. Most abnormal behavior is acquired and maintained according to the same principle as normal behavior.
2. Assessment is continuous and focuses on the current determinants of behavior.
3. People are best described by what they think, feel, and do in specific life situations.
4. Treatment is derived from the theory and experimental findings of scientific psychology.
5. Treatment methods are precisely specified and replicable.
6. Treatment is individually tailored to different problems and different people.
7. Treatment goals and methods are mutually contracted with the client.
8. Research evaluates the effects of specific techniques on specific problems.
9. Outcome is evaluated in terms of the initial induction of behavior change, its generalization to real-life settings, and its maintenance over time. (O'Leary & Wilson, 1987, as cited in Prochaska & Norcross, 2007, p. 260)

Social learning theory maintains that all behavior is influenced by the same principles of learning. Its evolutionary formulation has been in three principal steps: classical conditioning, operant conditioning, and cognitive behaviorism.

Initially researched by Wilson (2000), classical conditioning is a process of developing patterns of behavior through responses to environmental stimuli or specific behavioral consequences. In Pavlov's research, food (the conditioned stimulus) naturally produced salivation (an involuntary response) in dogs when it was placed before them. A bell (the unconditioned stimulus) when rung did not. However, after the bell was repeatedly paired with the food, the dogs would salivate to a ringing bell even if food was not offered. This learned response to a previously unconnected stimulus provided a different understanding to behavioral problems like overeating, substance abuse, and many anxiety-related disorders (Gambrill, 1994).

The next step in the evolution of learning theory and its application to mental health treatment was taken by B. F. Skinner (1976) in his development of the operant conditioning model. The major premise of operant conditioning is that future behavior is determined by the consequences of present behavior. That is, all behaviors have consequences on the environment and the consequences reinforce the response. Major concepts are positive and negative reinforcements, discrimination, extinction, generalization, and punishment. Operant behavioral approaches are used frequently with disciplining children and dealing with temper tantrums, generalized fears, and classroom and other misbehaviors.

The third, and most recent, step in the evolution of social learning theory and its application to therapy is cognitive behaviorism (Bandura, 1977). Here, learning occurs through modeling behaviors that the observer considers desirable. Learning also occurs by watching others engage in behaviors and how they are reinforced for that behavior. For example, young people may or may not acquire the habit of alcohol consumption because they have seen and heard friends bragging about how cool it is to drink (modeling); whether the youth actually imbibes is the result of watching friends drink and their consumptive behavior. In this instance, he or she got polluted. He or she retched and moaned, ruining the party (negative reinforcement for not drinking is vomit). A youth who cannot stand to vomit decides not to imitate his sick friend. Last, learning occurs as a result of efficacy ("It is important to me that I do [or not] emulate this behavior").

## General Effectiveness of Behavior Theory

Many research studies support the general applicability and effectiveness of behavioral therapies (Prochaska & Norcross, 2007). Currently, the service delivery environment, with its focus on outcome indicators and evidence-based practice, owes a great debt to behaviorists, who remain the most proficient group of practitioners in measuring intervention outcomes (Granvold, 1994).

More controlled outcome research has been conducted on behavior therapy than on any other psychotherapy. Behavior theory points toward the new emphasis in social sciences on empiricism (observable evidence) in evaluating the outcomes of intervention with children, adults, couples, and families. Indeed, the surge in the therapy movement toward efficiency, research-supported methods, and evaluation of the outcome can be credited to the behaviorists. Prochaska and Norcross (2007) write that behaviorists were committed to time-efficient, evidence-based interventions and were adherents of brief therapy before it became fashionable. For example, in a 1983 study by Norcross and Wogan (cited in Prochaska and Norcross, 2007), behavior therapists reported seeing clients less frequently and for a shorter duration than psychotherapists of other persuasions; and only 7% of their clients, on average, were seen more than a year.

Concerning the effectiveness of behavior therapy with children, Weisz, Hawley, and Doss (2004) statistically examined 236 published randomized trials on treatment for youth (3–18 years) from 1962 to 2002. They found that across various outcome measures 80% of treated youngsters were more improved after treatment than those not treated. Behavioral treatments proved more effective than nonbehavioral treatments regardless of client age. The authors revealed that several meta-analyses have been undertaken on adults, couples, and families concerning the effectiveness of behavior therapy and have produced similar results. Even though the authors cited many instances of the effectiveness of behavioral interventions with children, adults, couples and families and with specific disorders, they did not offer effectiveness data specifically for African Americans or other diverse people.

## Major Theorists, Normal Target Population, and African Americans

B. F. Skinner (1938), a Harvard University psychologist, developed the operant conditioning model that is concerned more with the consequences of a behavioral response than with the initial stimulus and changing the contingencies that control behavior. John B. Watson (Brown, 1965) is distinguished as the first behaviorist to outline the basic tenets of behaviorism in a psychology article. Albert Bandura (1977) is eminent for his scientific research concerning modeling and behavior. He stressed the importance of both environmental reinforcers and internal process as operative to modeling. It must be noted that these behaviorists were European American males, and their research and worldview were austerely Eurocentric in epistemology and orientation.

According to Ivey, Andrea, Ivey, and Simek-Morgan (2002), the worldview of behaviorism is cited as emphasizing freedom, shape and control of behavior, individual rights, collaboration in treatment, and self-efficacy. This opinion applies without question to the target population of predominantly Americans of European descent. Although behavior theory has been centrally concerned with concrete changes and empowerment of consumers, it should be noted that it has not substantially addressed cultural, multicultural, or African American issues despite important theoretical contributions made by Cheek (1976) and Kantrowitz and

Ballou (1992). Cheek, a pioneer in assertive training, was one of the first behaviorists to generalize behavior theory specifically to counseling and psychotherapy with African Americans. He demonstrated the validity of traditional behavioral concepts with African American clients and was an early proponent of "didactic assertive training." Cheek supplies a culturally relevant view to behavioral therapy. He points out that assertive behavior varies between African American and White cultures, and that both groups need to understand the frame of reference of the other (Ivey et al., 2002).

Kantrowitz and Ballou (1992, as cited in Prochaska & Norcross, 2007) suggest that the behavioral focus on individual skill training can neglect social issues and support dominant group values. For example, they indicate that assertiveness training is an example of evidence-based treatment and will probably meet with the approval of sexually harassed women, and the social norm of women's duty to protect themselves is not seriously questioned. Their distress may be temporarily reduced by assertiveness training, but the social status quo of the dominant society is also protected; therefore necessary social change does not occur.

## Applicability for African Americans

The effectiveness of behavior therapy is documented in the literature and has been used clinically with African Americans. The authors believe this is due in part to the type of behaviors, methods employed, and utilization of baseline and evidence-based data to assess the interventions for evidence of changed behaviors. Additionally, the process of intervention in behavior theory is quite systematic and, therefore, can be more generalized than most other psychotherapies. Clearly, a wide array of behavior therapies that apply the principles of behavior theory are applicable and used with African Americans; however, what is not as clear is whether research studies and analyses have been conducted substantially to prove efficacy and effectiveness with African Americans. Empirically, more research in behavioral therapies has yielded a great deal of effective therapies, some of which have been and are being used with African Americans for the treatment of stress, anxiety, depression, weight reduction, HIV/AIDS intervention, PTSD, addictions, and drug dependence. However, so far the data and research studies do not abundantly support evidence-based practice as effective treatment or its applicability with African Americans as with European Americans.

Modification of the use of traditional behavioral counseling and the primary focus of a Eurocentric worldview to include an Africentric worldview would prove to be more culturally relevant and effective for African Americans. The Africentric worldview, unlike the Eurocentric worldview, which primarily emphasizes individuality and self-efficacy, focuses more on group or collectivity, oneness of being, balance, and harmony of all things. Nobles (1973) argues that the African view of self is contingent on the existence of others. Thus, a major criticism of behavior theory from a cultural perspective is the primary exclusion of an African view of self and an Africentric worldview in theory and intervention. The authors believe that, without this incorporation of an Africentric worldview, it is doubtful that behavior theory works effectively and culturally with African Americans, especially with those who are more in tune with group culture and values. Second, behavior theory is expounded as being centrally concerned with concrete changes and empowerment of consumers, but the question is, empowerment of what group of consumers? Although behavior theory has been established as effective and the effectiveness has been generalized to include African Americans, there is a paucity of research articles and studies that specifically state that behavior theory is effective for African Americans.

There is a need for more theory and methods in the behavior theory that do not adapt and apply Eurocentric psychotherapy with African Americans and other cultural groups. The orientation and use of the theory with African Americans could take into account more of the culture and worldview of African Americans and, according to Cheek (1976), should not seek to "make African Americans White." He suggests that assertiveness training does not seek to have African Americans behave or think like Whites or to have women think like men but rather to recognize the perspective and worldview of different groups. As noted earlier in the chapter, his pioneering work demonstrates how the behavioral approach can be effectively used with African American clients when modified to meet their unique style and life experiences. Thus, more research studies like those conducted by Cheek could establish the behaviorists' claim of overall effectiveness of the theory with clients, and specifically African Americans. In order for behavior theory to be more effective with African Americans and other cultural groups, those utilizing the theory must acquire knowledge about the values, beliefs, and worldviews of persons from different cultural backgrounds, like African Americans, in order to work ethically, effectively, and respectfully with them.

## TRANSPERSONAL THEORY

Transpersonal psychology joins theories, psychological concepts, and methods with the subject and practices of the spiritual disciplines. Spirituality emphasizes the dynamic and evolutionary processes through which we seek purpose (Barker, 2007). Issues considered in transpersonal psychology include peak experiences, mystical experiences, systemic trance, and spiritual self development (Hartman & Zimberoff, 2004).

Mainstream psychotherapeutic systems have largely ignored human spiritual and religious experience. One of the hallmarks of transpersonal theory is that it seeks out and joins insights on human nature and healing from a wide variety of cultures and recognizes the role of the cultural context in the experience of individuals and groups. According to transpersonal theory, there are developmental stages beyond the adult ego that involve experiences of connectedness with experiences considered outside the boundaries of the ego (Kasprow & Scotton, 1999).

Spirituality in the social work profession is associated with the attempt to find meaning and purpose in life through relationships with self, others, or a higher power. Spirituality is also understood to include beliefs people have about reality beyond the material world. Spirituality is often an overlooked aspect of culture (the acknowledgment of language, art, customs, music, religion, and even food). One implication is that culture can be displayed in all aspects of daily living. Spirituality and religion are representations of culture that serve as sources of comfort and renewal, strength, and empowerment. Additionally, if we view culture as a mechanism for survival in the social environment, the importance of considering each element, including spirituality, is necessary to embrace and celebrate culture.

## Principles of Transpersonal Approaches and Cultural Diversity

Transpersonal approaches are concerned with accessing and integrating developmental stages beyond the adult ego and with fostering higher human development. Because of this concern, most transpersonal theories deal extensively with matters relating to human values and spiritual experience (Kasprow & Scotton, 1999). Transpersonal psychiatry does not promote any particular belief system but acknowledges that spiritual experiences and transcendent states are universal human experiences widely reported across cultures and, therefore, worthy of rigorous, scientific study. Inattention to these experiences and their roles in both psychopathology and healing constitutes a common limitation in conventional psychotherapeutic practice (Kasprow & Scotton, 1999).

Transpersonal psychology requires us to challenge our culturally defined views of mental health and psychotherapy and to draw cross-cultural insights into counseling and education. A core practice for transpersonal psychology includes meditation, mindfulness, and contemplation. Although ritual has not been identified as a core practice in transpersonal psychology, it is important in many cultural and religious traditions that promote spiritual values. For many cultures, ritual is the central means of discovering and developing intrapersonal, interpersonal, and transpersonal connections. Ritual provides a way of communicating with the unconscious, with each other, with the collective, and with the spirit (Davis, 2000). It gives us a deeper meaning to our actions and relationships. It also offers a sense of sanctuary within the ritual arena for exposing and exploring deep, possibly difficult experiences.

The role of cultural diversity is becoming well established in transpersonal psychology. One of the most important contributions of multicultural counseling theory and research to the mental health field has been the conceptual move from a narrow focus on the individual to a view of self in a cultural context (Burke, Chawin, & Miranti, 2005). This shift has prompted recognition of spiritual and healing systems original to racial-ethnic American cultures. Standards for multicultural counseling competencies include a call for practitioners to be knowledgeable.

## Major Theorists

Transpersonal philosophy can be traced back to philosophies and religious traditions as well as humanistic and transpersonal schools of psychology. The earliest use of the word *transpersonal* is attributed to William James (1929), who used it in his 1905 lecture notes at Harvard University (Kasprow & Scotton, 1999). Abraham Maslow (1971) is also considered a theorist within the transpersonal movement. Although his work regarding human peak experiences grew out of the humanistic movement of the 1960s, eventually "transpersonal" came to be associated with a school of psychology within the humanistic movement (Washburn, 1995).

Carl Jung (1938) was the first clinician to attempt to validate a spiritual approach to the practice of depth psychology. Jung was among the first to examine spiritual experience cross-culturally, and his study of Eastern mysticism, African shamanism, and Native American religion helped define the uniqueness of human spiritual experience and its relevance to psychological health (Washburn, 1995).

Maslow continued this theme with his naturalistic study of people he considered to be self-actualized. He found consistent descriptions of the characteristics of enlightened people across cultures and concluded that human beings have an instinctive, biology-based drive toward spiritual self-actualization. He characterized this as a state of deep altruism, periodic mystical peak experiences producing a sense of union, and freedom from conditioned thought and behavior (Washburn, 1995). Ken Wilber (1984), a transpersonal theorist, elaborated on a developmental model that incorporated not only the usual stages of human development suggested by Freud, Jung, and others but also the transpersonal stage (Washburn, 1995). Wilber identified 10 stages of human development. He then presented a vision-logic stage characterized by the integration of mind and body and associated with new capacities for the direct intuition of intricate patterns. There were also four transpersonal stages: the psychic, in which individual consciousness extends beyond the boundaries of the empirical ego, producing feelings of empathic understanding; the subtle, in which consciousness gains access to original forms; the causal, in which observing consciousness merges with what is observed; and the last stage, in which one has a willingness and ability to travel among all the stages because one is free of attachment to even the highest states (Washburn, 1995).

## Applicability for African Americans

Transpersonal theory can be applied in many ways, including teaching, organizational development, and health care. Its most common applications, however, are in counseling and psychotherapy. Transpersonal psychology includes transpersonal and mystical experiences, peak experiences, and spiritual emergencies. Transpersonal process refers to the techniques and strategies used. Aspects of a transpersonal context include holding in view the client's intrinsic health, being mindful and present centered regardless of the particular content or processes, viewing psychotherapy as both an act of service and an act of work on oneself, and recognizing the interconnectedness and individuality in the counseling situation (Davis, 2000).

One of the major challenges therapists face in attempting to integrate religion and spirituality into counseling for African Americans comes from within the field of psychotherapy itself. A core practice for transpersonal psychology includes meditation, mindfulness, breathing techniques, contemplation, and psychotropic medications. According to limited research, these methods have been success-ful. Although these methods can be used for self-regulation, relaxation, and pain control or for self-exploration and self-therapy, they have been used for gaining a wider perspective of one's true self.

Although ritual has not been identified as a core practice in transpersonal psychology, it is central in many cultural and religious traditions that promote spiritual values. There are several possibilities for the role of transpersonal psy-chology in relation to psychology and spiritual wisdom traditions, and they are not necessarily mutually exclusive. The context of transpersonal counseling is applicable to many educational or therapeutic situations and the issues that bring people to counseling or psychotherapy. It can also be practiced in settings such as schools, educational advising, individual private and agency practice, and com-munity development. Transpersonal psychology is not a specific set of beliefs or a religion but rather an orientation that is compatible with most educational and psychological approaches. As a result, a transpersonal approach in educational settings can support students' belief systems and practices.

## CONCLUSION

The power of African spiritual traditions is perceived in the transforming value they have had for generations. From slavery through more than 100 years of posteman-cipation inequities, spiritual survival has been possible through African and Afri-can American traditions of communalism, religion, music and dance, folklore and storytelling, and social change movements (Myers, 1988). These are inseparable from one another and are woven into what is experienced as spirituality in Afri-can American culture. These cultural patterns constitute important resources for counseling. Psychology and counseling can expand toward a richer accounting of the full range of human experience and potential while incorporating practices that speak more directly to the depth of our nature. The spiritual disciplines can incorporate insights and skills about human development, healing, and growth to deal more skillfully with the psychological issues that arise with spiritual devel-opment in many cultures.

Spirituality is another culturally relevant coping factor for African Ameri-cans. Faith-based institutions are a source of spirituality that represent a primary basis of support for African Americans. However, transpersonal theory continues to be underexplored. Culturally relevant research and practice continue to be a challenge to all helping professionals. Transpersonal psychology requires us to challenge our culturally defined views of mental health and psychotherapy and to draw cross-cultural insights into its practices and applications. African American culture is rich with religious and spiritual traditions and practices; however, research has been limited.

Competent psychotherapeutic practice requires that we acknowledge the variety of ways to connect with client systems (Barker, 2007). Transpersonal psychology values some dimensions of diversity, including race, culture, gender, age, sexual preference, social class, and biodiversity; however, more research is needed. Effective psychotherapeutic practice cannot ignore the diversity of spiritual and religious paradigms represented in the African American community, in the United States, and in the world.

## REFERENCES

Addams, M. V. (2002). African American dreaming and the beast of racism: The cultural unconscious in Jungian analysis. *Psychoanalysis and Psychology, 19*(1), 182–198.

ya Azibo, D. A. (1996). Personality, clinical, and social psychological research on Blacks: Appropriate research frameworks. In D. A. ya Azibo (Ed.), *African psychology in historical perspective and related commentary* (pp. 203–234). Trenton, NJ: Africa World Press.

Bandura, A. (1977). *Social learning theory*. Englewood Cliffs, NJ: Prentice Hall.

Barker, S. (2007). The integration of spirituality and religion content in social work education: Where we've been, Where we're going. *Social Work and Christianity, 34*(2), 146–166.

Boykin, A. W., & Toms, F. D. (1985). Black child socialization: A conceptualization, framework. In H. P. McAdoo & J. L. McAdoo (Eds.), *Black children: Social, educational, and parental environments* (pp. 33–52). Beverly Hills, CA: Sage.

Brown, R. (1965). *Social psychology*. New York: Free Press.

Budge, E. A. (1994). *Legends of the Egyptian Gods: Hieroglyphic texts and translations*. New York: Dover.

Burke, M., Chawin, J., & Miranti, J. (2005). *Religious and spiritual issues in counseling: Applications across diverse populations*. New York: Brunner-Rouledge.

Bynum, E. B. (1999). *The African unconscious: Roots of ancient mysticism and modern psychology*. New York: Teachers College Press.

Cheek, D. (1976). *Assertive Black ... puzzled White*. San Luis Obispo, CA: Impact.

Chein, I. (1972). *The science of behavior and the image of man*. New York: Basic Books.

Davis, J. (2000). We keep asking ourselves, what is transpersonal psychology? *Guidance and Counseling, 15*(3), 3–8.

Freud, A. (1966). *The writings of Anna Freud: Introduction to psychoanalysis: Lectures for child analysts and teachers, 1922–1935, Vol. 1*. New York: International Universities Press.

Freud, S. (1939). *Moses and monotheism*. New York: Vintage Books.

Gambrill, E. (1994). Concepts and methods of behavioral treatment. In D. K. Granvold

(Ed.), *Cognitive and behavioral treatment: Methods and applications* (pp. 32–62). Pacific Grove, CA: Brooks/Cole.

Gay, P. (1988). *Freud: A life for our times.* New York: Norton.

Granvold, D. (Ed.). (1994). *Cognitive and behavioral treatment: Methods and applications.* Pacific Grove, CA: Brooks/Cole.

Hartman, D., & Zimberoff, D. (2004). Corrective emotional experience in the therapeutic process. *Journal of Heart Centered Therapies, 7*(2), 3–84.

Hill, M. O. (1997). C. G. Jung in the heart of darkness. *Spring Journal, 61,* 125–133.

Ivey, A., Andrea, M., Ivey, M., & Simek-Morgan, L. (2002). *Theories of counseling and psychotherapy: A multicultural perspective* (5th ed.). Boston: Pearson.

James, W. (1929). *Varieties of religious experience.* New York: Random House.

Jenkins, A. (2001). Humanistic psychology and multiculturalism: A review and reflection. In J. F. T. Bugental, J. Pierson, & K. Schneider (Eds.), *The handbook of humanistic psychology: Leading edges in theory, research, and practice* (pp. 11–24). Thousand Oaks, CA: Sage.

Jourard, S. M. (1961). Sex in marriage. *Journal of Humanistic Psychology, 27*(1), 23–29.

Jung, C. G. (1938). *Psychology and religion.* New Haven, CT: Yale University Press.

Kambon, K. K. (1992). *The African personality in America: An African-centered framework.* Tallahassee, FL: NUBIAN Nation.

Kantrowitz, R., & Ballou, M. (1992). A feminist critique of cognitive-behavior behavioral therapy. In L. S. Brown & M. Ballou (Eds.), *Personality and psychopathology: Feminist reappraisals* (pp. 70–87). New York: Guilford Press.

Karenga, M. (1990). *The book of coming forth by day: The ethics of the declarations of innocence.* Los Angeles: University of Sankore Press.

Kasprow, M., & Scotton, B. (1999). A review of transpersonal theory and its application to the practice of psychotherapy. *Journal of Psychotherapy Practice and Research, 8,* 12–23.

Kazdin, A. E. (2001). *Behavior modification in applied settings* (6th ed.). Pacific Groves, CA: Brooks/Cole.

King, R. (2001). *Melanin: A key to freedom.* Chicago.: Lushena Books,.

Leary, J. D. (2005). *Post traumatic slave syndrome: America's legacy of enduring injury and healing.* Milwaukie, OR: Uptone Press.

Maslow, A. H. (1967). A theory of metamotivation: The biological rooting of the value-life. *Journal of Humanistic Psychology, 27*(2), 93–127.

Maslow, A. H. (1971). *The farther reaches of human nature.* New York: Viking Compass.

May, R. (1965). Relation of existential to humanistic psychology. *American Association for Humanistic Psychology Newsletter, 3*(2), 5–6.

Moustakas, C. (1962). Honesty, idiocy, and manipulation. *Journal of Humanistic Psychology, 23*(3), 1–15.

Myers, L. (1988). *Understanding an Afro-centric world view: Introduction to an optimal psychology.* Dubuque, IA: Kentall/Hunt.

Nobles, W. W. (1973). Psychological research and the Black self-concept: A critical review. *Journal of Social Issues, 29*(1), 11–31.

Pasteur, A. B., & Toldson, I. L. (1982). *Roots of soul: The psychology of Black expressiveness.* Garden City, NY: Anchor Press/Doubleday.

Perls, F. S. (1973). *The gestalt approach and eye witness to therapy.* Palo Alto, CA: Science & Behavior Books.

Prochaska, J. O., & Norcross, J. C. (2007). *Systems of psychotherapy: A transtheoretical analysis* (6th ed.). Belmont, CA: Thomson/Brooks/Cole.

Rickman, J. (Ed.). (1957). *A general selection from the works of Sigmund Freud*. New York: Liveright.

Sampson, E. E. (1988). The debate on individualism: Indigenous psychologies of the individual and their role in personal and social functioning. *American Psychologist, 43,* 15–22.

Skinner, B. F. (1938). *The behavior of organisms*. New York: Appleton-Century.

Skinner, B. F. (1976). *About behaviorism*. New York: Vintage.

Sutich, A. J. (1949). The growth-experience and the growth-centered attitude. *Journal of Psychology, 28*(3), 293–301.

Washburn, M. (1995). *The ego and the dynamic ground: A transpersonal theory of human development* (2nd ed., rev.). Albany, NY: State University of New York Press.

Weisz, J. R., Hawley, K., & Doss, A. (2004). Empirically tested psychotherapies for youth internalizing and externalizing problems and disorders. *Child and Adolescent Psychiatric Clinics of North America, 13,* 729–815.

Wilber, K. (1984). The developmental spectrum and psychopathology: Treatment modalities. *Journal of Transpersonal Psychology, 16,* 137–166.

Wilson, G. T. (2000). Behavior therapy. In R. J. Corsini & D. Wedding (Eds.), *Current psychotherapies* (6th ed., pp. 205–240). Itasca, IL: Peacock.

Winthrop, H. (1962). Humanistic psychology and intentional community. *Journal of Humanistic Psychology, 23*(3), 42–55.

# 7

## Pharmacotherapy in African Americans

### David C. Henderson

Race and ethnicity have a significant impact on psychiatric diagnosis and treatment. Moreover, treatment approaches and responses as well as prognosis are often different for disparate diagnoses. Historically, few minority populations have been included in large clinical trials, or analysis was not performed to understand similarities and differences between groups for major psychiatric illnesses such as depression, schizophrenia, bipolar disorder, or even attention-deficit/hyperactivity disorder (Corbie-Smith, St. George, Moody-Ayers, & Ransohoff, 2003; Lawson, 1986; Mark, Palmer, Russo, & Vasey, 2003). As a result, effective treatment approaches for White populations have been applied to minority populations with little evidence of effectiveness, safety, and tolerability.

A growing body of evidence suggests that many ethnic groups may differ in the rates at which certain medications are metabolized, which may impact safety, tolerability, and efficacy. Data suggest that genetic polymorphism variability for the cytochrome P450 (CYP450) enzymes may play a key role. In the future, genetics testing may allow for a better understanding of individual patients' rates of metabolism at various P450 enzymes, which will impact choice of medication and dosing.

## NONBIOLOGICAL FACTORS

Although there is a tremendous overlap of symptoms (e.g., aggression, agitation, anxiety, mood swings, psychotic thinking, anger, impulsivity) among schizophrenia, bipolar disorder, major depression, posttraumatic stress disorder, and intermittent explosive disorder, the diagnosis depends heavily on clinicians' interpretation of symptoms. For patients, there may be real differences in symptom expression; for example, protective wariness, common in different ethnic groups as well as immigrant populations, may be interpreted as paranoia (Adebimpe, 1981; Adebimpe, Klein, & Fried, 1981; Neighbors, Jackson, Campbell, & Williams, 1989; Strakowski et al., 1996). In addition, African Americans may seek medical or psychiatric attention later in the course of their illness and present with a more severe illness and worse prognosis.

Cultural differences allow psychiatric illnesses to present in a variety of ways. Performing a cross-cultural evaluation of the meanings of bizarre delusions, hallucinations, and psychotic-like symptoms remains a clinical challenge. An adequate understanding of a patient's sociocultural and religious background is required to determine whether symptoms are bizarre enough to yield a diagnosis of schizophrenia.

In addition to the potential biological differences, a number of nonbiological factors also influence drug metabolism, response, safety, and tolerability that require attention (see Figure 7.1). Factors such as language issues, communication styles (paucity of speech and content, poor eye contact), differences in cultural beliefs, and expectations may have a significant impact on the clinical encounter and affect outcome. Physician, clinician, and institutional biases should not be underestimated in this context and may affect a number of areas, including eliciting and interpreting symptoms, psychiatric diagnosis, and treatment recommendations (type of psychotherapy, if at all, and choice of psychotropic medications).

In the context of medical practice in the United States, patients from certain ethnic groups are often misdiagnosed, which leads to poor treatment outcomes. For instance, African American patients with affective disorders (major depression with psychosis, bipolar disorder) are more likely to be misdiagnosed as having schizophrenia because of biases in the health care system and the individual clinician (DelBello, Lopez-Larson, Soutullo, & Strakowski, 2001; Strakowski et al., 1996, 2003). Additionally, certain groups and communities, including African Americans, may have a tremendous mistrust of the health care system, frequently causing patients to procrastinate seeking attention and thus presenting with more severe, late-stage illnesses (Skeate, Jackson, Birchwood, & Jones, 2002).

Poor treatment adherence is one of the most frequent reasons for lack of response or for relapse in many psychiatric disorders. Adherence may be affected by a number of factors, including medication side effects, incorrect dosing, poor therapeutic alliance, shame regarding the need for medication to treat a mental problem, concern about potential medication addiction, lack of money or resources, and substance abuse. Additionally, it may be difficult for patients to inform their clinicians that they did not comply with the recommendations. Clinicians must provide a clear, understandable explanation of treatment and medication expectations to improve adherence rates.

- Psychiatric misdiagnosis
- Mistrust of the health care system (seek attention at later stage of illness)
- Difference in cultural beliefs and expectations (perception of illness and its treatment)
- Traditional and alternative healing (herbal medicines, traditional healers)
- Adherence (affected by side effects, incorrect dosing, poor therapeutic alliance, shame, lack of community support, lack of financial resources, substance abuse)
- Social support systems
- Language issues
- Communication styles
- Physician, clinician, and institutional biases
- Clinicians do not explain psychotropic medications to patients (what to expect, how long treatment needed, addictiveness of medications)

**FIGURE 7.1.** Nonbiological factors that have an impact on the effectiveness and safety of psychotropic medications.

Attention to the specificity of questions asked will improve response accuracy. Asking more detailed questions such as "Are you taking the medication every day?", "What time of day do you take the medication and how many pills do you take?", and "What color are the pills?" should allow a more accurate assessment of adherence. It is common for patients to take the medication differently from the way it was prescribed. More specific questions will allow for a more accurate report on compliance.

## ETHNOPSYCHOPHARMACOLOGY

A systematic approach that incorporates ethnopharmacological principles will allow for appropriate individual care. During the assessment of a patient's symptoms, it is important to consider the patient's own beliefs, expectations, and history of help-seeking behaviors as well as the nature of the support system and the use of "alternative" treatments (including herbal medicines) and healing methods. The choice of medications to treat a psychiatric disorder is based on the patient's medical history, concurrent medications, use of diet and food supplements or herbal medicines, and previous experience with psychotropic medications. Medications must be explained to patients and incorporated into their worldview. Taking a few minutes to address common side effects, expectations, and length of treatment will improve compliance and outcomes. The patient and family (when appropriate) should be involved in all treatment decisions.

## PHARMACOLOGY

Pharmacokinetics determines steady-state concentrations of drugs and their metabolites. Pharmacokinetics of medications deal with metabolism, blood levels, absorption, distribution, and excretion. However, other pharmacokinetic variables (e.g., conjugation, plasma protein binding, and oxidation by the CYP isoenzymes) exist. The activity of liver enzymes is controlled genetically, although environmental factors can alter activity. Understanding how pharmacokinetics and environmental factors relate to different populations will help to predict side effects, blood levels, and potential drug–drug interactions. Pharmacokinetics may be influenced by a number of factors (e.g., genetics, age, gender, total body weight, environment, diet, toxins, drug use and alcohol, and other disease states). Environmental factors include use of medications, drugs, herbal medicines, steroids, caffeine, alcohol, constituents of tobacco, dietary factors, as well as sex hormones.

## Cytochrome P450

Most medications are metabolized in two phases. Phase I primarily involves oxidation and is mediated through CYP450 enzymes. Phase II enzymes are transferases and allow endogenous substances to conjugate with drugs and their metabolites. There are a number of CYP450 isoenzymes that are involved with the metabolism of psychotropic drugs. Some of the P450 enzymes are inducible (CYP3A4); some psychotropic agents, such as carbamazepine and St. John's wort, may increase the activity level of such enzymes; and grapefruit juice may inhibit this enzyme. Understanding the CYP450 system will allow for predictions of potential drug interactions and side effects based on known demographic factors for individual patients.

### CYP2D6

The CYP450 enzyme 2D6 (debrisoquine hydroxylase) is an important step in the metabolic pathway for many medications and is often responsible for drug–drug interactions. It is a low-capacity enzyme with high affinity (more easily saturated) and is highly polymorphic. CYP2D6 metabolizes many antidepressants, including the tricyclic (TCAs) and heterocyclic antidepressants and the selective serotonin reuptake inhibitors (SSRIs). CYP2D6 also plays a role in metabolizing antipsychotics, including clozapine, haloperidol, perphenazine, risperidone, aripiprazole, thioridazine, and sertindole.

Individuals can be classified as poor metabolizers, intermediate or slow metabolizers, extensive metabolizers, and ultra-rapid metabolizers (Dahl, Johansson, Bertilsson, Ingelman-Sundberg, & Sjoqvist, 1995; Dahl, Yue, et al., 1995; Leathart, et al., 1998).

Rates of CYP2D6 vary among the world's populations, poor metabolization from 0.5 to 2.4% in Asian populations, 3 to 7.3% in Caucasians, 3.1% in Mexican Americans, 3.6% in Nicaraguans, and 1.9% in Tanzanians. The rates for African Americans and Blacks have been found to range from 2 to 8% (Bradford, 2002; Bradford, Gaedigk, & Leeder, 1998; Gaedigk, Bradford, Marcucci, & Leeder,

2002; Gaedigk, Ndjountche, Gaedigk, Leeder, & Bradford, 2003; Gaedigk, Ryder, Bradford, & Leeder, 2003). CYP2D6*4 (CYP2D6B) appears to be responsible for poor metabolization among Caucasians. CYP2D6*17 and CYP2D6*10 are found in individuals of African and Asian origin, respectively, and are responsible for lower enzyme (intermediate or slow metabolizers) (Dahl, Johansson, et al., 1995; Dahl, Yue, et al., 1995; Leathart et al., 1998; Lin, 1996; Lin, Poland, Wan, Smith, & Lesser, 1996). One study found CYP 2D6*17 in 33% of African Americans and a reduced capacity to metabolize dextromethorphan, a CYP2D6 probe drug (Bradford, 2002; Bradford et al., 1998) Additionally, approximately 33–37% of Asians are considered slow metabolizers compared with 34% of Nicaraguans (Agundez, Ramirez, Hernandez, Llerena, & Benitez, 1997; Dahl, Yue, et al., 1995). The potential for adverse events is quite high, because numerous drugs are metabolized through the P450 2D6 enzymes system, including TCAs (imipramine), SSRIs (fluoxetine, paroxetine), venlafaxine, nefazodone, beta-blockers, codeine, and antipsychotic agents (haloperidol, risperidone, perphenazine, thioridazine, sertindole, clozapine). Poor and slow metabolizers at the 2D6 appear to have higher rates of extrapyramidal symptoms and tardive dyskinesia from antipsychotic agents, higher risk of venlafaxine cardiovascular toxicity, and longer psychiatric hospitalizations (Chou et al., 2000; Reggiani et al., 2000; Zabrocka, Woszczek, Borowiec, Rabe-Jablonska, & Kowalski, 1999).

Another category for 2D6 metabolism is the "superextensive metabolizers or ultrarapid metabolizers." High rates of this category are seen with Ethiopians (29%), Saudi Arabians (19%), and Spaniards (10%), whereas Europeans (1%) and American Caucasians (3.5%) have relatively low rates. Superextensive metabolizers are often resistant to standard pharmacotherapy, have frequent psychiatric hospitalizations because of the poor response, are at greater risk of opiate addiction, and are more likely to be considered poorly compliant because blood levels of psychotropic medications are often very low at therapeutic doses (Chou et al., 2000; Reggiani et al., 2000; Zabrocka et al., 1999).

### CYP2C9

The CYP2C9 isoenzyme is involved in the metabolism of ibuprofen, naproxen, phenytoin, warfarin, and tolbutamide. Approximately 18–22% of Asians and African Americans are poor metabolizers of these drugs (Kidd et al., 2001; Ozawa et al., 1999; Shu et al., 2001; Tabrizi et al., 2002). Poor metabolizers at this enzyme system are at high risk for toxic effects of potentially dangerous drugs such as phenytoin and warfarin.

### CYP2C19

CYP2C19 is involved in the metabolism of diazepam, barbiturates, citalopram, clomipramine, imipramine, diazepam, mephenytoin, and propranolol; it is inhibited by fluoxetine and sertraline. The rates of poor metabolizers of this enzyme are approximately 3–6% in Caucasians, 4–18% in African Americans, and 18–23% in Asians (Masimirembwa, Bertilsson, Johansson, Hasler, & Ingelman-Sundberg, 1995). Another important enzyme is the CYP2C19, of which approximately 13–23% of East Asians (Chinese, Japanese, and Koreans) are poor metabolizers, compared with 3–5% of Whites, 4% of African Americans, and 19% of older African Americans (Pollock et al., 1991). Drugs metabolized through this enzyme system include diazepam, imipramine, amitriptyline, clomipramine, citalopram, sertraline, propranolol, and omeprazole.

## CYP3A4

Although ethnic or racial differences in metabolism at the 3A enzyme system have not been fully evaluated (Chowbay, Cumaraswamy, Cheung, Zhou, & Lee, 2003; Hsieh et al., 2001), a number of substances have been found to either inhibit or induce this enzyme, including medications such as fluoxetine, fluvoxamine, nefazodone, norfluoxetine, clozapine, haloperidol, diltiazem, verapamil, gestodene, erythromycin, itraconazole, ketoconazole, and ritonavir. Grapefruit juice and corn have also been found to inhibit this enzyme system. This is clinically relevant because there are populations that consume corn as a regular part of their diet, including some Asian groups, Mexicans, and Mexican Americans. Many years ago, the popular grapefruit juice diet led to many U.S. patients having side effects with medications that were previously well tolerated.

Additionally, there is a CYP3A4 G variant that is more common among African American men compared with White men. Among African American men, the GG (odds ratio, 11.9) and AG (odds ratio, 9.3) genotype was associated with a risk of aggressive prostate cancer (Bangsi et al., 2006).

### Use of Herbal Medications

Even more complicated is the widespread use of herbal medicines. African Americans may prefer herbal or "natural" medicines to artificial or synthetic medications. Herbal medicines pose significant dangers because most have not been well studied, so little is known regarding potential drug interactions. However, numerous case reports are emerging in the literature. Even common herbal products containing licorice have been found to induce P450 1A2, leading to decreased blood levels of theophylline, digoxin, amitriptyline, and phenytoin.

## IMPACT OF PSYCHOTROPIC MEDICATIONS ON AFRICAN AMERICANS

### Antidepressants

Overall, the trend in underdiagnosing depression in different ethnic populations as well in underprescribing SSRIs (in favor of TCAs) in African Americans and

Hispanic patients continues (Melfi, Croghan, Hanna, & Robinson, 2000). There are few studies examining the safety and effectiveness of SSRIs in different ethnic groups. Tsoi, Tan, and Kok (1995) reported a study of 19 Asian (Chinese and Indian) patients who satisfied the *Diagnostic and Statistical Manual of Mental Disorders* (third edition, revised; American Psychiatric Association, 1987) criteria for major depressive episode were treated with fluoxetine, 20 mg daily for 12 weeks. There was significant improvement in depressive symptoms and no serious side effects, changes in weight, temperature, blood pressure, and pulse rate throughout the 12 weeks. However, one study (Strickland, Stein, Lin, Risby, & Fong, 1997) reported significant adverse events in African American women taking 20 mg of paroxetine or fluoxetine and found a lower therapeutic dose compared with White subjects. African American patients have also been found to respond faster to TCAs and at lower doses, while also experiencing neurotoxicity at higher rates (Livingston, Zucker, Isenberg, & Wetzel, 1983). Patients who are poor or slow metabolizers via the CYP2D6 system will exhibit higher blood levels and require lower doses of TCAs and SSRI antidepressants.

## Lithium

Lithium also is a drug that must be used with additional caution in certain populations. It has a narrow therapeutic window and the consequences of toxicity can be severe, including central nervous system effects and renal toxicity. Lithium can be fatal in overdose secondary to renal toxicity. Long-term use also may lead to renal insufficiency or renal failure. African Americans have a greater risk of neurotoxicity from lithium, a fact that is greatly underrecognized. African Americans' sodium–lithium countertransport activity (millimeters of lithium per red blood cell) is significantly lower compared with that of White, South Asian, and Chinese patients (Hardman, Croft, Morrish, Anto-Awoakye, & Lant, 1998; Strickland, Lin, Fu, Anderson, & Zheng, 1995). Caution must be used when treating African Americans with lithium, including awareness of potential drug interactions with antihypertensive agents such as diuretics, which are commonly prescribed for this population.

## Antipsychotic Agents

Many antipsychotic agents are metabolized, in part, through the CYP2D6 system. Evidence from differences in CYP450 enzyme activity suggests that Asian and African American patients should receive lower doses of many antipsychotic agents (Lin, 1996; Lin et al., 1989, 1996). However, African Americans routinely receive higher doses, are more likely to receive depot injections, experience higher rates of involuntary psychiatric hospitalizations, and have significantly higher rates of seclusion-restraint application while in psychiatric hospitals (Jeste, Lindamer, Evans, & Lacro, 1996) compared with Whites in the United States (Diaz & De Leon, 2002; Walkup et al., 2000). DelBello and colleagues (2001) also found that African American adolescents with bipolar disorder were nearly twice as likely to receive antipsychotic agents (86% vs. 45%). The biases of the health care system are clearly evident.

Additionally, many African Americans have a significantly lower baseline White blood cell count (benign neutropenia) than non–African Americans. This may prevent trials or cause early discontinuation of clozapine in this population, although the risk of agranulocytosis appears to be the same as for other populations (Moeller et al., 1995). Asians are likely to experience the most extrapyramidal side effects, followed by African Americans (Lin et al., 1989).

The newer atypical antipsychotic agents offer some promise because they are associated with fewer extrapyramidal side effects. However, some of these agents appear to impair glucose metabolism by causing insulin resistance (unrelated to weight gain), cause significant weight gain, and are associated with hyperlipidemia (Henderson, Cagliero, et al., 2005). Of greatest concern is the onset of diabetic ketoacidosis after initiating one of these agents, as reported in numerous studies in the literature. Of note, many of the patients were African American, a group at greater baseline risk for diabetes. In populations with higher rates of obesity, Type 2 diabetes mellitus, and cardiovascular disease (such as African Americans, Hispanics, Asians, and Native Americans), the use of atypical antipsychotics may even increase the risk for development of these disorders. In fact, in one longitudinal study in clozapine-treated patients, African American and Hispanic patients had a dramatically elevated hazard ratio, compared with White patients, for both new-onset diabetes mellitus and death from myocardial infarction (Henderson, Nguyen, et al., 2005). Although there appears to be a spectrum of effect, care should be taken when prescribing these medications in populations at high risk for diabetes mellitus, obesity, and cardiovascular disease.

## CASE EXAMPLE

Ms. Z., a 49-year-old African American woman with a 3-year history of multiple psychiatric hospitalizations for major depression with psychotic features, was referred for consultation and potential treatment. The reason for the multiple hospitalizations was determined to be poor compliance with psychotropic medications. During the past 3 years and as a result of her recurrent episode, she experienced multiple job losses (as a health care professional) as well as severed relationships with family and friends. She explained that the medications that she received, although effective, had intolerable side effects. So she would stop them once she felt better or was out of the hospital. Her condition would then deteriorate to a full relapse requiring hospitalization several weeks later. Upon further questioning, it appeared that each drug (fluoxetine, duloxetine, venlafaxine, paroxetine, and perphenazine, and risperidone) she was prescribed (repeatedly) was metabolized through the CYP2D6. Her clinician suspected that Ms. Z. was a slow metabolizer at the CYP2D6 and changed her medication to an antidepressant (bupropion XL) that is not extensively metabolized through the CYP2D6 enzyme. The dose was titrated to 300 mg/day, and Ms. Z. experienced complete remission from her depression (with minimum side effects), remained episode free (and hospitalization free), and has been consistently employed full time for more than 24 months.

## CONCLUSIONS

A systematic approach that incorporates ethnopharmacological principles will allow for appropriate individual care for African Americans (see Figure 7.2):

• During the assessment of symptoms, it is important to consider patients' beliefs and understanding of their problems as well as expectations of treatment. It is critical that health care providers understand the role of shame and stigma and how it will impact not only patients' engagement with the health care system but also their utilization of services and support within their community.

• Patients' history of help-seeking behaviors should be assessed, which will allow targeted interventions. Understanding their support system, including family, friends, and religious organizations, will help patients to best utilize potential strengths as they work to resolve their psychiatric problems.

### Assessment
• Conduct a diagnostic evaluation regardless of previous diagnosis (structured may be beneficial).
• Use a cultural formulation for diagnosis: careful elicitation of beliefs, expectations, history of help seeking, nature of the support system, use of "alternative" treatment and healing methods.

### Choice of Medication
• Take a complete medical history, including concurrent medications, diet, and food supplements/herbs.
• Be aware of potential differences in drug metabolism.
• Choose a medication with a safer side-effect profile for the individual patient.
• Involve the patient and family in treatment decisions.
• Inform the patient about side effects and when he or she should expect to respond.
• Educate the patient about the illness and length of treatment.

### Patient Monitoring
• Start at a lower dose and titrate the medication slowly.
• Increase gradually as tolerated.
• Involve family if appropriate.
• If side effects are intolerable, lower dose or choose drug metabolized through a different route.
• If no response, check compliance, raise dose, monitor levels, add inhibitors, switch medications, or augment with another medication when only a partial response has been achieved.

**FIGURE 7.2.** An ethnopharmacological approach to the care of African American patients. This approach takes into account the patients' personal and cultural history and potential genetic variation that affects medication metabolism.

• Patients should always be asked about the use of "alternative" treatments (including herbal medicines) and healing methods, and their use must be assessed based on the treatment plan with psychotropic medications. Herbal medications and supplements do not always have to be discontinued; however, they should be used cautiously when combined with psychotropic medications. In general, a search within the medical literature and the Internet is important to gain information regarding potential herbal medication–psychotic drug interactions.

• The choice of medications to treat a psychiatric disorder is based on the patients' medical history, concurrent medications, use of diet and food supplements or herbal medicines, and previous experience with psychotropic medications. Medications must be explained to patients and incorporated into their "worldview." Taking a few minutes to address common side effects, expectations, and length of treatment will improve compliance and outcomes. Patients and family members (when appropriate) should be involved in all treatment decisions.

• To reduce the risk of adverse events, start psychotropic medication at a low dose and gradually increase toward the therapeutic range as tolerated. Some (but not all) patients will metabolize psychotropic medications at slower rates, thereby experiencing side effects at unexpected doses. Maintaining a simple medication regimen—and when possible a once-a-day dosing— will help to improve adherence. The use of multiple psychotropic drugs increases the potential for drug interactions, confusion, and adverse events and is indicated only when the beneficial effects outweigh these risks.

• Understanding these differences across populations as well as how particular agents are metabolized may allow clinicians to correctly prescribe lower doses for an individual patient or to switch to another agent that is metabolized through a different route or enzyme system.

• Future research and direction should focus on the inclusion of African Americans in clinical trials to best understand dosing, efficacy, safety, and tolerability of psychotropic medications. New drugs that are approved by the U.S. Food and Drug Administration should be adequately studied in African Americans before being marketed. Studies should measure blood levels of the medications and conduct a genetic analysis of P450 enzymes to determine the best and safest dose for psychotropic medications in African Americans.

• Genetic testing for P450 enzymes is currently available; however, it remains too expensive for clinical use. Over the next 10 years, it is likely that genetic screening of P450 enzyme activity will be routine and allow clinicians to appropriately dose medications based on the enzyme that metabolizes it as well as patients' own genetically determined activity level.

• The general recommendation is to start psychotropic medications at lower doses than what is recommended and increase slowly, watching for efficacy as well side effects. This approach may significantly reduce adverse events and improve adherence.

## REFERENCES

Adebimpe, V. R. (1981). Overview: White norms and psychiatric diagnosis of Black patients. *American Journal of Psychiatry, 138*(3), 279–285.

Adebimpe, V. R., Klein, H. E., & Fried, J. (1981). Hallucinations and delusions in Black psychiatric patients. *Journal of the National Medical Association, 73*(6), 517–520.

Agundez, J. A., Ramirez, R., Hernandez, M., Llerena, A., & Benitez, J. (1997). Molecular heterogeneity at the CYP2D gene locus in Nicaraguans: Impact of gene-flow from Europe. *Pharmacogenetics, 7*(4), 337–340.

American Psychiatric Association. (1987). *Diagnostic and statistical manual of mental disorders* (3rd., rev.). Washington, DC: Author.

Bangsi, D., Zhou, J., Sun, Y., Patel, N. P., Darga, L. L., Heilbrun, L. K., et al. (2006). Impact of a genetic variant in CYP3A4 on risk and clinical presentation of prostate cancer among White and African-American men. *Urology Oncology, 24*(1), 21–27.

Bradford, L. D. (2002). CYP2D6 allele frequency in European Caucasians, Asians, Africans and their descendants. *Pharmacogenomics, 3*(2), 229–243.

Bradford, L. D., Gaedigk, A., & Leeder, J. S. (1998). High frequency of CYP2D6 poor and "intermediate" metabolizers in Black populations: A review and preliminary data. *Psychopharmacology Bulletin, 34*(4), 797–804.

Chou, W. H., Yan, F. X., de Leon, J., Barnhill, J., Rogers, T., Cronin, M., et al. (2000). Extension of a pilot study: Impact from the cytochrome P450 2D6 polymorphism on outcome and costs associated with severe mental illness. *Journal of Clinical Psychopharmacology, 20*(2), 246–251.

Chowbay, B., Cumaraswamy, S., Cheung, Y. B., Zhou, Q., & Lee, E. J. (2003). Genetic polymorphisms in MDR1 and CYP3A4 genes in Asians and the influence of MDR1 haplotypes on cyclosporin disposition in heart transplant recipients. *Pharmacogenetics, 13*(2), 89–95.

Corbie-Smith, G., St. George, D. M., Moody-Ayers, S., & Ransohoff, D. F. (2003). Adequacy of reporting race/ethnicity in clinical trials in areas of health disparities. *Journal of Clinical Epidemiology, 56*(5), 416–420.

Dahl, M. L., Johansson, I., Bertilsson, L., Ingelman-Sundberg, M., & Sjoqvist, F. (1995). Ultrarapid hydroxylation of debrisoquine in a Swedish population. Analysis of the molecular genetic basis. *Journal of Pharmacology and Experimental Therapeutics, 274*(1), 516–520.

Dahl, M. L., Yue, Q. Y., Roh, H. K., Johansson, I., Sawe, J., Sjoqvist, F., et al. (1995). Genetic analysis of the CYP2D locus in relation to debrisoquine hydroxylation capacity in Korean, Japanese and Chinese subjects. *Pharmacogenetics, 5*(3), 159–164.

DelBello, M. P., Lopez-Larson, M. P., Soutullo, C. A., & Strakowski, S. M. (2001). Effects of race on psychiatric diagnosis of hospitalized adolescents: A retrospective chart review. *Journal of Child Adolescent Psychopharmacology, 11*(1), 95–103.

Diaz, F. J., & De Leon, J. (2002). Excessive antipsychotic dosing in 2 U.S. state hospitals. *Journal of Clinical Psychiatry, 63*(11), 998–1003.

Gaedigk, A., Bradford, L. D., Marcucci, K. A., & Leeder, J. S. (2002). Unique CYP2D6 activity distribution and genotype-phenotype discordance in Black Americans. *Clinical Pharmacology Therapeutics, 72*(1), 76–89.

Gaedigk, A., Ndjountche, L., Gaedigk, R., Leeder, J. S., & Bradford, L. D. (2003). Discovery of a novel nonfunctional cytochrome P450 2D6 allele, CYP2D642, in African American subjects. *Clinical Pharmacology Therapeutics, 73*(6), 575–576.

Gaedigk, A., Ryder, D. L., Bradford, L. D., & Leeder, J. S. (2003). CYP2D6 poor metabolizer status can be ruled out by a single genotyping assay for the -1584G promoter polymorphism. *Clinical Chemistry, 49*(6, Pt. 1), 1008–1011.

Hardman, T. C., Croft, P., Morrish, Z., Anto-Awoakye, K., & Lant, A. F. (1998). Kinetic characteristics of the erythrocyte sodium-lithium countertransporter in Black normotensive subjects compared with three other ethnic groups. *Journal of Human Hypertension, 12*(1), 29–34.

Henderson, D. C., Cagliero, E., Copeland, P. M., Borba, C. P., Evins, E., Hayden, D., et al. (2005). Glucose metabolism in patients with schizophrenia treated with atypical antipsychotic agents: A frequently sampled intravenous glucose tolerance test and minimal model analysis. *Archives of General Psychiatry, 62*(1), 19–28.

Henderson, D. C., Nguyen, D. D., Copeland, P. M., Hayden, D. L., Borba, C. P., Louie, P. M., et al. (2005). Clozapine, diabetes mellitus, hyperlipidemia, and cardiovascular risks and mortality: Results of a 10-year naturalistic study. *Journal of Clinical Psychiatry, 66*(9), 1116–1121.

Hsieh, K. P., Lin, Y. Y., Cheng, C. L., Lai, M. L., Lin, M. S., Siest, J. P., et al. (2001). Novel mutations of CYP3A4 in Chinese. *Drug Metabolism and Disposition, 29*(3), 268–273.

Jeste, D. V., Lindamer, L. A., Evans, J., & Lacro, J. P. (1996). Relationship of ethnicity and gender to schizophrenia and pharmacology of neuroleptics. *Psychopharmacology Bulletin, 32*(2), 243–251.

Kidd, R. S., Curry, T. B., Gallagher, S., Edeki, T., Blaisdell, J., & Goldstein, J. A. (2001). Identification of a null allele of CYP2C9 in an African-American exhibiting toxicity to phenytoin. *Pharmacogenetics, 11*(9), 803–808.

Lawson, W. B. (1986). Racial and ethnic factors in psychiatric research. *Hospital and Community Psychiatry, 37*(1), 50–54.

Leathart, J. B., London, S. J., Steward, A., Adams, J. D., Idle, J. R., & Daly, A. K. (1998). CYP2D6 phenotype–genotype relationships in African-Americans and Caucasians in Los Angeles. *Pharmacogenetics, 8*(6), 529–541.

Lin, K. M. (1996). Psychopharmacology in cross-cultural psychiatry. *Mount Sinai Journal of Medicine, 63*(5–6), 283–284.

Lin, K.-M., Poland, R. E., Nuccio, I., Matsuda, K., Hathuc, N., Su, T. P., et al. (1989). A longitudinal assessment of haloperidol doses and serum concentrations in Asian and Caucasian schizophrenic patients. *American Journal of Psychiatry, 146*, 1307–1311.

Lin, K. M., Poland, R. E., Wan, Y. J., Smith, M. W., & Lesser, I. M. (1996). The evolving science of pharmacogenetics: Clinical and ethnic perspectives. *Psychopharmacology Bulletin, 32*(2), 205–217.

Livingston, R. L., Zucker, D. K., Isenberg, K., & Wetzel, R. D. (1983). Tricyclic antidepressants and delirium. *Journal of Clinical Psychiatry, 44*(5), 173–176.

Mark, T. L., Palmer, L. A., Russo, P. A., & Vasey, J. (2003). Examination of treatment pattern differences by race. *Mental Health Services Research, 5*(4), 241–250.

Masimirembwa, C., Bertilsson, L., Johansson, I., Hasler, J. A., & Ingelman-Sundberg, M. (1995). Phenotyping and genotyping of S-mephenytoin hydroxylase (cytochrome P450 2C19) in a Shona population of Zimbabwe. *Clinical Pharmacology Therapeutics, 57*(6), 656–661.

Melfi, C. A., Croghan, T. W., Hanna, M. P., & Robinson, R. L. (2000). Racial variation in antidepressant treatment in a Medicaid population. *Journal of Clinical Psychiatry,* *61*(1), 16–21.

Moeller, F. G., Chen, Y. W., Steinberg, J. L., Petty, F., Ripper, G. W., Shah, N., et al. (1995). Risk factors for clozapine discontinuation among 805 patients in the VA hospital system. *Annals of Clinical Psychiatry, 7*(4), 167–173.

Neighbors, H. W., Jackson, J. S., Campbell, L., & Williams, D. (1989). The influence of racial factors on psychiatric diagnosis: A review and suggestions for research. *Community Mental Health Journal, 25*(4), 301–311.

Ozawa, S., Schoket, B., McDaniel, L. P., Tang, Y. M., Ambrosone, C. B., Kostic, S., et al. (1999). Analyses of bronchial bulky DNA adduct levels and CYP2C9, GSTP1 and NQO1 genotypes in a Hungarian study population with pulmonary diseases. *Carcinogenesis, 20*(6), 991–995.

Pollock, B. G., Perel, J. M., Kirshner, M., Altieri, L. P., Yeager, A. L., & Reynolds, C. F., III. (1991). S-mephenytoin 4-hydroxylation in older Americans. *European Journal of Clinical Pharmacology, 40*(6), 609–611.

Reggiani, K., Vandel, P., Haffen, E., Sechter, D., Bizouard, P., & Vandel, S. (2000). Secondaires extrapyramidaux effets de l'évaluation et la traitement neuroleptique antidépresseurs: Les facteurs de risque potentiels par le CYP2D6 polymorphisme génétique [Extrapyramidal side effects of neuroleptic and antidepressant treatment: Assessment of potential risk factors through CYP2D6 genetic polymorphism]. *Encephale, 26*(1), 62–67.

Shu, Y., Cheng, Z. N., Liu, Z. Q., Wang, L. S., Zhu, B., Huang, S. L., et al. (2001). Interindividual variations in levels and activities of cytochrome P-450 in liver microsomes of Chinese subjects. *Acta Pharmacologica Sinica, 22*(3), 283–288.

Skeate, A., Jackson, C., Birchwood, M., & Jones, C. (2002). Duration of untreated psychosis and pathways to care in first-episode psychosis. Investigation of help-seeking behaviour in primary care. *British Journal of Psychiatry Supplement, 43,* s73–s77.

Strakowski, S. M., Flaum, M., Amador, X., Bracha, H. S., Pandurangi, A. K., Robinson, D., et al. (1996). Racial differences in the diagnosis of psychosis. *Schizophrenia Research, 21*(2), 117–124.

Strakowski, S. M., Keck, P. E., Jr., Arnold, L. M., Collins, J., Wilson, R. M., Fleck, D. E., et al. (2003). Ethnicity and diagnosis in patients with affective disorders. *Journal of Clinical Psychiatry, 64*(7), 747–754.

Strickland, T. L., Lin, K. M., Fu, P., Anderson, D., & Zheng, Y. (1995). Comparison of lithium ratio between African-American and Caucasian bipolar patients. *Biological Psychiatry, 37*(5), 325–330.

Strickland, T. L., Stein, R., Lin, K. M., Risby, E., & Fong, R. (1997). The pharmacologic treatment of anxiety and depression in African Americans. Considerations for the general practitioner. *Archives of Family Medicine, 6*(4), 371–375.

Tabrizi, A. R., Zehnbauer, B. A., Borecki, I. B., McGrath, S. D., Buchman, T. G., & Freeman, B. D. (2002). The frequency and effects of cytochrome P450 (CYP) 2C9 polymorphisms in patients receiving warfarin. *Journal of American College Surgery, 194*(3), 267–273.

Tsoi, W. F., Tan, C. T., & Kok, L. P. (1995). Fluoxetine in the treatment of depression in Asian (Chinese and Indian) patients in Singapore. *Singapore Medical Journal, 36*(4), 397–399.

Walkup, J. T., McAlpine, D. D., Olfson, M., Labay, L. E., Boyer, C., & Hansell, S. (2000). Patients with schizophrenia at risk for excessive antipsychotic dosing. *Journal of Clinical Psychiatry, 61*(5), 344–348.

Zabrocka, M., Woszczek, G., Borowiec, M., Rabe-Jablonska, J., & Kowalski, M. L. (1999). [CYP2D6 gene polymorphism in psychiatric patients resistant to standard pharmacotherapy]. *Psychiatria Polska, 33*(1), 91–100.

# 8

# Engaging African Americans in Outpatient Mental Health Interventions

REGINALD SIMMONS
GRETCHEN CHASE VAUGHN

**H**istorically, most African Americans[1] in the United States have survived—and even thrived—despite the emotional and behavioral vestiges of slavery, racial segregation, discrimination, and lack of access to services through sheer determination and perseverance. The often-repeated African American folk saying "make a way out of no way" was both a badge of honor and a hymn of resignation in response to countless obstacles. This legacy in the African American community leaves the notion of seeking help for emotional and behavioral issues a culturally unfamiliar, if not taboo, concept to many. Engagement, then, becomes a key issue when providing behavioral health treatment for African Americans and other ethnic minority groups. The literature suggests that culture and race impact every aspect of the process of treatment engagement (Davey & Watson, 2008; Sue & Chu, 2003).

---

[1]We use an inclusive racial–ethnic–cultural definition of the term *African American* to encompass individuals who are the direct descendents of slaves brought involuntarily to the United States as well as Blacks who came to this country as immigrants or refugees largely from Africa, the Caribbean, and so on. We recognize, however, that much of the published literature does not distinguish between subgroups of African Americans in the United States, so caution should be used when generalizing to any specific subgroup.

# PROBLEM RECOGNITION

## Externally Assessed Need/Prevalence of Mental Illness

In the United States, it is estimated that approximately 30% of Americans are in need of mental health services (Messias, Eaton, Nestadt, Bienvenu, & Samuels, 2007). Researchers have studied ethnic differences in mental health prevalence rates for the past three decades. U.S. epidemiological studies in the late 1980s and 1990s such as the Epidemiologic Catchment Area Study (ECA) and the National Comorbidity Survey (NCS) resulted in mixed findings, leading researchers to conclude that the rates of mental health problems are similar for Blacks and Whites after controlling for socioeconomic differences (U.S. Department of Health and Human Services [USDHHS], 2001). The prevalence data from later studies indicated that African Americans had lower rates of mental health disorders (Sue & Chu, 2003). Only prevalence rates for some specific mental illnesses or symptoms (such as lifetime incidence of phobias/dysthymic disorders or somatization of physical illness) have been found to be higher for African Americans (Snowden, 2001; USDHHS, 2001). These findings of equivalent or lower prevalence of behavioral health disorders in the African American community are surprising given the high percentage of African Americans who fall into high-risk, high-need groups such as those who are poor, homeless, uninsured, incarcerated, exposed to violence, and so on (USDHHS, 2001). In the most recently published report from the secretary of Health and Human Services (National Center for Health Statistics, 2007), the percentage of Blacks or African American adults who experienced some psychological distress in the past 30 days was 3.5% in 2001–2002, 3.4% in 2003–2004, and 3.7% in 2005–2006. The paradox is that, despite similar or lower prevalence rates, the impact of mental illness on African Americans appears to be more severe or disabling, particularly when combined with low socioeconomic status (USDHHS, 1999). However, authors of these large-scale national surveys acknowledge that lifetime and projected risk estimates are likely to be conservative because of biases that include underreporting behaviors as a result of stigma, exclusion of institutionalized or marginal populations (psychiatric patients, incarcerated and homeless persons), as well as inaccuracies of self-report and recollection (Kessler et al., 2005). It is reasonable to conclude that many segments of the African American population in the United States, particularly African American males and immigrants, are underrepresented or absent from census data and household surveys. This noninclusion of African American subpopulations and lack of relevant cultural context in epidemiological studies and diagnostic assessments developed to externally assess need ultimately result in misdiagnosis and missed opportunities for treatment. Understanding the underlying cultural and contextual issues and assumptions that impact African Americans is fundamental to understanding both externally assessed and internally perceived need and why the recognition of mental health problems is so complex.

## Internally Perceived Need

"Help seeking is most likely to occur when a mental health problem is recognized as undesirable and when it is deemed not apt to go away on its own" (Cauce et al., 2002, p. 459). The perception of the severity of one's mental health problems is an intrinsically subjective issue compounded by the additional dimension of perception of need based on cultural beliefs/norms. African Americans frequently underestimate the impact of mental health problems. Symptoms are often labeled "the blues" or "nerves." Cultural norms and beliefs about the reasons for symptoms may lead African Americans to attribute the problem to physical rather than psychological causes. Even when a mental health problem is recognized as urgent, African Americans may take an activist stance, labeled "John Henryism" by James, LaCroix, Kelimbaum, and Strogatz (1984), which is the belief that problems can be dealt with through heroic striving and hard work, "picking up oneself up by the bootstraps" (Bonham, Sellers, & Neighbors, 2004). There is also the belief that the need to seek therapy results in "weakness" and "diminished pride" (Thompson, Bazile, & Akbar, 2004). Some families and cultures are less distressed by or have other explanations (spiritual, environmental) for certain mental health symptoms and may take longer to perceive the need for outside help (Cauce et al., 2002).

## CONTEXT: SYSTEMS IMPACT ON ACCESS AND QUALITY OF SERVICES

Overall, only one-third of the general population in need of mental health services receives it; however, the percentage of African Americans who receive treatment is half that of Whites (Davey & Watson, 2008; Diala et al., 2000; USDHHS, 2001). Health disparities are commonly defined as differences/inequities in health processes or health outcomes between groups. The landmark reports released by U.S. Surgeon General David Satcher (USDHHS, 1999) documented many of the key factors that contribute to the disparities in mental health care and the ongoing unmet mental health needs of African Americans. These disparities are influenced by a number of factors, including race, socioeconomic status, health care financing, health care quality, physical environment, cultural norms, community environment, and individual/family choices in health care management.

The economic pressure of paying for the ever-increasing cost of health care in the United States has a profound impact on access to mental health services. Approximately 20% of African Americans are uninsured, 51% have private insurance, and 26% have insurance through Medicaid (USDHHS, 2008). Even those who are insured confront the barriers of lack of parity of insurance coverage for mental health services, misdiagnosis, and lack of culturally competent or African American providers. Privately insured African Americans were less likely to receive outpatient mental health services, whereas there was no difference for African Americans and Whites whose health care was covered by Medicaid (Snowden, 2001). Because of the combined effect of lower socioeconomic status, environmental stressors, and institutional racism, poor African Americans suffer from the impact of mental illness more than poor Whites (Snowden, 2001). "This disparity does not stem from a greater prevalence rate or severity of illness in African Americans, but from a lack of culturally competent care, and receiving less or poor quality care" (American Psychiatric Association, 2008, p. 1). African Americans were more likely to receive mental health treatment in public sector "safety net" settings that typically are underresourced and lack state-of-the-art health technology resources that improve the quality of care. However, insurance and financial hardship do not fully explain difference in service use.

## CULTURE: IMPACT ON THE INITIATION OF HELP SEEKING

African Americans perceive and act upon mental health problems within a context that may either promote or hinder engagement in formal mental health services. The decision to seek help may be the result of a coercive process. African Americans are more frequently confronted with a situation in which they have been coerced to initiate mental health treatment through the judicial, educational, or child welfare systems. African American adolescents with a mental health disorder are more likely to end up in the juvenile justice system and to enter mental health care involuntarily than White adolescents (Cauce et al., 2002). Mental health professionals and other authorities such as police officers, judges, and business owners are not exempt from bias when making decisions as to whether an individual exhibiting deviant behavior is referred for treatment versus punishment. This results in African Americans being coerced into systems that are inappropriate for their needs. Voluntarily seeking help may be inhibited for multiple reasons. African Americans may have a higher threshold for distress, may have alternative religious or spiritual explanations for deviant behavior, or may be too stressed by the needs of daily living to seek treatment (Davey & Watson, 2008; Snowden, 2003). Moreover, the additional burden of stigma toward persons with mental illness may be particularly high in the African American community (Bell, 2001). African Americans have traditionally coped with and made decisions about treating the symptoms of mental illness using formal and informal family, religious, and social networks. The extended family system and trusted community members have traditionally been the first networks from which African Americans seek help (McMiller & Weisz, 1996). Cauce and colleagues (2002) found that African American youth are more likely than White youth to seek help from a family member when they disclose a mental health problem. The Black Church has historically been a multifaceted institution that has established a high level of respect and trust in the community while providing instrumental social and political support to its members. African American pastors as spiritual advisors and leaders frequently act as gatekeepers to provide consultation and referrals to families regarding mental health issues (Taylor, Chatters, & Levin, 2004). Studies have also found that individuals who contact clergy first are less likely to seek professional help (Neighbors, Musick, & Williams, 1998). African American civic/service organizations, along with fraternities and sororities, are also a potential source of support, particularly for the middle class. These institutions have customarily been the first place for help seeking given historical misdiagnosis, discrimination, and financial barriers to culturally competent care. However, these and other social networks may function both as a barrier (impede access because of cultural norms of mistrust, secrecy, or stigma) and a bridge (providing instrumental support such as transportation, child care, and emotional support) to engagement into more formal mental health services (Boyd-Franklin, 1989).

## TREATMENT INITIATION AND RETENTION

The process of engagement into therapeutic treatment involves at least two phases: (1) initiating the first help-seeking call and visit and (2) sustaining participation in the treatment process after the first visit. African Americans are more likely to use mental health services inconsistently, seek treatment later, stop treatment early, and receive poorer quality care (Kazdin, Stolar, & Marciano, 1995; Snowden, 2003; Thompson et al., 2004; USDHHS, 2001). African American children in need of mental health services were less likely to have received treatment in the past 6 months than White children (USDHHS, 2001). In a study of racial differences in the use of professional mental health care, Diala and colleagues (2000) found that prior to using mental health services African Americans had positive attitudes about seeking care, but those who needed and used mental health services were less likely to use them again compared with Whites. Research has found generally that inpatient services are overutilized and outpatient services are both over- and underutilized depending on the setting and problem (Thompson et al., 2004). Also less use of outpatient services and more frequent use of crisis-oriented health care services by African Americans results in the likelihood that mental health care will be concentrated in more restrictive/intensive settings (e.g., emergency room, inpatient hospitalization) (Snowden, 2001, 2003).

African Americans have a preference for particular styles and venues for treatment (e.g., in a primary care setting vs. specialized care setting, where the provider takes the time to establish a relationship of mutual respect and trust). There is a preference among African Americans for providers who are from the same ethnic group or who are culturally competent to interact on a cultural level; however, it did not impact willingness to engage in mental health treatment (Snowden, 2003; USDHHS, 2001). African Americans who had a high level of cultural mistrust were more likely to terminate therapy early, and their level of stigma concerning mental illness was higher than other ethnic groups (Thompson et al., 2004).

Thompson and colleagues (2004) reported that African Americans participating in focus groups revealed fears that therapists had inadequate knowledge of their culture and daily struggles to avoid bias and stereotyping. In summary, factors that impede African Americans in need of treatment from obtaining it fall into several categories:

- Structural: later referrals for treatment, resulting in higher levels of inpatient hospitalization, higher rate of involuntary referrals/commitments, and fewer specialized mental health services in African American communities.
- Provider: more frequent misdiagnosis, bias, lack of cultural competency, and fewer providers from the same ethnicity and cultural background.
- Individual/cultural: delayed problem recognition and initiation of treatment, fear of stigma and discrimination, historical and cultural mistrust of mental health providers, etc. (Breland-Noble, Bell, & Nicolas, 2006; Snowden, 2001).
- Historical racism and bias: from scientific reports that falsified the levels of "insanity" among northern free Blacks, to the act of running away from slavery mislabeled as a disease, to the Tuskegee syphilis study.

The remaining sections of this chapter describe best practices in engaging African Americans into outpatient mental health intervention. Davey and Watson (2008) developed an integrated public policy and mental health framework that sought to advance a culturally sensitive understanding of key variables that influence African American engagement into therapy. Of the variables that comprise this comprehensive model, we describe how the variables from the person–environment interaction construct, which consists of the relationships between the local social networks and the individual, are both extremely powerful influences on the help-seeking behavior of African Americans as well as worthy targets of efforts to increase engagement of African Americans in mental health intervention. However, the authors also imply that, in addition to addressing the person–environment interaction, efforts to improve engagement of ethnic minority clients should also seek to improve the provider behavior and practice of engaging ethnic minority clients in a culturally sensitive manner. Additionally, relationship building, collaboration, and needs assessment have been deemed essential components of effective outreach and engagement with underserved communities of color (Lerner, 1995; Vera, Buhin, Montgomery, & Shin, 2005).

Therefore, the following sections lay out best practices in community collaboration and needs assessment that recognizes and utilizes the powerful relationship between the individual and local networks to foster community trust of a provider. It is community trust that will enable providers to receive referrals of African American clientele. Moreover, the following sections also describe best practices in relationship building that will improve provider behavior and practice of engaging African Americans into mental health intervention once referrals are received.

## COMMUNITY COLLABORATION

African Americans are overrepresented in receipt of mental health services, but Snowden (2001) and Gayles, Alston, and Staten (2005) understand this occurrence is due to a high percentage of African American referrals via "coercive processes" such as mandates or recommendations to take part in mental health services from social service, child welfare, and legal agencies. Clients referred in this manner may associate counseling with punishment and/or government, which may exacerbate resistance, mistrust, and delay engagement.

Social service providers and clinicians are usually sophisticated in linking with agencies via formal contractual arrangements or informal agreements to receive referrals of a coercive nature. However, there is less sophistication regarding appropriate means of receiving referrals directly from the African American community via collaboration with local networks trusted by the community. The potential benefit is substantial. By receiving referrals directly from the community, it is possible to intervene early in the manifestation of problems, thus increasing the likelihood of treatment effectiveness, decreasing the likelihood of formal involvement in social service and governmental (e.g., juvenile justice and criminal justice), and decreasing the overrepresentation of African Americans in higher levels of medical care such as emergency department visits and inpatient hospitalization (Snowden, 2001). When African American clients have choice via insurance or private pay, it is the social capital and trust that a provider has within the African American community that will determine whether they will choose to be served by the provider or not.

## The Importance of Local Networks to African American Help Seeking

Primary medical care is often the first point of engagement for African Americans in need of mental health care (Davey & Watson, 2008; McMiller & Weisz, 1996). However, Davey and Watson (2008) note that some have questioned the quality of care in primary care settings when addressing serious mental health issues. Moreover, African Americans are more likely to drop out before being referred by a primary care physician to mental health treatment (Davey & Watson, 2008; Hu, Snowden, Jerrell, & Nguyen, 1991). When physicians do refer to mental health services, African American clients often do not follow up with the referral (Davey & Watson, 2008).

Interestingly, studies suggest that, although African Americans first receive formal mental health treatment at primary medical care settings, the majority first seek help from local networks (Davey & Watson, 2008; McMiller & Weisz,

1996; Snowden, 1998). McMiller and Weisz (1996) found that African American parents were only 0.37 times as likely as White parents to consult professionals as the first step in help seeking. Before formal involvement with a service provider, the majority of help-seeking efforts by African Americans involved contact with local networks such as family and community members. On the other hand, the majority of White help-seeking efforts involved contact with professionals.

Because of the preference to first seek help from local networks, providers seeking to increase African American utilization of outpatient mental health services should expand outreach efforts beyond the professional level to engage those local network leaders trusted by African Americans (Davey & Watson, 2008; McMiller & Weisz, 1996; Snowden, 2001). However, the literature consistently indicates the literature that these networks are often placed in the same category of care, as if each is similar in form and function. For example, Davey and Watson (2008) and Farris (2006) found that family, friends, school, and church were included in the category of local networks, although each type of support is qualitatively different in role and function. In this chapter, we classify African American local networks into two categories: culturally specific formal local networks and culturally specific informal networks.

## Culturally Specific Formal Local Networks

It is important that agencies strive to form relationships with culturally specific formal local networks in the African American community such as fraternal organizations and churches. These entities are culturally specific because they either originated in the African American community (fraternal organizations) or were adapted from mainstream institutions, modified for compatibility with the unique interests, needs, and culture of the African American community (churches). They are considered formal instead of informal because their organizational structure resembles that of mainstream formal supports by having a staff hierarchy or chain of command, clearly defined roles and responsibilities, organization at the national and local levels, and specific rules of operation, and many are selective in their membership. These institutions began developing in the late 18th century during the American Revolution period. They are well recognized, highly regarded, and known for their role in supporting the interests of the African American community long before African Americans were allowed access to mainstream institutions.

The oldest African American fraternal organization is the Prince Hall Masonic Order, founded in 1787 as African Lodge No. 459 by Prince Hall, a free man who emigrated from Barbados. By the late 19th century, African American voluntary/fraternal organizations and benevolent secret societies included not only parallel Euro-American groups such as the Elks and Masons but also independent orders with a national membership of hundreds of thousands (Trotter, 2004). In the beginning of the 20th century, African American Greek organizations were formed on both historically Black and White college campuses by students who were excluded from White fraternal organizations (Parks, 2008). Ironically, although these organizations were often denigrated or ignored by historians as crude, exaggerated imitations of parallel White civic organizations, many of the rituals and traditions actually are derived from African secret societies (Trotter, 2004). These organizations have helped to shape African American identity and culture; maintained cultural history and traditions; and uplifted the community and protected members from racism and poverty. They also promoted mutual self-help and philanthropy, assisted in circumventing racial exclusion, supported movements for social change and justice, established lifelong fictive kin bonds (brotherhood/sisterhood), and promoted the formation of other African American institutions (e.g., Black churches, schools).

Farris (2006) elaborates on the potential benefit of mental health providers linking with African American churches. The church has historically been defined as an institution that was and is instrumental to social and political movements that benefited African Americans. In essence, the church is viewed as an instrumental means of giving and receiving support to African Americans. It is not uncommon for churches to have multiple ministries that involve providing social support to African Americans in need across social issues (i.e., housing assistance, food pantries, HIV/AIDS intervention, financial services). The church is perceived by nine of 10 African Americans as fulfilling multifaceted roles in their communities and as having an encouraging influence on their lives (Taylor, Ellison, Chatters, Levin, & Lincoln, 2000). Both Farris and Taylor and colleagues have specifically indicated the relevance of providers forming relationships with church pastors, who often are sought out to address mental health concerns instead of formal mental health providers. The tendency to seek help from pastors may be related to factors such as mental health treatment expense, access, lack of insurance coverage, and nonrequirement of insurance copayments (Taylor et al., 2004). Moreover, often a meaningful, trusting personal pastor–congregant relationship has already been established that facilitates help seeking. Neighbors (as cited in Farris, 2006) emphasized that pastors are strongly rooted in the African American community in a way that mental health professionals will never be, and they are as accessible as other sources of informal support, including family and friends.

Although African American pastors may be well suited to address many of the concerns of their congregation, they may require support to appropriately address pervasive or serious mental health concerns. Alternatively, mental health providers may benefit from learning how to address religious/spiritual concerns. Farris recommends that program leadership seek a mutual collaboration with pastors. Service providers can offer in-service training for clergy and church leaders on how to identify when a person may need a referral to formal mental health services. In turn, pastors could train service providers in religious beliefs and practices that may influence experiences of personal and family problems. Such a collaboration acknowledges and supports the strength of both religious and mental health service involvement, which can be an effective mechanism for meeting the needs of many African American clients.

### Culturally Specific Informal Local Networks

Snowden (1999) and Davey and Watson (2008) emphasize the importance of providers linking with trusted natural helpers in the Black community, who can be gatekeepers to mental health treatment. These popular and influential local networks include hairdressers, barbershops, and local merchants, to name a few. Hammond (2008) experienced success in engaging African American men by partnering with barbers in the Black community. The collaboration involved offering free haircuts in return for participation in a study on racism-related stress. The Ethnic Diversity Task Force (EDTF) of the Connecticut Psychological Association (CPA) has partnered with hairstylists in an urban city to develop their MindStylz intervention (CPA Ethnic Diversity Task Force, 2008).

Supported by the American Psychological Association's Ethnic Minority Recruitment, Retention, and Training in Psychology grant as well as the CPA Educational Foundation, the goal of MindStylz is to provide training to local hairstylists and barbers of color on (1) recognition of mental health issues and signs among their clientele, (2) appropriate referrals for mental health services, and (3) making such referrals to mental health professionals who work with African American providers. The EDTF chose to partner with hairstylists in recognition of the fact that African Americans often share details of their lives with trusted personal service providers whom they have known for many years. Therefore, hairstylists and barbers are often among the first to hear of a person's problems. By collaborating with these natural helpers, MindStylz creates another avenue for African Americans to access mental health services. Of course, communities may vary in the type and number of natural helpers. However, the work of the provider is to find out from community members to whom or where people turn to talk freely about the issues in their lives.

Mental health providers stand to gain greatly by collaborating with trusted, culturally specific local networks, both formal and informal. By recognizing the value and importance of these support networks, providers can earn respect in the community and gain a reputation for both acknowledging the assets of the African American community and collaborating with those assets to effectively serve the community.

## Community-Informed Needs Assessment

A provider can benefit from incorporating a local institution's knowledge of community needs into the design of specific interventions (Vera et al., 2005). This may involve speaking to knowledgeable members of the African American community via one-on-one discussions, interviews, and focus groups (Breland-Noble & King, 2008). Furthermore, to ensure that an intervention continually addresses the needs of the community, a provider should have a mechanism in place for regularly assessing its effectiveness. This is essential because of the often-changing needs of disadvantaged African American communities, which may require different services or alteration in how they are delivered. This can be accomplished in several ways, such as seeking feedback via satisfaction surveys or periodic focus groups with service recipients. If the provider has a board, then installation of community residents as board members can help ensure ongoing relevance of services and demonstrate a commitment to integrating a community perspective into the decision-making process.

Providers can be aware of community needs by having staff who know and reside in the community and attending to patterns in presenting problems of one's clientele. For example, in response to a growing client base that was manifesting symptoms related to trauma exposure, the Clifford Beers Child Guidance Clinic in New Haven, Connecticut, adopted an intervention called trauma-focused cognitive-behavioral therapy (TF-CBT), which enhanced the agency's ability to meet the needs of its clientele. TF-CBT is an evidence-based treatment approach designed to help children, adolescents, and their caretakers overcome trauma-related difficulties. The agency implemented system changes to make intake a trauma-informed process that also enhanced collaboration and engagement with consumers. Universal trauma screening and assessment instruments were incorporated into the intake session, along with a follow-up intake session where the results are reviewed by the clinician and consumer to facilitate treatment planning.

This systems change process at the Clifford Beers Child Guidance Clinic began with an assessment period that incorporated consumer and staff feedback through observation, surveys, interviews, and meetings. The agency then conducted a pilot intake study to compare rates of successful intake completion as well as no-show and cancellation rates with those of the previous year. Consumers were then asked to give feedback on their experience via telephone surveys. They found an increase in successful intake completion and first-session attendance and received favorable feedback from consumers. It is important that agencies be nimble in their ability to respond to the pressing needs of disadvantaged communities, which are disproportionately African American (Snowden, 2001). The Clifford Beers Child Guidance Clinic demonstrated how both quantitative and qualitative data can be used to assess and respond to the needs of its clientele.

As previously discussed, cultural mistrust is embedded in many African American communities, and deservedly so given the history of maltreatment or inappropriate receipt of services by supposedly well-meaning helping institutions. This dynamic, as well as an often-negative perception of mental health services, has precipitated an underutilization of outpatient mental health (Snowden, 2001).

## CLIENT RELATIONSHIP BUILDING

### Structural Characteristics of the Provider

#### Organizational Climate

Studies have suggested that perceptions of the program and staff are the most significant motivators of a client's willingness to participate (Pinto et al., 2007; Roberts & Nishimoto, 2006). The provider setting should be culturally welcoming, displaying positive, affirming images and messages that represent the culture. This would help convey the message to members of the African American community that they are welcome and would serve as a noticeable contrast to the culture-neutral settings of many government social service agencies. Regarding staff, client perception of staff attitude predicts length of time in treatment, treatment completion, and motivation to participate (Roberts & Nishimoto, 2006). Roberts and Nishimoto (2006) suggest that it is important for helping professionals to be aware of their own "attitudes, behaviors, and feelings" when working with a client population (p. 68). Providers must convey respectful and positive attitudes toward their clients in order to build trust and rapport.

Pinto and colleagues (2007) found that client perception of the ability of a provider to be helpful and a perception of provider staff as friendly were important motivators to participation in a clinical program. CHAMPS, the program evaluated by Pinto and colleagues, built activities around meals and other forms of recreation that may have been perceived as fun, a practice other programs have found to be successful in engaging low-income, inner-city African American families, particularly those who experience multiple stressors (Frazier, Abdul-Adil, Atkins, Gathright, & Jackson, 2007). As Boyd-Franklin (1987) has indicated, low-income African American families often experience multiple stressors that negatively impact quality of life. Program activities that are fun and have a social component can serve an important role in alleviating stress as well as a means for people experiencing similar problems to interact and find additional social support.

An intervention that values enhancement of social support may be particularly of interest to low-income African Americans because the degree of social support in one's life has been found related to mental health service use (Harrison, McKay, & Bannon, 2004). In many disadvantaged communities, families can be isolated, and efforts to decrease this isolation can be of particular value. Events that bring people together around activities perceived as fun can be a powerful motivator for program participation for people who encounter significant stressors on a regular basis. For instance, in an effort to attract parents to a parenting intervention in a predominately African American community in Chicago, a school-based mental health service program, Positive Attitudes for Learning in School (PALS), held "parenting parties," events with a set amount of time dedicated to socializing and a set amount of time dedicated to skill building (Frazier et al., 2007). This combination of fun and skill building increased participation among low-income African American parents, which Frazier and colleagues (2007) attributed, in part, to the socialization component of the program. Indeed, even the title of "parenting party" implies a positive, fun, and uplifting event compared with the more common, but more stigmatizing and demoralizing, "parent training" or "parenting groups."

Similarly, the Clifford Beers Child Guidance Clinic implemented "Family Night," a more informal approach to invite parents, extended family members, and friends to join supportive activities that (1) enhance their involvement in the clinic's services and (2) empower them to become a voice for recovery at the clinic and in the community. Clinicians are also invited to attend with their family members. Entertainment and activities such as circus acts, storytelling, music, dance, and crafts are provided, along with time for families and clinicians to interact informally, which can serve to increase client–clinician rapport. In addition to serving as a forum for social support and interaction, the event reinforces the concept of self-care for both families and clinicians who are coping/working with trauma as a priority in the agency. It also presents an opportunity to engage families in other services offered by the agency.

Studies suggest that respectful provider attitudes and settings that are positive, nurturing, and fun are more likely to attract African American individuals and families, particularly those who experience multiple challenges in their daily lives. By facilitating positive events that foster socialization not just among the potential clients but also between clients and staff, the program is perceived as one that truly values and invests in the client, which facilitates the development of a trusting relationship.

### Ethnic Compatibility of Staff

Breland-Noble and colleagues (2006) suggest that a dearth of African American mental health professionals contributes to African American underutilization of mental health services. Allen-Meares and Burman (1999) further indicate that ethnic differences between client and therapist may contribute to challenges in initial engagement. Clients may be more open to someone of similar ethnicity because of a perception that the therapist may be able to relate to their experience as a fellow ethnic minority (Allen-Meares & Burman, 1999; Rodriguez, 2008). Providers who have successfully engaged culturally diverse clientele have emphasized the relevance of having staff who are culturally and linguistically compatible with the target population in order to facilitate rapport development (Frazier et al., 2007; Simmons et al., 2008). Therefore, providers seeking to serve the African American community may benefit from aggressively recruiting African American helping professionals.

This, however, can be challenging. Providers who experience some success often use nontraditional recruitment strategies such as advertising available positions in community newspapers popular among African Americans. Another strategy is to link with local and national professional organizations popular among African American helping professionals such as National Association of Black Social Workers or the Association of Black Psychologists. Providers may also strive to form relationships with historically Black colleges and universities (HBCUs) that graduate a significant number of young African American professionals to engage students nearing graduation and in need of a job or internship. The provider may be able to collaborate with the HBCU to develop internships for students, fostering a "pipeline" for later employment. If there are no HBCUs within close proximity, the provider may want to make a similar connection with African American student organizations at predominantly White colleges and universities. African American student organizations at colleges specific to helping professions such as social work, counseling, or psychology are not uncommon, and such relationships can be instrumental in developing a culturally diverse workforce, which may convey a message to the community served that diversity is valued by the provider.

## Flexible Office Hours and Staffing Patterns

In addition to recruiting staff who are ethnically similar to the clients served, providers can improve the likelihood of their staff forming relationships with African American clients by establishing nontraditional office hours. This is imperative for a number of reasons. Transportation is a frequent barrier to service involvement among low-income African Americans (McKay et al., 2004). For instance, some may rely on public transportation, which is an additional burden of time and expense. Likewise, some families may rely on one car to serve the needs of multiple working adults, again restricting opportunities for daytime appointments.

Many African American adults are employed outside of the typical 9 to 5 workday, in "second-shift" (beginning in early evening) or "third-shift" (beginning in the late evening or early morning) jobs. These shifts are particularly common among industries that employ a high percentage of African Americans, such as manufacturing and health care. These adults may require either evening appointments, coming for therapy before they begin their shift, or early-morning appointments, after finishing a shift.

It is common in some occupational fields, such as civil service, a prodigious employer of African Americans, to have shifting days off. In order to accommodate this, a provider can exercise flexibility in scheduling clients for different times and days. This flexibility would benefit those families who are unable to come before, after, or during work but are committed enough to therapy to be willing to come on days off. Toward this end, clinics may want to explore weekend hours, which can accommodate those families who are not able to attend during the week despite best efforts.

By implementing these or related alternative staffing patterns, providers are better able to meet the needs of clients who require nontraditional hours. Agencies that strive to remove as many barriers to treatment access as possible will facilitate increased show rates and ability for clinicians to form viable relationships with their clients. Moreover, agencies may earn a reputation in the community as one that strives to accommodate the families in a culturally responsive and respectful manner, versus expecting families to comply with a structure that does not take into account their reality.

### Child Care Arrangements

Relying on extended kinship for support is a strength of the African American community (Boyd-Franklin, 1989). When resources do not allow enrollment in professional child care, which can be costly, many families are able to rely on relatives or neighbors to provide care. However, this option may not always be available, limiting the opportunity for an adult or family to attend therapy. This may be particularly salient for single-parent families or families in which one parent works second or third shift and is not always available to care for children. Providers who offer child care will build viable clinical caseloads for their clinical staff and increase service attendance, which would be conducive to client relationship building.

## Interpersonal Characteristics of the Provider

### Engaging in Collaborative and Active Problem Solving

African Americans, particularly those of low income, often face substantial, multiple barriers to involvement in mental health services. It is essential for a provider to identify these barriers at first contact and work actively with each family to address them. When possible, it is important to provide some immediate means of addressing the difficulty even before the first in-person session. For example, a caregiver may call in distress, but during the course of the conversation the provider learns that the client has recently lost transportation to work, much less to therapy. The provider must work during this initial contact to identify with the client a means of addressing this barrier. By focusing on the immediate resolution of these barriers, the client may gain trust in the provider's ability to be of service. Boyd-Franklin (1989) states how low-income African American families often experience multiple systems in their lives involuntarily. Often these providers prove stressful and disempowering to the family because of their tendency to place mandates on the family without their input. Also, the agencies may not communicate with each other, resulting in a family having multiple mandates from multiple agencies, which may prove overwhelming and impede the ability to invest in outpatient therapy. The family may also be demoralized by the treatment received by these agencies, which may assume a deficit-based model of viewing the family.

To counteract this, it is important that the provider identify and emphasize strengths during the first contact with the family and to acquaint them with the collaborative nature of the therapeutic process by focusing on the problems that they want to address and change (Boyd-Franklin, 1989). Even simply recognizing the strength required to request help while dealing with multiple stressors can be empowering to the client. It is important to emphasize during first contact that the situation can improve, and that, when the client comes to the session, "we" will work to immediately address these stressors. The use of "we" indicates that the therapeutic process will be collaborative, and that the family will have input into the treatment process in an empowering fashion, providing hope for the family, which may increase their investment in attending the first session.

During the first session, it is imperative to identify and develop immediate interventions to address stressors that were not amenable to intervention at intake. These stressors may include delinquent utility or housing payments, legal entanglements, or child welfare issues, to name a few. This again serves to engender in the family a sense that the provider is invested in making their overall lives better, which helps to build trust. The therapist must be prepared to be active, including meeting with other agency stakeholders involved with the family and linking the family with supportive services. In essence, the provider has to be willing to either engage in case management or link the family with a trusted entity that can provide case management. Without addressing immediate stressors, via case management and efforts to coordinate with multiple systems that are involved in the client's life, the family's ability to invest in mental health intervention will be challenged (Boyd-Franklin, 2003). This form of active approach may be novel to many therapists, and it can be labor intensive. However, it is often necessary in order to engage overwhelmed and underresourced African American clients effectively.

Mary McKay has developed and tested an engagement intervention for urban youth that exemplifies a collaborative and active problem-solving approach to engagement (McKay, Stoewe, McCadam, & Gonzales, 1998). Clients who received this intervention demonstrated significantly greater initial mental health outpatient therapy attendance rates and ongoing service use than those who experienced the usual intake procedures. McKay has since replicated these results and has developed and implemented a protocol to train mental health providers who serve urban communities in this effective engagement intervention (Cavaleri et al., 2006; McKay et al., 2004).

McKay's two-step model of engagement, as described in McKay and colleagues (2004), involves:

- Step 1: Initial telephone contact that is designed to help the primary caretaker invest in the help-seeking process by (1) clarifying for both the caregiver and the provider the need for child mental health care, (2) maximizing the caregiver's investment and efficacy in relation to help seeking, (3) identifying attitudes about and previous experiences with mental health that might dissuade the adult from bringing the child for services, and (4) using active problem solving to develop strategies to overcome concrete obstacles to involvement in therapy, such as lack of time, transportation, and child care issues.

- Step 2: First face-to-face interview session that seeks to (1) clarify the helping process for the client, (2) develop the foundation for a collaborative working relationship with the client, (3) identify concrete, practical concerns that can be immediately addressed, and (4) develop a plan to overcome barriers to ongoing involvement with the agency.

When training professionals in this model, McKay emphasizes identifying and addressing both family-based barriers to treatment involvement, such as previous experiences with mental health services, transportation, racism, perceptions of services and staff, and lack of time, as well as environmental-based barriers to treatment common in urban communities, such as issues of safety, community violence, and poverty. In essence, McKay emphasizes use of active problem solving and a multisystemic perspective when engaging African American disadvantaged families, which has demonstrated positive results.

### Taking Time to Build Trust and Rapport

Cultural mistrust can exist not only because of a historical legacy of racism and slavery (Breland-Noble et al., 2006; Dana, 2002; Sue & Chu, 2003; Whaley, 2001) but also as a result of the counseling being mandated or highly recommended via a coercive process involving governmental legal or social welfare agencies (Davey & Watson, 2008; Gayles et al., 2005; Snowden, 2001). Clients referred in this manner may associate counseling with punishment or government, which may encourage resistance, mistrust, and delay engagement. The task of the clinician is to allay concerns and earn clients' trust and confidence. Any source of reluctance should be addressed as part of the assessment and treatment-planning process (McMiller & Weisz, 1996).

It is imperative that the clinician empower clients to let them tell their story (Cooper-Patrick et al., 1999; McKay et al., 2004; Nunez & Robertson, 2006). According to Nunez and Robertson (2006, p. 375), "The gap between patient and provider expectations and communication is not new ... patients often want to be heard, understood, and to have physicians understand the larger context of their lives." The communication during the interaction with a helping professional is key to whether African Americans will attend additional sessions with a therapist or follow-up on a referral to a helping professional (Davey & Watson, 2008).

### Addressing Racial/Cultural Differences

There exists a dearth of mental health providers of color available to serve African American clients in many communities. When African Americans do enter into therapy, it is often with therapists who are of a different race. Allen-Meares and Burman (1999), in their comprehensive review of cross-cultural therapeutic relationships with African Americans, state that the degree of familiarity or differences between the client and therapist can either promote a therapeutic alliance or derail it. One such difference is race/culture. Allen-Meares and Burman discuss factors key to establishing cross-cultural therapeutic relationships with African Americans, one of which is the degree to which therapists acquire a working knowledge of the historical and cultural context that "comprises the existence of living as an African-American in the United States" (p. 2). Inherent in this knowledge is an understanding of the relationship between historical systemic and intentional oppression and current disparities in well-being that exist disproportionately in the African American community.

The importance of knowledge acquisition applies not just to cross-racial therapeutic dyads but also to dyads that differ by social class or cultural experience (i.e., therapist is African American but raised in affluent suburbs vs. an African American client raised in a disadvantaged community of a large urban area). In the latter case, the African American therapist should not assume that he or she understands the world of the client, but instead should express an openness and desire to learn from the client. Such authenticity often will be appreciated by a client.

Additionally, therapists should develop an ability to assess one's own biases and worldviews as well as the ability to see the world through their clients' cultural lens versus their own. This particular degree of self-exploration can be challenging and is best accomplished through supervision and training with someone skilled in culturally responsive intervention. This may involve the therapist being willing to process with African American clients any perceptions of the role of racism in their presenting problems, perceptions that are particularly prevalent among male clients (Gayles et al., 2005). Therapists are encouraged to query this, which may send the message to clients that talking about perceived racism is sanctioned in the therapeutic relationship. Otherwise, the clients may not be willing to discuss perceived racism, even if it is a key issue for them.

Allen-Meares and Burman (1999) suggest that therapists must exhibit empathy, nonjudgmental positive regard, genuineness, and acceptance in efforts to establish rapport. It is imperative that therapists be collaborative versus hierarchical in their interaction with clients, which can convey a sense of respect and value of the clients and their perspective.

Therapists can establish cross-racial and cross-cultural therapeutic relationships with African American clients. The authors of the current chapter seek to make readers aware of certain practices key to cross-cultural or cross-racial therapeutic engagement. Yet we discourage providers with no previous training in cross-racial or cross-cultural therapeutic engagement to attempt it solely based on reading this chapter. As is the case for acquisition of other therapeutic skills, cross-cultural and cross-racial engagement with African

American clients requires a commitment to acquiring the requisite awareness, knowledge, and skills (Sue & Torino, 2005) through competent supervision and training.

## CONCLUSION

Although the need exists, African Americans are underrepresented in less expensive but preventive voluntary outpatient mental health intervention. Instead, they are often coerced into outpatient mental health intervention, which impedes client investment, or are admitted to costly higher levels of care after the mental health issue has severely impeded functioning. It has been argued that if there were greater voluntary utilization of outpatient mental health services, there would be an increased likelihood that mental health issues of African Americans could be ameliorated before damaging their lives and their families.

There exist historical, structural, and cultural factors that impact African American help seeking as well as provider practices that impede engagement once African Americans seek mental health services. These factors have been well documented by multiple scholars, yet what has not been as well developed is the articulation of effective engagement practices that take these factors into consideration. Such an articulation is the focus of this chapter. The authors present a bilevel approach to effective outreach and engagement that builds upon previous scholarship.

One level involves collaborating with trusted local networks of African American communities and demonstrating active involvement in the community. These endeavors can facilitate the acquisition of community trust often necessary for client referrals. A second level involves utilizing culturally and contextually appropriate practices for building a relationship with a client once a referral is received, starting with the all-important first contact between the provider and the client.

The strategies described are designed to be utilized by any individual, group, or agency mental health provider who has a willingness to improve their service to the African American community. Given the implications of continued underidentification and/or delayed identification of mental health needs, coercive means of mental health involvement, and overutilization of expensive higher levels of care by African Americans, it is imperative that the mental health field invest in improving the involvement of African Americans in quality preventive outpatient mental health intervention.

## ACKNOWLEDGMENT

We wish to acknowledge the contribution of Rachel Tirnady, MA, of the Criminology and Criminal Justice Department of Central Connecticut State University, who provided instrumental research support.

# REFERENCES

Allen-Meares, P., & Burman, S. (1999). Cross-cultural therapeutic relationships: Entering the world of African-Americans. *Journal of Social Work Practice, 13*, 49–57.

American Psychiatric Association. (2008). *Let's talk facts about mental health in the African American community.* Arlington, VA: Author.

Bell, C. (2001). Multiple stigmas keep Blacks away from MH system. *Psychiatric News, 36*(20), 19.

Bonham, V. L., Sellers, S. L., & Neighbors, H. W. (2004). John Henryism and self-reported physical health among high-socioeconomic status African-American men. *American Journal of Public Health, 94*, 737–738.

Boyd-Franklin, N. (1987). The contribution of family therapy models to the treatment of Black families. *Psychotherapy, 24*, 621–629.

Boyd-Franklin, N. (1989). Five key factors in the treatment of Black families. In G. W. Saba, B. M. Karrer, & K. V. Hardy (Eds.), *Minorities and family therapy* (pp. 53–69). Philadelphia: Haworth Press.

Boyd-Franklin, N. (2003). *Black families in therapy: Understanding the African American experience* (2nd ed.). New York: Guilford Press.

Breland-Noble, A. M., Bell, C., & Nicolas, G. (2006). The development of an evidence-based family intervention for increasing participation in psychiatric clinical care and research in depressed African American adolescents. *Family Process, 45*(2), 153–169.

Breland-Noble, A. M., & King, J. L. (2008, August). *Treatment engagement with African-American adolescents and families: Evidence from the African American Knowledge Organized for Mindfully Healthy Adolescents (AAKOMA) Project.* Paper presented at the 116th Annual Convention of the American Psychological Association, Boston.

Cauce, A. M., Domenech-Rodriguez, M., Paradise, M., Cochran, B. N., Shea, J. M., Srebnik, D., et al. (2002). Cultural and contextual influences in mental health help seeking: A focus on ethnic minority youth. *Journal of Consulting and Clinical Psychology, 70*, 44–55.

Cavaleri, M. A., Gopalan, G., McKay, M. M., Appel, A., Bannon, W. M., Bigley, M. F., et al. (2006). Impact of a learning collaborative to improve child mental health service use among low-income urban youth and families. *Best Practices in Mental Health, 2*, 67–79.

Connecticut Psychological Association Ethnic Diversity Task Force. (2008). *MindStylz training protocol.* Unpublished manuscript.

Cooper-Patrick, L., Gallo, J. J., Powe, N. R., Steinwachs, D. M., Eaton, W. W., & Ford, D. E. (1999). Mental health service utilization by African-Americans and Whites. *Medical Care, 37*, 1034–1045.

Dana, R. H. (2002). Mental health services for African-Americans: A cultural/racial perspective. *Cultural Diversity and Ethnic Minority Psychology, 8*, 3–18.

Davey, M., & Watson, M. (2008). Engaging African Americans in therapy: Integrating a public policy and family therapy perspective. *Contemporary Family Therapy, 30*, 31–47.

Diala, C., Muntaner, C., Walrath, C., Nickerson, K., LaVeist, T., & Leaf, P. (2000). Racial differences in attitudes toward professional mental health care and in the use of services. *American Journal of Orthopsychiatry, 70*, 455–464.

Farris, K. (2006). The role of African-American pastors in mental health care. *Journal of Human Behavior in the Social Environment, 14*, 159–182.

Frazier, S. L., Abdul-Adil, J., Atkins, M. S, Gathright, T., & Jackson, M. (2007). Can't have one without the other: Mental health providers and community parents reducing barriers to services for families in urban poverty. *Journal of Community Psychology, 35*, 434–446.

Gayles, T. A., Alston, R. J., & Staten, D. (2005). Understanding mental illness among African-American males: Risk factors and treatment parameters. In D. A. Harley & J. M. Dillard (Eds.), *Contemporary mental health issues among African-Americans* (pp. 49–60). Alexandria, VA: American Counseling Association.

Hammond, W. (2008, August). *Racism-related stress, masculinity ideology, depression, and African-American men.* Paper presented at the 116th Annual Convention of the American Psychological Association, Boston.

Harrison, M. E., McKay, M. M., & Bannon, W. M. (2004). Inner-city child mental health service use: The real question is why youth and families do not use services. *Community Mental Health Journal, 40*, 119–131.

Hu, T., Snowden, L., Jerrell, J., & Nguyen, T. (1991). Ethnic populations in public mental health: Services choice and level of use. *American Journal of Public Health, 81*, 1429–1434.

James, S. A., LaCroix, A. Z., Kelimbaum, D. C., & Strogatz, D. S. (1984). John Henryism and blood pressure differences: The role of occupational stressors. *Journal of Behavioral Medicine, 7*, 259–279.

Kazdin, A. E., Stolar, M. J., & Marciano, P. L. (1995). Risk factors for dropping out of treatment among White and Black families. *Journal of Family Psychology, 9*, 402–417.

Kessler, R. C., Berglund, P., Demler, O., Jin, R., Merikangas, K., & Walters, E. (2005). Lifetime prevalence and age-of-onset distributions of DSM-IV disorders in the National Comorbidity Survey replication. *Archives of General Psychiatry, 62*, 593–602.

Lerner, R. M. (1995). *America's youth in crisis: Challenges and options for programs and policies.* Thousand Oaks, CA: Sage.

McKay, M. M., Hibbert, R., Hoagwood, K., Rodriguez, J., Murray, L., Legerski, J., et al. (2004). Integrating evidence-based engagement interventions into "real world" child mental health settings. *Brief Treatment and Crisis Intervention, 4*, 177–186.

McKay, M. M., Stoewe, J., McCadam, K., & Gonzales, J. (1998). Increasing access to child mental health services for urban children and their care givers. *Health and Social Work, 23*, 9–15.

McMiller, W. P., & Weisz, J. R. (1996). Help-seeking preceding mental health clinic intake among African-American, Latino, and Caucasian youths. *Journal of the American Academy of Child and Adolescent Psychiatry, 35*, 1086–1094.

Messias, E., Eaton, W., Nestadt, G., Bienvenu, J., & Samuels, J. (2007). Psychiatrists' ascertained treatment needs for mental disorders in a population-based sample. *Psychiatric Services, 58*(3), 373–377.

National Center for Health Statistics. (2007). *Health, United States, 2007 with chartbook on trends in the health of Americans.* Washington, DC: U.S. Government Printing Office.

Neighbors, H. W., Musick, M. A., & Williams, D. R. (1998). The African American minister as a source of help for serious personal crises: Bridge or barrier to mental health care? *Health Education and Behavior, 25*, 759–778.

Nunez, A., & Robertson, C. (2006). Cultural competencies in clinical medicine: The patient encounter. In D. Satcher, R. J. Pumies, & N. W. Woelff (Eds.), *Multicultural medicine and health disparities* (pp. 371–388). New York: McGraw-Hill.

Parks, G. S. (2008). *Black Greek letter organizations in the 21st century: Our fight has just begun.* Lexington: University Press of Kentucky.

Pinto, R. M., McKay, M. M., Baptiste, D., Bell, C., Madison-Boyd, S., Paikoff, R., et al. (2007). Motivation and barriers to participation of ethnic-minority families in a family-based HIV prevention program. *Social Work in Mental Health, 5,* 187–201.

Roberts, A. C., & Nishimoto, R. (2006). Barriers to engaging and retaining African-American post-partum women in drug treatment. *Journal of Drug Issues, 36,* 53–76.

Rodriguez, M. D. (2008, August). *Criando con Amor: Promoviendo Armonia y Superacion— Findings from a randomized trial of a culturally-adapted PMTO intervention.* Paper presented at the 116th Annual Convention of the American Psychological Association, Boston.

Simmons, R., Ungemack, J., Sussman, J., Anderson, R., Adorno, S., Aguayo, J., et al. (2008). Bringing adolescents into substance abuse treatment through community-based outreach and engagement: The Hartford Youth Project. *Journal of Psychoactive Drugs, 40,* 41–54.

Snowden, L. R. (1998). Racial differences in informal help seeking for mental health problems. *Journal of Community Psychology, 26,* 429–438.

Snowden, L. R. (1999). African-American service use for mental health problems. *Journal of Community Psychology, 27,* 303–313.

Snowden, L. R. (2001). Barriers to effective mental health services for African Americans. *Mental Health Services Research, 3,* 181–187.

Snowden, L. R. (2003). Bias in mental health assessment and intervention: Theory and evidence. *American Journal of Public Health, 93,* 239–243.

Sue, D. W., & Torino, G. C. (2005). Racial-cultural competence: Awareness, knowledge, and skills. In R. T. Carter (Ed.), *Handbook of racial-cultural psychology and counseling: Training and practice* (Vol. 2, pp. 3–18). Hoboken, NJ: Wiley.

Sue, S., & Chu, R. (2003). The mental health of ethnic minority groups: Challenges posed by the supplement to the surgeon general's report on mental health. *Culture, Medicine and Psychiatry, 27,* 447–465.

Taylor, R., Chatters, L., & Levin, J. (2004). *Religion in the lives of African-Americans: Social, psychological, and health perspectives.* Thousand Oaks, CA: Sage.

Taylor, R., Ellison, C., Chatters, L., Levin, J., & Lincoln, K. (2000). Mental health services in faith communities: The role of clergy in Black churches. *Social Work, 45,* 73–87.

Thompson, V. L., Bazile, A., & Akbar, M. (2004). African Americans' perceptions of psychotherapy and psychotherapists. *Professional Psychology: Research and Practice, 35,* 19–26.

Trotter, J. (2004). African American fraternal associations in American history. *Social Science History, 28*(3), 355–366.

U.S. Department of Health and Human Services. (1999). *Mental health: A report of the surgeon general.* Rockville, MD: U.S. Department of Health and Human Services, Substance Abuse and Mental Health Services Administration, Center for Mental Health Services, National Institute of Mental Health, National Institutes of Health.

U.S. Department of Health and Human Services. (2001). *Mental health: Culture, race and ethnicity: A supplement to mental health: A report of the surgeon general* (Report No.

0-16-050892-4). Rockville, MD: U.S. Department of Health and human Services, Public Health Service, Office of the Surgeon General.

U.S. Department of Health and Human Services. (2008). *Summary health statistics for the U.S. population: National Health Interview Survey, 2006* (Vital and Health Statistics Series 10, No. 236). Rockville, MD: Centers for Disease Control and Prevention, National Center for Health Statistics.

Vera, E. M., Buhin, L., Montgomery, G., & Shin, R. (2005). Enhancing therapeutic interventions with people of color: Integrating outreach, advocacy, and prevention. In R. T. Carter (Ed.), *Handbook of racial-cultural psychology and counseling: Training and practice* (Vol. 2, pp. 477–491). Hoboken, NJ: Wiley.

Whaley, A. L. (2001). Cultural mistrust and mental health services for African-Americans: A review and meta-analysis. *Counseling Psychologist, 29*, 513–531.

# PART II

## Health Issues for African Americans

# 9

# Obesity

M. Kathleen Figaro
Rhonda BeLue
Bettina M. Beech

The increased global prevalence of obesity in both adults and children over the past 30 years represents a significant public health problem. Long-term effects of obesity, including Type 2 diabetes, cardiovascular disease, respiratory problems, and metabolic disorders, are estimated to cost billions of dollars worldwide (Finkelstein, Trogar, Cohen, & Dietz, 2009; Thorpe, 2009). The increase in obesity has been observed in all racial, ethnic, gender, and age groups in the United States. However, racial and ethnic minority populations, particularly African American women and girls, are disproportionately affected by obesity and many of its sequelae (Centers for Disease Control and Prevention [CDC], 2009).

Obesity arises from a complex interaction of biological, cultural, economic, environmental, and historical factors, and benefits from being studied multifactorially (Alonso, 2004). This chapter first provides an overview of the biology and genetics of obesity, and describes the epidemiological patterns in the general population and African Americans in particular. The socioeconomic, individual, familial, environmental, and cultural issues that serve as important influences in the obesogenic milieu of African Americans are then presented. Furthermore, the complications of obesity, barriers to weight loss, and the complex nature of multilevel interventions needed to address this epidemic in the African American community are comprehensively discussed. The chapter culminates with a discussion of prevention strategies, including policy considerations that show promise for reducing obesity's incidence and prevalence.

## ETIOLOGY: BIOLOGY AND GENETICS

### Definition, Measurement, and Diagnosis

In general, obesity is the result of an imbalance in energy intake and energy expenditure. Dietary and lifestyle habits, metabolic and neuroendocrine alterations, and heredity all interact to determine weight. Excessive fat accumulation in adipose tissue results from chronic consumption of foods and drinks in excess of energy expenditures. If the stored energy leads to weight that is 120–130% of the ideal or recommended weight for one's height, then the condition is termed *obesity*. Although criteria for overweight and obesity vary, body mass index (BMI) is routinely used, given the relative simplicity of measuring height and weight (Cameron & Demerath, 2002).

BMI is computed as weight in kilograms (body weight) divided by height in meters squared ($kg/m^2$). According to the World Health Organization (1998), *obesity* for adults is defined as a BMI of greater than or equal to 30. More specifically, Grade 1 overweight, commonly called *overweight*, is a BMI of $25–29.9 \, kg/m^2$. Grade 2 overweight/obesity is a BMI of $30–39.9 \, kg/m^2$, and Grade 3 obesity is a BMI of $40–59.9 \, kg/m^2$. Grade 4 obesity, or *supermorbid obesity*, is a BMI $> 60 \, kg/m^2$. BMI may be an inaccurate measure of obesity for those with increased muscle mass, such as athletes, and may conceal underlying excess adiposity for those with poor muscle mass, such as older adults. Consequently, several additional measurements (including waist circumference and waist-to-hip ratio) are significant in the diagnosis of obesity (Gallagher et al., 2000).

It is important to note that BMI is used differently with children than it is with adults. Because of changes in body fatness associated with growth, the interpretation of BMI is dependent on a child's age and gender, and can vary in its validity as a measurement of future risk (Freedman et al., 2005; Freedman & Sherry, 2009). In children, BMI-for-age is plotted according to sex-specific growth charts that account for gender differences associated with fat distribution and maturation. Currently, revised cutoff points for BMI values define overweight and obesity in youth. The new values established by the American Medical Association indicate that for children between 2 and 20 years of age, BMIs between the 85th and the 94th percentile define overweight, and a BMI at or over the 95th percentile defines obesity (Barlow & Expert Committee, 2007). Children with BMIs over these cutoff points do not necessarily have clinical complications or health risks related to obesity.

### Types of Obesity

There are two major types of obesity, which correspond to the popular notion of "apple-shaped" and "pear-shaped" body types. Patients with predominantly subcutaneous fat are more commonly "pear-shaped." Those with visceral fat or central obesity generally have increased abdominal girth and are "apple-shaped." Although there is substantial overlap between the two types, they are generally associated with different pathophysiology and so serve as simple markers and predictors of outcomes.

Hip, thigh, and buttock fat is largely inert from a pathophysiological and endocrine function standpoint. This fat is used largely for long-term energy reserves. This type of fat is more commonly found in African American women than in White women (Lovejoy, de la Bretonne, Lemperer, & Tulley, 1996). Central obesity is much more pathological. The visceral fat associated with this type causes an increase in inflammation and increases the subsequent risk of cardiovascular morbidity and mortality. Weight gain and development of visceral adiposity in both African American and White women are associated with greater risk for hypertension (Lloyd-Jones et al., 2005).

Several lifestyle factors have an impact on visceral adiposity. Cigarette smoking, physical inactivity, and low dietary fiber intake are strongly associated with increases in visceral adipose tissue. Two major disease processes are also associated with visceral adiposity: diabetes and heart disease. The risk for both conditions is termed *metabolic syndrome* and includes abdominal obesity, insulin resistance, glucose intolerance, hyperinsulinemia, hypertension, and hypertriglyceridemia. Those with this syndrome have a four-times-increased risk of heart disease and seven-times-increased risk of diabetes, compared to those without the condition (Guize et al., 2007).

## Pathophysiology

The pathophysiology of central obesity involves several derangements of adipokines, other inflammatory markers in the liver and muscle, and smooth muscle changes in the blood vessels. Adipose tissue is known to be a repository of various cytokines, especially interleukin-6 and tumor necrosis factor-alpha. Lipoprotein lipase (LPL) also facilitates fat storage in both fat and muscle cells. Estrogen and testosterone both influence the activity of LPL. In women, fat cells in the breasts, hips, and thighs produce large amounts of LPL. In men, fat cells in the abdomen produce the most LPL (Votruba & Jensen, 2007). In one study, lower LPL levels were found in Whites than in African Americans, although ethnicity had only a minor effect on the variance in plasma lipoprotein levels after age and other factors were considered (Despres et al., 2000). The less atherogenic profile in African Americans did not, however, translate into a lower risk of heart disease.

Several neurotransmitters are also involved in the regulation of weight. The most important of these is dopamine, which has been shown to have a tremendous effect on regulation of food intake and appetite (Stice, Spoor, Ng, & Zald, 2009). In addition, serotonin has effects on appetite. When extra serotonin is given to lab animals, they decrease their intake of food, rates of eating, and meal sizes (Simansky, 1995). Since depression and obesity are related, a disorder in either dopamine or serotonin levels may affect the ability to lose weight.

Concentrations of the anti-inflammatory hormone adiponectin are lower and insulin concentrations are higher in African Americans than in Whites, especially in older adults (Kanaya et al., 2006). African American men and women also have lower visceral and abdominal subcutaneous adiposity than do Whites (Katzmarzyk et al., 2010). Given this latter finding, the racial variation in the consequences of obesity are even more striking. Understanding why African American adults, who have lower visceral adiposity on average than Whites do, still have a higher risk for obesity-related disorders is an ongoing area of genetic and environmental research (Demerath, 2010).

## Genetic Contributions to Obesity Risk

Although more than 90% of human cases of obesity are polygenic, several monogenic obesity syndromes have influenced our knowledge about the pathogenesis of obesity. These include deletions in PPAR-gamma and leptin. PPAR-gamma is a transcription factor involved in adipocyte differentiation. Humans with mutations of the receptor described so far are severely obese or insulin-resistant (Kersten, Desvergne, & Wahli, 2000). Leptin gene mutations are associated with both overweight and hyperphagia, and thus can induce the metabolic syndrome in White subjects (Lakka et al., 2004). Similar studies have not been done in African Americans.

At least half a dozen quantitative trait loci on several chromosomes influencing obesity have been found across a number of populations and ethnic groups. No studies to date have been able to use a genetic marker to predict obesity definitively and reliably. In the future, genetic studies will be of importance to assess excess risk of obesity (Marti, Moreno-Aliaga, Hebebrand, & Martinez, 2004). Certainly the interaction between genetic makeup and environment complicates understanding the role of genes versus lifestyle and dietary habits in obesity. Energy balance most likely influences weight in combination with genetic susceptibility (Ogden, Yanovski, Carroll, & Flegal, 2007).

## Secondary Causes of Obesity

Several endocrine disorders are associated with obesity, including hypothyroidism, Cushing's syndrome (hypercortisolism), and polycystic ovarian syndrome (PCOS). Cushing's syndrome causes muscle and bone weakness; moodiness, irritability, or depression; sleep disturbances; high blood sugar; and menstrual disorders in women. PCOS is a common endocrine disorder of reproductive-age women, with an estimated prevalence of 4–8% (Knochenhauer, 1998). Women with PCOS are usually obese and intensely insulin-resistant, and display features of the metabolic syndrome. African American women are less likely to exhibit signs of PCOS than are White women (Knochenhauer, 1998). In addition, other endocrine disorders, such as growth hormone deficiency and insulinomas (tumors of the pancreas), can cause obesity.

Medication-related obesity is becoming more common and involves an array of drugs, some with psychoactive properties. These include phenothiazines, sodium valproate, carbamazepine, tricyclic antidepressants, and lithium. In addition, several cancer and diabetes drugs are associated with weight gain, including glucocorticoids, megestrol acetate, thiazolidinediones, sulphonylureas, and even insulin itself. Almost all oral contraceptives are associated with increases in weight. For example, an estimated 10% of adolescent girls ages 15–19 years use Depo-Provera, a long-acting contraceptive, as their contraceptive method (U.S. Census Bureau, 2001). Depo-Provera use among obese women is associated with an increasing rate of weight gain with longer duration of use. Depo-Provera is more commonly used among African American adolescent girls and has contributed to the increase in obesity among this age group (Bonny et al., 2006).

## EPIDEMIOLOGY

About 65% of the U.S. adult population is overweight, and above 30% of these are obese (CDC, 2010a). In the United States, there has been a threefold increase in the number of obese individuals in the past 30 years, with the percentage increasing from approximately 10% to 33% of adults between the ages of 25 and 64. In 2007–2008, the prevalence of obesity was 32.2% among adult men and 35.5% among adult women (Flegal, Carroll, Ogden, & Curtin, 2010). Within that context, obesity rates increased to over 40% among African American adults (CDC, 2010b).

Over the past two decades, the prevalence of children who are obese has doubled, while the number of obese adolescents has tripled. According to the National Health and Nutrition Examination Survey, 31.9% of children and adolescents are overweight (BMI at or above the 85th percentile), and 16.3% are obese (BMI at or above the 95th percentile) (Ogden, Carroll, & Flegal, 2008). African American and Hispanic girls are at particular risk for higher BMI-for-age than their non-Hispanic White counterparts (Ogden et al., 2008). Despite these worrisome statistics, the most recent data from the CDC indicate a slowing of this epidemic among preschoolers. Data from the CDC's Pediatric Nutrition Surveillance System indicates that among low-income children 2–4 years old, the prevalence of obesity increased from 12% in 1998 to 14.5% in 2003, but rose only to 14.6% in 2008 (CDC, 2009). These promising epidemiological outcomes provide support for maintaining an intense focus on reducing rates of pediatric obesity in the United States.

According to a 2007 National Center for Health Statistics report, 23.8% of African American girls ages 12–19 are overweight, compared with 14.6% of White girls the same age (Ogden et al., 2008). These changes will have tremendous future consequences, as obesity at younger ages is associated with more negative health consequences. Prepubescent African American girls are generally leaner than comparable White girls, but by age 20 African American women are considerably heavier than their White counterparts. Therefore, the racial disparity in adiposity appears to evolve during adolescence, not prior to it (Kimm et al., 2001).

About four out of five African American women are overweight or obese. African American women are 70% more likely to be obese than non-Hispanic White women, with 44% of African American women and 25% of White women obese (Ogden et al., 2007). Both age and childbearing have an impact on obesity rates in African American women (Gunderson et al., 2004). In addition to the increase in weight, the height of African American women has been declining both in absolute terms (by 0.56 inches) and relative to that of White women in the past decade, making the potential BMI averages even greater (Komlos, 2010).

The relation between obesity and income among African American women seems to have changed during the past decade. The increase in obesity prevalence is highest in the high-income group for all racial/ethnic groups. Among African American women, the increase in prevalence of obesity in the lowest income group was from 42.1% to 51%, compared to an increase from 28.8% to 45.5% in the highest income group (Ogden et al., 2007). Young African American women from low-education families are still at the greatest risk of obesity. However, young African American men from similar families are at the lowest risk (Robinson, Gordon-Larsen, Kaufman, Suchindran, & Stevens, 2009).

This pattern may just represent a transition, as the rates of obesity in African American men may simply lag behind those in African American women. Forces such as peer group influence and gender-related physical activity choices may be more important than within-family dynamics in explaining the gender difference in obesity prevalence in African American young adults. This pattern makes intervening in families of low socioeconomic status (SES) more challenging, as young African American men and women demonstrate different tendencies toward obesity despite experiencing similar familial socioeconomic situations.

Older African Americans are also more commonly overweight than their White counterparts and experience significant morbidity associated with that excess weight (Bowman, 2009). Because obesity can be underappreciated in this age group, its importance for morbidity is probably underrecognized in older adults. Attitudes among older African Americans suggest that pain is an important cause for decreased activity and subsequent weight gain. Sciatic nerve and arthritic pain in the limbs and back, common in this population, may present limitations to exercise (Lavizzo-Mourey et al., 2001). More prospective weight loss studies in this age group are needed.

## INDIVIDUAL FACTORS AND RESILIENCY

It is important to note that while physical activity is part of the solution to obesity, a Cochrane Database meta-analysis found that exercise alone leads to little weight loss (Shaw, Gennat, O'Rourke, & Del Mar, 2006). In combination with diet, however, exercise results in an average of 3 pounds of weight loss when compared to no exercise/no diet (Shaw et al., 2006). As average BMIs increase in the population, this level of weight loss will not be sufficient to ensure adequate improvements in community health. Many of the reported ethnic differences in obesity and its complications in the United States are markers for differences in education, SES, cultural standards, and utilization of preventive and clinical treatments. In developing interventions, the impact of the above-mentioned nonclinical factors is incredibly great in comparison to the simple physiological derangements of obesity. Behavior is at least as important as physiology.

There are several behavioral factors that have a direct influence on energy balance, and that are associated with excess obesity risk for African Americans in an obesogenic environment. Heesch, Brown, and Blanton (2000) found that physical activity was less common among African American women who lived in rural areas, smoked, and had lower levels of education. African Americans, especially women, are likely to underestimate their body size (Potti, Milli, Jeronis, Gaughan, & Rose, 2009) and to prefer slightly larger body sizes than White women do. Furthermore, African American women are less affected by peer pressure from thinner women to lose weight (Chandler-Laney et al., 2009).

Compared to their White counterparts, young African American women, are more likely to focus on the health consequences of food choices and of obesity, rather than obesity's effects on body size and aesthetics (Malpede et al., 2007). Studies have found that African American women experience less obesity-related social stigma than Whites do. With less external pressure to lose weight among African American women, and more internal focus on health than on the ideal of thinness, the low perceived value of weight loss can impede the use of their financial resources to achieve this goal.

A qualitative study (Thomas, Moseley, Stallings, Nichols-English, & Wanger, 2008) found several factors relating to African American women's weight preferences. Issues included (1) disagreement with the thin "standard"; (2) dislike of physical activity, due to the effect of perspiration on hair and appearance; and (3) lack of access to physical activity programs. In regard to the first issue, African American women in another study were also less likely to internalize the ideal of thinness or to perceive the romantic appeal of thinness (Vaughan, Sacco, & Beckstead, 2008). The factors above can influence desire to reduce food intake and increase energy expenditures among African American women. Accordingly, addressing these factors will be crucial to developing successful programs. Such programs should deal with the need to maintain hair and appearance; use a resilient self-image to advantage, avoid targeting thinness as a goal, focus on the health consequences of weight, and increase access to exercise facilities for African American women. These targeted messages during interventions for African American women may increase the interventions' effectiveness.

Over the past few decades, the increase in the consumption of sugar-sweetened soft drinks, especially among those with lower SES, has paralleled an increase in obesity. Americans increased their caloric intake from soft drinks from 3% of their total energy intake in the 1980s to 7% in the early 2000s, with an increase of calories per day from 50 kcal to 144 kcal (Nielsen & Popkin, 2004). Similarly,

19- to 39-year-olds increased their intake of energy from soft drinks from 4% to 10% of their total intake.

In multiethnic studies, overweight adolescents have been found to consume more savory snacks, watch more television, and drink more fruit juices (Rennie, Johnson, & Jebb, 2005; Singh et al., 2009). Regardless of racial/ethnic group, adolescents tend to consume high amounts of sugar-sweetened beverages (SSBs); however, African American youth consume relatively high quantities of SSBs daily (Lim et al., 2009). Consumption of fast foods is also associated with weight gain and subsequent insulin resistance, although the association is weaker in African Americans than in Whites (Pereira et al., 2005).

Excessive SSB consumption is believed to increase the risk of obesity through a variety of mechanisms. The leading hypothesis is that energy consumed in liquid form is less satisfying than energy in solid foods and leads to overconsumption of large portion sizes of SSBs. These factors have been inconsistently found to be related to obesity, mostly because data are more often cross-sectional and trials are few (Wolff & Dansinger, 2008). More prospective studies with accurate measures of predictors of SSB intake and weight gain will provide better evidence on which to base interventions to achieve long-term behavioral change in African American youth (Ebbeling et al., 2006). However, if serious inroads to decreasing obesity in African American youth are to be made, the reduction of SSB ingestion, especially at school, will be an important step.

## FAMILIAL, CULTURAL, AND ENVIRONMENTAL INFLUENCES

Families are the first level of the ecological context for individuals throughout their lives. Specifically, families form the first environment in which beliefs, values, and social attitudes influence individual development and behavior. Parental lifestyle behaviors are powerful influences on children's health behaviors. Strong social bonds between parents and children increase the likelihood that children will internalize the values and norms about weight exemplified by their parents (Birch et al., 2001; Davidson, Francis, & Birch, 2005). Parents may influence their children by serving as role models for children's food and physical activity behaviors; communicating their views and selectively reinforcing or discouraging behaviors; and influencing children's access to food and physical activity (Birch et al., 2001; Davidson et al., 2005). In addition, parents' attitudes are thought to affect their children indirectly through the foods purchased for and served in the household (Wardle, 1995).

The concept of *feeding styles* has been introduced into the literature to explain parental attitudes toward children around eating within a general parenting style framework. Two recent studies involving low-income families suggested that African American parents, in comparison to White and Hispanic parents, were more often "indulgent" in their dietary parenting styles. They were more likely to allow their children to eat freely, to provide high-calorie food choices, and not to "demand" that the children eat nutritious foods. In the case of preschoolers, too little "demandingness" did not allow adequate intake of fruits and vegetables, and was associated with too many calories consumed during the evening hours (Hennessy, Hughes, Goldberg, Hyatt, & Economos, 2010; Hoerr et al., 2009). The indulgent feeding style was also associated with overweight in preschoolers (Hughes, Shewchuk, Baskin, Nicklas, & Qu, 2008). Depending on their feeding styles, African American families, especially those with limited incomes and access to fresh fruits and vegetables, may inadvertently predispose their children to obesity.

Parental weight status significantly affects familial lifestyle behaviors. Baseline data from a 5-year longitudinal study of family health behaviors indicated that mothers and fathers from obesogenic families reported significantly higher levels of total energy and dietary fat intake, and significantly lower levels of physical activity, than did parents from nonobesogenic families (Davidson et al., 2005). Interestingly, follow-up data indicated distinct similarities in behavioral patterns over time, with parents from obesogenic families reporting less healthy dietary and physical activity practices than those of their nonobesogenic counterparts. Although parents in both groups gained weight over time, the nonobesogenic families appeared to adopt obesity-reducing practices more often than the obesogenic families adopted health-promoting behaviors (Davidson et al., 2005). Girls from obesogenic families had greater increases in their BMI scores over time, had a higher percentage of body fat, and consumed diets higher in fat than girls from nonobesogenic families. The majority of these studies have been conducted with White families; few longitudinal studies of this nature have been documented with African American families.

Gender effects were also noted in findings from the National Longitudinal Study of Adolescent Health. The direct influence of a mother's obesity on her son's body weight was found to be limited to the younger ages, although the indirect influences continue to be felt into young adulthood. In contrast, a father's obesity affects his son's weight from childhood to young adulthood (Crossman, Sullivan, & Benin, 2006). Collectively, these findings illuminate the negative effects for youth living in obesity-promoting environments.

Structural aspects of neighborhoods and communities also contribute to the epidemic of obesity in African American communities. Lack of structures that facilitate energy expenditure contributes to obesity among African American families. African Americans often live in neighborhoods characterized by low sidewalk connectivity (McAlexander, Banda, McAlexander, & Lee, 2009), lack of green spaces (Casagrande, Whitt-Glover, Lancaster, Odoms-Young, & Gary, 2009), and lack of other exercise facilities. Many African American families live in communities that have been found to have a disproportionate presence of fast-food chains and unhealthy-food outdoor advertising.

Television and magazine advertisements aimed at African Americans disproportionately features unhealthy food products. Black faces are also more frequently used to advertise products with negative health impact than are White faces (Duerksen et al., 2005). A recent study found that 24% of African Americans lived in neighborhoods with a low availability of healthy food, compared with 5% of Whites (Franco et al., 2009). Segregation's effects on population and economic characteristics, physical infrastructure, and social processes work in tandem to increase the likelihood that African American neighborhoods in urban environments will bear a disproportionate burden of fast-food restaurants (Kwate, 2008). These social and economic forces form a powerful recipe for obesity, hypertension, heart disease, and diabetes. Increasing supermarket access, places to exercise, and neighborhood safety will be promising strategies to reduce obesity-related complications in the African American community.

## COMPLICATIONS

Obesity influences several body systems: It causes declines in musculoskeletal, cardiac, liver, intestinal, endocrine, and reproductive functions. Obesity, especially chronic obesity, is associated with an excess in joint-related abnormalities and arthritis. In weight-bearing joints such as hips, knees, and ankles, weight gain is associated with an increase in symptoms, and weight loss to near normal/recommended weight is associated with improvement. Obstructive sleep apnea, obesity hypoventilation syndrome (Pickwickian syndrome), increased predisposition to respiratory infections, and increased incidence of bronchial asthma are all related to the anatomic and skeletal changes that occur with obesity (Parameswaran, Todd, & Soth, 2006).

Several metabolic disorders are associated with obesity, including insulin resistance, hyperinsulinemia, Type 2 diabetes mellitus, hypertension, and dyslipidemia (high total cholesterol, high triglycerides, high low-density lipoproteins, and/or low high-density lipoproteins). Type 2 diabetes involves a complex set of metabolic derangements leading to insulin resistance. Almost 80% of the risk of diabetes may be attributed to the effect of inactivity and obesity (Stein & Colditz, 2004). A person's probability of developing diabetes doubles for every 20% increase over desirable body weight (Narayan, Boyle, Thompson, Gregg, & Williamson, 2007). Given that African Americans have a greater prevalence of obesity than Whites do, it is not surprising that they have twice the risk for diabetes (Brancati, Kao, Folsom, & Szklo, 2000).

Significant weight gain or weigh loss strongly influences blood pressure. Obesity is associated with excess risk for hypertension and the increased risk of stroke that accompanies it. The benefits in blood pressure reduction from weight loss in hypertensive patients are also well known. Even if an ideal weight is not reached, weight loss can be beneficial for reducing risk factors, such as blood pressure (Ogden et al., 2007). African Americans have a higher prevalence of hypertension than either Hispanics or non-Hispanic Whites (Kurian & Cardarelli, 2007). There appears to be an effect of race on the obesity–hypertension relationship. Whether the greater prevalence and degree of obesity completely explain the higher prevalence of hypertension in older African Americans is not known (Okosun, Boltri, Anochie, & Chandra, 2004).

Obesity is also a major contributor to metabolic dysfunctions involving lipid and glucose. Dyslipidemia, hypertension, and atherosclerosis are all associated with obesity and cardiac disease. In addition, the inflammatory changes that occur with visceral obesity cause insulin resistance, hypertension, and thrombosis. Central obesity also promotes the release of adipokines, which cause blood vessel plaques, in the bloodstream as a result of excess visceral fat. The actions of leptin and resistin, proteins secreted by fat cells, increase the risk for heart disease. African Americans generally have a less arthrogenic plasma lipid pattern than Whites do, but still have higher rates of coronary heart disease and stroke (Despres et al., 2000). It is not clear why these racial differences are not protective in African Americans. Perhaps the lipid threshold at which their risk increases is at a lower level of triglycerides and a higher level of high-density-lipoprotein cholesterol.

Several cancers are associated with obesity, including prostate, breast, and ovarian cancers. Being overweight or obese is associated with an increased risk of breast cancer among postmenopausal women. Several biological reasons for this have been posited, including increased levels of serum sex hormones; increased insulin and insulin-like growth factor; and increased inflammatory markers. Proportions of breast cancers at advanced stages are highest among overweight and obese women (Kerlikowske et al., 2008). African American women have four times more triple-negative (tumor receptor status) breast cancers than obese non-AA women do, and this association varies with age. Therefore, factors other than whole-body obesity must be important in determining African American women's risk for breast cancer (Stead et al., 2009).

African American women who are breast cancer survivors have a high risk for adverse health effects related to obesity, both before and after their treatment for the disease (Cui et al., 2002). Qualitative studies with African American breast cancer survivors suggest that weight gain is a stressor that generates further concerns about health; that the perceived inability to control weight is a further source of frustration (Hughes Halbert et al., 2008); and that barriers to successful weight control include pain, fatigue, lack of time, and lack of knowledge about what to eat and how to prepare healthy foods (Stolley, Sharp, Wells, Simon, & Schiffer, 2006).

Although the more accepting self-image of African American women has traditionally been protective against eating disorders, there has been a steady increase in binge-eating disorder among African American women (Smolak & Striegel-Moore, 2001). Body image is a less significant predictor of obesity in African American women (Flynn & Fitzgibbon, 1998). However, stressors including economic and other social barriers may influence bulimic and binge-eating disorders, leading to excess weight (Talleyrand, 2006).

Obesity is associated with excess rates of depression, as well as with significant social stigma. Both a decrease in physicians' respect for obese patients and a decreased sense of self-worth have been noted in recent studies (Huizinga, Cooper, Bleich, Clark, & Beach, 2009). Social anthropologists have suggested that the combined challenges of racism and sexism faced by African American women can have an impact on their health and well-being. African American women also typically take on multiple roles within their families (such as economic providers and heads of households), and are therefore more likely to face stresses associated with these roles. Furthermore, African American women are commonly social-ized to appear strong, resilient, and self-sufficient, despite environmental stres-sors they may be experiencing (Talleyrand, 2006).

African Americans and Hispanic Americans generally experience excess mor-tality at higher BMIs than non-Hispanic White Americans. The optimal BMI in terms of life expectancy is about 23–25 for Whites and 23–30 for African Ameri-cans (Durazo-Arvizu, McGee, Cooper, Liao, & Luke, 1998). The ideal BMI for Asians is actually lower than that for Whites. Coexisting obesity and smoking are associated with even greater risks than those for premature mortality. BMI-related increase in risk begins at a 1- to 3-kg/m$^2$ higher BMI for African Americans than for Whites. For White adults with Grade 3 obesity (BMIs of 40–59.9 kg/m$^2$), life expectancy is reduced by as much as 20 years in men and by about 5 years in women (Fontaine, Redden, Wang, Westfall, & Allison, 2003).

## EVIDENCE-BASED INTERVENTIONS

In most clinical interactions between a physician and an obese individual, there is a balance between the "ideal" body weight and the personal goals of the patient. These two goals must be reconciled if there is to be significant progress in weight loss. The possibility of bingeing, purging, lack of satiety, food-seeking behavior, and other abnormal feeding habits must be identified because management of these habits is crucial to the success of any weight management program. Special stages in life, such as pregnancy and childhood status, require more complex goal setting.

### Interventions for Children and Adolescents

Although clinical treatment approaches for pediatric obesity have been effective in the short term; the positive long-term outcomes of treatment approaches are limited (Epstein, Myers, Raynor, & Saelens, 1998; Harrell et al., 1998). In 2007, however, an expert committee recommended a "systematic intensification of efforts, tailored to the capacity of the clinical office, the motivation of the family, and the degree of obesity, with the most aggressive treatment stage being consid-ered only for those who have not responded to other interventions" (Barlow & Expert Committee, 2007).

Not surprisingly, prevention remains Stage 1 of this treatment protocol. Family members are encouraged to consume at least five servings of fruits and vegetables, minimize sugar intake, limit television viewing to no more than 2 hours daily, engage in at least 1 hour of physical activity daily, and eat meals as a family. Furthermore, cultural tailoring of each of these recommendations is suggested. Increasing in intensity, Stage 2 includes structured weight management, meal plans, and supervised physical activity. Comprehensive, multidisciplinary interventions are recommended as needed, with Stage 3 including a tertiary care intervention to follow if needed. Pharmacotherapy, in combination with lifestyle modification, should be considered in obese children after failure of an intensive lifestyle modification alone. Pharmacotherapy is indicated earlier in overweight children with cardiovascular complications or a strong family history of Type 2 diabetes (August et al., 2008).

Few pharmaceutical therapies have received approval from the U.S. Food and Drug Administration (FDA) for the treatment of adolescent obesity. Orlistat has been proven both safe and effective for weight reduction in overweight adolescents, and sibutramine has also been proven effective in reducing weight in this population. Safety and efficacy have only been determined for 2 and 4 years for sibutramine and orlistat, respectively; therefore, concerns about the potential for severe adverse effects (especially in adolescents) require further investigation (Gogakoa, Tzotzas, & Krassas, 2009).

Bariatric surgery for morbidly obese adolescents in the United States has almost quadrupled in recent years, from about 200 in 2000 to nearly 800 in 2003 (Tsai, Inge, & Burd, 2007). To date, adolescent bariatric surgery has resulted in sustained weight loss; however, the potential for complications remains, including possible impacts on neuronal development and on bone growth (Gogakoa et al., 2009). Few African American youth have utilized bariatric surgery.

## Adult Weight Management/Behavior Management

Behavioral aspects of weight management include weekly weight checks, food journals, and monitoring of daily food intake. Behavioral changes for obese individuals includes eating breakfast soon after awakening and eating balanced meals at regular intervals thereafter; incorporating physical activity into the day; and scheduling the week to include rest, play, and social interactions along with work, school, and family responsibilities. Behavior modification in general and cognitive-behavioral therapy in particular have been found to be effective for short-term weight loss in those both with and without an eating disorder (Munsch et al., 2007; Werrij et al., 2010). Generally, however, follow-up over the long term shows that the majority of people regain weight close to pretreatment levels.

Behavior therapy in obesity can identify cravings and weaken or disconnect triggering events that lead to overeating. However, the effectiveness of behavior therapy alone against obesity is modest, compared with the effects of exercise and caloric restriction (Mun, Blackburn, & Matthews, 2001). Both calorie restriction and increase in physical activity or exercise influence weight. Diet-only and diet-plus-exercise interventions are associated with partial weight regain over a 2-year span of time. Diet-plus-exercise programs provide greater long-term weight loss than diet-only interventions (Wu, Gao, Chen, & van Dam, 2009). Maintenance of weight loss for greater than 2 years is associated with successful longer-term weight stabilization (Wing & Phelan, 2005).

## Calorie Restriction

The primary lifestyle changes for combating obesity are decreasing caloric intake and increasing exercise behavior. Very-low-calorie diets (VLCDs) are best used in an established, comprehensive program. VLCDs involve reducing caloric intake to 800 kcal/d or less. They can achieve weight loss of as much as 30 pounds over 12 weeks (Yancy, Olsen, Guyton, Bakst, & Westman, 2004). VLCDs are less appropriate for children, adolescents, or older-adult subjects than for middle-aged adults. They are also not used in people with significant cardiac, renal, hepatic, psychiatric, or cerebrovascular disease. Thus they are of limited value for persons with some of the most common complications of obesity.

VLCDs are associated with profound initial weight loss, much of which is from muscle mass loss in a few weeks (Saris, 2001). These diets are associated with notable short-term weight loss (sometimes less than 15% of baseline weight) and are associated with improved blood pressure and glycemic control, but they cannot be sustained longer than 3–6 months. The greater initial weight loss with a VLCD produces better long-term results if the VLCD period is actively followed up with a program including nutritional education, behavioral therapy, and increased physical therapy. Compliance beyond a few weeks is poor, and the cost of these types of programs is prohibitive for those of low SES.

Low-calorie diets (LCDs), the types that dietitians and most commonly prescribe, are usually high in fiber and have a low concentrated sweet content (Strychar, 2009). These diets underlie most of the popular commercial weight loss programs, such as those advocated by Jenny Craig and Weight Watchers. The basic goal is to keep a detailed dietary inventory, estimate mean daily caloric intake, and decrease it by 10–15%. Although the meals in these programs are based on regular, everyday foods at a decreased portion size, meal replacement shakes, bars, prepackaged meals, and frozen entrees can be used to replace major macronutrients. High-protein and low-fat LCDs have been found to be effective for weight loss in adults (Brehm, Seeley, Daniels, Daniels, & D'Alessio, 2003; Johnston, Tjonn, & Swan, 2004), but no more effective than high-protein, low-carbohydrate diets (Meckling, O'Sullivan, & Saari, 2004). The difference is that low-carbohydrate diets noticeably improve biomarkers for diabetes and the metabolic syndrome (Samaha et al., 2003), even at a 1-year follow-up (Stern et al., 2004).

## Exercise

Exercise is vital to any weight management program because it helps build muscle mass and increases basal metabolic rates (Shaw et al., 2006). Exercise also helps reduce body fat and decreases the amount of muscle mass loss that typically results from weight loss. Consistent moderate exercise is also important in maintaining weight and in improving overall cardiac fitness. Aerobic isotonic exercise is most important for those who are most obese. Anaerobic isometric exercise, including resistance training, can be added after the aerobic goals are achieved. Physical exercise goals are for at least 150 minutes a week of aerobic exercise, such as walking, swimming, or stair climbing. Even if people exercise regularly and do not lose weight, they can reduce the central obesity associated with diabetes and heart disease. Diet associated with exercise produces a 20% greater initial weight loss than dieting alone, so addition of exercise to LCDs has the potential to increase the diets' effectiveness (Curioni & Lourenço, 2005).

## Medical and Surgical Treatments for Adults

### Oral Medications

Several drugs have shown promise in reducing weight in mild to moderate obesity, at least in the short term. Since drug-induced weight loss is never more than 10% of baseline weight, these medications are only appropriate for those with Grade 1 or 2 overweight/obesity (Bray & Tartaglia, 2000). Sibutramine is a centrally acting appetite suppressant that inhibits reuptake of noradrenalin, serotonin, and dopamine. In the Sibutramine Trial of Obesity Reduction and Maintenance, participants were able to maintain a 9% weight loss for as long as 18 months after the start of therapy (James et al., 2000). Orlistat blocks the action of pancreatic lipase, reducing triglyceride absorption (Heck, Yanovski, & Calis, 2000). Two major clinical trials have shown sustained weight loss of 9–10% over 2 years. Weight losses with sibutramine and orlistat are 4.5 and 2.9 kg, respectively (Li et al., 2005).

Both these drugs can produce serious side effects, such as high blood pressure in the blood vessels of the lungs and heart disease. An interim analysis of the Sibutramine Cardiovascular Outcome Trial recently found that sibutramine increased morbidity from cardiovascular disease. For this reason, it has been taken off the market in Europe and is not recommended for those with a history of cardiac disease (FDA, 2010). Moreover, both sibutramine and orlistat are costly prescription drugs that are not readily available to those who are either uninsured or underinsured.

Metformin has become a very effective drug for obese people with symptoms of prediabetes (elevated fasting glucose or glucose intolerance). Several studies show that metformin used for up to 3 years not only decreases the likelihood that prediabetes will progress to diabetes, but causes significant weight loss (Levri et al., 2005; Lilly & Gowin, 2009). Metformin is effective regardless of age and may also have a role in the treatment of other conditions associated with insulin resistance, including PCOS. Metformin's effects on glucose metabolism were studied in African Americans at risk for Type 2 diabetes. Subjects were randomly assigned to receive either metformin (500 mg daily) or placebo; metformin-treated individuals had a modest weight reduction and better liver metabolism of glucose (Schuster, Gaillard, Rhinesmith, Habash, & Osei, 2004). Metformin has been found to be as effective as orlistat in reducing weight and BMI, but inferior to sibutramine (Desilets, Dhakal-Karki, & Dunican, 2008).

Drugs acting on sympathetic tone, such as amphetamines, have been used successfully in the past to encourage weight loss (Bray & Tartaglia, 2000). Ephedrine and caffeine both act by increasing energy expenditure, but they are associated with the potential for tachycardia, hypertension, and palpitations. They are associated with more weight loss when used in combination than when used alone. They cause 60–75% of their weight loss effect by decreasing food intake. Given their lower cost, they are more commonly used by those of low SES.

Other medications for other indications that are sometimes used for weight loss include topiramate, selective serotonin reuptake inhibitors (SSRIs), and other antidepressants. Topiramate, a seizure medication, is associated with loss of as much as 15–18% of baseline body weight, but its severe side effects (e.g., drowsiness, paresthesias, memory loss, and confusion) limit its utility (Bray & Tartaglia, 2000). SSRIs are sometimes used for their anorexic side effect, which leads to mild weight loss; animal studies have also linked serotonin to appetite. Two other antidepressants, bupropion and venlafaxine, also cause mild weight loss (Li et al., 2005). Lastly, activation of the cannabinoid type 1 receptor is associated with increased appetite (Black, 2004). This pathway is a current target for new drugs to treat obesity, including rimonabant (Van Gaal et al., 2005).

### Surgical Treatments: Gastric Bypass and Beyond

Gastric bypass has become a more common treatment of obesity because it can cause loss of over 50–70% excess weight. Surgery is more effective than most LCDs (Mun et al., 2001). The long-term health benefits after bariatric surgery include improved cardiovascular-related and diabetes-related outcomes. These improvements in comorbidities are associated with a decrease in mortality that ranges from 24 to 40%, compared to that for patients treated with weight loss medications (Sjöström et al., 2007). The mortality after gastric bypass is also decreased in comparison to that for control subjects who have not attempted weight loss; however, the procedure is still associated with excess deaths from suicide and accidents, compared to those in the same control subjects (Adams et al., 2007).

Bariatric procedures vary not only in the time until weight loss is achieved or in the mechanisms that effect weight reduction, but also in their effects on glycemic control. After placement of an adjustable gastric band, improvements in glycemic control are dependent on weight loss, and obese patients with diabetes may not see appreciable improvements in blood glucose control for some time. However, after Roux-en-Y gastric bypass (RYGB), most diabetic patients see an improvement in their glycemic control before any weight loss occurs. This is likely because the RYGB may cause extensive improvements in the neuroendocrine system of the gastrointestinal tract. RYGB almost immediately enhances insulin sensitivity and beta-cell responsiveness to glucose, and increases levels of glucagon-like peptide 1, in part because of incretin increases (Kashyap et al., 2010).

The complications of all weight loss surgeries remain numerous; they include vitamin deficiencies, pain with eating, osteoporosis, and late reoperations, as well as inflammation in the transverse mesocolon, ascites, and common bile duct stones (Longitudinal Assessment of Bariatric Surgery Consortium, 2009). Because of the risks of major surgery and the morbidity associated with gastric bypass, further refinements are occurring in surgical approaches to weight loss. For instance, patients with a BMI of more than 50 kg/m² lose more weight after laparoscopic duodenal switch than after laparoscopic RYGB (Søvik et al., 2010). Thus, though this surgery is more invasive, it may be more appropriate for those with morbid or supermorbid obesity.

The prevalence of obesity and obesity-related disorders is on the rise in African American young adults, adolescents, and even in children. Primary prevention through diet and exercise will need to be carefully applied to alleviate the need for any surgical intervention. If obesity is halted early enough, surgery many not be not necessary. Long-term studies on large cohorts that include African Americans are still not available for gastric surgical procedures. Because these procedures are not typically covered by private insurance companies, they are not sustainable solutions for those of low and moderate SES. However, until we see more success with primary prevention to avoid supermorbid obesity or to develop effective medications for Grade 3 and Grade 4 obesity, bariatric surgery will remain an important intervention.

## BARRIERS TO WEIGHT LOSS

Throughout an individual's life, barriers to weight loss or maintenance of normal weight exist. Repeated failed attempts to lose weight are common, and this failure may be accompanied by guilt, hopelessness, and poor self-esteem. Factors that influence individuals' resiliency to these and other stressors are primarily related to increasing their sense of familial and community connection. Building resiliency in African Americans and their communities will require patience and a focus on long-term, communal solutions. Prevention and intervention strategies should be based on evidence-based practices that are tailored to individuals' race, ethnicity, culture, and gender (Fisher et al., 2007).

### Addiction and Binge Eating

Reward and addiction are related to intake of food, and thus potentially to obesity. Dopamine D2 receptor levels are decreased in obese individuals and vary in proportion to their BMIs. This deficiency may drive the overingestion of food to obtain levels similar to those of normal weight (Wang et al., 2001). Brain dopamine and obesity are linked in that dopamine is associated with both alcohol and drug use. It is also associated with both short-term and long-term hunger. These reward pathways are likely to influence the drive to eat, probably through influencing dopamine levels in the nucleus accumbens.

Serotonin- and catecholamine-containing brain neurons are also under dietary control. The injection of insulin and the consumption of a single protein-free high-carbohydrate meal both elevate brain tryptophan and serotonin levels. The addition of protein to the meal suppresses the increases in brain tryptophan and serotonin (Wurtman & Fernstrom, 1975). High-carbohydrate and high-protein foods can cause substantial differences in plasma tryptophan ratio, and thus probably in brain tryptophan concentrations and serotonin synthesis (Wurtman et al., 2003).

Addiction is related to eating in African Americans only inasmuch as we know that African American women are prone to binge eating, and that this disordered eating is associated with excess weight (Striegel-Moore, Wilfley, Pike, Dohm, & Fairburn, 2000). A study also showed that African American women with binge-eating disorder have higher rates of sexual abuse, physical abuse, and bullying by peers—but not discrimination—than healthy African American women do (Striegel-Moore, Dohm, Pike, Wilfley, & Fairburn, 2002). Studies that intervene in addictive eating patterns such as binge eating have not been done in African American women. Interventions that can address the impact of abuse or bullying on eating behavior could improve our ability to facilitate weight loss in the sub-population that experiences these symptoms.

## Depression

Depression is characterized by symptoms of low mood, sadness, helplessness, loss of interest and pleasure in activities, and feelings of worthlessness or guilt. Other symptoms include difficulty concentrating, weight gain or loss, irritability, withdrawal, isolation, thoughts of death, and physical symptoms such as pain (American Psychiatric Association, 2000). Although African American and White women have similar rates of depression in the general population, African American women are less likely to seek treatment and are less likely to be diagnosed with depression when they do seek treatment (O'Malley, Forrest, & Miranda, 2003). Clinical guidelines that stress changes in lifestyle for obesity will be less effective if they do not include strategies for mediating the impact of stress, depression, racism, and discrimination on African Americans. Untreated depressive symptoms are associated with nonadherence to weight loss goals (Teixeira et al., 2004). The treatment of obesity will probably need to include interventions that treat depression in African Americans and mobilize resources in the community, such as progressive churches, grassroots groups, and political organizations.

Approximately 25% increased rates of depression have been found in severely obese people (Simon et al., 2006). One explanation for this may be found in studies suggesting a biological link between depression and increased adiposity/weight gain, possibly mediated through changes in dopamine levels and the reward centers of the brain (Morton, Cummings, Baskin, Barsh, & Schwartz, 2006). Depression has been found to be related to visceral obesity in women (Everson-Rose et al., 2009). Weight loss often leads to improved depression scores (Dixon, Dixon, & O'Brien, 2003). Depression is more commonly seen in obese women and teenagers, and is less likely to be diagnosed in obese men (Linde et al., 2004). Depression, especially in younger women, is associated with weight gain. Depression has been associated with poor weight loss outcomes (Dixon et al., 2003; McGuire, Wing, Klem, Lang, & Hill, 1999). Bariatric surgery patients with poorly managed depression or anxiety are at greater risk for weight regain within the first 5 postoperative years (Ames, Patel, Ames, & Lynch, 2009). More studies are needed to address the links between obesity and depression, especially in African Americans.

## PREVENTION

In general, obesity prevention efforts operate at four levels: *primordial, primary, secondary,* and *tertiary* (World Health Organization, 1998; World Health Organization Expert Committee, 1990). Primordial prevention focuses on the underlying conditions leading to exposure to the causative factors of obesity (Fuster, 2005). Primary prevention is aimed at reducing the number of new cases of obesity (incidence), or completely preventing the development of obesity. These efforts usually include lifestyle-based, nonmedical interventions (Fox & Trautman, 2009). Secondary prevention is aimed at reducing the number of those who are already overweight/obese (prevalence), or controlling existing obesity to reduce the severity of the problem. These types of prevention efforts focus on normalizing body fat and body weight, as well as on long-term weight maintenance. Finally, tertiary prevention is aimed at reducing the degree of morbidity associated with overweight/obesity.

### Prevention in Childhood

Childhood obesity is difficult to treat successfully. At this time, there are no "gold standard" treatment protocols or other interventions to address this issue. This dearth of interventions, combined with concerns about the potential negative effects of dieting during childhood, necessitates a focus on prevention to slow and ultimately reverse the obesity epidemic. Systematic literature reviews have identified several known modifiable and immutable risk factors for pediatric obesity: parental obesity, birthweight, dietary factors, physical inactivity, timing of puberty, degree of exposure to toxic environmental factors, behavioral variables, and psychosocial factors (Campbell, Waters, O'Mera, & Summerbell, 2001; Doak, Heitman, Summerbell, & Lissner, 2009; Summerbell et al., 2005).

Childhood obesity prevention interventions typically target one or more of the modifiable risk factors. Despite the disturbing obesity trends among African American youth, surprisingly few intervention studies developed for this group have been reported in the scientific literature (Alio et al., 2006). Furthermore, the vast majority of this literature focuses on low-income populations, providing an incomplete assessment of the heterogeneity of issues in communities of color.

### Physical Activity Approaches

Barriers to regular physical activity among racial/ethnic minority children range from environmental and socioeconomic barriers to preferences for sedentary activities (Burnet et al., 2008). Opportunities for regular physical activity in safe environments can pose a challenge for disadvantaged pediatric populations. Furthermore, time for physical activity in schools has been greatly reduced during the school day, and competitive sports (which often eliminate many youth from participation) are the dominant models from middle school onward. High amounts of leisure time may therefore be spent in sedentary behaviors such as television viewing, where frequent exposure to advertisements for high-calorie, low-nutrient foods is likely (Grier & Kumanyika, 2008).

There is a dearth of interventions to increase physical activity among African American youth. A recently published systematic review of physical activity interventions found only 14 studies that targeted African American children and adolescents; most of these studies reported null results (Whitt-Glover & Kumanyika, 2009). However, a few promising approaches have emerged. A 14-week after-school program for 5- to 10-year-olds (51% female, 91% African American) significantly improved cardiovascular fitness, body composition, and some dietary habits (Topp et al., 2009). Students participated three times each week in 90-minute sessions involving track-and-field activities. Nutrition education was aimed at changing attitudes, perceptions, and beliefs about obesity and fast-food consumption. The findings from this pilot study provide a preliminary basis for assessing the efficacy of the intervention in a larger, more rigorously conducted intervention.

### Dietary Approaches

Nutrition is a major determinant of body size, and eating occurs within particular social and cultural environments. Since young children rely on their parents and family members for their nutrition, changes in the home food environment have a positive impact on obesity (Hudson, 2008). Dietary risk factors that predispose to obesity include lack of infant breastfeeding; frequent intake of SSBs and fruit juice (Ebbeling et al., 2006); large portion sizes; frequency of fast-food consumption and intake of fried foods; and infrequent intake of fruits and vegetables. African American children are disproportionately exposed to each of the aforementioned risk factors. For example, several studies suggest that breastfeeding may be protective against the development of obesity in childhood (August et al., 2008). However, in general, African American mothers tend to bottle-feed their infants (Woo, Dolan, Morrow, Geraghty, & Goodman, 2008).

Portion sizes have increased tremendously in the past 20 years (Young & Nestle, 2003). Several national reports, including the 2001 U.S. Surgeon General's call to action on obesity prevention, have emphasized the need to address portion size as a factor in the obesity epidemic (U.S. Department of Health and Human Services, 2001). The toxic food environments in many low-income and minority communities predispose many African American children to consume the large portion sizes offered in fast-food restaurants. Value menu pricing offers a higher volume of low-nutrient, calorie-dense foods for a minimal cost.

Few intervention studies have been specifically designed for African American youth, and the vast majority have been tailored for girls. The Girls health Enrichment Multi-site Studies (GEMS), funded by the National Heart, Lung, and Blood Institute, focused on obesity prevention with 8- to 10-year-old African American girls (Obarzanek & Pratt, 2003). These unique interventions, conducted at four field centers, were 12-week pilot studies examining approaches to preventing weight gain in African American girls at risk for obesity (Rochon et al., 2003). Details of each of these studies are presented elsewhere (Baranowski, Baranowski, Cullen, Thompson, & Nicklas, 2003; Beech et al., 2003; Kumanyika, Obarzanek, Robinson, & Beech, 2003; Robinson et al., 2003; Story et al., 2003). Although the GEMs research was not powered to detect changes in BMI, the interventions were successful in reducing the consumption of SSBs (Beech et al., 2003) and decreasing television viewing (Robinson et al., 2003).

## Prevention and Management in Adulthood

Although prevention and treatment of childhood obesity among African American children are imperative for protecting the health and life expectancy of future generations of African Americans, interventions for African American adults are also vital—not only to support parents in preventing childhood obesity, but to improve adults' overall health, including the prevention of diabetes and other chronic consequences of obesity. Lifestyle interventions to optimize energy balance may include dietary interventions to reduce energy intake and/or exercise-based programs aimed at increasing energy expenditure.

Whitt-Glover, Hogan, Lang, and Heil (2008) implemented a church-based program to increase physical activity among sedentary African Americans. They found that after 12 weeks, the 87 participants increased both moderate-intensity and vigorous-intensity physical activity, as well as number of steps walked over the course of a week. Thompson, Berry, and Nasir (2009) conducted a review of church-based weight management programs among African Americans. Specifically, they found that after the 16 interventions reviewed in their study, participants demonstrated significant weight loss ranging from 2 to 10 pounds. In their overview of effective interventions to increase physical activity in African Americans, Whitt-Glover and Kumanyika (2009) have highlighted the importance of a structured exercise component to success. They did not note an increased rate of success for culturally adapted programs, however.

Kumanyika and colleagues (2009) conducted a 2-year weight loss program (Supporting Healthy Activity and eating Right Everyday, or SHARE) for African American adults and their families/friends. Index participants enrolled either alone (*n* = 63) or with one or two family members (*n* = 130). Participants were randomly assigned to either a high- or low-social-support treatment condition; the vast majority (90%) were women. Grounded in social support frameworks, the intervention concepts and approaches were adapted from large evidence-based trials such as the Diabetes Prevention Program and Look Ahead. Over a 6-month period, group intervention sessions were held weekly for 90 minutes, augmented by periodic personal sessions for problem solving. Despite the fact that the SHARE program was theoretically sound and culturally tailored, differences between the intervention conditions were not found. Interestingly, however, greater weight loss in the index participants was associated with greater partner participation and weight loss.

## The Importance of Church- and Community-Based Interventions

As noted above, church-based programs have generally been shown to be effective in weight reduction among African Americans. The church setting may provide an effective and culturally appropriate way to deliver information and interventions related to health and nutrition program (Kennedy et al., 2005). For example, a randomized church-based clinical trial designed to promote fruit and vegetable intake among African Americans showed that using motivational techniques grounded in a spiritual, church-based framework could significantly increase intake of these healthy foods (Resnicow et al., 2004, 2005).

Energy balance strategies targeting obesity among African Americans may benefit from the emphasis of social interaction at the community and family levels (Burnet et al., 2008; Low, Grothe, Wofford, & Bouldin, 2007; Parham & Scarinci, 2007). Several types of community- and family-based interventions have been found to be successful. For example, a national program called Sisters Together: Move More, Eat Better is administered through community organizations. This program contains a guide that helps community leaders through the process of planning, promotion, implementation, and evaluation. The program is funded by the National Institute of Diabetes and Digestive and Kidney Diseases. The Sisters Together programs helps African American women and their families to improve their eating and exercise habits (Curtis, Brown, & Gill, 2008).

Other nationwide community-based initiatives have targeted different aspects of improving energy balance. A program funded by the Robert Wood Johnson Foundation, Active Living by Design (ALBD), promotes community-based innovations designed to alter social and physical environments to promote physical activity (Bussel, Leviton, & Orleans, 2009). For example, the ALBD program in Buffalo, New York, called the Healthy Communities Initiative (HCI), targets African American neighborhoods. The initiative's goals are to "develop and maintain an effective partnership to promote physical activity, increase community awareness of the benefits of active living, increase access to opportunities for physical activity, enhance policy and organizational supports, and improve built and natural environments to support active living in the campus and its surrounding neighborhoods." The HCI has been successful in making changes to the built environment that encourage physical activity in target neighborhoods (Lovasi, Hutson, Guerra, & Neckerman, 2009).

Lastly, community-based interventions involving African American community establishments have been successful in improving obesogenic behavior. Yancey and colleagues (2006) conducted a culturally adapted, community-based trial among 366 healthy, obese African American women. The trial was administered through local African American–owned fitness establishments and included social support, health education components, and a free gym membership. Modest improvements in body composition were found. The free gym membership was the most potent component.

## RECOMMENDED BEST PRACTICES

In summary, this chapter describes approaches for both the prevention and treatment of obesity. Although behavioral strategies to increase physical activity and decrease caloric intake work in the short term, longer-term studies that show significant and lasting weight loss are less common, especially in African Americans. Most studies show evidence and promise for promotion of weight loss in a communal context (Faith, Fontaine, Baskin, & Allison, 2007). Thus they include several components of the ecological model: They address individual, family, and environmental effects on adherence to dietary and exercise regimens to reduce weight and maintain weight loss.

On the basis of the research reviewed in this chapter, we make several recommendations regarding interventions to promote weight loss in obese African Americans:

1. Early intervention is crucial to avoid the metabolic and cardiovascular complications associated with excess weight.

2. Greater consideration should be given to medical/surgical interventions, given the lack of evidence for the efficacy of behavioral approaches as a long-term solution.

3. Obese children and adolescents must be prioritized for intervention, to give them the best chances of avoiding the long-term complications of obesity.

4. Obesity interventions in the African American community must continue to balance the individual person and his or her family and community context.

5. Additional research is needed on the sustainability, the long-term effects, and the potential for more widespread use of obesity-related interventions among African Americans.

6. Additional studies specific to African Americans, with a focus on men and older adults, are needed to inform longer-term weight loss programs.

Multiple interventions for obesity exist, but most are not sufficiently successful to provide an evidence-based practice approach for African Americans. However, we have discussed several factors influencing behavioral and medical management. Findings from these approaches suggest that successful interventions include two or more components of the ecological model. Resource availability has thus far limited the implementation of interventions using all levels of the model. The best methods of delivery in any environment will be culturally conscious, cost-effective, and sustainable for long-term weight loss.

## REFERENCES

Adams, T., Gress, R., Sherman, C., Halverson, R., Simper, S., Rosamond, W., et al. (2007). Long-term mortality after gastric bypass surgery. *New England Journal of Medicine, 357,* 753–761.

Alio, A., Salihu, H., Berrings, T., Gramling, M., Burton, J., Gayles, J., et al. (2006). Obesity research and the forgotten African American child. *Ethnicity and Disease, 16*(2), 569–575.

Alonso, Y. (2004). The biopsychosocial model in medical research: The evolution of the health concept over the last two decades. *Patient Education and Counseling, 53*(2), 239–244.

American Psychiatric Association (2000). *Diagnostic and statistical manual of mental disorders* (4th ed., text rev.). Washington, DC: Author.

Ames, G., Patel, R., Ames, S., & Lynch, S. (2009). Weight loss surgery: Patients who regain. *Obesity and Weight Management, 5*(4), 154–161.

August, G., Caprio, S., Fennoy, I., Freemark, M., Kaufman, F., Lustig, R., et al. (2008). Prevention and treatment of pediatric obesity: An Endocrine Society clinical practice guideline based on expert opinion. *Journal of Clinical Endocrinology and Metabolism, 93*(12), 4576–4599.

Baranowski, T., Baranowski, T., Cullen, K., Thompson, D., & Nicklas, T. (2003). The Fun, Food, and Fitness Project (FFFP): The Baylor GEMS pilot study. *Ethnicity and Disease, 13*(1, Suppl. 1), S30–S39.

Barlow, S., & Expert Committee. (2007). Expert committee recommendations regarding the prevention, assessment, and treatment of child and adolescent overweight and obesity: Summary report. *Pediatrics, 120*(Suppl. 4), S164–S192.

Beech, B., Klesges, R., Kumanyika, S., Murray, D., Klesges, L., McClanahan, B., et al.

(2003). Child- and parent-targeted interventions: The Memphis GEMS pilot study. *Ethnicity and Disease, 13*(1, Suppl. 1), S40–S53.

Birch, L., Fisher, J., Grimm-Thomas, K., Markey, C., Sawyer, R., & Johnson, S. (2001). Confirmatory factor analysis of the Child Feeding Questionnaire: A measure of parental attitudes, beliefs and practices about child feeding and obesity proneness. *Appetite, 36*, 201–210.

Black, S. (2004). Cannabinoid receptor antagonists and obesity. *Current Opinion in Investigational Drugs, 5*, 389–394.

Bonny, A., Ziegler, J., Harvey, R., Debanne, S., Secic, M., & Cromer, B. (2006). Weight gain in obese and nonobese adolescent girls initiating depot medroxyprogesterone, oral contraceptive pills, or no hormonal contraceptive method. *Archives of Pediatrics and Adolescent Medicine, 160*, 40–45.

Bowman, S. (2009). Socioeconomic characteristics, dietary and lifestyle patterns, and health and weight status of older adults in NHANES, 1999–2002: A comparison of Caucasians and African Americans. *Journal of Nutrition for the Elderly, 28*(1), 30–46.

Brancati, F. L., Kao, W. L., Folsom, A. R., & Szklo, M. (2000). Incident Type 2 diabetes mellitus in African American and White adults: The Atherosclerosis Risk in Communities study. *Journal of the American Medical Association, 283*(17), 2253–2259.

Bray, G., & Tartaglia, L. (2000). Medicinal strategies in the treatment of obesity. *Nature, 404*, 672–677.

Brehm, B., Seeley, R., Daniels, S., Daniels, S., & D'Alessio, D. (2003). A randomized trial comparing a very low carbohydrate diet and a calorie-restricted low fat diet on body weight and cardiovascular risk factors in healthy women. *Journal of Clinical Endocrinology and Metabolism, 88*, 1617–1623.

Burnet, D., Plaut, A., Ossowski, K., Ahmad, A., Quinn, M., Radovick, S., et al. (2008). Community and family perspectives on addressing overweight in urban, African American youth. *Journal of General Internal Medicine, 23*(2), 175–179.

Bussel, J., Leviton, L., & Orleans, C. (2009). Active living by design: Perspectives from the Robert Wood Johnson Foundation. *American Journal of Preventive Medicine, 37*(Suppl. 2), S309–S312.

Cameron, N., & Demerath, E. (2002). Critical periods in human growth and their relationship to diseases of aging. *American Journal of Physical Anthropology, 119*(Suppl. 35), 159–184.

Campbell, K., Waters, E., O'Mera, S., & Summerbell, C. (2001). Interventions for preventing obesity in childhood: A systematic review. *Obesity Reviews, 2*(3), 149–157.

Casagrande, S., Whitt-Glover, M., Lancaster, K., Odoms-Young, A., & Gary, T. (2009). Built environment and health behaviors among African Americans: A systematic review. *American Journal of Preventive Medicine, 36*(2), 174–181.

Centers for Disease Control and Prevention (CDC). (2009). Obesity prevalence among low-income, preschool-aged children—United States, 1998–2008. *Morbidity and Mortality Weekly Report, 58*(28), 769–773.

Centers for Disease Control and Prevention (CDC). (2010a). *Obesity: Halting the epidemic by making health easier.* Atlanta, GA: Author. Retrieved February 11, 2010, from *www.cdc.gov/nccdphp/publications/AAG/pdf/obesity.pdf*

Centers for Disease Control and Prevention (CDC). (2010b). *Prevalence of overweight, obesity and extreme obesity among adults: United States, trends 1976–1980 through*

*2005–2006.* Atlanta, GA: Author. Retrieved January 21, 2010, from *www.cdc.gov/nchs/ products/pubs/pubd/hestats/overweight/overweight_adult.htm*

Chandler-Laney, P., Hunter, G., Ard, J., Brock, D., Gower, B., & Roy, J. (2009). Perception of others' body size influences weight loss and regain for European American but not African American women. *Health Psychology, 28*(4), 414–418.

Crossman, A., Sullivan, D., & Benin, M. (2006). The family environment and American adolescents' risk of obesity as young adults. *Social Science and Medicine, 63,* 2255–2267.

Cui, Y., Whiteman, M., Langenberg, P., Sexton, M., Tkaczuk, K., Flaws, J., et al. (2002). Can obesity explain the racial difference in stage of breast cancer at diagnosis between Black and White women? *Journal of Women's Health and Gender-Based Medicine, 11*(6), 527–536.

Curioni, C., & Lourenço, P. (2005). Long-term weight loss after diet and exercise: A systematic review. *International Journal of Obesity, 29*(10), 1168–1174.

Curtis, L., Brown, Z., & Gill, J. (2008). Sisters Together: Move More, Eat Better: A community-based health awareness program for African-American women. *Journal of the National Black Nurses Association, 19*(2), 59–64.

Davidson, K., Francis, L., & Birch, L. (2005). Reexamining obesigenic families: Parents' obesity-related behaviors predict girls' change in BMI. *Obesity Research, 13,* 1980–1990.

Demerath, E. (2010). Causes and consequences of human variation in visceral adiposity. *American Journal of Clinical Nutrition, 91,* 1–2.

Desilets, A., Dhakal-Karki, S., & Dunican, K. (2008). Role of metformin for weight management in patients without Type 2 diabetes. *Annals of Pharmacotherapy, 42*(6), 817–826.

Despres, J., Couillard, C., Gagnon, J., Bergeron, J., Leon, A., Rao, D., et al. (2000). Race, visceral adipose tissue, plasma lipids, and lipoprotein lipase activity in men and women. The Health, Risk Factors, Exercise Training, and Genetics (HERITAGE) family study. *Arteriosclerosis, Thrombosis, and Vascular Biology, 20,* 1932–1938.

Dixon, J., Dixon, M., & O'Brien, P. (2003). Depression in association with severe obesity: Changes with weight loss. *Archives of Internal Medicine, 163,* 2058–2065.

Doak, C., Heitman, B., Summerbell, C., & Lissner, L. (2009). Prevention of childhood obesity: What type of evidence should we consider relevant? *Obesity Reviews, 10*(3), 350–356.

Duerksen, S., Mikail, A., Tom, L., Patton, A., Lopez, J., Amador, X., et al. (2005). Health disparities and advertising content of women's magazines: A cross-sectional study. *BioMed Central Public Health, 5,* 85.

Durazo-Arvizu, R., McGee, D., Cooper, R., Liao, Y., & Luke, A. (1998). Mortality and optimal body mass index in a sample of the U.S. population. *American Journal of Epidemiology, 147,* 739–749.

Ebbeling, C., Feldman, H., Osganian, S., Chomitz, V., Ellenbogen, S., & Ludwig, D. (2006). Effects of decreasing sugar-sweetened beverage consumption on body weight in adolescents: A randomized, controlled pilot study. *Pediatrics, 117,* 673–680.

Epstein, L., Myers, M., Raynor, H., & Saelens, B. (1998). Treatment of pediatric obesity. *Pediatrics, 101*(Suppl. 3), S554–S570.

Everson-Rose, S., Lewis, T., Karavolos, K., Dugan, S., Wesley, D., & Powell, L. (2009).

Depressive symptoms and increased visceral fat in middle-aged women. *Psychosomatic Medicine, 71*(4), 410–416.

Faith, M., Fontaine, K., Baskin, M., & Allison, D. (2007). Toward the reduction of population obesity: Macrolevel environmental approaches to the problems of food, eating, and obesity. *Psychological Bulletin, 133*(2), 205–226.

Finkelstein, E., Trogar, J., Cohen, J., & Dietz, W. (2009). Annual medical spending attributable to obesity: Payer- and service-specific estimates. *Health Affairs, 28*(5), 822–831.

Fisher, E., Brownson, C., O'Toole, M., Shetty, G., Anwuri, V., Fazzone, P., et al. (2007). The Robert Wood Johnson Foundation Diabetes Initiative: Demonstration projects emphasizing self-management. *The Diabetes Educator, 33,* 83–94.

Flegal, K., Carroll, M., Ogden, C., & Curtin, L. (2010). Prevalence and trends in obesity among US adults, 1999–2008. *Journal of the American Medical Association, 303*(3), 235–241.

Flynn, K., & Fitzgibbon, M. (1998). Body images and obesity risk among Black females: A review of the literature. *Annals of Behavioral Medicine, 20,* 13–24.

Fontaine, K., Redden, D., Wang, C., Westfall, A., & Allison, D. (2003). Years of life lost due to obesity. *Journal of the American Medical Association, 289*(2), 187–193.

Food and Drug Administration (FDA). (2010). Follow-up to the November 2009 early communication about an ongoing safety review of sibutramine, marketed as Meridia. Retrieved February 10, 2010, from *www.fda.gov/Drugs/DrugSafety/PostmarketDrugSafetyInformationforPatientsandProviders/DrugSafetyInformationforHeathcareProfessionals/ucm198206.htm*

Fox, R., & Trautman, D. (2009). The epidemic of childhood obesity: A case for primary prevention. *Bariatric Nursing and Surgical Patient Care, 4*(3), 169–172.

Franco, M., Diez-Roux, A., Nettleton, J., Lazo, M., Brancati, F., Caballero, B., et al. (2009). Availability of healthy foods and dietary patterns: The Multi-Ethnic Study of Atherosclerosis. *American Journal of Clinical Nutrition, 89*(3), 897–904.

Freedman, D., Khan, L., Serdula, M., Dietz, W., Srinivasan, S., & Berenson, G. (2005). Racial differences in the tracking of childhood BMI to adulthood. *Obesity Research, 13,* 928–935.

Freedman, D., & Sherry, B. (2009). The validity of BMI as an indicator of body fatness and risk among children. *Pediatrics, 124*(Suppl. 1), S23–S34.

Fuster, V. (2005). Childhood: A critical focus for primordial prevention research. *Cardiovascular Medicine, 2*(3), 113.

Gallagher, D., Heymsfield, S., Heo, M., Jebb, S., Murgatroyd, P., & Sakamoto, Y. (2000). Healthy percentage body fat ranges: An approach for developing guidelines based on body mass index. *American Journal of Clinical Nutrition, 72*(3), 694–701.

Gogakoa, A., Tzotzas, T., & Krassas, G. (2009). Recent concepts of pharmacotherapy and bariatric surgery for childhood obesity: An overview. *Pediatric Endocrinology Review, 7*(2), 83–94.

Grier, S., & Kumanyika, S. (2008). The context for choice: Health implications of targeted food and beverage marketing to African Americans. *American Journal of Public Health, 98*(9), 1616–1629.

Guize, L., Thomas, F., Pannier, B., Bean, K., Jego, B., & Benetos, A. (2007). All-cause mortality associated with specific combinations of the metabolic syndrome according to recent definitions. *Diabetes Care, 30,* 2381–2387.

Gunderson, E., Murtaugh, M., Lewis, C., Quesenberry, C., West, D. S., & Sidney, S. (2004). Excess gains in weight and waist circumference associated with childbearing: The Coronary Artery Risk Development in Young Adults Study (CARDIA). *International Journal of Obesity, 28,* 525–535.

Harrell, J., Gansky, S., McMurray, R., Bangdiwala, S., Frauman, A., & Bradley, C. (1998). School-based interventions improve heart health in children with multiple cardio-vascular disease risk factors. *Pediatrics, 102,* 371–380.

Heck, A., Yanovski, J., & Calis, K. (2000). Orlistat, a new lipase inhibitor for the management of obesity. *Pharmacotherapy, 20*(3), 270–279.

Heesch, K., Brown, D., & Blanton, C. (2000). Perceived barriers to exercise and stage of exercise adoption in older women of different racial/ethnic groups. *Women's Health, 30*(4), 61–76.

Hennessy, E., Hughes, S., Goldberg, J., Hyatt, R., & Economos, C. (2010). Parent behavior and child weight status among a diverse group of underserved rural families. *Appetite, 54*(2), 369–377.

Hoerr, S., Hughes, S., Fisher, J., Nicklas, T., Liu, Y., & Shewchuk, R. (2009). Associations among parental feeding styles and children's food intake in families with limited incomes. *International Journal of Behavioral Nutrition and Physical Activity, 13*(6), 55.

Hudson, C. (2008). Being overweight and obese: Black children ages 2–5 years. *ABNF Journal, 19*(3), 89–91.

Hughes, S., Shewchuk, R., Baskin, M., Nicklas, T., & Qu, H. (2008). Indulgent feeding style and children's weight status in preschool. *Journal of Developmental and Behavioral Pediatrics, 29*(5), 403–410.

Hughes Halbert, C., Weathers, B., Esteve, R., Audrain-McGovern, J., Kumyanika, S., DeMichele, A., et al. (2008). Experiences with weight change in African American breast cancer survivors. *The Breast Journal, 14*(2), 182–187.

Huizinga, M., Cooper, L., Bleich, S., Clark, J. M., & Beach, M. (2009). Physician respect for patients with obesity. *Journal of General Internal Medicine, 24*(11), 1236–1239.

James, W., Astrup, A., Finer, N., Hilsted, J., Kopelman, P., Rössner, S., et al. (2000). Effect of sibutramine on weight maintenance after weight loss: A randomised trial. STORM Study Group. Sibutramine Trial of Obesity Reduction and Maintenance. *Lancet, 356,* 2119–2125.

Johnston, C., Tjonn, S., & Swan, P. (2004). High-protein, low-fat diets are effective for weight loss and favorably alter biomarkers in healthy adults. *Journal of Nutrition, 134*(3), 586–591.

Kanaya, A. M., Wassel Fyr, C., Vittinghoff, E., Havel, P. J., Cesari, M., Nicklas, B., et al. (2006). Serum adiponectin and coronary heart disease risk in older Black and White Americans. *Journal of Clinical Endocrinology and Metabolism, 91*(12), 5044–5050.

Kashyap, S., Daud, S., Kelly, K., Gastaldelli, A., Win, H., Brethauer, S., et al. (2010). Acute effects of gastric bypass versus gastric restrictive surgery on beta-cell function and insulinotropic hormones in severely obese patients with Type 2 diabetes. *International Journal of Obesity, 34*(3), 462–471.

Katzmarzyk, P., Bray, G., Greenway, F., Johnson, W., Newton, J., Ravussin, E., et al. (2010). Racial differences in abdominal depot-specific adiposity in White and African American adults. *American Journal of Clinical Nutrition, 91,* 7–15.

Kennedy, B., Paeratakul, S., Champagne, C., Ryan, D., Harsha, D., McGee, B., et al. (2005). A pilot church-based weight loss program for African-American adults using church members as health educators: A comparison of individual and group intervention. *Ethnicity and Disease, 15*(3), 373–378.

Kerlikowske, K., Walker, R., Miglioretti, D., Desai, A., Ballard-Barbash, R., & Buist, D. (2008). Obesity, mammography use and accuracy, and advanced breast cancer risk. *Journal of the National Cancer Institute, 100,* 1724–1733.

Kersten, S., Desvergne, B., & Wahli, W. (2000). Roles of PPARs in health and disease. *Nature, 405,* 421–424.

Kimm, S., Barton, B., Obarzanek, E., McMahon, R., Sabry, Z., Waclawiw, M., et al. (2001). Racial divergence in adiposity during adolescence: The NHLBI Growth and Health Study. *Pediatrics, 107*(3), e34.

Knochenhauer, E. S. (1998). Prevalence of the polycystic ovary syndrome in unselected Black and White women of the Southeastern United States: A prospective study. *Journal of Clinical Endocrinology and Metabolism, 83*(9), 3078–3082.

Komlos, J. (2010). The recent decline in the height of African-American women. *Economics and Human Biology, 8*(1), 58–66.

Kumanyika, S., Obarzanek, E., Robinson, T., & Beech, B. (2003). Phase 1 of the Girls health Enrichment Multi-site Studies (GEMS): Conclusion. *Ethnicity and Disease, 13*(1, Suppl. 1), S88–S91.

Kumanyika, S., Wadden, T., Shults, J., Fassbender, J., Brown, S., Bowman, M., et al. (2009). Trial of family and friend support for weight loss in African American adults. *Archives of Internal Medicine, 169*(19), 1795–1804.

Kurian, A., & Cardarelli, K. (2007). Racial and ethnic differences in cardiovascular disease risk factors: A systematic review. *Ethnicity and Disease, 17*(1), 143–152.

Kwate, N. (2008). Fried chicken and fresh apples: Racial segregation as a fundamental cause of fast food density in Black neighborhoods. *Health Place, 14*(1), 32–44.

Lakka, T., Rankinen, T., Weisnagel, S., Chagnon, Y., Lakka, H., Ukkola, O., et al. (2004). Leptin and leptin receptor gene polymorphisms and changes in glucose homeostasis in response to regular exercise in nondiabetic individuals: The HERITAGE family study. *Diabetes, 53*(6), 1603–1608.

Lavizzo-Mourey, R., Cox, C., Strumpf, N., Edwards, W., Lavizzo-Mourey, R., Stinemon, M., et al. (2001). Attitudes and beliefs about exercise among elderly African Americans in an urban community. *Journal of the National Medical Association, 83*(12), 475–480.

Levri, K., Slaymaker, E., Last, A., Yeh, J., Ference, J., D'Amico, F., et al. (2005). Metformin as treatment for overweight and obese adults: A systematic review. *Annals of Family Medicine, 3,* 457–461.

Li, Z., Maglione, M., Tu, W., Mojica, W., Arterburn, D., Shugarman, L., et al. (2005). Meta-analysis: Pharmacologic treatment of obesity. *Annals of Internal Medicine, 142,* 532–546.

Lilly, M., & Gowin, M. (2009). Treating prediabetes with metformin: Systematic review and meta-analysis. *Canadian Family Physician, 55*(4), 363–369.

Lim, A., Zoellner, J., Lee, J., Burt, B., Sandretto, A., Sohn, W., et al. (2009). Obesity and sugar-sweetened beverages in African American preschool children: A longitudinal study. *Obesity, 17*(6), 1262–1268.

Linde, J., Jeffery, R., Levy, R., Sherwood, N., Utter, J., Pronk, N., et al. (2004). Binge eating disorder, weight control self-efficacy, and depression in overweight men and women. *International Journal of Obesity, 28,* 418–425.

Lloyd-Jones, D., Sutton-Tyrrell, K., Patel, A., Matthews, K., Pasternak, R., Everson-Rose, S., et al. (2005). Ethnic variation in hypertension among premenopausal and peri-menopausal women: Study of women's health across the nation. *Hypertension, 46,* 689–695.

Longitudinal Assessment of Bariatric Surgery Consortium. (2009). Perioperative safety in the longitudinal assessment of bariatric surgery. *New England Journal of Medicine, 361,* 445–454.

Lovasi, G., Hutson, M., Guerra, M., & Neckerman, K. (2009). Built environments and obesity in disadvantaged populations. *Epidemiology Review, 31,* 7–20.

Lovejoy, J., de la Bretonne, J., Lemperer, M., & Tulley, R. (1996). Abdominal fat distribution and metabolic risk factors: Effects of race. *Metabolism, 45,* 1119–1124.

Low, A., Grothe, K., Wofford, T., & Bouldin, M. (2007). Addressing disparities in cardiovascular risk through community-based interventions. *Ethnicity and Disease, 17*(Suppl. 2), S55–S59.

Malpede, C., Greene, L., Fitzpatrick, S., Jefferson, W., Shewchuk, R., Baskin, M., et al. (2007). Racial influences associated with weight-related beliefs in African American and Caucasian women. *Ethnicity and Disease, 17*(1), 1–5.

Marti, A., Moreno-Aliaga, M., Hebebrand, J., & Martínez, J. (2004). Genes, lifestyles and obesity. *International Journal of Obesity, 28*(Suppl. 3), S29–S36.

McAlexander, K., Banda, J., McAlexander, J., & Lee, R. (2009). Physical activity resource attributes and obesity in low-income African Americans. *Journal of Urban Health, 86*(5), 696–707.

McGuire, M. T., Wing, R. R., Klem, M. L., Lang, W., & Hill, J. O. (1999). What predicts weight regain in a group of successful weight losers? *Journal of Consulting and Clinical Psychology, 67*(2), 177–185.

Meckling, K., O'Sullivan, C., & Saari, D. (2004). Comparison of a low-fat diet to a low-carbohydrate diet on weight loss, body composition, and risk factors for diabetes and cardiovascular disease in free-living, overweight men and women. *Journal of Clinical Endocrinology and Metabolism, 89,* 2717–2723.

Morton, G., Cummings, D., Baskin, D., Barsh, G., & Schwartz, M. (2006). Central nervous system control of food intake and body weight. *Nature, 443,* 289–295.

Mun, E., Blackburn, G., & Matthews, J. (2001). Current status of medical and surgical therapy for obesity. *Gastroenterology, 120*(3), 669–681.

Munsch, S., Biedert, E., Meyer, A., Michael, T., Schlup, B., Tuch, A., et al. (2007). A randomized comparison of cognitive behavioral therapy and behavioral weight loss treatment for overweight individuals with binge eating disorder. *International Journal of Eating Disorders, 40*(2), 102–113.

Narayan, K., Boyle, J., Thompson, T., Gregg, E., & Williamson, D. (2007). Effect of BMI on lifetime risk for diabetes in the U.S. *Diabetes Care, 30*(6), 1562–1566.

Nielsen, S., & Popkin, B. (2004). Changes in beverage intake between 1977 and 2001. *American Journal of Preventive Medicine, 27,* 205–210.

Obarzanek, E., & Pratt, C. (2003). Girls health Enrichment Multi-site Studies (GEMS): A new approach to obesity prevention among African American girls. *Ethnicity and Disease, 13*(1, Suppl. 1), S1–S5.

Ogden, C., Carroll, M., & Flegal, K. (2008). High body mass index for age among US children and adolescents, 2003–2006. *Journal of the American Medical Association, 299*(20), 2401–2405.

Ogden, C., Yanovski, S., Carroll, M., & Flegal, K. (2007). The epidemiology of obesity. *Gastroenterology, 132,* 2087–2102.

Okosun, I. S., Boltri, J. M., Anochie, L. K., & Chandra, K. M. (2004). Racial/ethnic differences in prehypertension in American adults: Population and relative attributable risks of abdominal obesity. *Journal of Human Hypertension, 18*(12), 849–855.

O'Malley, A. S., Forrest, C. B., & Miranda, J. (2003). Primary care attributes and care for depression among low-income African American women. *American Journal of Public Health, 93*(8), 1328–1334.

Parameswaran, K., Todd, D., & Soth, M. (2006). Altered respiratory physiology in obesity. *Canadian Respiratory Journal, 13*(4), 203–210.

Parham, G., & Scarinci, I. (2007). Strategies for achieving healthy energy balance among African Americans in the Mississippi Delta. *Preventing Chronic Disease, 4*(4), A97.

Pereira, M., Kartashov, A., Ebbeling, C., Van Horn, L., Slattery, M., Jacobs, D., et al. (2005). Fast-food habits, weight gain, and insulin resistance (the CARDIA study): 15-year prospective analysis. *Lancet, 365,* 36–42.

Potti, S., Milli, M., Jeronis, S., Gaughan, J., & Rose, M. (2009). Self-perceptions of body size in women at an inner-city family-planning clinic. *American Journal of Obstetrics and Gynecology, 200*(5), e65–e68.

Rennie, K., Johnson, L., & Jebb, S. (2005). Behavioural determinants of obesity. *Best Practice and Research: Clinical Endocrinology and Metabolism, 19,* 343–358.

Resnicow, K., Campbell, M., Carr, C., McCarty, F., Wang, T., Periasamy, S., et al. (2004). Body and Soul: A dietary intervention conducted through African-American churches. *American Journal of Preventive Medicine, 27*(2), 97–105.

Resnicow, K., Jackson, A., Blissett, D., Wang, T., McCarty, F., Rahotep, S., et al. (2005). Results of the Healthy Body Healthy Spirit Trial. *Health Psychology, 24*(4), 339–348.

Robinson, T., Killen, J., Kraemer, H., Wilson, D., Matheson, D., & Haskell, W. L. (2003). Dance and reduced TV viewing to prevent weight gain in African American girls: The Stanford GEMS study. *Ethnicity and Disease, 13*(1, Suppl. 1), S65–S77.

Robinson, W., Gordon-Larsen, P., Kaufman, J., Suchindran, C., & Stevens, J. (2009). The female–male disparity in obesity prevalence among Black American young adults: Contributions of sociodemographic characteristics of the childhood family. *American Journal of Clinical Nutrition, 89*(4), 1204–1212.

Rochon, J., Klesges, R., Story, M., Robinson, T., Baranowski, T., Obarzanek, E., et al. (2003). Common design elements of the Girls health Enrichment Multi-site Studies (GEMS). *Ethnnicity and Disease, 13*(1, Suppl. 1), S6–S14.

Samaha, F., Samaha, M., Iqbal, N., Seshadri, P., Prakash, S., Chicano, K., et al. (2003). A low-carbohydrate as compared with a low-fat diet in severe obesity. *New England Journal of Medicine, 348*(21), 2074–2081.

Saris, W. (2001). Very-low-calorie diets and sustained weight loss. *Obesity Research, 9,* s295–S301.

Schuster, D., Gaillard, T., Rhinesmith, S., Habash, D., & Osei, K. (2004). Impact of metformin on glucose metabolism in nondiabetic, obese African Americans: A placebo-controlled, 24-month randomized study. *Diabetes Care, 27,* 2768–2769.

Shaw, K., Gennat, H., O'Rourke, P., & Del Mar, C. (2006). Exercise for overweight or obesity. *Cochrane Database of Systematic Reviews,* Issue 4 (Article No. CD003817), DOI: 10.1002/14651858.CD003817.pub3.

Simansky, K. (1995). Serotonergic control of the organization of feeding and satiety. *Behavioural Brain Research, 73*(1–2), 37–42.

Simon, G. E., Von Korff, M., Saunders, K., Miglioretti, D. L., Crane, P. K., van Belle, G., et al. (2006). Association between obesity and psychiatric disorders in the US adult population. *Archives of General Psychiatry, 63*, 824–830.

Singh, A., Chinapaw, J., Brug, J., Kremers, S., Visscher, T., & van Mechelen, W. (2009). Ethnic differences in BMI among Dutch adolescents: What is the role of screen-viewing, active commuting to school, and consumption of soft drinks and high-caloric snacks? *International Journal of Behavioral Nutrition and Physical Activity, 6*, 23.

Sjöström, L., Narbro, K., Saelens, B., Sjöström, C., Karason, K., Larsson, B., et al. (2007). Effects of bariatric surgery on mortality in Swedish obese subjects. *New England Journal of Medicine, 357*, 741–752.

Smolak, L., & Striegel-Moore, R. (2001). Challenging the myth of the golden girl: Ethnicity and eating disorders. In R. Striegel-Moore & L. Smolak (Eds.), *Eating disorders: Innovative directions in research and practice* (pp. 111–132). Washington, DC: American Psychological Association.

Søvik, T. T., Taha, O., Aasheim, E. T., Engström, M., Kristinsson, J., Björkman, S., et al. (2010). Randomized clinical trial of laparoscopic gastric bypass versus laparoscopic duodenal switch for superobesity. *British Journal of Surgery, 97*(2), 160–166.

Stead, L., Lash, T., Sobieraj, J., Chi, D., Westrup, J., Charlot, M., et al. (2009). Triple-negative breast cancers are increased in Black women regardless of age or body mass index. *Breast Cancer Research, 11*(2), R18.

Stein, C., & Colditz, G. (2004). The epidemic of obesity. *Journal of Clinical Endocrinology and Metabolism, 89*(6), 2522–2525.

Stern, L., Iqbal, N., Seshadri, P., Chicano, K., Daily, D., McGrory, J., et al. (2004). The effects of low-carbohydrate versus conventional weight loss diets in severely obese adults: One-year follow-up of a randomized trial. *Annals of Internal Medicine, 140*, 778–785.

Stice, E., Spoor, S., Ng, J., & Zald, D. (2009). Relation of obesity to consummatory and anticipatory food reward. *Physiology and Behavior, 97*(5), 551–560.

Stolley, M., Sharp, L., Wells, A., Simon, N., & Schiffer, L. (2006). Health behaviors and breast cancer: Experiences of urban African American women. *Health Education and Behavior, 33*(5), 604–624.

Story, M., Sherwood, N. E., Himes, J. H., Davis, M., Jacobs, D. R., Jr., Cartwright, Y., et al. (2003). An after-school obesity prevention program for African-American girls: The Minnesota GEMS pilot study. *Ethnicity and Disease, 13*(1, Suppl. 1), S1–S64.

Striegel-Moore, R., Dohm, F., Pike, K., Wilfley, D., & Fairburn, C. (2002). Abuse, bullying, and discrimination as risk factors for binge eating disorder. *American Journal of Psychiatry, 159*(11), 1902–1907.

Striegel-Moore, R., Wilfley, W., Pike, K., Dohm, F., & Fairburn, C. (2000). Recurrent binge eating in Black American women. *Archives of Family Medicine, 9*, 83–87.

Strychar, I. (2009). Diet in the management of weight loss. *Canadian Medical Association Journal, 174*(1), 56–63.

Summerbell, C., Waters, E., Edmunds, L., Kelly, S., Brown, T., & Campbell, K. (2005). Interventions for preventing obesity in children. *Cochrane Database of Systematic Reviews,* Issue 3 (Article No. CD001871), DOI:10.1002/14651858.CD001871. pub2.

Talleyrand, R. (2006). Potential stressors contributing to eating disorder symptoms in African American women: Implications for mental health counselors. *Journal of Mental Health Counseling, 28*(4), 338–352.

Teixeira, P., Going, S., Houtkooper, L., Cussler, S., Metcalfe, L., Blew, R., et al. (2004). Pretreatment predictors of attrition and successful weight management in women. *International Journal of Obesity, 28*, 1124–1133.

Thomas, A., Moseley, G., Stallings, R., Nichols-English, G., & Wagner, P. (2008). Perceptions of obesity: Black and White differences. *Journal of Cultural Diversity, 15*(4), 174–180.

Thompson, E., Berry, D., & Nasir, L. (2009). Weight management in African-Americans using church-based community interventions to prevent Type 2 diabetes and cardiovascular disease. *Journal of the National Black Nurses Association, 20*(1), 59–65.

Thorpe, K. (2009). The future costs of obesity: National and state estimates of the impact of obesity on direct health care expenses. United Health Foundation and the American Public Health Association and Partnership for Prevention. Retrieved February 16, 2010, from *www.fightchronicdisease.org/pdfs/CostofObesityReport-FINAL.pdf*

Topp, R., Jacks, D., Wedig, T., Newman, J., Tobe, L., & Hollingsworth, A. (2009). Reducing risk factors for childhood obesity: The Tommie Smith youth athletic initiative. *Western Journal of Nursing Research, 31*, 715.

Tsai, W., Inge, T., & Burd, R. (2007). Bariatric surgery in adolescents: Recent national trends in use and in-hospital outcome. *Archives of Pediatric and Adolescent Medicine, 161*(3), 217–221.

U.S. Census Bureau. (2001). *Statistical abstract of the United States: 2000.* Washington, DC: Author. Retrieved February 10, 2010, from *www.census.gov/prod/2001pubs/statab/sec02.pdf*

U.S. Department of Health and Human Services. (2001). *The Surgeon General's call to action to prevent and decrease overweight and obesity.* Rockville, MD: Public Health Service, Office of the Surgeon General.

Van Gaal, L., Rissanen, A., Scheen, A., Ziegler, O., Rössner, S., & RIO-Europe Study Group. (2005). Effects of the cannabinoid-1 receptor blocker rimonabant on weight reduction and cardiovascular risk factors in overweight patients: 1-year experience from the RIO-Europe study. *Lancet, 365*, 1389–1397.

Vaughan, C., Sacco, W., & Beckstead, J. (2008). Racial/ethnic differences in body mass index: The roles of beliefs about thinness and dietary restriction. *Body Image, 5*(3), 291–298.

Votruba, S., & Jensen, M. (2007). Sex differences in abdominal, gluteal, and thigh LPL activity. *American Journal of Physiology: Endocrinology and Metabolism, 292*(6), e1823–e1828.

Wang, G., Volkow, N., Logan, J., Pappas, N., Wong, C., Wei, Z., et al. (2001). Brain dopamine and obesity. *Lancet, 357*, 354–357.

Wardle, J. (1995). Parental influences on children's diets. *Proceedings of the Nutrition Society, 54*, 747–758.

Werrij, M., Jansen, A., Mulkens, S., Elgersma, H., Ament, A., & Hospers, H. (2009). Adding cognitive therapy to dietetic treatment is associated with less relapse in obesity. *Journal of Psychosomatic Research, 67*(4), 315–324.

Whitt-Glover, M., Hogan, P., Lang, W., & Heil, D. (2008). Pilot study of a faith-based physical activity program among sedentary Blacks. *Preventing Chronic Disease, 5*(2), A51.

Whitt-Glover, M., & Kumanyika, S. (2009). Systematic review of interventions to increase physical activity and physical fitness in African-Americans. *American Journal of Health Promotion, 23*(6), S33–S56.

Wing, R., & Phelan, S. (2005). Science-based solutions to obesity: What are the roles of academia, government, industry, and health care? Long-term weight loss mainte-nance. *American Journal of Clinical Nutrition, 82*(1), 222S–225S.

Wolff, E., & Dansinger, M. (2008). Soft drinks and weight gain: How strong is the link? *Medscape Journal of Medicine, 10*(8), 189.

Woo, J., Dolan, L., Morrow, A., Geraghty, S., & Goodman, E. (2008). Breastfeeding helps explain racial and socioeconomic status disparities in adolescent adiposity. *Pediat-rics, 121*(3), e458–e465.

World Health Organization. (1998). *Obesity: Preventing and managing the global epi-demic.* Geneva: Author. Retrieved February 10, 2010, from *www.nutritionsociety.org/ documents/20051116reading3Clin.pdf*

World Health Organization Expert Committee. (1990). *Prevention in childhood and youth of adult cardiovascular diseases: Time for action.* Geneva: World Health Organization. Retrieved February 10, 2010, from *whqlibdoc.who.int/trs/WHO_TRS_792.pdf*

Wu, T., Gao, X., Chen, M., & van Dam, R. (2009). Long-term effectiveness of diet-plus-exercise interventions vs. diet-only interventions for weight loss: A meta-analysis. *Obesity Reviews, 10*(3), 313–323.

Wurtman, R., & Fernstrom, J. (1975). Control of brain monoamine synthesis by diet and plasma amino acids. *American Journal of Clinical Nutrition, 28*, 638–647.

Wurtman, R., Wurtman, J., Regan, M., McDermott, J., Tsay, R., & Breu, J. (2003). Effects of normal meals rich in carbohydrates or proteins on plasma tryptophan and tyrosine ratios. *American Journal of Clinical Nutrition, 77*(1), 128–132.

Yancey, A., McCarthy, W., Harrison, G., Wong, W., Siegel, J., & Leslie, J. (2006). Chal-lenges in improving fitness: Results of a community-based, randomized, controlled lifestyle change intervention. *Journal of Women's Health, 15*(4), 412–429.

Yancy, W., Olsen, M., Guyton, J., Bakst, R., & Westman, E. (2004). A low-carbohydrate, ketogenic diet versus a low-fat diet to treat obesity and hyperlipidemia. *Annals of Internal Medicine, 140*, 769.

Young, L., & Nestle, M. (2003). Expanding portion sizes in the US marketplace: Impli-cations for nutrition counseling. *Journal of the American Dietetic Association, 103*, 231–234.

# 10

# Asthma

MICHELLE M. CLOUTIER

## EPIDEMIOLOGY OF ASTHMA

### Asthma Prevalence and Severity

Asthma is one of the leading chronic diseases worldwide in people of all ages but especially in children, second only to dental caries as a cause of chronic disease. Industrialized countries with a Western lifestyle have high and rising rates of asthma (Al Frayh, Shakoor, Gad, Rab, & Hasnian, 2001; Celedón et al., 2001; Manfreda et al., 2001). Between 1980 and 1998, the number of individuals with asthma in the United States more than doubled, from 6.7 million to an estimated 17.3 million (Mannino et al., 1998). In 2005, 8.9% of children, or 6.5 million, in the United States were reported to have current asthma (Akinbami, 2006). In 2006, this number had increased to 6.8 million, or 9.4% (National Center for Health Statistics, 2006). For adults in the United States in 2000, the lifetime and current self-reported asthma prevalence rates based on the Behavioral Risk Factor Surveillance System were 10.5% and 7.2%, respectively (Centers for Disease Control and Prevention [CDC], 2001).

Asthma disproportionately affects underrepresented minority populations, with African Americans and (some) Hispanics having higher rates than other ethnic groups (Akinbami, 2006; Akinbami & Schoendorf, 2002; CDC, 2001; Lee, Haselkorn, Chipps, Miller, & Wenzel, 2006; Mannino et al., 1998). In addition to race/ethnicity, risk factors contributing to the development of asthma include maternal *in utero* exposures and environmental factors, gender, low socioeconomic status (SES), aeroallergen sensitization, elevated endotoxin exposure, eczema,

213

family history of asthma, maternal smoking, and reduced maternal intake of foods containing vitamin E and zinc during pregnancy (Devereux et al., 2006; Ehrlich et al., 1996; Park, Gold, Spiegelman, Burge, & Milton, 2001; Ramsey, Celedón, Stredl, Weiss, & Cloutier, 2005; Sporik, Holgate, Platts-Mills, & Cogswell, 1990; Squillace et al., 1997).

Differences in asthma severity also exist between and within minority populations. For example, Puerto Rican Hispanic children have more asthma, and of greater severity, than Black children, who have more severe disease than non-Hispanic Whites, who have more severe disease than Mexican Hispanics (Peat et al., 1996; Ramsey et al., 2005; Sears, 1997; Sporik et al., 1990; Squillace et al., 1997). Previous studies have estimated that 66–75% of individuals with asthma have mild disease, although a more recent study, designed to identify adults and parents of children with asthma, suggests that more than 75% of individuals have an asthma burden consistent with moderate to severe persistent disease (Auerbach, Springer, & Godfrey, 1993; Fuhlbrigge et al., 2002). In addition to race/ethnicity, other factors found to be associated with greater asthma severity include endotoxin exposure, gender, and disparities in health care (Halterman, Aligne, Auinger, McBride, & Szilagyi, 2000; Rizzo et al., 1997).

## Asthma Morbidity and Mortality

Asthma-related morbidity and mortality are high. In 2005 in the United States, there were approximately 450,000 hospitalizations (2002 data), 1.8 million emergency department (ED) visits, and approximately 12.8 million physician office visits among persons of all ages (National Center for Health Statistics, 2006). In 2004, asthma in children accounted for 7 million ambulatory visits, 750,000 ED visits, and 198,000 hospitalizations (Akinbami, 2006).

In the United States, asthma morbidity disproportionately affects non-White children living in urban areas and children living in poverty (Gold & Wright, 2005). Black children have high rates of ED and outpatient visits for asthma and hospitalizations for asthma (Akinbami, 2006; Gold & Wright, 2005; Mannino et al., 1998). Compared with White children, Black children have a 260% higher ED visit rate, a 250% higher hospitalization rate, and a 350% higher death rate from asthma. In 2002, adult African Americans with asthma had an ED visit rate of 380%, hospitalization rate of 225%, and mortality rate more than 200% higher than non-Hispanic Whites (CDC, 2002; Warman, Silver, & Stein, 2001).

Greater asthma severity is associated with increased resource utilization (Halterman et al., 2000) and higher costs. Between 1985 and 1994, the total costs of asthma in the United States had risen 54% to $10.7 billion (Weiss, Sullivan, & Lyttle, 2000). By 1998, the total costs were $12.7 billion (Weiss & Sullivan, 2001). A more recent estimate of the total annual cost of asthma was nearly $18 billion for hospital care and $5 billion in indirect costs (Asthma and Allergy Foundation of America, 2006). No other single disease accounts for a larger proportion of health care costs (Doan, Grammer, Yarnold, Greenberger, & Patterson, 1996).

In one study, on average, 6.4% of a family's yearly income was spent caring for a child's asthma; for low-income families, this was 10% of their yearly income (Marion, Creer, & Reynolds, 1985).

Asthma is a leading cause of school and work absenteeism. In 2003 children ages 5 to 17 years missed 12.8 million days of school and adults with asthma missed 10.1 million workdays (Akinbami, 2005). Children with asthma miss more school days than children without asthma (Parcel, Gilman, Nader, & Bunce, 1979). African American children also report more days of restricted activity, more symptomatic nights with asthma than Whites, and more absent school days per year than Whites (Zoratti et al., 1998). African American adults report higher rates of episodes of poor asthma control and asthma exacerbations even when controlling for SES and disease severity (McCoy et al., 2006).

In 2005 asthma accounted for 3,884 deaths (National Center for Health Statistics, 2006). Although overall death rates from asthma have declined in the United States since 1999, the death rate for Black children has remained relatively level, increasing the disparity in death rates. African Americans make up 12.7% of the U.S. population but account for 26% of asthma deaths (CDC, 2002; Mannino et al., 1998). Although death from childhood asthma is rare, the death rate increased by 3.4% per year from 1980 to 1998, with adolescents having the highest mortality (Akinbami & Schoendorf, 2002). In 2004, 186 children in the United States died from asthma (Akinbami, 2006). Asthma mortality rates vary by age, geographical region, and race/ethnicity (Mannino et al., 1998; Sly & O'Donnell, 1997; Weiss & Wagener, 1990), and several studies have suggested that Black race/ethnicity, low SES, and low levels of education may independently be associated with an elevated risk for asthma mortality (Grant, Lyttle, & Weiss, 2000). Similar to adults, the disparity in asthma mortality between Black and White children is increasing (Akinbami, 2006).

## BIOLOGICAL/GENETIC FACTORS

The disparities in asthma prevalence and severity in African Americans cannot be explained entirely by environmental, social, cultural, or economic factors (Collins, 2004). Genetic variations clearly affect susceptibility to asthma. However, the exact nature and extent of this genetic variation are not clear because there are limited linkage and association studies in non-European populations. In addition, genetic predisposition is probably caused by particular patterns of polymorphisms in multiple genes involved in the allergic response. In the Collaborative Study on the Genetics of Asthma (CSGA), there was no overlap between six novel and previously reported chromosomal regions and asthma in European Americans, African Americans, and Hispanic Americans, suggesting distinct genes in each of the groups or a unique gene–environment interaction (CGSA, 1997). Another study found a number of target candidate genes and polymorphisms in host defense genes that have been associated with both asthma and treatment pathways (Barnes, Grant, Hansel, Gao, & Dunston, 2007).

In African American families, two novel genetic regions—5p15 and 17p11.1-q11.2—have been associated with asthma (Caggana et al., 1999). Others have found a gene–gene interaction between the IL-13 gene, a pro-inflammatory cytokine that lies on chromosome 5q31-33 and is produced by activated T cells in response to allergen exposure and its receptor IL-4R$\alpha$ genes in African Americans (Battle et al., 2007). A single-nucleotide polymorphism (SNP) in the promoter region of IL-13 has also been associated with allergic asthma in African Americans (Moissidis et al., 2005). Another gene on chromosome 5 in the family of the T-cell immunoglobulin domain and mucin domain proteins may also contribute to asthma susceptibility in African Americans. These genes encode cell surface glycoproteins, are selectively expressed on activated CD4[+] T cells, and are involved in the development and regulation of TH2-immune responses (P.-S. Gao et al., 2005). Other studies suggest a complex gene–environment interaction recently demonstrated by a functional variant in the CD14 gene in which domestic endotoxin levels conferred either risk or protection (Barnes et al., 2007). There is even some suggestion that overlying these complex gene–environment and gene–gene interactions may be developmentally regulated responses. For example, in utero cat exposure may confer immunity while a similar exposure in early childhood may result in sensitization (Karjalainen et al., 2005; Owenby, Johnson, & Peterson, 2002).

Genetic susceptibility to complex traits that affect African Americans may also be related to selective pressures associated with the out-of-Africa expansion. For example, in African Caribbean and African American families, a haplotype involving the myosin light chain kinase, a multifunctional protein involved in regulation of airway hyperreactivity, was associated with decreased risk of asthma but increased risk of sepsis (L. Gao et al., 2007). Thus, one haplotype that is protective in one condition may be deleterious in another.

In terms of treatment responses, T-lymphocyte responses to corticosteroids may be less in African Americans than in Whites, making them more susceptible to a poorer response to inhaled corticosteroids (ICSs) and increased mortality and morbidity (Federico, Covar, Brown, Leung, & Spahn, 2005). In addition, genetic variations in the beta$_2$-adrenergic receptor (ADRB2) have been found (Barnes, 1995). The ADRB2 regulates bronchomotor tone and mediates the action of beta$_2$-agonists on airway smooth muscle. It is dysfunctional in asthma. Association studies have demonstrated that African Americans who are homozygous for an SNP at loci 523 on chromosome 5q31-33 have greater asthma severity than heterozygotes or other individuals with asthma (Lima et al., 2006). Furthermore, certain polymorphisms in the ADRB2 associated with down-regulation of the receptor and decreased responsiveness to beta-adrenergic drugs, and the length of a poly-C repeat in the 3′ untranslated region of the ADRB2 associated with lower levels of lung function are more common in African Americans than other ethnic groups (Hawkins et al., 2006; Litonjua, 2006).

## INDIVIDUAL FACTORS
## INFLUENCING RISK AND RESILIENCY

Health-related quality of life, which considers the effect of health on physical and social function and overall well-being, has been shown to be reduced in individuals with asthma, especially Blacks (Mancuso, Rincon, McCulloch, & Charlson, 2001; Wisnivesky, Leventhal, & Halm, 2005). Black race and asthma have been associated with poorer mental health status and asthma-specific quality of life, although SES was a significant confounder of the effect (Erickson, Iribarren, Tolstykh, Blanc, & Eisner, 2007). In this same study, Black patients reported, and pharmacy-dispensing records confirmed, a higher frequency of the use of short-acting inhaled beta-agonists compared with Whites but no association between race and use of controller medications or referral to an asthma specialist. Other studies, however, have found that African Americans do not fill as many asthma prescriptions, especially for controller medications, and are more likely not to fill a controller medication prescription compared with other minorities and non-Hispanic Whites (Cloutier, Jones, Hinckson, & Wakefield, 2008; Krishnan et al., 2001). Additionally, depression and low self-efficacy are independent factors associated with quality of life (Cloutier et al., 2008; Mancuso, Peterson, & Charlson, 2000; Mancuso et al., 2001). Maternal depression is associated with increased asthma morbidity possibly because of decreased adherence to therapy secondary to forgetfulness and difficulty using metered-dose inhalers (MDIs) (Bartlett et al., 2004).

Nonadherence to medications, ICSs in particular, has been associated with poorer asthma outcomes, including higher rates of ED visits and hospitalizations (Williams et al., 2004). Medication adherence for a variety of diseases is lower in African Americans compared with Whites (Bosworth et al., 2006; Schectman, Nadkarni, & Voss, 2002). At all income tertiles, African Americans with asthma have lower ICS adherence than Whites, which is not explained by location of residence (Williams et al., 2007). African Americans use fewer ICSs than oral steroids and are less frequently seen by an asthma specialist compared with Caucasians even when financial barriers are reduced by participation in a health maintenance organization (Zoratti et al., 1998). In addition, among African Americans with asthma, adherence to ICS medication increased with increasing age and decreased with increasing crime rate in the area of residence for both violent and property crimes.

Several studies have demonstrated differences in use of asthma therapy by different ethnic groups. Specifically, minority children were more likely to use short-acting reliever medication in lieu of controller therapies (Halterman et al., 2000; Ledogar, Penchaszadeh, & Garden, 2000; Wisnivesky et al., 2005). Others have demonstrated that children with greater asthma severity used fewer anti-inflammatory drugs regardless of caretaker sociodemographic factors (Warman et al., 2001). Although controller therapy is underprescribed by clinicians, even when prescribed, African Americans are less likely to report a controller prescription, and this discordance is related to the caregiver's beliefs about treatment (Riekert et al., 2003). Increased asthma morbidity has been linked to inadequate access to medical care, but in the Canadian context of universal access to medical care, children from homes with greater socioeconomic disadvantage had more asthma symptoms, including nocturnal cough and exercise-induced asthma (Ernst, Demissie, Joseph, Locher, & Becklake, 1995). Finally, some of the differences in therapy may be related to differences in how symptoms are reported. In a small study of African American and Caucasian adults with asthma, African Americans were less likely to report nocturnal awakenings, dyspnea, or chest pain compared with Caucasians (Trochtenberg, BeLue, Piphus, & Washington, 2008).

Individual factors such as income and educational attainment are known to contribute to disparities in part through issues related to access to health care and health literacy in addition to environmental exposures, suboptimal treatment, genetic and behavioral differences, and health care provider shortcomings. Inadequate health literacy is associated with a greater likelihood of hospitalization for asthma exacerbations in the previous year and improper MDI (Wittich, Mangan, Grad, Wang, & Gerald, 2007) technique, but is not associated with difficulty learning or retaining instructions about the discharge regimen (Paasche-Orlow et al., 2005). African Americans with acute asthma are also more likely to present for emergency care with greater obstruction than Whites and with a history of greater reliance on inhaled bronchodilators as a result of a self-imposed "wait-and-see" course of action (El-Ekiaby et al., 2006). Their response to inhaled bronchodilator therapy in the ED, however, is similar to that of Whites, and in controlled studies there are no racial differences in immediate outcomes or hospitalizations when standardized treatments are used.

Other individual factors associated with asthma severity or morbidity include obesity (Luder, Melnik, & DiMaio, 1998). In young African American and White men and women who were monitored for 10 years, incident asthma was more common in women and was associated with the highest and lowest baseline and change in body mass index (Beckett et al., 2001). In addition, the weight gain appeared to precede a diagnosis of asthma and was not explained by lower physical activity. Obesity is also associated with an increased risk of new-onset asthma in boys and in nonallergic children (Camargo, Field, Colditz, & Speizer, 1999; Gilliland et al., 2003). Unlike most asthma, however, obesity-related asthma is more likely to be nonatopic (Kelley, Mannino, Homa, Savage-Brown, & Holguin, 2005). Other nutritional individual risk factors for the development of asthma include a diet high in polyunsaturated fats—a possible link with the Western lifestyle—and a history of ear infections (Eldeirawi & Persky, 2004); breastfeeding and having older siblings are protective factors against asthma (Haby, Peat, Marks, Woolcock, & Leeder, 2001).

## Gender Disparities

In childhood, asthma is more prevalent in boys than girls, but in adults asthma prevalence and severity are greater in women than men (Cloutier, Wakefield, Hall,

& Bailit, 2002). Gender, however, influences both the diagnosis and the treatment of asthma. Women with asthma have greater morbidity and excess mortality than men. The excess morbidity in women is unexplained but dissimilar environmental exposure, host susceptibility factors, and improper inhaler technique may be important in the gender-related differences. In the Epidemiology and Natural History of Asthma: Outcomes and Treatment Regimens study (Lee et al., 2006), females had more steroid bursts, had more unscheduled office visits, and missed more workdays than males.

Gender differences in asthma care also exist, with boys receiving more, and earlier, care. In the Tucson Childhood Respiratory Study, boys with asthma symptoms were more likely than girls to see a specialist physician, were more likely to be labeled as having asthma even after adjusting for symptom frequency, and had a shorter lag time between the first episode of wheezing and the diagnosis of asthma (A. L. Wright, Stern, Kauffmann, & Martinez, 2006). Similar results were found in a Swiss study in which boys received significantly better treatment for asthma symptoms than girls (Kuhni & Sennhauser, 1995). Women with asthma also appear to have higher morbidity than men.

Asthma is one of the most common complications of pregnancy and, when uncontrolled, is associated with premature delivery, low birthweight, fetal death, and pregnancy-induced hypertension (Carroll et al., 2005; National Asthma Education and Prevention Program, 2005). African American women have the highest incidence of preterm labor and pregnancy-induced hypertension, and African American women with asthma have the highest incidence of preterm labor and are more likely than Whites to experience infection of the amniotic cavity (MacMullen, Tymkow, & Shen, 2006).

## FAMILY FACTORS INFLUENCING RISK AND RESILIENCY

Systematic differences in family perceptions of the presence and attributes of usual source of care vary by race/ethnicity. Access to health care is limited in individuals with no medical insurance coverage, and Black children with asthma are more likely than their White counterparts to lack health insurance, an issue that is more problematic for near-poverty than for in-poverty families (Weinick, Weigers, & Cohen, 1998). Despite the provision of insurance, however, disparities in care and the location of care can remain (Ernst et al., 1995). Data from the 1996–2000 Medical Expenditure Panel Survey Household Component suggest that, compared with Whites, Blacks are less likely to identify a usual source of health care, and if a usual source is identified, it is more likely to be a hospital clinic or outpatient department (Greek, Kieckhefer, Kim, Joesch, & Baydar, 2006). Even privately insured Black children report fewer physician visits, a greater likelihood of lack of continuity of care, and less use of physician offices and greater use of EDs for care compared with middle-class White children (Weitzman, Byrd, & Auinger, 1999). Blacks more than Hispanics also report difficulty in getting appointments on short notice. Despite these problems, Blacks report satisfaction with staff and overall quality of care.

Patient–physician interaction is an important determinant of asthma outcomes. Patients with no regular source of care have been shown to have worse asthma control (Eggleston et al., 1998; Haas, Cleary, Guadagnoli, Fanta, & Epstein, 2001; Halfon & Newacheck, 1993), whereas minority patients with a regular source of care are more likely to receive ICSs and spacers (Halm, Wisnivesky, & Leventhal, 2005) and to have improved outcomes (Wisnivesky et al., 2005). Disparities in asthma care continue for minority populations and women. Compared with Whites with asthma, even primarily college-educated (60%), insured African American adults with moderate or severe asthma use fewer daily ICSs, receive less asthma self-management and trigger-avoidance education by their primary care physician, and are less unlikely to be referred for specialist care (Krishnan et al., 2001). This same study found that women were less likely than men to use an ICS daily and to receive care from an asthma specialist. Although treatment bias by clinicians has been suggested as a possible reason for underprescribing of ICSs in African Americans, several studies have demonstrated that Black children are no more or less likely to be prescribed an ICS than children of other ethnicities/race (Cloutier, 2008; Smith & Pawar, 2007). Even when patients are prescribed appropriate therapy, many patients, in particular African American adults and children with asthma, are less likely than Whites to use ICSs (Cloutier et al., 2008; Legorreta et al., 1998; Rand et al., 2000).

## SOCIAL AND COMMUNITY FACTORS INFLUENCING RISK AND RESILIENCY

There are many environmental factors and exposures that are important in a complex gene–environment disease such as asthma. Health disparities are created in part when the capacity to control disease becomes available but this new capacity is distributed unequally. Contributing to disparities in asthma are social and community-based inequities regarding SES, housing quality, population density, stresses related to urban living, lack of family and community support, environmental tobacco smoke exposure, and rodent- and cockroach-infested living areas (Aligne, Auinger, Byrd, & Weitzmann, 2000; Ernst et al., 1995; Grant et al., 2000; Mannino et al., 1998; Sly & O'Donnell, 1997; von Maffei et al., 2001; Warman et al., 2001; Weiss & Wagener, 1990). Disparities also exist at other levels, including geographical differences in asthma prevalence and, as previously mentioned, differences in access to medical care, medical services utilization, knowledge about asthma, diagnosis and treatment of asthma, prescription of medications by clinicians, and parental use of these medications (Auerbach et al., 1993; Centers for Disease Control and Prevention, 2001; Haby, Peat, Marks, Woolcock, & Leeder, 2001; Park et al., 2001; Rizzo et al., 1997; Venn et al., 2001; R. J. Wright, Cohen, Carey, Weiss, & Gold, 2002).

Race is an imperfect surrogate for biology and one that has certain social, cultural, educational, and economic variables that influence the health of minority populations and disparities. In addition, socioeconomic variables, regardless of race, influence health. For example, numerous studies have demonstrated that children residing in urban communities, regardless of ethnicity, are at significantly increased risk for asthma compared with non-urban-dwelling children (Aligne et al., 2000). Factors contributing to this higher prevalence and to greater disease severity include the physical characteristics of the environment, and in particular the inner-city environment, such as outdoor air pollution (especially diesel); crowding, which may predispose to viral infections; poor housing stock, resulting in the potential for increased indoor aeroinhalant exposures; the presence of a humidifying device and a gas range or oven; and increased tobacco smoke exposure (Aligne et al., 2000; von Maffei et al., 2001). Use of nonbiomass fuels such as kerosene and gas has also been associated with wheezing and eczema (Venn et al., 2001).

These factors, however, do not explain all of the asthma-related disparities among inner-city dwellers. Community-level stressors such as poverty, unemployment or underemployment, limited social capital, and high crime or violence exposure may also be important (Williams et al., 2007; Wright, 2006). Exposure to violence could affect and limit resources needed to manage asthma, influence an individual's behavior, reduce compliance with therapy, and increase family dysfunction (Strunk, Mrazek, Fuhrmann, & LaBrecque, 1985; Wright et al., 2002). Neighborhood violence has been associated with asthma symptom days in children, an effect at least partially mediated by poorer medication adherence (R. J. Wright et al., 2004). Caretaker stress has been shown to be associated with wheezing in a genetically predisposed prospective birth cohort (R. J. Wright et al., 2002). Psychological stress and feelings of lack of control over health have been associated with lower SES and altered immune responses in adolescents with asthma (Chen, Fisher, Bacharier, & Strunk, 2003). An association between higher levels of community violence and increased caretaker-reported asthma symptoms in children 5 to 12 years of age enrolled in the National Cooperative Inner City Asthma Study (NCICAS) has also been demonstrated (R. J. Wright et al., 2004). In adults, area crime is a predictor of adherence in African American patients even after adjusting for multiple measures of SES (Williams et al., 2007).

## EVIDENCE-BASED TREATMENT INTERVENTIONS

Numerous interventions designed to reduce asthma incidence, morbidity, and mortality have been investigated. Overall, however, these interventions have done little to substantially reduce morbidity, and none have consistently been shown to reduce incidence. We now discuss some of the more effective interventions to date.

## Effective Interventions

### Inhaled Corticosteroid Therapy

Of all of the interventions, only one group of interventions has consistently been shown to reduce asthma morbidity: those that increase the use of ICSs, which are most effective in improving asthma symptoms and in reducing hospitalizations and ED visits (Cloutier, Hall, Wakefield, & Bailit, 2005; Donahue et al., 1997; Haahtela et al., 1991; Wennergren, Kristjansson, & Strannegard, 1996). ICSs may also be effective in reducing asthma mortality (Suissa, Ernst, Benayoun, Baltzan, & Cai, 2000). Use of ICSs has been shown to vary among racial/ethnic groups, and several studies have shown that they are especially underused in children (Donahue et al., 2000; Joseph, Havstad, Ownby, Johnson, & Tilleym, 1998; Lieu et al., 2002). A cross-sectional study of 3,671 children and adults from 1989 to 1998 found that differences in prescribing rates for ICSs between minorities and nonminorities have resolved for Black but not for Hispanic adults (Ferris, Kuhlthau, Ausiello, Perrin, & Kahn, 2006). However, this study did not control for asthma severity; thus, although the rates of ICS prescription were similar, the burden of asthma, namely severity, was greater for minorities, suggesting possible continued underuse in minorities. Furthermore, the use of ICSs in children, especially minority children, has continued to lag behind ICS use in adults, and this difference would also have been greater had disease severity been considered. Finally, ICS use varies by care setting: lower in managed-care settings compared with private insurance settings (Ferris et al., 2006).

Guidelines for the diagnosis and management of asthma have been developed in both the United States and internationally (Global Initiative for Asthma, 1995; National Institutes of Health, National Heart, Lung, and Blood Institute, 1997, 2001) These guidelines are a mechanism for providers to systematically manage asthma in a standardized way. They have been demonstrated to be effective when used by specialists (Laforest et al., 2006; Wu et al., 2001) and primary care clinicians (Cloutier et al., 2005; Cloutier, Wakefield, Sangeloty-Higgins, Delaronde, & Hall, 2006). Unfortunately, these guidelines have not been universally adopted by primary care physicians. One program that has demonstrated sustained success in reducing hospitalizations, ED visits, and urgent care outpatient visits in large numbers of both Medicaid and privately insured children with asthma is Easy Breathing (Cloutier et al., 2005, 2006), a disease management program for primary care clinicians based on the National Asthma Education and Prevention Program asthma guidelines. To date, the program has screened more than 85,000 children in Connecticut and has identified more than 22,000 children with physician-confirmed asthma who are receiving guideline-appropriate treatment for their asthma. Results have been sustained for more than 8 years. For Black children specifically, Easy Breathing decreased hospitalization rates by 53%, ED visits for asthma by 27% and urgent care outpatient visits by 12% (Cloutier et al., 2008). Smaller studies with both children and adults have also demonstrated the effectiveness of appropriate asthma therapy administered by a clinician in reducing medical services utilization; some of these programs are combined with home interventions and intensive patient education with written asthma treatment plans (Kelly et al., 2000; Lieu et al., 1997; Mayo, Richman, & Harris, 1990; Pauley, Magee, & Cury, 1999).

Improved asthma management and increased ICS therapy can be achieved in settings other than the primary care physician's office. Using an ED follow-up clinic, Teach demonstrated reduced medical services utilization over a 6-month period in children who used the ED as a primary source of care (Teach, Crain, Quint, Hylan, & Joseph, 2006). Unlike other ED studies that enhanced follow-up with the child's primary care physician (Smith et al., 2004; Zorc et al., 2003), this study prescribed ICSs and gave families a written asthma treatment plan, suggesting that appropriate therapy, regardless of where it is prescribed, is key to reducing ED visits and hospitalizations. Using a clinical pharmacist, Kelso and colleagues (1996) demonstrated improved outcomes for African Americans who utilized the ED as their primary source of care.

School-based mobile clinics (Brito et al., 2000; Liao, Morphew, Amaro, & Galant, 2006) have also been successful in reaching children with asthma and getting them onto appropriate therapy. Likewise, community-based programs (e.g., the Harlem Children's Zone Asthma Initiative) that combine improved therapy with home visits and outreach have been successful in reducing ED utilization in children with asthma (Nicholas et al., 2005).

## Patient Education

Asthma education, whether by a nurse or a physician, has been shown to increase the number of symptom-free days and improve functional health status and disease-specific quality of life (Blixen, Hammel, Murphy, & Ault, 2001; Cote et al., 1997; Kamps et al., 2003; Pauley et al., 1999; Tatis, Remache, & DiMango, 2005). Most of the studies that have utilized asthma education as the intervention, however, have coupled it with pharmacotherapy. For example, in adults with asthma, the combination of high-dose beclomethasone (> 1,000 mcg/day) and asthma education compared to low-dose beclomethasone alone reduced ED visits and improved quality of life (Kelso et al., 1996). In another study using physicians and nurse educators, however, Kamps and colleagues (2003) demonstrated improvements in asthma control in association with a reduction in the daily ICS dose. They suggested that these improvements may have been mediated by improved inhaler technique, and education may have improved appropriate use of the prescribed medications. A 30-minute one-on-one educational program with a teach-to-goal strategy has also been shown to reduce deficiencies in asthma medication knowledge, MDI technique, and mastery of the discharge regimen in a study of predominantly urban-dwelling African American adults and was especially beneficial in individuals with low health literacy (Paasche-Orlow et al., 2005). For many of these studies, however, it is difficult to sort out the benefits attributable to improved therapy and to patient education. Low-income African American adults respond well to an educational intervention (Ford, Marvella, Havstad, Tilley, & Bolton, 1997), but asthma care among low-income African American patients is complicated by attitudes reflecting acceptance of inadequate care (Haire-Joshu, Fisher, Munro, & Wedner, 1993). Studies that did not change therapy were not nearly as successful as those described previously (Blixen et al., 2001).

In addition to the physician's office, asthma education can also be provided in public health clinics (D. Evans et al., 1997). Training public health staff improved access to care, follow-up, and quality of care (increased ICS use), but the effects were modest (D. Evans et al., 1997). In the NCICAS, the asthma intervention consisted of a social worker-driven, individual family intervention. Investigators found decreased symptom days in a clinical trial of urban-dwelling children, but it was difficult to translate this research study to a community setting (R. Evans et al., 1999; Wood, Tumiel-Berhalter, Owen, Taylor, & Kattan, 2006).

School-based programs, many of which are modeled on Open Airways, have been used to enhance knowledge and self-efficacy among children (Evans, Clark, & Feldman, 1990; Homer, 1998; Levy, Heffner, Stewart, & Beeman, 2006). One school-based program that combined Open Airways and case management by nurses in a low-income primarily African American school district in Tennessee demonstrated fewer school absences and fewer ED visits and hospital days compared with a control group (Levy et al., 2006). The program was replicated the following year in a new group of schools and is currently being expanded. A novel study that used a multimedia, culturally sensitive, tailored, Web-based educational program targeted to urban high school students demonstrated decreased asthma symptoms, school days missed, and hospitalization compared with a control condition at an estimated program delivery cost of $6.66 per participating student (Joseph et al., 2007).

The results of these studies suggest that education coupled with appropriate asthma therapy can be successful and can be accomplished in both traditional medical settings and in less traditional community settings.

## Possibly Effective Interventions

### Addition of Long-Acting Bronchodilators

Numerous studies and meta-analyses have demonstrated that long-acting bronchodilators such as salmeterol and formoterol can improve asthma control and reduce asthma symptoms in individuals whose asthma is not well controlled with ICSs (Shrewsbury, Pyke, & Britton, 2000). These long-acting bronchodilators are more effective than increasing the dose of the inhaled corticosteroid and are steroid-sparing; that is, there is no loss of control when the ICS dose is reduced (Busse et al., 2003; Greenstone et al., 2005; Masoli, Weatheral, Holt, & Beasley, 2005). However, in a prospective study of 60,000 adults with a history of asthma and no prior exposure to a long-acting bronchodilator, an increase in mortality, especially among African American participants, was observed (Nelson et al., 2006). Although more than half of these individuals were using long-acting bronchodilators as monotherapy (not the recommended use), this study was the catalyst for the U.S. Food and Drug Administration Black box warning regarding long-acting bronchodilators.

### Improving Adherence to Therapy

Adherence to inhaled corticosteroids is poor in all patient groups but especially in African Americans. Individual factors such as depression and patient attitudes toward ICSs (the concept that the benefits outweigh the risks) are mutable factors influencing adherence, but whether treatment of these factors improves adherence is not clear. Apter and colleagues (2003) demonstrated that some previously demonstrated factors such as patient–physician perceived adequacy of communication were not predictors of adherence, and that immutable factors such as social disparity (household income, commercial insurance) are the most important factors influencing the effect of race/ethnicity on adherence. Results from these studies suggest that interventions to enhance adherence may be especially difficult to design.

Coupled to adherence is the importance of understanding the cultural context of health and illness. A lack of concordance between the patient's and the clinician's view of health may lead to poor adherence, which could result in frustration, mistrust, and dissatisfaction. A qualitative analysis of in-depth interviews with Black women with asthma found strong fundamental Christian practices and beliefs for asthma's cause and control (George, 1999). Adherence to chronic asthma therapy for individuals who believe that communion with a higher spiritual forces makes all things possible could be difficult. For these individuals, an increase in prayer, church attendance, and good deeds is a more appropriate asthma management strategy than daily anti-inflammatory therapy. Strategies to bridge these differing views include eliciting the patient's cultural worldview of ill health and its concomitant therapy (Kleinman, Eisenberg, & Good, 1978). In addition, a study of Black children from Baltimore found that an ongoing relationship with a single health care provider is the most important factor that determined whether a child took ICS therapy, although alone it was not sufficient to guarantee that families received regular asthma primary care (Eggleston et al., 1998; Rand et al., 2000). Thus, in this study, the quality of the relationship between the health care provider and the patient was paramount to improving adherence and follow-up (Resch, Hill, & Ernst, 1997).

Three cognitive-behavioral factors are believed to affect the management of childhood asthma: asthma knowledge, practice problem-solving skills, and caretaker expectations regarding asthma. Interventions solely designed to improve asthma knowledge have not been especially successful in controlling asthma symptoms or reducing asthma morbidity (Clark et al., 1986; Howland, Bauchner, & Adair, 1988). In the NCICAS, in which more than two-thirds of the participants were African American children, caregivers who demonstrated ineffective problem-solving strategies had greater asthma morbidity, whereas positive caregiver expectations were associated with better functional status (Wade, Holden, Lynn, Mitchell, & Ewart, 2000). Whether interventions to increase problem-solving skills will reduce asthma morbidity is not known.

### Decreasing Environmental Exposures

Sensitization to cockroach has been reported to be a strong predictor of ED visits, hospitalizations, and asthma-related quality of life (Halterman et al., 2000; Wisnivesky et al., 2005), especially in children (Rosenstreich et al., 1997). In the NCICAS report, children who were sensitized to cockroach and exposed to high levels of cockroach allergen in their homes had higher hospitalization rates, more unscheduled asthma visits, and worse asthma control (Kattan et al., 1997). Cockroach allergen reduction strategies in association with dust mite reduction strategies were successful in reducing asthma-associated morbidity in these children (Morgan et al., 2004). This study, however, had many other elements, including education and improving therapy, thus making it difficult to sort the effect of the environmental intervention from other elements of the program.

The Childhood Asthma Prevention Study (CAPS), a home-based secondary prevention intervention study of wheezing infants and their low-income caregivers (Klinnert et al., 2005), used an environmental support intervention to decrease allergen and environmental tobacco smoke (ETS) exposure, coupled with maternal education in asthma prevention and management and intervention in maternal mental health, parenting, and social stressors. Although the intervention significantly reduced cockroach exposure and ETS exposure, especially in individuals with low resources, and enhanced knowledge and asthma management skills, CAPS had no effect on respiratory symptom frequency or medical services utilization. As the authors acknowledge, this failure to improve outcomes raises questions about the usefulness of this intensive intervention in decreasing wheezing episodes in low-income families.

### Community-Level Interventions to Improve Asthma

Asthma interventions are more effective when adapted to ethnic, social, and economic characteristics of specific populations (de Oliveria, Faresin, Bruno, de Bittencourt, & Fernandes, 1999). The Moving to Opportunity study (Katz, Kling, & Liebman, 2001) provided vouchers to families living in areas of poverty (> 40% poverty census tracts) and public housing to move to apartments in neighborhoods with census tract poverty levels of less than 10%. Families with asthma who moved to the apartments in the "better" neighborhoods reported improved asthma in their children, independent of other risk factors. Asthma Coaches and the Neighborhood Asthma Coalition (NAC), who work with families not only on asthma management but also life stressors, including violence, safety, landlord issues, and employment, have been successful in engaging typically difficult-to-engage subjects (Brown et al., 2002; Fisher, Strunk, Sussman, Sykes, & Walker, 2004). The NAC study of African American children 5 to 14 years of age with at least one acute care incident in the previous year used parent and child educational programs, promotional activities, and individualized support by trained neighborhood residents. Of the 100 subjects randomized to the intervention, 66% had appreciable contact with the program (i.e., attendance at a promotional or educational activity or experiencing face-to-face contact with the Change Asthma with Social Support worker). Acute care visit rates decreased both for the intervention and the control groups over the 3 years of the program, with no significant between-group differences. Subjects, however, with high participation in the NAC-sponsored activities, including individuals with social isolation, experienced reductions in acute care rates, suggesting a dose–response relationship.

Most of the environmental intervention studies in general were labor intensive and involved relatively small numbers of individuals. They have not been reproduced and require further study of both their effectiveness and their cost.

### *Interventions to Prevent the Development of Asthma*

Currently, there are no known strategies to prevent the development of asthma. Treatment with ICSs in preschool children at high risk for asthma does not appear to prevent the subsequent development of asthma (Guilbert et al., 2006). Although use of ICSs improves symptoms and asthma control, it does not improve ultimate lung growth or lung function (Childhood Asthma Management Program Research Group, 2000).

Efforts to eliminate ETS exposure by the developing fetus and infant may reduce asthma prevalence (Caudri et al., 2007; Gilmour, Jaakkola, London, Nel, & Rogers, 2006). Studies to reduce allergen exposure and prevent sensitization have found mixed results. High-dose endotoxin exposure associated with farm animal exposure is associated with lower rates of asthma and may be effective, while the induction of tolerance associated with high-dose exposure to cat and dog dander before and during pregnancy and after birth has been associated with decreased sensitization to cat and dog, respectively (Owenby et al., 2002). Whether breast-feeding is protective in the development of asthma especially in mothers with a history of atopic disease is controversial (Benn et al., 2004; Oddy, 2004; Rothenbacher, Weyermann, Beermann, & Brenner, 2005).

## RECOMMENDED BEST PRACTICES

The use of ICSs in individuals with persistent disease improves quality of life, increases symptom-free days, and reduces medical services utilization but does not improve ultimate lung function (Childhood Asthma Management Program Research Group, 2000). Prescribing an ICS is essential to reduce asthma morbidity, but this treatment is not sufficient if not used regularly. Even though some studies have shown that the patient-perceived adequacy of communication does not predict adherence, efforts to understand the barriers to ICS use by patients and to improve the clinician–patient interaction are needed. Exploring a patient's beliefs and concerns about the safety and benefits of medication is important as fear of adverse effects influences adherence. Equally important is patient education, especially regarding appropriate use of medications. There is probably no single intervention that will successfully address patient beliefs and practices, but individualized interventions will be needed.

In the area of education, the evidence suggests that master's-degree social workers can partner with health care professionals to address issues surrounding asthma care for children, but collaboration between team members and community partners is critical to success (Williams & Redd, 2006).

Of all pediatric-specific programs, Open Airways, an asthma education program for children, has clearly been shown to improve asthma knowledge, self-efficacy, and asthma and general self-care practices in African American schoolchildren (Velsor-Friedrich, Pigott, & Srof, 2005).

## REFERENCES

Akinbami, L. J. (2005). *Asthma prevalence, health care use and mortality—United States, 2003.* Retrieved August 10, 2007, National Center for Health Statistics website: *www. CDC.gov.nchs/data/hestat/asthma03-05/asthma03-05.htm.*

Akinbami, L. J. (2006, December 12). The state of childhood asthma, United States, 1980–2005. *Advance Data from Vital and Health Statistics* (No. 381). Retrieved December 23, 2009, from National Center for Health Statistics website: *www.cdc.gov/nchs/data/ad/ad381.pdf.*

Akinbami, L. J., & Schoendorf, K. (2002). Trends in childhood asthma: Prevalence, health care utilization, and mortality. *Pediatrics, 110*(2), 315–322.

Al Frayh, A. R., Shakoor, Z., Gad, E. L., Rab, M. O., & Hasnain, S. M. (2001). Increased prevalence of asthma in Saudi Arabia. *Annals of Allergy, Asthma, and Immunology, 86*(3), 292–296.

Aligne, C. A., Auinger, P., Byrd, R. S., & Weitzman, M. (2000). Risk factors for pediatric asthma: Contributions of poverty, race and urban residence. *American Journal of Respiratory and Critical Care Medicine, 162,* 873–877.

Apter, A. J., Boston, R. C., George, M., Norfleet, A. L., Tenhave, T., Coyne, J. C., et al. (2003). Modifiable barriers to adherence to inhaled steroids among adults with asthma: It's not just Black and White. *Journal of Allergy and Clinical Immunology, 111,* 1219–1226.

Asthma and Allergy Foundation of America. (2006). *Asthma facts and figures.* Landover, MD: Author. Retrieved January 29, 2008, *www.aafa.org/display.cfm?id=8&sub=42.*

Auerbach, I., Springer, C., & Godfrey, S. (1993). Total population survey of the frequency and severity of asthma in 17 year old boys in an urban area of Israel. *Thorax, 48,* 139–141.

Barnes, K. C., Grant, A. V., Hansel, N. N., Gao, P., & Dunston, G. M. (2007). African

Americans with asthma: Genetic insights. *Proceedings of the American Thoracic Society, 4*, 58–68.

Barnes, P. J. (1995). Beta-adrenergic receptors and their regulation. *American Journal of Respiratory and Critical Care Medicine, 152*, 838–860.

Bartlett, S. J., Krishnan, J. A., Riekert, K. A., Butz, A. M., Malveaux, F. J., & Rand, C. S. (2004). Maternal depressive symptoms and adherence to therapy in inner-city children with asthma. *Pediatrics, 113*, 229–237.

Battle, N. C., Choudry, S., Tsai, H.-J., Eng, C., Kumar, G., Beckman, K. B., et al. (2007). Ethnicity-specific gene-gene interaction between IL-13 and IL-4Rα among African Americans with asthma. *American Journal of Respiratory and Critical Care Medicine, 175*, 881–887.

Beckett, W. S., Jacobs, J., David, R., Yu, X., Iribarren, C., & Williams, O. D. (2001). Asthma is associated with weight gain in females but not males, independent of physical activity. *American Journal of Respiratory and Critical Care Medicine, 164*(11), 2045–2050.

Benn, C. S., Wohlfahrt, J., Aaby, P., Westergaard, T., Benfeldt, E., Michaelsen, K. F., et al. (2004). Breastfeeding and risk of atopic dermatitis, by parental history of allergy, during the first 18 months of life. *American Journal of Epidemiology, 160*(3), 217–223.

Blixen, C. E., Hammel, J. P., Murphy, D., & Ault, V. (2001). Feasibility of a nurse-run asthma education program for urban African-Americans: A pilot study. *Journal of Asthma, 38*(1), 23–32.

Bosworth, H. B., Dudley, T., Olsen, M. K., Voils, C. I., Powers, B., Goldstein, M. K., et al. (2006). Racial differences in blood pressure control: Potential explanatory factors. *American Journal of Medicine, 119*, e9–e15.

Brito, B., Wurm, G., Delamater, A. M., Grus, C. L., Lopez-Hernandez, C., Applegate, E. B., et al. (2000). School-based identification of asthma in a low-income population. *Pediatric Pulmonology, 30*, 297–301.

Brown, J. V., Bakeman, R., Celano, M. P., Demi, A. S., Kobrynski, L., & Wilson, S. R. (2002). Home-based asthma education of young low-income children and their families. *Journal of Pediatric Psychology, 27*, 677–688.

Busse, W., Koenig, S. M., Oppenheimer, J., Sahn, S. A., Yancey, S. W., Reilly, D., et al. (2003). Steroid sparing effects of fluticasone 100 mcg and salmeterol 50 mcg administered twice daily in a single product in patients previously controlled with fluticasone 250 mcg twice daily. *Journal of Allergy and Clinical Immunology, 111*(1), 57–65.

Caggana, M., Walker, K., Reilly, A. A., Conroy, J. M., Duva, S., & Walsh, A. C. (1999). Population-based studies reveal differences in the allelic frequencies of two functionally significant human interleukin-4 receptor polymorphisms in several ethnic groups. *Genetics Medicine, 1*(6), 267–271.

Camargo, C. A., Field, A. E., Colditz, G. A., & Speizer, F. E. (1999). Body mass index and asthma in children age 9–14. *American Journal of Respiratory and Critical Care Medicine, 159*, A150.

Carroll, K. N., Griffin, M. R., Gebretsadik, T., Shintani, A., Mitchel, E., & Hartert, T. V. (2005). Racial differences in asthma morbidity during pregnancy. *Obstetrics and Gynecology, 106*(1), 66–72.

Caudri, D., Wijga, A., Gehring, U., Smit, H. A., Brunekreef, B., Kerkhof, M., et al. (2007). Respiratory symptoms in the first 7 years of life and birth weight at term: The PIAMA birth cohort. *American Journal of Respiratory and Critical Care Medicine, 175*(10), 1078–1085.

Celedón, J. C., Palmer, L. J., Weiss, S. T., Wang, B., Fang, Z., & Xu, X. (2001). Asthma, rhinitis, and skin test reactivity to aeroallergens in families of asthmatic subjects in Anqing, China. *American Journal of Respiratory and Critical Care Medicine, 163*, 1108–1112.

Centers for Disease Control and Prevention. (2001). Self-reported asthma prevalence among adults—United States, 2000. *Morbidity and Mortality Weekly Report, 50*(32), 682–686.

Centers for Disease Control and Prevention. (2005). *Asthma prevalence, health care use and mortality*. Atlanta, GA: Author. Retrieved May 15, 2008, from *cdc.gov/nchs/products/ pubs/pubd/hestats/asthma/asthma.htm*.

Chen, E., Fisher, E. B., Bacharier, L. B., & Strunk, R. C. (2003). Socioeconomic status, stress and immune markers in adolescents with asthma. *Psychosomatic Medicine, 65*, 984–992.

Childhood Asthma Management Program Research Group. (2000). Long-term effects of budesonide or nedocromil in children with asthma. *New England Journal of Medicine, 343*(15), 1054–1063.

Clark, N. M., Feldman, C. H., Evans, D., Levison, M. J., Wasilewski, Y., & Mellins, R. B. (1986). The impact of health education on frequency and cost of health care use by low income children with asthma. *Journal of Allergy and Clinical Immunology, 78*, 108–115.

Cloutier, M. M. (2008). Considerations in culturally directed asthma disease management programs. *Disease Management and Health Outcomes, 16*(2), 95–105.

Cloutier, M. M., Hall, C. B., Wakefield, D. B., & Bailit, H. (2005). Use of asthma guidelines by primary care providers reduces hospitalizations and emergency department visits in poor, minority, urban children. *Journal of Pediatrics, 146*, 591–597.

Cloutier, M. M., Jones, G. A., Hinckson, V., & Wakefield, D. B. (2008). Effectiveness of an asthma management program in reducing disparities in care in urban children. *Annals of Allergy, Asthma, and Immunology, 100*, 545–550.

Cloutier, M. M., Wakefield, D. B., Hall, C. B., & Bailit, H. (2002). Childhood asthma in an urban community: Prevalence, care system and treatment. *Chest, 122*, 1571–1579.

Cloutier, M. M., Wakefield, D. B., Sangeloty-Higgins, P., Delaronde, S., & Hall, C. B. (2006). Asthma guideline use by pediatricians in private practices and asthma morbidity. *Pediatrics, 118*(5), 1880–1887.

Collaborative Study on the Genetics of Asthma. (1997). A genome-wide search for asthma susceptibility loci in ethnically diverse populations. *Nature Genetics, 15*, 389–392.

Collins, F. S. (2004). What we do and don't know about "race," "ethnicity," genetics and health at the dawn of the genome era. *Nature Genetics, 36*(11, Suppl.), S13–S15.

Cote, J., Cartier, A., Robichaud, P., Boutin, H., Malo, J.-L., Rouleau, M., et al. (1997). Influence on asthma morbidity of asthma education programs based on self-management plans following treatment optimization. *American Journal of Respiratory and Critical Care Medicine, 155*, 1509–1514.

de Oliveria, M. A., Faresin, S. M., Bruno, V. W., de Bittencourt, A. R., & Fernandes, A. L. G. (1999). Evaluation of an educational programme for socially deprived asthma patients. *European Respiratory Journal, 14*, 908–914.

Devereux, G., Turner, S., Craig, L., McNeill, G., Martindale, S., Harbour, P., et al. (2006).

Low maternal vitamin E intake during pregnancy is associated with asthma in 5-year-old children. *American Journal of Respiratory and Critical Care Medicine, 174,* 499–507.

Doan, T., Grammer, L., Yarnold, P., Greenberger, P., & Patterson, R. (1996). An intervention program to reduce the hospitalization, cost of asthmatic patients requiring intubation. *Annals of Allergy, Asthma, and Immunology, 76,* 513–518.

Donahue, J. G., Fuhlbrigge, A. L., Finkelstein, J. A., Fagan, J., Livingston, J. M., Lozano, P., et al. (2000). Asthma pharmacotherapy and utilization by children in 3 managed care organizations. The pediatric asthma care patient outcomes research team. *Journal of Allergy and Clinical Immunology, 106*(6), 1108–1114.

Donahue, J. G., Weiss, S. T., Livingston, J. M., Goetsch, M. A., Greineder, D. K., & Platt, R. (1997). Inhaled steroids and the risk of hospitalization for asthma. *Journal of the American Medical Association, 277,* 887–891.

Eggleston, P. A., Malveaux, F. J., Butz, A. M., Huss, K., Thompson, L., Kolodner, K., et al. (1998). Medications used by children with asthma living in the inner city. *Pediatrics, 101*(3, pt. 1), 349–354.

Ehrlich, R., Du Toit, D., Jordaan, E., Zwarenstein, M., Potter, P., Volmink, J., et al. (1996). Risk factors for childhood asthma and wheezing. Importance of maternal and household smoking. *American Journal of Respiratory and Critical Care Medicine, 88,* 154–681.

Eldeirawi, K., & Persky, V. (2004). History of ear infections and prevalence of asthma in a national sample of children aged 2 to 11 years. *Chest, 125*(5), 1685–1692.

El-Ekiaby, M., Brianas, L., Skowronski, M. E., Coreno, A. J., Galan, G., Kaeberlein, R. J., et al. (2006). Impact of race on the severity of acute episodes of asthma and adrenergic responsiveness. *American Journal of Respiratory and Critical Care Medicine, 174,* 508–513.

Erickson, S. E., Iribarren, C., Tolstykh, I. V., Blanc, P. D., & Eisner, M. D. (2007). Effect of race on asthma management and outcomes in a large, integrated managed care organization. *Archives of Internal Medicine, 167*(17), 1846–1852.

Ernst, P., Demissie, K., Joseph, L., Locher, U., & Becklake, M. R. (1995). Socioeconomic status and indicators of asthma in children. *American Journal of Respiratory and Critical Care Medicine, 152*(2), 570–575.

Evans, D., Clark, N. M., & Feldman, C. H. (1990). School-based health education for children with asthma: Some issues for adherence research. In S. Shumaker, S. Schron, & J. K. Ockene (Eds.), *The handbook for health behavior change* (pp. 144–152). New York: Springer.

Evans, D., Mellins, R., Lobach, K., Ramos-Bonoan, C., Pinkett-Heller, M., Wiesemann, S., et al. (1997). Improving care for minority children with asthma: Professional education in public health clinics. *Pediatrics, 99*(2), 157–164.

Evans, R., Gergen, P. J., Mitchell, H., Kattan, M., Kercsmar, C., Crain, E., et al. (1999). A randomized, clinical trial to reduce asthma morbidity among inner city children: Results of the National Cooperative Inner-City Asthma Study. *Journal of Pediatrics, 135*(3), 332–338.

Federico, M. J., Covar, R. A., Brown, E. E., Leung, D. Y. M., & Spahn, J. D. (2005). Racial differences in T-lymphocyte response to glucocorticoids. *Chest, 127,* 571–578.

Ferris, T. G., Kuhlthau, K., Ausiello, J., Perrin, J., & Kahn, R. (2006). Are minority children the last to benefit from a new technology?: Technology diffusion and inhaled corticosteriods for asthma. *Medical Care, 44*(1), 81–86.

Fisher, E. B., Strunk, R. C., Sussman, L. K., Sykes, R. K., & Walker, M. S. (2004). Community organization to reduce the need for acute care for asthma among African American children in low-income neighborhoods: The Neighborhood Asthma Coalition. *Pediatrics, 114,* 116–123.

Ford, M., Marvella, E., Havstad, S., Tilley, B., & Bolton, M. (1997). Health outcomes among African American and Caucasian adults following a randomized trial of an asthma education program. *Ethnicity Health, 2*(4), 329–339.

Fuhlbrigge, A. L., Adams, R. J., Guilbert, T. W., Grant, E. N., Lozano, P., Janson, S. L., et al. (2002). The burden of asthma in the United States. Level and distribution are dependent on interpretation of the National Asthma Education and Prevention Program guidelines. *American Journal of Respiratory and Critical Care Medicine, 166,* 1044–1049.

Gao, L., Grant, A. V., Rafaels, N., Stockton-Porter, M., Watkins, T., Gao, P., et al. (2007). Polymorphisms in the myosin light chain kinase gene that confer risk of severe sepsis are associated with a lower risk of asthma. *Journal of Allergy and Clinical Immunology, 119,* 1111–1118.

Gao, P.-S., Mathias, R. A., Plunkett, B., Togias, A., Barnes, K. C., Beaty, T. H., et al. (2005). Genetic variants of the T-cell immunoglobulin mucin 1 but not the T-cell immunoglobulin mucin 3 gene are associated with asthma in an African American population. *Journal of Allergy and Clinical Immunology, 115,* 982–988.

George, M. (1999, May). *Patient perception of disease causality: Explanatory models for asthma in two African-American women.* Paper presented at the international meeting of the American Thoracic Society, San Diego, CA.

Gilliland, F., Berhane, K., Islam, T., McConnell, R., Gauderman, W., Gilliland, S. S., et al. (2003). Obesity and the risk of newly diagnosed asthma in school-age children. *American Journal of Epidemiology, 158*(5), 406–415.

Gilmour, M. I., Jaakkola, M. S., London, S. J., Nel, A. E., & Rogers, C. A. (2006). How exposure to environmental tobacco smoke, outdoor air pollutants and increased pollen burden influences the incidence of asthma. *Environmental Health Perspectives, 114*(4), 627–633.

Global Initiative for Asthma. (1995). *Global strategy for asthma management and prevention. NHLBI/WHO workshop report.* Washington, DC: National Institutes of Health, National Heart, Lung and Blood Institute.

Gold, D. R., & Wright, R. J. (2005). Population disparities in asthma. *Annual Review of Public Health, 26,* 89–113.

Grant, E. N., Lyttle, C. S., & Weiss, K. B. (2000). The relation of socioeconomic factors and racial/ethnic differences in US asthma mortality. *American Journal of Public Health, 90,* 1923–1925.

Greek, A. A., Kieckhefer, G. M., Kim, H., Joesch, J. M., & Baydar, N. (2006). Family perceptions of the usual source of care among children with asthma by race/ethnicity, language and family income. *Journal of Asthma, 43,* 61–69.

Greenstone, I. R., Ni Chromin, M. N., Masse, V., Danish, A., Magdalinos, H., Zhang, X., et al. (2005). Combination of inhaled long-acting beta2-agonists and inhaled steroids versus higher dose of inhaled steroids in children and adults with persistent asthma. *Cochrane Database of Systematic Reviews*, Issue 4 (Article No. CD005533), DOI: 10.1002/14651858.CD005533.

Guilbert, T. W., Morgan, W. J., Zeiger, R. S., Mauger, D. T., Boehmer, S. J., Szefler, S. J., et al. (2006). Long-term inhaled corticosteroids in preschool children at high risk for asthma. *New England Journal of Medicine, 354*(19), 1985–1997.

Haahtela, T., Jarvinen, M., Kava, T., Kiviranta, K., Koskinen, S., Lehtonen, K., et al. (1991). Comparison of a beta 2-agonist, terbutaline, with an inhaled corticosteroid, budesonide, in newly detected asthma. *New England Journal of Medicine, 325*(6), 388–392.

Haas, J. S., Cleary, P. D., Guadagnoli, E., Fanta, C., & Epstein, A. M. (2001). The impact of socioeconomic status on the intensity of ambulatory treatment and health outcomes after hospital discharge for adults with asthma. *Journal of General Internal Medicine, 9*, 121–126.

Haby, M. M., Peat, J. K., Marks, G. B., Woolcock, A. J., & Leeder, S. R. (2001). Asthma in preschool children: Prevalence and risk factors. *Thorax, 56*(8), 589–595.

Haire-Joshu, D., Fisher, E. B., Munro, J., & Wedner, H. J. (1993). A comparison of patient attitudes toward asthma self-management among acute and preventive care settings. *Journal of Asthma, 30*, 359–371.

Halfon, N., & Newacheck, P. (1993). Childhood asthma and poverty: Differential impacts of utilization of health services. *Pediatrics, 91*(1), 56–61.

Halm, E., Wisnivesky, J., & Leventhal, H. (2005). Quality and access to care among a cohort of inner city adults with asthma: Who gets guideline concordant care? *Chest, 128*(4), 1943–1950.

Halterman, J. S., Aligne, C. A., Auinger, P., McBride, J. T., & Szilagyi, P. G. (2000). Inadequate therapy for asthma among children in the United States. *Pediatrics, 105*(1, pt. 3), 272–276.

Hawkins, G. A., Tantisira, K., Meyers, D. A., Ampleford, E. J., Moore, W. C., Klanderman, B., et al. (2006). Sequence, haplotype and association analysis of ADRb2 in a multiethnic asthma case-control study. *American Journal of Respiratory and Critical Care Medicine, 174*, 1101–1109.

Homer, S. D. (1998). Using the Open Airways curriculum to improve self-care for third grade children with asthma. *Journal of School Health, 68*(8), 329–333.

Howland, J., Bauchner, H., & Adair, R. (1988). The impact of pediatric asthma education on morbidity. *Chest, 80*, 506–511.

Joseph, C. L., Havstad, S. L., Ownby, D. R., Johnson, C. C., & Tilleym, B. C. (1998). Racial differences in emergency department use persist despite allergist visits and prescriptions filled for antiinflammatory medications. *Journal of Allergy and Clinical Immunology, 101*, 484–490.

Joseph, C. L., Peterson, E., Havstad, S., Johnson, C. C., Hoerauf, S., Stringer, S., et al. (2007). A Web-based, tailored asthma management program for urban African-American high school students. *American Journal of Respiratory and Critical Care Medicine, 175*(9), 888–895.

Kamps, A., Brand, P., Kimpen, J., Maille, A., Overgoor-van de Groes, A., van Helsdingen-Peek, L., et al. (2003). Outpatient management of childhood asthma by paediatrician or asthma nurse: Randomised controlled study with one year follow up. *Thorax, 58*(11), 968–973.

Karjalainen, J., Virta, M., Pessi, T., Hulkkonen, J., Nieminen, M. M., & Hurme, M. (2005).

Childhood cat exposure-related tolerance is associated with IL1A and IL10 polymorphisms. *Journal of Allergy and Clinical Immunology, 116*(1), 223–225.

Kattan, M., Mitchell, H., Eggleston, P., Gergen, P., Crain, E., Redline, S., et al. (1997). Characteristics of inner-city children with asthma: The National Cooperative Inner-City Asthma Study. *Pediatric Pulmonology, 24*(4), 253–264.

Katz, L. F., Kling, J. R., & Liebman, J. B. (2001). Moving to opportunity in Boston: Early results of a randomized mobility experiment. *Quality Journal of Economics, 116*, 2.

Kelley, C. F., Mannino, D. M., Homa, D. M., Savage-Brown, A., & Holguin, F. (2005). Asthma phenotypes, risk factors, and measures of severity in a national sample of US children. *Pediatrics, 115*, 726–731.

Kelly, C. S., Morrow, A. L., Shults, J., Nakas, N., Strope, G. L., & Adelman, R. D. (2000). Outcomes evaluation of a comprehensive intervention program for asthmatic children enrolled in Medicaid. *Pediatrics, 105*, 1029–1035.

Kelso, T. M., Abou-Shala, N., Heiker, G. M., Ahreart, K. L., Portner, T. S., & Self, T. H. (1996). Comprehensive long-term management program for asthma: Effect on outcomes in adult African Americans. *American Journal of Medical Science, 311*, 272–280.

Kleinman, A., Eisenberg, L., & Good, B. (1978). Culture illness, and care: Critical lessons from anthropologic and cross-cultural research. *Annals of Internal Medicine, 88*(2), 251–258.

Klinnert, M. D., Liu, A. H., Pearson, M. R., Ellison, M. C., Budhiraja, N., & Robinson, J. L. (2005). Short-term impact of a randomized multifaceted intervention for wheezing infants in low-income families. *Archives of Pediatrics and Adolescent Medicine, 159*(1), 75–82.

Krishnan, J. A., Diette, G. B., Skinner, E. A., Clark, B. D., Steinwachs, D., & Wu, A. W. (2001). Race and sex differences in consistency of care with national asthma guidelines in managed care organizations. *Archives of Internal Medicine, 161*(13), 1660–1668.

Kuhni, C. E., & Sennhauser, F. H. (1995). The Yentl syndrome in childhood asthma: Risk factors for undertreatment in Swiss children. *Pediatric Pulmonology, 19*(3), 156–160.

Laforest, L., Van Ganse, E., Devouassoux, G., Chretin, S., Osman, L., Bauguil, G., et al. (2006). Management of asthma in patients supervised by primary care physicians or by specialists. *European Respiratory Journal, 27*(1), 42–50.

Ledogar, R. J., Penchaszadeh, A., & Garden, C. C. (2000). Asthma and Latino cultures: Different prevalence reported among groups sharing the same environment. *American Journal of Public Health, 90*(6), 929–935.

Lee, J., Haselkorn, T., Chipps, B., Miller, D., & Wenzel, S. (2006). Gender differences in IgE-mediated allergic asthma in the epidemiology and natural history of asthma: Outcomes and treatment regimens (TENOR) study. *Journal of Asthma, 43*, 179–184.

Legorreta, A., Christian-Herman, J., O'Connor, R., Hasan, M., Evans, R., & Leung, K. M. (1998). Compliance with national asthma management guidelines and specialty care: A health maintenance organization experience. *Archives of Internal Medicine, 158*(5), 457–464.

Levy, M., Heffner, B., Stewart, T., & Beeman, G. (2006). The efficacy of asthma case management in an urban school district in reducing school absences and hospitalizations for asthma. *Journal of School Health, 76*(6), 320.

Liao, O., Morphew, T., Amaro, S., & Galant, S. P. (2006). The Breathmobile: A novel comprehensive school-based mobile asthma care clinic for urban underprivileged children. *American School Health Association, 76*(6), 313–317.

Lieu, T. A., Lozano, P., Finkelstein, J. A., Chi, F. W., Jensvold, N. G., Capra, A. M., et al. (2002). Racial/ethnic variation in asthma status and management practices among children in managed Medicaid. *Pediatrics, 109*(5), 857–865.

Lieu, T. A., Quesenberry, C. P., Capra, A. M., Sorel, M. E., Martin, K. E., & Mendoza, G. R. (1997). Outpatient management practices associated with reduced risk of pediatric asthma hospitalization and emergency department visits. *Pediatrics, 100*, 334–341.

Lima, J. J., Holbrook, J. T., Wang, J., Sylvester, J. E., Blake, K. V., Blumenthal, M. N., et al. (2006). The C523A ß2-adrenergic receptor polymorphism associates with markers of asthma severity in African Americans. *Journal of Asthma, 43*, 185–191.

Litonjua, A. A. (2006). The significance of [beta]2-adrenergic receptor polymorphisms in asthma. *Pulmonary Medicine, 12*(1), 12–17.

Luder, E., Melnik, T. A., & DiMaio, M. (1998). Association of being overweight with greater asthma symptoms in inner city Black and Hispanic children. *Journal of Pediatrics, 132*, 699–703.

MacMullen, N. J., Tymkow, C., & Shen, J. J. (2006). Adverse maternal outcomes in women with asthma: Differences by race. *American Journal of Maternal Child Nursing, 31*(4), 263–268.

Mancuso, C. A., Peterson, M. G., & Charlson, M. E. (2000). Effects of depressive symptoms on health-related quality of life in asthma patients. *Journal of General Internal Medicine, 15*, 301–310.

Mancuso, C. A., Rincon, M., McCulloch, C. E., & Charlson, M. E. (2001). Self-efficacy, depressive symptoms, and patients' expectations predict outcomes in asthma. *Medical Care, 39*, 1326–1338.

Manfreda, J., Becklake, M. R., Sears, M. R., Chan-Yeung, M., Dimich-Ward, H., Siersted, H. C., et al. (2001). Prevalence of asthma symptoms among adults aged 20–44 years in Canada. *Canadian Medical Association Journal, 164*(7), 995–1001.

Mannino, D. M., Homa, D. M., Pertowski, C. A., Ashizawa, A., Nixon, L. L., Johnson, C. A., et al. (1998). Surveillance for asthma—United States, 1960–1995. *Morbidity and Mortality Weekly Report, 47*(1), 1–27.

Marion, R., Creer, T., & Reynolds, R. (1985). Direct and indirect costs associated with the management of childhood asthma. *Annals of Allergy, 54*, 31–34.

Masoli, M., Weatheral, M., Holt, S., & Beasley, R. (2005). Moderate dose inhaled corticosteroids plus salmeterol versus higher doses of inhaled corticosteroids in symptomatic asthma. *Thorax, 60*, 730–734.

Mayo, P. H., Richman, J., & Harris, H. W. (1990). Results of a program to reduce admissions for adult asthma. *Annals of Internal Medicine, 112*, 864–871.

McCoy, K., Shade, D. M., Irvin, C. G., Mastronarde, J. G., Hanania, N. A., Castro, M., et al. (2006). Predicting episodes of poor asthma control in treated patients with asthma. *Journal of Allergy and Clinical Immunology, 118*, 1226–1233.

Moissidis, I., Chinoy, B., Yanamandra, K., Napper, D., Thurman, T., Bocchini, J., et al. (2005). Association of IL-13, RANTES, and leukotriene C4 synthase gene promoter polymorphisms with asthma and/or atopy in African Americans. *Genetics in Medicine, 7*(6), 406–410.

Morgan, W. J., Crain, E. F., Gruchalla, R. S., O'Connor, G. T., Kattan, M., Evans, R., et al.

(2004). Results of a home-based environmental intervention among urban children with asthma. *New England Journal of Medicine, 351*(11), 1068–1080.

National Asthma Education and Prevention Program. (2005). Managing asthma during pregnancy: Recommendations for pharmacologic treatment–Update 2004. Retrieved December 23, 2009, from www.nhlbi.nih.gov/health/prof/lung/asthma/astpreg/astpreg_qr.pdf.

National Center for Health Statistics. (2006). *Asthma.* Atlanta, GA: Centers for Disease Control and Prevention. Retrieved May 15, 2008, from *www.cdc.gov/nchs/fastats/asthma.htm.*

National Institutes of Health, National Heart, Lung and Blood Institute. (1997). *Guidelines for the diagnosis and management of asthma* (NIH Publication No. 97-4053). Washington, DC: U.S. Department of Health and Human Services.

National Institutes of Health, National Heart, Lung and Blood Institute. (2001). *Guidelines for the diagnosis and management of asthma-update on selected topics, 2002* (NIH Publication No. 01-4057). Washington, DC: U.S. Department of Health and Human Services.

Nelson, H. S., Weiss, S. T., Bleecker, E. R., Yancey, S. W., Dorinsky, P. M., & SMART Study Group. (2006). The salmeterol multicenter asthma research trial (SMART): A comparison of usual pharmacotherapy for asthma or usual pharmacotherapy plus salmeterol. *Chest, 129,* 15–26.

Nicholas, S. W., Jean-Louis, B., Ortiz, B., Northridge, M., Shoemaker, K., Vaughan, R., et al. (2005). Addressing the childhood asthma crisis in Harlem: The Harlem Children's Zone Asthma Initiative. *American Journal of Public Health, 95*(2), 245–249.

Oddy, W. H. (2004). A review of the effects of breastfeeding on respiratory infections, atopy, and childhood asthma. *Journal of Asthma, 41*(6), 605–621.

Owenby, D. R., Johnson, C. C., & Peterson, E. L. (2002). Exposure to dogs and cats in the first year of life and risk of allergic sensitization at 6 to 7 years of age. *Journal of the American Medical Association, 288,* 963–972.

Paasche-Orlow, M. K., Riekert, K. A., Bilderback, A., Chanmugam, A., Hill, P., Rand, C. S., et al. (2005). Tailored education may reduce health literacy disparities in asthma self-management. *American Journal of Respiratory and Critical Care Medicine, 172,* 980–986.

Parcel, G. S., Gilman, S. C., Nader, P. R., & Bunce, H. A. (1979). A comparison of absentee rates of elementary school children with asthma and non-asthmatic schoolmates. *Pediatrics, 64,* 878–881.

Park, J., Gold, D. R., Spiegelman, D. L., Burge, H. A., & Milton, D. K. (2001). House dust endotoxin and wheeze in the first year of life. *American Journal of Respiratory and Critical Care Medicine, 163,* 322–328.

Pauley, T. R., Magee, M. J., & Cury, J. D. (1999). Results of pharmacy managed, physician directed program to reduce emergency department visits in a group of inner city adult asthma patients. *Annals of Pharmacology and Therapeutics, 29,* 5–9.

Peat, J. K., Tovey, E., Toelle, B. G., Haby, M. M., Gray, E. J., Mahmic, A., et al. (1996). House dust mite allergens. A major risk factor for childhood asthma in Australia. *American Journal of Respiratory and Critical Care Medicine, 153*(1), 141–146.

Ramsey, C. D., Celedón, J. C., Stredl, D. L., Weiss, S. T., & Cloutier, M. M. (2005). Predictors of disease severity in children with asthma in Hartford, Connecticut. *Pediatric Pulmonology, 39*(3), 268–275.

Rand, C. S., Butz, A. M., Kolodner, K., Huss, K., Eggleston, P., & Malveaux, F. (2000). Emergency department visits by urban African American children with asthma. *Journal of Allergy and Clinical Immunology, 105*(1), 83–90.

Resch, K., Hill, S., & Ernst, E. (1997). Use of complementary therapies by individuals with arthritis. *Clinical Rheumatology, 16,* 391–395.

Riekert, K. A., Butz, A. M., Eggleston, P. A., Huss, K., Winkelstein, M., & Rand, C. S. (2003). Caregiver-physician medication concordance and undertreatment of asthma among inner-city children. *Pediatrics, 111,* e214–e220.

Rizzo, M. C., Naspitz, C. K., Fernandez-Caldas, E., Lockey, R. F., Mimica, I., & Sole, D. (1997). Endotoxin exposure and symptoms in asthmatic children. *Pediatric Allergy and Immunology, 8,* 121–126.

Rosenstreich, D. L., Eggleston, P., Kattan, M., Baker, D., Slavin, R. G., Gergen, P., et al. (1997). The role of cockroach allergy and exposure to cockroach allergen in causing morbidity among inner-city children with asthma. *New England Journal of Medicine, 336*(19), 1356–1363.

Rothenbacher, D., Weyermann, M., Beermann, C., & Brenner, H. (2005). Breastfeeding, soluble CD14 concentration in breast milk and risk of atopic dermatitis and asthma in early childhood: Birth cohort study. *Clinical and Experimental Allergy, 35*(8), 1014–1021.

Schectman, J. M., Nadkarni, M. M., & Voss, J. D. (2002). The association between diabetes metabolic control and drug adherence in an indigent population. *Diabetes, 25,* 1015–1021.

Sears, M. R. (1997). Epidemiology of childhood asthma. *Lancet, 350,* 1015–1020.

Shrewsbury, S., Pyke, S., & Britton, M. (2000). Meta-analysis of increased dose of inhaled steroid or addition of salmeterol in symptomatic asthma (MASMA). *British Medical Journal, 320,* 1368–1373.

Sly, R. M., & O'Donnell, R. (1997). Stabilization of asthma mortality. *Annals of Allergy Asthma and Immunology, 78,* 347–354.

Smith, M. J., & Pawar, V. (2007). Medical services and prescription use for asthma and factors that predict inhaled corticosteroid use among African-American children covered by Medicaid. *Journal of Asthma, 44,* 357–363.

Smith, S. R., Jaffe, D. M., Fisher, E. B., Trinkaus, K. M., Highstein, G., & Strunk, R. C. (2004). Improving follow-up for children with asthma after an acute emergency department visit. *Journal of Pediatrics, 145,* 772–777.

Sporik, R., Holgate, S. T., Platts-Mills, T. A., & Cogswell, J. J. (1990). Exposure to house-dust mite allergen (Der p 1) and the development of asthma in childhood. A prospective study. *New England Journal of Medicine, 323*(8), 502–507.

Squillace, S. P., Sporik, R. B., Rakes, G., Couture, N., Lawrence, A., Merriam, S., et al. (1997). Sensitization to dust mites as a dominant risk factor for asthma among adolescents living in central Virginia. Multiple regression analysis of a population-based study. *American Journal of Respiratory and Critical Care Medicine, 156*(6), 1760–1764.

Strunk, R. C., Mrazek, D. A., Fuhrmann, G., & LaBrecque, J. F. (1985). Physiologic and psychological characteristics associated with deaths due to asthma in childhood: A case-controlled study. *Journal of the American Medical Association, 254*(9), 1193–1198.

Suissa, S., Ernst, P., Benayoun, S., Baltzan, M., & Cai, B. (2000). Low-dose inhaled corticosteroids and the prevention of death from asthma. *New England Journal of Medicine, 343,* 332–336.

Tatis, V., Remache, D., & DiMango, E. (2005). Results of a culturally directed asthma intervention program in an inner-city Latino community. *Chest, 128*(3), 1163–1167.

Teach, S. J., Crain, E. F., Quint, D. M., Hylan, M. L., & Joseph, J. G. (2006). Improved asthma outcomes in a high-morbidity pediatric population: Results of an emergency department-based randomized clinical trial. *Archives of Pediatrics and Adolescent Medicine, 160*(5), 535–541.

Trochtenberg, D. S., BeLue, R., Piphus, S., & Washington, N. (2008). Differing reports of asthma symptoms in African Americans and Caucasians. *Journal of Asthma, 45*(2), 165–170.

Velsor-Friedrich, B., Pigott, T., & Srof, B. (2005). A practitioner-based asthma intervention program with African American inner-city school children. *Journal of Pediatric Health Care, 19*, 163–171.

Venn, A. J., Yemaneberhan, H., Bekele, Z., Lewis, S. A., Parry, E., & Britton, J. (2001). Increased risk of allergy associated with the use of kerosene fuel in the home. *American Journal of Respiratory and Critical Care Medicine, 164*, 1660–1664.

von Maffei, J., Beckett, W. S., Belanger, K., Triche, E., Zhang, H., Machung, J. F., et al. (2001). Risk factors for asthma prevalence among urban and non-urban African American children. *Journal of Asthma, 38*(7), 555–564.

Wade, S. L., Holden, G., Lynn, H., Mitchell, H., & Ewart, C. (2000). Cognitive-behavioral predictors of asthma morbidity in inner-city children. *Journal of Developmental and Behavioral Pediatrics, 21*, 340–345.

Warman, K. L., Silver, E. J., & Stein, R. E. K. (2001). Asthma symptoms, morbidity, and antiinflammatory use in inner-city children. *Pediatrics, 108*(2), 277–282.

Weinick, R. M., Weigers, M. E., & Cohen, J. W. (1998). Children's health insurance, access to care and health status: New findings. *Health Affairs, 17*, 127–136.

Weiss, K. B., & Sullivan, S. D. (2001). The health economics of asthma and rhinitis. Assessing the economic impact. *Journal of Allergy and Clinical Immunology, 107*, 3–8.

Weiss, K. B., Sullivan, S. D., & Lyttle, C. S. (2000). Trends in the cost of illness for asthma in the United States, 1985–1994. *Journal of Allergy and Clinical Immunology, 106*, 493–499.

Weiss, K. B., & Wagener, D. K. (1990). Changing patterns of asthma mortality: Identifying target populations at high risk. *Journal of the American Medical Association, 264*, 1683–1687.

Weitzman, M., Byrd, R. S., & Auinger, P. (1999). Black and White middle class children who have private health insurance in the United States. *Pediatrics, 104*, 151–157.

Wennergren, G., Kristjansson, S., & Strannegard, I. L. (1996). Decrease in hospitalization for treatment of childhood asthma with increased use of antiinflammatory treatment, despite an increase in prevalence of asthma. *Journal of Allergy and Clinical Immunology, 97*, 742–748.

Williams, L. K., Joseph, C. L., Peterson, E. L., Moon, C., Xi, H., Krajenta, R., et al. (2007). Race-ethnicity, crime and other factors associated with adherence to inhaled corticosteroids. *Journal of Allergy and Clinical Immunology, 119*(1), 168–175.

Williams, L. K., Pladevall, M., Xi, H., Peterson, E. L., Joseph, C., Lafata, J. E., et al. (2004). Relationship between adherence to inhaled corticosteroids and poor outcomes among adults with asthma. *Journal of Allergy and Clinical Immunology, 114*(6), 1288–1293.

Williams, S. G., & Redd, S. C. (2006). From research to reality: From the National Cooperative Inner-City Asthma Study to the inner-city asthma implementation. *Annals of Allergy, Asthma, and Immunology, 97*(Suppl. 1), S4–S5.

Wisnivesky, J. P., Leventhal, H., & Halm, E. A. (2005). Predictors of asthma-related health care utilization and quality of life among inner-city patients with asthma. *Journal of Allergy and Clinical Immunology, 116*(3), 636–642.

Wittich, A. R., Mangan, J. M., Grad, R., Wang, W., & Gerald, L. B. (2007). Pediatric asthma: Caregiver health literacy and the clinician's perception. *Journal of Asthma, 44*, 51–55.

Wood, P., Tumiel-Berhalter, L., Owen, S., Taylor, K., & Kattan, M. (2006). Implementation of an asthma intervention in the inner city. *Annals of Allergy, Asthma, and Immunology, 97*(Suppl. 1), S20–S24.

Wright, A. L., Stern, D. A., Kauffmann, F., & Martinez, F. D. (2006). Factors influencing gender differences in the diagnosis and treatment of asthma in childhood: The Tucson Children's Respiratory Study. *Pediatric Pulmonology, 41*(4), 318–325.

Wright, R. J. (2006). Health effects of socially toxic neighborhoods: The violence and urban asthma paradigm. *Clinics in Chest Medicine, 27*(3), 413–421.

Wright, R. J., Cohen, S., Carey, V., Weiss, S. T., & Gold, D. R. (2002). Parental stress as a predictor of wheezing in infancy. A prospective birth-cohort study. *American Journal of Respiratory and Critical Care Medicine, 165*, 358–365.

Wright, R. J., Mitchell, H., Visness, C. M., Cohen, S., Stout, J., Evans, R., et al. (2004). Community violence and asthma morbidity: The Inner-City Asthma Study. *American Journal of Public Health, 94*(4), 625–632.

Wu, A. W., Young, Y., Skinner, E. A., Diette, G. B., Huber, M., Peres, A., et al. (2001). Quality of care and outcomes of adults with asthma treated by specialists and generalists in managed care. *Archives of Internal Medicine, 161*, 2554–2560.

Zoratti, E., Havstad, S., Rodriguez, J., Robens-Paradise, Y., Lafata, J., & McCarthy, B. (1998). Health services use by African-Americans and Caucasians with asthma in a managed care setting. *American Journal of Respiratory and Critical Care Medicine, 158*, 371–377.

Zorc, J. J., Scarfone, R. J., Li, Y., Hong, T., Harmelin, M., Grunstein, L., et al. (2003). Scheduled follow-up after a pediatric emergency department visit for asthma: A randomized trial. *Pediatrics, 111*(3), 495–502.

# 11

## Diabetes

M. Kathleen Figaro
Verla M. Vaughan
Freida Hopkins Outlaw

$\mathbf{D}$iabetes mellitus is a complex of disorders causing increased amounts of glucose in the blood (hyperglycemia) and urine (Nathan, 2002). This hyperglycemia can lead to serious damage to many of the body's systems over time, especially the nerves and blood vessels (Nathan, 1993). There are two primary types of diabetes, both reflecting different problems with regulation of glucose and insulin levels in the body: Either the beta cells of the pancreas do not produce insulin (Type 1) or that the body cannot effectively use the insulin it produces (Type 2).

The prevalence of all types of diabetes in 2007 was 24 million, or 8% of the U.S. population (Centers for Disease Control and Prevention [CDC], 2005). Type 1 diabetes mellitus (T1DM) has an overall incidence of approximately 15 cases per 100,000 individuals annually in the United States and is increasing (Diamond Project Group, 2006). Whites are affected more often than African Americans, who have the lowest overall incidence of T1DM. Males are as likely to have the disease as females (Dorman & Bunker, 2000). T1DM is diagnosed primarily in childhood, adolescence, or early adulthood; the peak incidence occurs before age 20.

Type 2 diabetes mellitus (T2DM) is often called "sugar" in African American communities. It has disproportionately affected this community for more than half a century. T2DM is currently diagnosed in approximately 1.5 million Americans of African descent and is thought to be undiagnosed in another 730,000 members of this group (American Diabetes Association [ADA], 2000). Both African American men and women are at twice the risk of T2DM compared with their White counterparts, with a rate of 6.5% for the total population: 5.6% in Whites but 10% in African Americans (CDC, 2005; Cowie et al., 2006). The prevalence of T2DM in children is 4.1 per 1,000 12- to 19-year-olds in the United States (ADA, 2000). Its prevalence is rising in all populations but is especially marked in African American youth.

A third type of diabetes, gestational diabetes mellitus (GDM), develops during some pregnancies but usually disappears afterward. It increases a woman's chance of developing T2DM later by 17–63% and, untreated, increases negative outcomes of pregnancy by as much as 59% (Kjos & Buchanan, 1999; Langer, Yogev, Most, & Xenakis, 2005). GDM is more common among women of African descent than White women, in part because they are more likely to be overweight or obese during pregnancy.

These three types of diabetes are all associated with psychosocial complications. There is a clear bidirectional association between T2DM and depression (Golden et al., 2008), although the reasons for this are not entirely understood. However, understanding that link is likely a particularly important part of the solution to the epidemic of diabetes in the African American community. As part of our focus on African Americans and diabetes, we discuss T2DM, socioeconomic status (SES), race and ethnicity, and depression.

Major depressive disorder is characterized by symptoms of depressed mood, sadness, helplessness, loss of interest and pleasure in activities, and feelings of worthlessness or guilt. Other symptoms include difficulty concentrating, weight gain or loss, irritability, withdrawal, isolation, thoughts of death, and physical symptoms such as pain (American Psychiatric Association, 2000). Depression affects more than 21 million children and adults in the United States (U.S. Department of Health and Human Services, 2006). Those with diabetes and serious mental illness such as major depression suffer worse clinical and social outcomes of the disease (CDC, 2004b). Although African American and White women have similar rates of depression in the general population, African American women are less likely to seek treatment, and when they do, they are less likely to be diagnosed with depression (O'Malley, Forrest, & Miranda, 2003). Thus, depression is common in T2DM in women and is likely an underrecognized source of diabetes outcomes disparities for African American women.

## EXPLANATORY MODEL

The developmental ecological systems model provides a framework for conceptualizing T2DM and the associated clinical depression in African Americans from five levels of behavioral influence: individual, interpersonal, organizational, community or cultural group, and policy (Fisher et al., 2002, 2005, 2007). The model provides a specific theory-driven approach to address the interrelated levels of behavioral influence of T2DM on African Americans. For example, as a group, African Americans are disproportionately diagnosed with T2DM and experience a disparity in mortality and morbidity related to the disease (Harris, Eastman, Cowie, Flegal, & Eberhardt, 1999). The developmental ecological systems model allows us to explore T2DM in African Americans from the biological to the health policy level.

There is great heterogeneity in the African American community. We focus on low-resource African American individuals, families, and communities because they are most at risk for T2DM, and their vulnerabilities require them to develop greater resilience. This chapter emphasizes interventions that encompass the individual and the community. Because T2DM requires significant self-care interventions with a holistic approach that include clinical treatment, behavioral change and community support are important. These types of interventions—collaborative, resource rich, and available to those with private and public insurance—will likely be most effective.

## BIOLOGICAL/GENETIC FACTORS

Individuals with T1DM produce very little or no insulin and require daily injections of insulin to survive. Common symptoms of T1DM include excessive thirst, constant hunger, excessive urination, unexplained weight loss, labored breathing, visual changes, drowsiness, fatigue, or exhaustion. These symptoms may occur suddenly and generally before the age of 30. The relatively sudden loss of insulin within the body comes from an immune reaction that kills the beta cells of the pancreas (ADA, 2003). This disorder can be fatal in children if not recognized early.

T1DM occurs mostly in children and young adults but may develop in older adults. It is usually diagnosed by measuring islet cell antibodies or C-peptide levels, which are high and low, respectively. In general, although African Americans are less likely to have T1DM, they suffer higher mortality from its complications (Bosnyak et al., 2005). Among African Americans, T1DM has an incidence rate of approximately five to eight per 100,000, although some recent studies show an increase in prevalence (Lipman et al., 2006).

T1DM is associated with an increased risk for coronary artery disease (CAD) and loss of vision and kidney function. Poor blood sugar control has been shown to increase these risks. African Americans with T1DM have a higher relative risk of losing vision in at least one eye (Roy & Skurnick, 2007), dialysis (Roy, 2004), and CAD compared with Whites (Cleary et al., 2006; Hozawa, Folsom, Sharrett, & Chambless, 2007). People with T1DM are generally at higher risk of CAD, and the excess risk seems to be higher than in those with T2DM.

Most people (90–95%) with diabetes mellitus have Type 2 (ADA, 2007). People with T2DM cannot use their body's insulin effectively, although they usually produce excess insulin at the onset of disease. Generally, those who are diagnosed with T2DM are older than 40; however, younger people increasingly have Type 2, as obesity increases and physical activity decreases in these age groups (CDC, 2004a). People with T2DM may initially have less obvious symptoms compared with those with Type 1. They may have mild symptoms such as fatigue that mimic depression. Many have no symptoms and are only diagnosed after many years of mild hyperglycemia. As a consequence, 30–40% of people with T2DM are not aware that they have this serious condition (Gregg et al., 2004). They can manage their condition with lifestyle measures, oral medications, and ultimately insulin in order to achieve good metabolic control (Krentz & Bailey, 2005). Metabolic control is generally considered to be hemoglobin A1C (A1C) measures of 7% or less (ADA, 2007).

T2DM is strongly associated with inactivity and obesity (Jeon, Lokken, Hu, & van Dam, 2007; Rana, Li, Manson, & Hu, 2007). About 65% of the U.S. adult population is overweight, and more than 30% of these are obese (Flegal, Carroll, Ogden, & Johnson, 2002). A body mass index (BMI) between 25 and 30 is considered overweight and above 30, obese. A person's probability of developing T2DM doubles for every 20% increase over desirable body weight (Narayan, Boyle, Thompson, Gregg, & Williamson, 2007). Obesity is also associated with greater insulin resistance and higher A1C levels. Almost 80% of the risk of disease may be attributed to inactivity and obesity (Stein & Colditz, 2004). T2DM is also related to the intake of concentrated sweets, excess caloric intake, and subsequent inflammation (Basciano, Federico, & Adeli, 2005; Hu et al., 2001; Schulze et al., 2004). The prevalence of Type 2 diabetes is greater in the African American community than would be predicted on the basis of obesity alone.

A series of environmental changes, including industrialization and migration to cities, appears to confer increased risk of T2DM and other cardiovascular diseases as a result of inactivity and obesity (Koya & Egede, 2007). Sedentary behavior is also related to the metabolic syndrome, a disorder that is, in essence, a prediabetic state. This cluster of abnormalities includes abdominal obesity, insulin resistance, glucose intolerance, hyperinsulinemia, hypertension, and hypertriglyceridemia. The metabolic syndrome, in turn, leads to a four-time greater risk of heart disease and seven-time greater risk of diabetes compared with those without the condition (Guize et al., 2007). Although fewer African Americans, proportionally, meet the definition of metabolic syndrome, this population is more insulin resistant and has higher blood glucose levels than Whites at similar levels of adiposity; they also have higher blood pressures and, among women, are more likely to have abdominal obesity (Butler et al., 2006; R. A. Williams et al., 2006).

Hypertension appears to confer an independent risk for T2DM, especially in African Americans (Douglas, 1990). The combination of hypertension and T2DM confers additional risk for renal failure. African Americans thus have a disproportionate risk of renal failure from T2DM: four times the prevalence rates for Whites and 2.6 times the rate when controlling for the presence of diabetes (Lea & Nicholas, 2002). Having low high-density lipoprotein cholesterol and high triglyceride levels are also risk factors for T2DM (Festa et al., 1999). All together, disorders of blood pressure, cholesterol, and glucose make T2DM a metabolic disorder.

Because of the association between obesity and metabolic disorders, the increased incidence of childhood obesity is a disturbing current public health trend (Ogden, Carroll, & Flegal, 2008). It is linked to subsequent metabolic abnormalities such as elevated blood pressure, lipids, lipoproteins, and insulin levels in adulthood (Dietz, 1998). Childhood obesity will increase the lifetime risk of both CAD and T2DM. In particular, adolescent T2DM is more common among African Americans (SEARCH for Diabetes in Youth Study Group, 2006). African Americans are already at high risk for chronic disease; increased obesity and T2DM will only add to the current burden of health disparities.

Both Type 1 and Type 2 diabetes are associated with genetic susceptibilities and environmental triggers. Genes related to immunological functions likely play a role in the development of T1DM (Yoon & Jun, 2001), and racial differences in the proportion of these major histocompatibility genes may account for the lower rates in African Americans. Several studies show seasonal and temporal differences in incidence of T1DM that suggest environmental and even infectious causes (Jordan, Lipton, Stupnicka, Cruickshank, & Fraser, 1994; Lipton, Drum, Li, & Choi, 1999). The inability to find single-gene defects in most cases of T1DM suggests a polygenic cause (Dorman & Bunker, 2000). In addition, family members of those with T1DM have been shown to have increased markers for oxidative stress; this could predispose them to both the renal and coronary complications associated with T1DM (Matteucci & Giampietro, 2007).

For T2DM, research has implicated multiple genes that determine insulin secretion and resistance (Wolford & Vozarova de Courten, 2004). One hypothesis states that the genetic predisposition to T2DM may stem from a lower beta cell mass at birth or previous beta cell toxicity, which leads to hyperglycemia and further beta cell deterioration (Leahy, 2005). However, the complex inheritance patterns and substantial environmental interaction have limited discovery of the genes involved in T2DM (Alberti et al., 2004). Only a small percentage of cases can be explained by a single-gene defect such as the condition known as maturity-onset diabetes of the young (Pinterova et al., 2007).

Mutations of several genes are under investigation, including CD36, peroxisome proliferator-activated receptor gamma, Calpain 10, GLUT1, insulin and insulin receptor genes, mitochondrial DNA, and the glucagon receptor (Alberti et al., 2004; Cheng, 2005; Love-Gregory et al., 2008). More severe gestational diabetes in African Americans (and increased risk for T2DM) has been associated with a defective gene for insulin (Bell et al., 1990). Some investigators have postulated a thrifty gene that, when combined with excess caloric intake and decreased caloric expenditure, can predispose people to T2DM (Watve & Yajnik, 2007). The thought was that African Americans more commonly have this gene variant, which puts them at higher risk for T2DM. Little evidence currently exists to support this theory (Paradies, Montoya, & Fullerton, 2007).

In 2006, a variant in a gene called TCF7L2 that predisposes people to Type 2 T2DM was identified that increased risk by 80% in those with two alleles of the abnormal gene (Florez et al., 2006). This risk was not replicated in the Pima Indian population (Guo et al., 2007) but was duplicated in a small sample of African Americans (Sale et al., 2007). Further study of the impact of genes will hopefully include greater percentages of high-risk populations such as African Americans and Pima Indians. We do not yet know whether T2DM is substantially different genetically between African Americans and Whites or, more likely, whether the expression of the disease is more aggressive because of social and cultural factors.

In summary, physical inactivity and obesity confer great risk for T2DM, the most common type of diabetes. The recent increase in prevalence of T2DM appears to be related to both environmental and lifestyle factors. The risk of T2DM is relatively low before age 30 and, then increases with age. African American men and women show marked relative increased risk for T2DM and its complications compared with White men and women. The risks for T2DM appear to be similar to those for other metabolic disorders such as cardiovascular disease since T2DM is a metabolic disorder. Genetic factors play a role in the susceptibility to both T1DM and T2DM but may not account for the majority of differences in prevalence seen in the different racial groups. If we approach diabetes using the ecological model, then we first need to address how the individual experiences the risk for disease and develops resilience in the face of that risk.

## INDIVIDUAL RISK FACTORS/RESILIENCY

For T2DM, the central theme for individuals is modifying, when possible, factors that increase risk, such as overweight, sedentary lifestyle, and poor dietary habits; some factors for T2DM, such as age and family history, cannot be modified. In addition, cultural factors such as diet, choice of leisure activities, health beliefs, and values impact the risk of T2DM as well as its progression (Baptiste-Roberts et al., 2007). These factors should be targeted for early intervention and prevention of T2DM, especially among high-risk groups such as African American children and adolescents.

Many African American men become overweight and sedentary as they age (CDC, 2004a). African American men of whatever SES are well known for underutilizing the health care system relative to other racial groups (Fiscella & Shin, 2005). African American men are less likely to see physicians for preventive care (Liburd, Namageyo-Funa, & Jack, 2007). Distrust of the health care system, deeply ingrained, culturally based stoic attitudes, and fatalistic beliefs may make African American men an especially difficult group to engage in diabetes prevention and treatment (Bonhomme & Braithwaite, 2003). In addition, few published papers consider masculinity, specifically Black masculinity, and how it may influence diabetes self-management behaviors (Jack, Toston, Jack, & Sims, 2010). This is an area ripe for additional research.

Some African American men may also become nonadherent with diabetes pharmacotherapy because of the side effects, which may lessen quality of life. The combination of T2DM and blood pressure medications many diabetic people take sometimes causes erectile dysfunction. This side effect, which impacts more than 50% of men with diabetes, is more common among African American men (Grover et al., 2006; Laumann et al., 2007). Because men in general have difficulty discussing sexuality, they are less likely to have treatment plans that include care for this important issue. It may be particularly useful to provide men with education regarding the natural history of diabetes and its treatment complications soon after their diagnosis. Men can also be reassured that there are positive sexual and psychological effects of successfully managing their diabetes and that they can adapt to life with erectile dysfunction. Cooper-Patrick and colleagues (1999) found that race-concordant doctor–patient relationships tended to promote more patient participation. Having an awareness of the perceived quality-of-life burden of diabetes treatments can improve communication between Black men with diabetes and their health care providers, whatever their race. However, this suggests that African American men might benefit from relationships with same-race physicians to improve their diabetes outcomes.

Obesity affects one-third of African American women. This condition exists for many cultural, economic, and medical reasons and greatly impacts the tendency for older Black women to be diagnosed with and suffer greater complications of diabetes. Older studies showed that African American women viewed obesity favorably (Allan, Mayo, & Michel, 1993) and had more positive body images at higher weight. This attitude and others associated with perceptions of femininity have likely contributed to the current prevalence of obesity in African American women. More recent evidence suggests that body satisfaction beliefs of women of both races are converging (Grabe & Hyde, 2006). However, this has occurred during the same time period that obesity has become much more prevalent among all Americans. The true impact of current obesity levels on the future life span and chronic disease burden is a currently underdocumented important factor in health care.

African American men in general have also moved from approving larger body sizes to becoming similar in their preferences to White men (Jones, Fries, & Danish, 2007; Powell & Kahn, 1995). Studies (Allan et al., 1993; DiGioacchino, Sargent, & Topping, 2001) suggest that obese African American women of lower SES continue to believe larger body sizes are more attractive. However, this finding does not hold among African American women of higher SES or with a college education. There are thus clear and significant within-group differences based on economic status. These data suggest that new interventions to reduce the risk of diabetes among obese African American women take SES into consideration. New valuation of smaller body sizes in certain African American women may make community-level messages regarding weight loss for better health more acceptable to them.

African American women are traditionally at risk of neglecting care of themselves when they prioritize taking care of others in their family. Being strong is a central concept for certain African American women (Beauboeuf-Lafontant, 2007). Although being strong may be associated with greater self-efficacy, it may also be associated with the tendency to delay treatment. A recent study suggests that both African American and White women experience great psychological stress from their diabetes treatment (Penckofer, Ferrans, Velsor-Friedrich, & Savoy, 2007). This stress can mitigate good food choices and be associated with binging behaviors. A recent study to induce weight loss in women with T2DM found that African American women lost less weight than White women and appeared to have a diminished benefit from the addition of the technique of motivational interviewing (West, DiLillo, Bursac, Gore, & Greene, 2007). However, African American women with better dietary restraint skills and greater self-efficacy beliefs regarding their ability have been shown to follow a diet more faithfully and demonstrate greater readiness to lose weight when necessary (Delahanty, Meigs, Hayden, Williamson, & Nathan, 2002).

Being diagnosed with T2DM is itself a major life stressor. It requires many physical and behavioral adjustments. The individual must learn about and maintain a complex regimen of dietary, exercise, and medical treatments. Work and school schedules often have to be changed. These added tasks can consume a lot of energy for patients and their family members, especially those with limited resources. There are immense psychological adjustments as well. These adjustments to being diagnosed with T2DM can predispose individuals to depression. Although this depression can be treated, it must first be diagnosed. Some studies suggest African Americans are less likely to be diagnosed with depression compared with White patients (O'Malley et al., 2003; Wagner, Tsimikas, Abbott, de Groot, & Heapy, 2007). In addition, communication difficulties in patient–provider relationships may impede identification of depressive symptoms among African Americans (Kogan, Brody, Crawley, Logan, & Murry, 2007).

Studies (R. J. Anderson, Freedland, & Clouse, 2001; Golden et al., 2008) suggest a reciprocal relationship between depression and T2DM. Those with T2DM are twice as likely to suffer from depression compared with those without the disease. Psychological factors and psychiatric conditions can affect the course of T2DM. Among people with T2DM, major depression is associated with increased risk of diabetic complications, lower treatment adherence, and poorer self-care of T2DM (Gonzalez et al., 2007; Kalsekar et al., 2006). The interaction between cardiovascular disorders and depression has also been previously documented (Lett et al., 2004; Whooley, 2006). Depression has been linked directly to an increased risk of neuropathy and to other factors (e.g., smoking and substance abuse; CDC, 2004b) that add to the risk of diabetic complications.

Thus, depression has direct and indirect links to both poor glycemic control and diabetes complications in both adults (Lustman, Griffith, Gavard, & Clouse,

1992) and adolescents (La Greca, Swales, Klemp, Madigan, & Skyler, 1995). T2DM and depression can predate one another. Therefore, when depression is diagnosed, it should be aggressively treated to prevent diabetes and its cardiovascular complications (Saydah, Brancati, Golden, Fradkin, & Harris, 2003). In those who already have diabetes, treatment of depression may lead to a better medical prognosis as well as improved quality of life.

Depression is associated with obesity, physical inactivity, and treatment noncompliance, factors that contribute to poor glycemic control in African Americans (Ciechanowski, Katon, Russo, & Hirsch, 2003; Lin et al., 2004). African Americans, with and without diabetes, face a number of barriers in the treatment of depression, including presenting psychological distress as somatic or physical symptoms, minimizing of their emotional complaints by providers, and fearing stigma from the diagnosis of depression (Das, Offson, McCurtis, & Weissman, 2006). Because those with depression may have worse outcomes, providers can focus interventions on patients with greater risks for poor outcomes such as African Americans and those of low SES. Clearly, barriers must be matched by resilience in those with diabetes and depression to improve the outcomes of both diseases.

Resilience is a dynamic process in which individuals display positive adaptation despite significant adversity or trauma (Brooks & Goldstein, 2003; Luthar & Cicchetti, 2000). Research suggests more positive health outcomes in those with greater resilience (Edward, 2005; Humphreys, 2003). People who cope well with the diagnosis of T2DM often have learned and can demonstrate resilience under adverse conditions. Resilience models advocate the development of protective factors by the individual that can be used to lessen the impact of T2DM.

To increase resilience, primary care providers can use an array of strategies such as educating their patients about diabetes self-care and building self-efficacy. For example, they can encourage patients to be active participants in acquiring the knowledge they need to control their T2DM. Providers can specifically encourage adherence to medication, exercise, and dietary changes that can decrease the risk for complications of T2DM. Providers may also emphasize that patients have control over their outcomes to some degree depending on their self-management behavior. This belief may be less common among African Americans than among Whites (Figaro, Elasy, BeLue, Speroff, & Dittus, 2009). Last, primary health providers who are treating individuals with T2DM can have a routine brief screening for depression in their treatment plan and include mental health providers as a part of their team for more complicated cases.

In summary, it is important for providers and educators to build resilience through learning tools that are culturally competent. Such skills can enable African American patients to believe that they can manage their T2DM. It will also allow them to build the support system of family and community to bolster their disease management success. The ecological model posits that although individuals play an important role in T2DM, self-care, disease prevention, and disease management are an individual, family, and community responsibility (Haignere, 1999).

## FAMILY FACTORS INFLUENCING RISK AND RESILIENCY

Families are the first level of the human ecology for the individual from birth and throughout their life span. They provide an essential context in which individuals exist. Specifically, families form the initial environment in which mutigenerational beliefs, values, social status, and lifestyle shape development and behavior.

The history of the African American family shows contextual support for individuals that may be used to increase resilience among those with T2DM. Very few studies have addressed the role of the family in promoting emotional health and adaptation to risks for T2DM in the African American community. It is true that African American families are disproportionately poor, with 20% living at the poverty level compared to 8% of White families and 12% of the total population (U.S. Department of Health and Human Services, 2006). Poverty is associated with long-term hardship, often experienced over many generations. Generational poverty produces disproportionate social and negative health problems that result in higher mortality and morbidity from diseases such as T2DM (Rhee et al., 2005; D. R. Williams & Collins, 1995). However, the strength of the multigenerational African American family is underrecognized and underutilized as a support system to improve individual resilience.

According to Fisher and colleagues (2002), family beliefs and values also greatly influence the individual's perceptions about the risk of developing an illness that is usually a combination of some knowledge, misinformation, and ignorance. There is evidence that individuals and their family members often underestimate their own risk status (Fisher et al., 2002) or are fatalistic, believing that the disease cannot be prevented or managed (Egede & Bonadonna, 2003; Figaro et al., 2009). Family history is a significant risk factor for the development of T2DM. For this reason, the family is an apt place to center efforts both to treat and prevent diabetes.

Poor African American families may place individual members at higher risk for developing T2DM for several reasons. Family meals that are generally high in salt, fat, and carbohydrates are often associated with cultural preference and social norms (Baptiste-Roberts et al., 2007). Families pass on these dietary preferences from generation to generation. Additionally, poverty limits families' ability to purchase expensive foods such as fruits, vegetables, lean poultry, and fish. For this reason, access to healthy, fresh food as well as the familial or cultural meanings of food need to be addressed in behavioral interventions.

African American children and adults are also less likely to exercise in communities that do not include sidewalks or that are dangerous. The responsibilities of families include protection of vulnerable members by stronger members. Parents are charged with limiting their children's exposure to risk in multiple ways.

Among these important tasks are to limit their risks to outside influences at unsafe parks, playgrounds, and community centers. These challenges to good self-care behavior for T2DM management act on both individual and family levels.

Some of the dietary habits of poor African American families are likely due to lack of access to healthy foods such as fresh fruits and vegetables in the inner city (Horowitz, Colson, Hebert, & Lancaster, 2004): Smaller urban markets often do not carry expensive produce. Alternatives such as community gardens, which serve as a source of produce and extra income for poorer inner-city residents, are starting up in major cities like New York City and Philadelphia (McMillan, 2008). Projects such as this may mitigate the impact of limited access to fresh foods on the diets of poor African American families. Interventions that increase the safety of public places in the inner city will have great influence on the physical activity levels of African American families who reside there. Increases in physical activity within the school system can also moderate the risks for childhood and adolescent obesity that fuels the current surge in T2DM in this community.

Poverty is also associated with being underinsured or uninsured. This can prevent African American families from accessing preventive health care (Agency for Healthcare Research Quality, 2006). For example, in 2002, 22% of African Americans lacked insurance coverage compared with 11% of White people (U.S. Census Bureau, 2003). Initiatives of universal health care as well as better funding for Medicaid can mitigate this important familial risk. Although generations of African American families have been underinsured (Schoen, Doty, Collins, & Holmgren, 2005), the current national focus on greater coverage for individuals and families should help improve their T2DM outcomes.

Because a family history of T2DM is a major risk factor for the disease, family-based behavioral and culturally specific interventions are important. For example, in African American families with a history of T2DM, members can embark on self-care programs that have been found to be effective in weight management. Programs are better when they also are developed specifically for African Americans. These programs are best when designed to consider their specific social, environmental, and financial situations. At present, there is a paucity of culturally specific programs that help to reduce risk factors associated with T2DM, such as obesity, in African Americans (Chin, Walters, Cook, & Huang 2007).

The outcomes associated with building resilience in families, including learning self-efficacy and competence, problem solving, and a sense of hope for the future, are very important. Research in the diabetes prevention literature suggests that families, one of the key components of the ecological model, must be active, engaged, and participatory for optimal individual benefit. When prevention and educational interventions are developed for African Americans with or at risk for T2DM, individuals should be placed in their larger family and community context (Fisher et al., 2002; Salmon, Booth, Phongsavan, Murphy, & Timperio, 2007).

African American women often are the head of nuclear and multigenerational families. This status requires resilience in the face of dicrimination. However, a study of depression in African American women with T2DM found that they were more sensitive to perceived invidious discrimination than men. These women's perceptions about racial discrimination were associated with their depressive symptoms (Meinert, Blehar, Peindl, Neal-Barnett, & Wisner, 2003). African American women often remain stoic for the good of their family. A history of strength and silence may help to understand how African American women can live with depression as they care for others in their family (Beauboeuf-Lafontant, 2007).

Family tradition and culture impact men's health as well and has relevance for T2DM risk and resilience. Men's usual cultural roles as part of a family often give women control over the family's diet. Interventions that allow men to assume greater control of their diets within families may allow them to shape family choices that decrease the risk of T2DM in future generations. African Americans, primarily men, are currently overrepresented in the criminal justice system. They make up more than 50% of the inmates and have a lifetime incarceration rate of 32% (Raphael, 2004). While incarcerated, men may find it difficult to control their diet. During incarceration, educating African Americans regarding better dietary skills might also improve T2DM outcomes in the aging prison population.

## SOCIAL AND COMMUNITY FACTORS

The ecological systems model emphasizes connections not only within the immediate environment, like the family, but also among systems, including communities and other social institutions and organizations. Together, they affect many factors related to the individual or families' lives, including their health status. Research suggests that sustained multigenerational pervasive and repetitive stressful events experienced by African Americans, such as poverty, discrimination, and racism, heighten their risk for chronic physical illnesses such as T2DM (Outlaw, 1993; Sanders-Thompson, 2002). Global health status varies by SES and race in an interconnected fashion (Williams & Collins, 2001). White Americans as a group are generally healthier and have higher incomes than African Americans. In fact, African Americans report poorer health than Whites, even when they have higher levels of income. Therefore, race and SES have a bidirectional influence on one another.

The collective social and cultural norms in many African American communities illustrate the interaction between gender and race. These norms are perpetuated by social and community-based cultural beliefs and practices that influence health disparities, such as T2DM in African American women. For example, T2DM is disproportionately a burden on the African American community. African Americans, especially women, are disproportionately poor, in part because of gender discrimination and institutionally and personally mediated racism.

Therefore, these women are overrepresented in every category of health inequality (U.S. Department of Health and Human Services, 2001; Williams & Collins, 2001), including T2DM. Recent studies have begun to identify racism and institutionalized discrimination as risk factors associated with poor health outcomes in African American women across socioeconomic strata. The more negative factors, such as poverty, that individuals encounter, the more likely they are to have negative outcomes, including in health status (Krueger & Chang, 2008; Powell, Hoffman, & Shahabi, 2001).

The Institute of Medicine (2003) addressed the issue of racial and ethnic disparities in health in their report *Unequal Treatment: Confronting Racial and Ethnic Disparities*. Among the many factors addressed, the lack of available culturally appropriate care emerged as a specific important contributing factor to racial and ethnic disparities. Sequist and colleagues (2008) found similar results in their recent study of patients in 90 physicians' practices. In this sample, income and health insurance status accounted for only 13–18% of racial differences in diabetes health outcomes. They found systemic differences between the rates of prescriptions for African Americans compared with Whites within the same doctor's practice. Finally, the lack of culturally competent diabetes care accounted for more than 70% of racial differences in patients treated by physicians in the same practice.

Potential sources of disparities in health and health care experienced by African Americans identified by the Institute of Medicine report were at the level of the individual patient, the environment, and the health care system. Although individual interventions are becoming more common, those that involve the provider–patient dyad and the family and larger community are less common. Taken together, these findings make a compelling case for developing culturally appropriate interventions to improve diabetes care in African Americans using the ecological model. This perspective requires health care providers, researchers, educators, and others to explore systemically the interrelatedness of individual, community, and public policy factors as ways to increase empowerment (Jenkins et al., 2004). The ecological model is very congruent with population-based public health approaches. Both link physical, emotional, cultural, and social environments to people's health (U.S. Department of health and Human Services, 2001).

Building resilience in African American communities will require that prevention and intervention strategies be based on evidence-based practices that are racially, ethnically, culturally, and gender specific (Fisher et al., 2007; Haignere, 1999). That is, clinical guidelines that stress changes in lifestyle are less effective if they do not include strategies for mediating the impact of stress, depression, racism, and discrimination on African Americans. Because untreated depressive symptoms are associated with nonadherence in diabetic patients (Ciechanowski et al., 2003), the focus will have to include interventions that treat the depression of African Americans and mobilize resources in the community such as progressive churches, grassroots, and political organizations.

# EVIDENCE-BASED TREATMENT INTERVENTIONS

Once diabetes is diagnosed, tight control leads to better outcomes in all racial, ethnic, and cultural groups. Compared with standard T1DM care, intensive therapy as administered in the Diabetes Control and Complications Trial showed remarkable decreases in important vascular outcomes. Glucose control was important to preventing complications. In particular, incidence of retinopathy, nephropathy, and neuropathy decreased for those in the intensive control group compared with the control group (Diabetes Control and Complications Trial Research Group, 1993). However, because only 2% of participants in the study were African American and participants had T1DM, not T2DM, the findings from the trial are less applicable.

The U.K. Prospective Diabetes Study confirmed in T2DM the importance of controlling the "ABC's": A1C (a long-term measure of glucose control) (Stratton et al., 2000), blood pressure (Adler et al., 2000), and cholesterol. With a decline in A1C, small blood vessel disease decreased as well. Better control of blood sugar was associated with better outcomes even when blood sugar levels approached normal nondiabetic levels. In this British study, 8% of participants were of African Caribbean descent; however, it is not clear how similar this population is to African Americans. Reichard, Nilsson, and Rosenqvist (1993) had already found that any sustained lowering of glucose in T2DM helps prevent complications related to the blockage of small blood vessels even when the individual has a history of poor control.

A more complex set of results was found in some recent randomized trials of glucose control in T2DM (Action to Control Cardiovascular Risk in Diabetes Study Group [ACCORD], 2008; Duckworth et al., 2009). High-risk T2DM patients were treated with either current standard therapy or intensive metabolic control. The ACCORD trial showed no effect on cardiovascular event rates with a slight increase in death rates with intense treatment. In the VA Diabetes Trial, patients had diabetes for an average of 8 years, with 40% having already had a cardiovascular complication, and experienced no benefit in the rates of cardiovascular events, death, or microvascular complications. The ADVANCE (Action in Diabetes and Vascular Disease: Preterax and Diamicron Modified Release Controlled Evaluation) study did show an advantage from intensive control for reduction of the macrovascular and microvascular complications, specifically renal disease (ADVANCE Collaborative Group et al., 2008). Unfortunately, the studies above all had low representation of subjects of African descent. However, the findings suggest that strict biological control of T2DM is possible, is best done early in the disease, and may not impact all disease outcomes equally.

Despite evidence that glucose control can prevent or delay T2DM complications and the many advances made in diabetes management, African Americans still have higher A1Cs and T2DM-related complications compared with Whites (CDC, 2005). A number of contributing factors have been associated with this differential in A1C values. Limitations in access to health care have been shown to impact T2DM outcomes negatively among African Americans. In a study by Cook, Dunbar, Panayioto, and Rhee (2005), only one-third of the predominantly African American participants had health insurance, and the lack of care without insurance was the main determinant of poor glycemic control.

Even with appropriate access to health care there is disparity in treatment for minority patients. Studies have suggested bias in treating African American patients (Hravnak, Whittle, Kelly, Sereika, & Conigliaro, 2007; Schneider, Zaslavsky, & Epstein, 2002). The magnitude of disparities between African American and White patients with T2DM is also associated with poverty. Barriers to medication adherence, such as the cost of drugs, resulted in higher A1C levels among African Americans compared to Whites and Latinos in a study by Heisler and colleagues (2007). In a study by Sambamoorthi, Olfson, Wei, and Crystal (2006), African Americans diagnosed with diabetes and depression were less likely to receive treatment for depression compared with Whites and, if treated, were more likely to receive the older medications for depression. These drugs may cause elevated blood sugar, unlike the newer medications, which do not cause this side effect.

The Standards of Medical Care for Diabetes (ADA, 2007) developed by expert panel consensus currently recommends that people with diabetes receive diabetes self-management education. This education should conform to national standards, including development of individualized dietary, self-testing, and exercise plans that take into consideration cultural differences. The ADA also recommends that patients with T2DM receive individualized medical nutritional therapy taught by registered dieticians who know medical nutrition requirements. Patients who never receive diabetes education show a fourfold increased risk of major diabetes complications (Nicolucci et al., 1996). The standards also recommend that patients with T2DM receive screening for depression without waiting for symptoms to appear or for psychological status to deteriorate. Although these standards apply to all patients, they are not equally and systematically applied to different ethnic groups. Moreover, in concert with the general standards, approaches unique to African Americans may help improve the application of known effective strategies. Effective application of such strategies will increase the chances of improving the lives of African Americans who bear a disproportionate burden of the T2DM epidemic.

Diabetes-related disparities have many causes. Discussed next are evidence-based interventions that may help to eliminate some of the disparities in diabetes among African Americans at the individual, family, health care provider, and health care organization levels. Regrettably, review of the literature revealed extensive documentation of the diabetes-related disparities among African Americans but fewer interventions addressing solutions. Evidence-based treatment options are widely available and compiled by the ADA (2007). The guideline recommendations for clinical practice are derived through a reasoned methodological process that includes meta-analyses and systematic reviews of evidence such as randomized controlled trials.

A systematic review of 43 diabetes intervention studies to reduce health care disparities was recently conducted by Peek, Cargill, and Huang (2007). Interventions were categorized as patient interventions, provider interventions, health care organizations interventions, and complex interventions. The patient interventions focused on self-care education in academic primary care centers and community health centers. Those patient programs that were culturally appropriate improved diabetes knowledge and self-care behaviors. They also preferentially lowered A1C in the intervention group compared with the control group and those undergoing interventions that were not culturally based.

The provider interventions occurred in public hospitals, academic internal medicine clinics, and community-based private physician practices. None of the provider interventions included a cultural component. Improvements resulted from provider processes of care such as patient feedback, computer-generated patient reminders, and increased use of practice guidelines.

When registered nurses were used as case managers for these studies, there were significant improvements in process measures such as A1C testing and in outcome measures such as diabetes management as well as hypertension and dyslipidemia. Intervention using a combination of a community health worker for community support and a registered nurse was more effective than interventions by the registered nurse or the community health worker alone. The findings suggest that registered nurses and community health workers are effective team members in delivering care for T2DM at the community level.

Multilevel interventions reviewed by Chin and colleagues (2007) included a combination of interventions such as diabetes registries, quality improvement measures, health care systems efforts, and community-based management programs. Studies they reviewed even suggested that generalized quality improvement efforts within the Veterans Administration system have diminished or eliminated diabetes health disparities among racial/ethnic minority populations (Heisler, Smith, Hayward, Klein, & Kerr, 2003). Overall, the richer the interventions and the greater number of components, the greater their effectiveness.

African American families are composed of large extended networks that provide support during illness. Social support plays a very important role in diabetes management for African Americans. A systematic review of social support among African American adults with T2DM found that they used informal social supports such as family members more than Whites for their diabetes management needs. Their self-care of diabetes improved because of these types of support. They received help with self-care activities such as foot care, diet supervision, medication assistance, and blood sugar monitoring (Ford, Tilley, & McDonald, 1998). Among African Americans, social support was related to an improvement in T2DM outcomes (Silliman, Bhatti, & Khan, 1996). The development of a treatment plan depends on a systematic assessment that should, whenever possible, involve not only individuals but also their families or other community members.

Evidence suggests that collaborative care in treating depression and T2DM is effective. Individuals with T2DM and comorbid depression who received collaborative care for treatment of depression improved compared with those who received usual care (Simon et al., 2007). Collaborative care consisted of a combination of treatments: antidepressant pharmacotherapy, structured psychotherapy, or the combination of both treatments. A study of older patients with T2DM and depression also found that collaborative care for depression was more effective than usual care (Katon et al., 2006). However, these studies have not focused on African Americans; similar studies in this community are warranted.

The survey of diabetes interventions just presented underscores the need for family-based, culturally appropriate interventions to improve diabetes outcomes for African Americans. As stated, despite the best evidence showing that glucose control can prevent and delay T2DM complications, African Americans still have higher A1Cs and rates of complications. Nonadherence to diabetes regimen, obesity, and lack of access to health care account for some, but not all, of the racial differences in A1C levels. Because these factors influence glycemic control in African Americans, they underscore the need to develop interventions based on the multiple levels of the ecological model.

## Psychopharmacology and T2DM

Depression represents a major impediment to successful treatment of T2DM; and poorly controlled T2DM may mimic depression. Several related psychological and behavioral factors such as depression, binge eating, and anxiety occur more frequently among those with or at high risk for T2DM (Delahanty et al., 2002). The increase in risk applies equally to persons with subclinical and clinical depression. The possibility of depression is greatest in patients with emotional problems associated with the disease itself, such as recurrent episodes of severe hypoglycemia, vascular insufficiency associated with lower extremity pain, and neuropathy (Lustman, Griffith, Freedland, & Clouse, 1997; Tolle, Xu, & Sadosky, 2006). Antidepressant medication is more effective than placebo in treating major depression in patients with T2DM and improves their glucose control (Katon et al., 2004). Finally, those with depression and diabetes require treatment for both disorders, and these medications can interact negatively with one another.

For instance, tricyclic antidepressants (TCAs), more commonly used in minority patients because of their lower cost (Sambamoorthi et al., 2006), tend to have more common and more serious side effects than other, newer types of antidepressant medications, such as selective serotonin reuptake inhibitors. These side effects include nausea, vomiting, seizures, and cardiac arrhythmias. TCAs are also associated with a higher risk of heart attack. These risks increase with age, use of other medications, and preexisting cardiovascular disease. TCAs may also affect blood sugar levels in those with a predisposition to diabetes as well as those with current diabetes. Use of TCAs often requires those with T2DM to perform more frequent blood glucose checks (Preskorn & Irwin, 1982).

Multiple studies show that dysregulation of both glucose and lipids occurs with atypical antipsychotic medications at a higher frequency than would be expected, even accounting for the weight gain associated with their use (Newcomer, 2005). In people with serious psychological disorders, newer, atypical antipsychotic drugs, which control disease symptoms, are associated with increased risk of hyperglycemia and subsequent T2DM (Lamberti et al., 2005; Sernyak, Gulanski, Leslie, & Rosenheck, 2003). Furthermore, studies suggest that psychological disorders are associated with an increased risk of adiposity and multiple adverse physiological effects, such as decreases in insulin sensitivity and changes in lipid levels. For instance, the point prevalence of T2DM in a study of nearly 500 patients was higher at the onset of treatment, about 14% (Lamberti et al., 2004). These findings are likely more common in African Americans, who have greater rates of obesity at the onset of treatment for serious psychological disorders.

Because depression is a risk factor for poor control of diabetes, it is imperative that it be treated (M. M. Williams, Clouse, & Lustman, 2006). Depression is more prevalent in women, but African American women are at particular risk for the complications resulting from poorly managed T2DM. In addition, when diagnosed with any serious mental illness, African American men and women may be at increased risk for obesity and T2DM because of the side effects of atypical antipsychotics as well as their BMI before treatment. These risks must be mitigated by appropriate use of psychopharmacological agents to improve diabetes outcomes. In summary, when mental disorders are managed more effectively, better diabetes-related outcomes are possible.

## Prevention of T2DM

T2DM can be delayed and, when diagnosed, is treatable with good outcomes. Short-term prevention of T2DM is possible. In the Diabetes Prevention Program for 3,000 high-risk individuals over a 3-year span, there was a 58% relative reduction in the progression to T2DM in the lifestyle change group and a 37% reduction in the medication group compared with controls. Within the lifestyle change group, 50% achieved the goal of maintaining at least 150 minutes of activity each week (DPP Research Group, 2002; Knowler et al., 2002). The Study to Prevent Non-Insulin-Dependent Diabetes Mellitus trial included patients with prediabetes and showed a reduction in cardiovascular events (Chiasson et al., 2002). In the Diabetes Reduction Assessment with Ramipril and Rosiglitazone Medication trial, the incidence rate of cardiovascular events did not differ between the rosiglitazone and placebo groups (Gerstein et al., 2006).

Several small trials have shown a significant effect on weight loss, glucose metabolism, and other markers of diabetes. Calorie restriction, whether by changes in behavior or from gastric bypass operation, leads to rapid improvement in fasting glucose levels and insulin resistance (Greenway, Greenway, & Klein, 2002). Levels of chemicals that influence weight such as postmeal adiponectin are influenced by surgery for weight loss (Ballantyne et al., 2005). Gastric bypass has the potential to correct abnormal glucose in those at risk for T2DM and to lower A1C in those with T2DM. Long-term studies on large cohorts are still not available. Because these procedures are not typically covered by insurance companies, they remain beyond the reach of those of low SES. They require long-term follow-up, including supplementation with vitamins that are not absorbed from the shortened small intestines.

It is still not clear whether people with impaired glucose control, or pre-diabetes, can benefit long term from treatments that lower blood glucose. In contrast, there are known benefits of glucose control to prevent the progression of complications in those with T2DM. Intervention trials in people with predia-betes suggest, but have not demonstrated, a benefit of glycemic control. Direct evidence is lacking for mass screening for T2DM, and evidence also fails to demonstrate benefits for screening special populations such as African Americans. Persons with hypertension benefit from screening, because blood pressure targets for persons with diabetes are lower than those without diabetes. In summary, intensive lifestyle, medication, and surgical interventions can reduce the progression of prediabetes to diabetes, but few data examine the effect of these interventions on long-term health outcomes (Norris, Kansagara, Bougatsos, & Fu, 2008).

Among all U.S. adults, only approximately one in five consume the recommended five servings of fruits and vegetables a day. Compared with Whites, African Americans eat greater amounts of dietary fat and lower amounts of fruits, vegetables, and dietary fiber; their fruit and vegetable intake is inadequate for the prevention of T2DM (CDC, 2005). Obesity, physiological stress, and associated changes in circulating enzymes, free fatty acids, and inflammatory mediators are central to the cardiovascular effects of prediabetes. Recently, intensive behavioral interventions using meal replacements and low-energy diets have enabled some severely obese persons to achieve a nonobese weight and maintain it for at least 5 years (J. W. Anderson, Conley, & Nicholas, 2007).

Many African Americans live in a less resourceful ecological context that negatively influences their social, institutional, and physical environments. These environments can pose challenges to preventive strategies. The diagnosis of pre-diabetes can also cause anxiety. In the Anglo-Danish-Dutch Study of Intensive Treatment in People with Screen Detected Diabetes in Primary Care study (Eborall et al., 2007), screening had little affect on participants' anxiety levels at 1 year follow-up. In a cross-sectional study, Skinner and colleagues (2005) showed that screening high-risk patients for T2DM was not associated with significant anxiety. However, both studies were performed in Europe, so neither had African American enrollment. The challenges must be considered when conceptualizing determinants of diet and physical activity. In addition to individual actions, family and social environments influence behavior. Finally, preventive interventions will include educational components but will also address the behavioral, emotional, and family/environmental challenges to management of T2DM. Future studies should focus on reversing the lifestyle behaviors that are the fundamental causes of prediabetes in African Americans as well as assessing the psychological consequences of labeling.

Race and gender are important to consider in the prevention of T2DM. Racial differences in potentially modifiable risk factors, particularly obesity, account for 48% of the excess risk in African American women (Brancati, Kao, Folsom, & Szklo, 2000). Preventive strategies for addressing weight control and T2DM risk need to address both calorie intake and expenditure. Health education strategies, including participatory development and teaching by peer educators, should be applied to address cultural relevance. They also need to promote lasting lifestyle changes. The most common areas of change that African American women identified in a recent study were in food purchasing, preparation, and portion size. Barriers to medical nutrition therapy identified included low income, time constraints, competing demands, and knowledge deficits (Galasso, Amend, Melkus, & Nelson, 2007).

A meta-analysis of 36 studies to determine whether ethnic disparities exist for diabetes-related preventive care found that rates for some T2DM preventive care measures were low for African Americans compared with Whites (Kirk et al., 2006). If individuals do not believe that T2DM complications are preventable and do not practice effective self-care, they will not comply with proven treatments that prevent or delay these complications. For this reason, promising interventions will include attention to the individual, family, and social contexts of persons with T2DM, all components of the ecological models. Processes addressed across approaches, at least to some degree, include behavioral skills such as coping and problem solving, adaptive family processes, and a consideration of the ecological context in which T2DM management occurs. In addition, consideration is given to the interface of T2DM management of challenges as well as social and cultural situations.

In summary, individual-, family-, and community-level interventions are all key in reducing diabetes-related health disparities. Although some barriers to care, such as lack of insurance, preferentially affect African Americans, the causes of disparities and priorities for addressing them are worth the effort to reduce poor outcomes. Successfully addressing these disparities will require focused community-based projects that are supported by local resources.

## RECOMMENDED BEST PRACTICES

Cultural competence will be of benefit to best practices for T2DM care, especially among those with depression (Haire-Joshu & Fleming, 2006). These best practices seem straightforward. However, their implementation in low-resource African American communities will require consideration of limitations and barriers for individuals, families, and communities. These include lack of access to (1) nutrition such as fresh fruits and vegetables, (2) transportation to doctors, (3) affordable weight reduction programs, and (4) safe spaces for recreation.

We have described several approaches for the prevention and treatment of T2DM. A consistent theme in these interventions is the influence of physical, behavioral, and emotional health on positive outcomes. Most studies show evidence and promise for promotion of all of these components. Interventions reviewed in this chapter primarily focus on two or more of the components of the ecological model. Interrelated and dynamic factors, such as individual, family, and environment, will likely impact adherence to self-care demands. On the basis of the findings from the studies reviewed, we make the following recommendations when developing and implementing interventions for those with T2DM, whether primarily preventive or treatment focused.

1. Tight metabolic control of T2DM early in the disease is best in order to obtain potentially better individual clinical outcomes.

2. Equal consideration should be given to biological and emotional/behavioral factors, especially depression, in treatment approaches.

3. In persons with T2DM, especially in African Americans who face mental health care disparities, there should be screening and assessment of depression to improve outcomes.

4. Interventions in the African American community must include components of the ecological model, considering the individual in his or her larger context.

5. For the greatest impact in the African American community, cultural competence is crucial for practitioners embarking on effective clinical practice and behavioral interventions.

6. Additional studies that are race specific and gender specific focusing on African Americans in their various context are sorely needed to inform clinical practice.

In sum, interventions in T2DM management have improved, but they are not sufficiently racially and ethnically specific to provide an evidence-based practice approach for African Americans. However, we have discussed several factors influencing emotional health and behavioral management in those with T2DM. Findings from these approaches suggest that successful interventions include two or more components of the ecological model. Cost constraints, availability of personnel, and other resources may limit the ability to implement at all levels of the model. Therefore, the best methods of delivery in a resource-poor environment include approaches that are culturally conscious and cost-efficient and can thus be sustained over time.

# REFERENCES

Action to Control Cardiovascular Risk in Diabetes Study Group. (2008). Effects of intensive glucose lowering in Type 2 diabetes. *New England Journal of Medicine, 358,* 2545–2559.

Adler, A. I., Stratton, I. M., Neil, H. A., Yudkin, J. S., Matthews, D. R., Cull, C. A., et al. (2000). Association of systolic blood pressure with macrovascular and microvascular complications of type 2 diabetes (UKPDS 36): Prospective observational study. *British Medical Journal, 321,* 412–419.

ADVANCE Collaborative Group, Patel, A., MacMahon, S., Chalmers, J., Neal, B., Billot, L., et al. (2008). Intensive blood glucose control and vascular outcomes in patients with type 2 diabetes. *New England Journal of Medicine, 358*(24), 2560–2572.

Agency for Healthcare Research Quality. (2006). *National healthcare disparities report, 2006.* Retrieved June 30, 2008, from *www.ahrq.gov/qual/nhdr06/nhdr06.htm.*

Alberti, G., Zimmet, P., Shaw, J., Bloomgarden, Z., Kaufman, F., & Silink, M. (2004). Type 2 diabetes in the young: The evolving epidemic: The international Diabetes Federation consensus workshop. *Diabetes Care, 27*(7), 1798–1811.

Allan, J. D., Mayo, K., & Michel, Y. (1993). Body size values of White and Black women. *Research in Nursing and Health, 16*(5), 323–333.

American Diabetes Association. (2000). Type 2 diabetes in children and adolescents. *Diabetes Care, 23*(3), 381–389.

American Diabetes Association. (2003). Report of the Expert Committee on the Diagnosis and Classification of Diabetes Mellitus. *Diabetes Care, 26*(Suppl. 1), S5–S20.

American Diabetes Association. (2007). Standards of medical care in diabetes. *Diabetes Care, 30*(Suppl. 1), S4–S41.

American Psychiatric Association. (2000). *Diagnostic and statistical manual of mental disorders* (4th ed., text rev.). Washington, DC: Author.

Anderson, J. W., Conley, S. B., & Nicholas, A. S. (2007). One hundred pound weight losses with an intensive behavioral program: Changes in risk factors in 118 patients with long-term follow-up. *American Journal of Clinical Nutrition, 86,* 301–307.

Anderson, R. J., Freedland, K. E., & Clouse, E. E. (2001). The prevalence of comorbid depression in adults with diabetes. *Diabetes Care, 24,* 1069–1078.

Ballantyne, G. H., Gumbs, A., Modlin, I. M., Baptiste-Roberts, K., Gary, T. L., Beckles, G. L., et al. (2005). Changes in insulin resistance following bariatric surgery and the adipoinsular axis: Role of the adipocytokines, leptin, adiponectin and resistin. *Obesity Surgery, 15*(5), 692–699.

Baptiste-Roberts, K., Gary, T. L., Beckles, G. L., Gregg, E. W., Owens, M., Porterfield, D., et al. (2007). Family history of diabetes, awareness of risk factors, and health behaviors among African Americans. *American Journal of Public Health, 97*(5), 907–912.

Basciano, H., Federico, L., & Adeli, K. (2005). Fructose, insulin resistance, and metabolic dyslipidemia. *Nutrition and Metabolism, 2*(1), 5.

Beauboeuf-Lafontant, T. (2007). You have to show strength: An exploration of gender, race, and depression. *Gender and Society, 21*(1), 28–51.

Bell, D. S., Barger, B. O., Go, R. C., Goldenberg, R. L., Perkins, L. L., Vanichanan, C. J., et al. (1990). Risk factors for gestational diabetes in Black population. *Diabetes Care, 13*(11), 1196–1201.

Bonhomme, J., & Braithwaite, R. (2003, November). *Characteristics of effective health outreach to African-American males: Overcoming healthcare underutilization.* Abstract presented at the 131st Annual Meeting of the American Public Health Association, Philadelphia.

Bosnyak, Z., Nishimura, R., Hagan Hughes, M., Tajima, N., Becker, D., Tuomilehto, J., et al. (2005). Excess mortality in Black compared with White patients with Type 1 diabetes: An examination of underlying causes. *Diabetes Medicine, 22*(12), 1636–1641.

Brancati, F. L., Kao, W. L., Folsom, A. R., & Szklo, M. (2000). Incident type 2 diabetes mellitus in African American and White adults—The Atherosclerosis Risk in Communities Study. *Journal of the American Medical Association, 283*(17), 2253–2259.

Brooks, R., & Goldstein, S. (2003). *The power of resilience: Achieving balance, confidence, and personal strength in your life.* New York: McGraw-Hill.

Butler, J., Rodondi, N., Zhu, Y. W., Figaro, K., Fazio, S., Vaughan, D., et al. (2006). Metabolic syndrome and the risk of cardiovascular disease in older adults. *Journal of American College of Cardiology, 47*(8), 1595–1602.

Centers for Disease Control and Prevention. (2004a). Prevalence of overweight and obesity among adults with diagnosed diabetes—United States, 1988–1994 and 1999–2002. *Morbidity and Mortality Weekly Report, 53*(45), 1066–1068.

Centers for Disease Control and Prevention. (2004b). Serious psychological distress among persons with diabetes—New York City, 2003. *Morbidity and Mortality Weekly Report, 53*(46), 1089–1092.

Centers for Disease Control and Prevention. (2005). *National diabetes fact sheet: general information and national estimates on T2DM in the United States, 2005.* Atlanta, GA: U.S. Department of Health and Human Services, Centers for Disease Control and Prevention. Retrieved July 1, 2008, from *www.cdc.gov/diabetes/pubs/factsheet05.htm.*

Centers for Disease Control and Prevention. (2008). *Number of people with diabetes increases to 24 million.* Atlanta, GA: Author. Retrieved July 1, 2008, from *www.cdc.gov/media/pressrel/2008/r080624.htm.*

Cheng, D. (2005). Prevalence, predisposition and prevention of type II diabetes. *Nutrition and Metabolism, 2,* 29.

Chiasson, J.L., Josse, R.G., Gomis, R., Hanefeld, M., Karasik, A., Laakso, M., et al. (2002). Acarbose for prevention of type 2 diabetes mellitus: The STOP-NIDDM randomised trial. *Lancet, 359,* 2072–2077.

Chin, M. H., Walters, A. E., Cook, S. C., & Huang, E. S. (2007). Interventions to reduce racial and ethnic disparities in health care. *Medical Care Research Reviews, 64*(5, Suppl.), 7S–28S.

Ciechanowski, P. S., Katon, W. J., Russo, J. E., & Hirsch, I. B. (2003). The relationship of depressive symptoms to symptom reporting, self-care and glucose control in diabetes. *General Hospital Psychiatry, 25,* 246–252.

Cleary, P. A., Orchard, T. J., Genuth, S., Wong, N. D., Detrano, R., Backlund, J. Y., et al. (2006). The effect of intensive glycemic treatment on coronary artery calcification in type 1 diabetic participants of the Diabetes Control and Complications Trial/Epidemiology of Diabetes Interventions and Complications (DCCT/EDIC) Study. *Diabetes, 55*(12), 3556–3565.

Cook, C., Dunbar, V., Panayioto, R., & Rhee, M. (2005). Limited health care access impairs glycemic control in low socioeconomic status urban African Americans with type 2 Diabetes. *Journal of Health Care for the Poor and Underserved, 16*(4), 734–746.

Cooper-Patrick, L., Gallo, J., Gonzales, J., Vu, H. T., Powe, N. R., Nelson, C., et al. (1999). Race, gender, and partnership in the patient-physician relationship. *Journal of the American Medical Association, 282,* 583–589.

Cowie, C. C., Rust, K. F., Byrd-Holt, D. D., Eberhardt, M. S., Flegal, K. M., Engelgau, M. M., et al. (2006). Prevalence of diabetes and impaired fasting glucose in adults in the U.S. population: National Health and Nutrition Examination Survey 1999–2002. *Diabetes Care, 29*(6), 1263–1268.

Das, A. K., Offson, M., McCurtis, H. L., & Weissman, M. M. (2006). Depression in African Americans: Breaking barriers to detection and treatment. *Journal of Family Practice, 55*(1), 30–39.

Delahanty, L. M., Meigs, J. B., Hayden, D., Williamson, D. A., & Nathan, D. M. (2002). Psychological and behavioral correlates of baseline BMI in the Diabetes Prevention Program (DPP). *Diabetes Care, 25*(11), 1992–1998.

Diabetes Control and Complications Trial Research Group. (1993). The effect of intensive treatment of diabetes on the development and progression of long-term complications in insulin-dependent diabetes mellitus. *New England Journal of Medicine, 329,* 977–986.

Diabetes Prevention Program Research Group. (2002). The Diabetes Prevention Program (DPP): Description of lifestyle intervention. *Diabetes Care, 25*(12), 2165–2171.

Diamond Project Group, (2006). Incidence and trends of childhood Type 1 diabetes worldwide 1990–1999. *Diabetic Medicine, 23*(8), 857–866.

Dietz, W. H. (1998). Health consequences of obesity in youth: Childhood predictors of adult disease. *Pediatrics, 101,* 518–525.

DiGioacchino, R. F., Sargent, R. J., & Topping, M. (2001). Body dissatisfaction among White and African American male and female college students. *Eating Behaviors, 2*(1), 39–50.

Dorman, J. S., & Bunker, C. H. (2000). HLA-DQ locus of the human leukocyte antigen complex and type 1 diabetes mellitus: A HuGE review. *Epidemiologic Reviews, 22*(2), 218–227.

Douglas, J. G. (1990). Hypertension and T2DM in Blacks. *Diabetes Care, 13*(11), 1191–1195.

Duckworth, W., Abraira, C., Moritz, T., Reda, D., Emanuele, N., Reaven, P. D., et al. (2009). Glucose control and vascular complications in veterans with type 2 diabetes (VADT). *New England Journal of Medicine, 360,* 129–139.

Eborall, H. C., Griffin, S. J., Prevost, A. T., Kinmonth, A., French, D. P., & Sutton, S. (2007). Psychological impact of screening for type 2 diabetes: Controlled trial and comparative study embedded in the ADDITION (Cambridge) randomised controlled trial. *British Medical Journal, 335,* 486.

Edward, K. (2005). Resilience: A protector from depression. *Journal of the American Psychiatric Nurses Association, 11*(4), 241–243.

Egede, L., & Bonadonna, R. J. (2003). Diabetes self-management in African Americans: An exploration of the role of fatalism. *Diabetes Educator, 29*(1) 105–115.

Festa, A., D'Agostino, R., Jr., Mykkanen, L., Tracy, R. P., Hales, C. N., Howard, B. V., et al. (1999). LDL particle size in relation to insulin, proinsulin, and insulin sensitivity. The Insulin Resistance Atherosclerosis Study. *Diabetes Care, 22*(10), 1688–1693.

Figaro, M. K., Elasy, T., BeLue, R., Speroff, T., & Dittus, R. (2009). Exploring socioeconomic variations in diabetes control strategies: Impact of outcome expectations. *Journal of the National Medical Association, 101*(1), 18–23.

Fiscella, K., & Shin, P. (2005). The inverse care law: Implications for healthcare of vulnerable populations. *Journal of Ambulatory Care Management. Community Health Centers, 28*(4), 304–312.

Fisher, E. B., Brownson, C. A., O'Toole, M. L., Shetty, G., Anwuri, V. V., Fazzone, P., et al. (2007). The Robert Wood Johnson Foundation Projects emphasizing self-management. *Diabetes Educator, 33*(1), 83–84.

Fisher, E. B., Brownson, C. A., O'Toole, M. L., Shetty, G., Anwuri, V. V., Glasgow, R. E., et al. (2005). Ecologic approaches to self-management: The case of diabetes. *American Journal of Public Health, 95,* 1523–1535.

Fisher, E. B., Walker, E., Bostrom, A., Fischoff, B., Haire-Joshu, D., & Johnson, S. (2002). Behavioral science research in the prevention of diabetes. *Diabetes Care, 25*(3), 599–606.

Flegal, K. M., Carroll, M. D., Ogden, C. L., & Johnson, C. L. (2002). Prevalence and trends in obesity among US adults, 1999–2000. *Journal of the American Medical Association, 288*(14), 1723–1727.

Florez, J. C., Jablonski, K. A., Bayley, N., Pollin, T. I., de Bakker, P. I., Shuldiner, A. R., et al. (2006). TCF7L2 polymorphisms and progression to diabetes in the Diabetes Prevention Program. *New England Journal of Medicine, 355*(3), 241–250.

Ford, M., Tilley, B., & McDonald, P. (1998). Social support among African-American adults with diabetes, Part 2: A review. *Journal of National Medical Association, 90*(7), 425–432.

Galasso, P., Amend, A., Melkus, G. D., & Nelson, G. T. (2007). One hundred pound weight losses with an intensive behavioral program: Changes in risk factors in 118 patients with long-term follow-up. *American Journal of Clinical Nutrition, 86,* 301–307.

Gerstein, H. C., Yusuf, S., Bosch, J., Pogue, J., Sheridan, P., Dinccag, N., et al. (2006). Effect of rosiglitazone on the frequency of diabetes in patients with impaired glucose tolerance or impaired fasting glucose: A randomised controlled trial. *Lancet, 368,* 1096–1105.

Golden, S. H., Lazo, M., Carnethon, M., Bertoni, A. G., Schreiner, P. J., Roux, A. V., et al. (2008). Examining a bidirectional association between depressive symptoms and diabetes. *Journal of the American Medical Association, 299*(23), 2751–2759.

Gonzalez, J. S., Safren, S. A., Cagliero, E., Wexler, D. J., Delahanty, L., Wittenberg, E., et al. (2007). Depression, self-care, and medication adherence in type 2 diabetes: Relationships across the full range of symptom severity. *Diabetes Care, 30,* 2222–2227.

Grabe, S., & Hyde, J. S. (2006). Ethnicity and body dissatisfaction among women in the United States: A meta-analysis. *Psychological Bulletin, 132*(4), 622–640.

Greenway, S. E., Greenway, F., III, & Klein, S. (2002). Effects of obesity surgery on non-insulin-dependent diabetes mellitus. *Archives of Surgery, 137*(10), 1109–1117.

Gregg, E. W., Cadwell, B. L., Cheng, Y. J., Cowie, C. C., Williams, D. E., Geiss, L., et al. (2004). Trends in the prevalence and ratio of diagnosed to undiagnosed diabetes according to obesity levels in the U.S. *Diabetes Care, 27*(12), 2806–2812.

Grover, S., Lowensteyn, I., Kaouache, M., Marchand, S., Coupal, L., DeCarolis, E., et al. (2006). The prevalence of erectile dysfunction in the primary care setting—Importance of risk factors for diabetes and vascular disease. *Archives of Internal Medicine, 166*(2), 213–219.

Guize, L., Thomas, F., Pannier, B., Bean, K., Jego, B., & Benetos, A. (2007). All-cause mortality associated with specific combinations of the metabolic syndrome according to recent definitions. *Diabetes Care, 30,* 2381–2387.

Guo, T., Hanson, R. L., Traurig, M., Muller, Y. L., Ma, L., Mack, J., et al. (2007). TCF7L2 is not a major susceptibility gene for type 2 diabetes in Pima Indians: Analysis of 3,501 individuals. *Diabetes, 56*(12), 3082–3088.

Haignere, C. S. (1999). Closing the ecological gap: The public/private dilemma. *Health Education Research, 14*(4), 507–518.

Haire-Joshu, D., & Fleming, C. (2006). An ecological approach to understanding contributions to disparities in T2DM prevention and care. *Current Diabetes Report, 6*(2), 123–129.

Harris, M. I., Eastman, R. C., Cowie, C. C., Flegal, K. M., & Eberhardt, M. (1999). Racial and ethnic differences in glycemic control of adults with type 2 diabetes. *Diabetes Care, 22,* 403–408.

Heisler, M., Faul, J. D., Hayward, R. A., Langa, K. M., Blaum, C., & Weir, D. (2007). Mechanisms for racial and ethnic disparities in glycemic control in middle-aged and older Americans in the health and retirement study. *Archives of Internal Medicine, 167*(17), 1853–1860.

Heisler, M., Smith, D. M., Hayward, R. A., Klein, S. L., & Kerr, E. A. (2003). Racial disparities in diabetes care processes, outcomes, and treatment intensity. *Medical Care, 41,* 1221–1232.

Horowitz, C. R., Colson, K. A., Hebert, P. L., & Lancaster, K. (2004). Barriers to buying healthy foods for people with diabetes: Evidence of environmental disparities. *American Journal of Public Health, 94*(9), 1549–1554.

Hozawa, A., Folsom, A. R., Sharrett, A. R., & Chambless, L. E. (2007). Absolute and attributable risks of cardiovascular disease incidence in relation to optimal and borderline risk factors: Comparison of African American with White subjects—Atherosclerosis Risk in Communities Study. *Archives of Internal Medicine, 167*(6), 573–579.

Hravnak, M., Whittle, J., Kelly, M., Sereika, S., & Conigliaro, J. (2007). Symptom expression in coronary heart disease revascularization recommendations for Black and White patients. *American Journal of Public Health, 97*(9), 1701–1708.

Hu, F. B., Manson, J. E., Stampfer, M. J., Colditz, G., Liu, S., Solomon, C. G., et al. (2001). Diet, lifestyle, and the risk of type 2 diabetes mellitus in women. *New England Journal of Medicine, 345*(11), 790–797.

Humphreys, J. (2003). Resilience in sheltered battered women. *Issues in Mental Health Nursing, 24,* 137–152.

Institute of Medicine. (2003). *Unequal treatment: Confronting racial and ethnic disparities in health care.* Washington, DC: National Academies Press.

Jack, L., Toston, T., Jack, N. H., & Sims, M. (2010). A gender-centered ecological framework targeting Black men living with diabetes: Integrating a "masculinity" perspective in diabetes management and education research. *American Journal of Men's Health, 4,* 7–15.

Jenkins, C. S., McNary, B. A., Carlson, M. G., King, C. L., Hossler, G., Magwood, K., et al. (2004). Reducing disparities for African Americans with diabetes: Progress made by the REACH 2010 Charleston and Georgetown diabetes coalition. *Public Health Reports, 119*(3), 322–330.

Jeon, C. Y., Lokken, R. P., Hu, F. B., & van Dam, R. M. (2007). Physical activity of moderate intensity and risk of type 2 diabetes: A systematic review. *Diabetes Care, 30*(3), 744–752.

Jones, L. R., Fries, E., & Danish, S. J. (2007). Gender and ethnic differences in body image and opposite sex figure preferences of rural adolescents. *Body Image, 4*(1), 103–108.

Jordan, O. W., Lipton, R. B., Stupnicka, E., Cruickshank, J. K., & Fraser, H. S. (1994). Incidence of type I diabetes in people under 30 years of age in Barbados, West Indies, 1982–1991. *Diabetes Care, 17*(5), 428–431.

Kalsekar, I. D., Madhavan, S. S., Amonkar, M. M., Makela, E. H., Scott, V. G., Douglas, S. M., et al. (2006). Depression in patients with type 2 diabetes: Impact on adherence to oral hypoglycemic agents. *Annals of Pharmacotherapy, 40*(4), 605–611.

Katon, W., Unutzer, J., Fan, M., Williams, J. W., Schoenbaum, M., Lin, E., et al. (2006). Cost effectiveness and net benefit of enhanced treatment of depression for older adults with diabetes and depression. *Diabetes Care, 29*(2), 265–270.

Katon, W. J., Von Korff, M., Lin, E. H. B., Simon, G., Ludman, E., Russo, J., et al. (2004). The Pathways Study: A randomized trial of collaborative care in patients with diabetes and depression. *Archives of General Psychiatry, 61*(10), 1042–1049.

Kirk, J. K., D'Agostino, R. B., Jr., Bell, R. A., Passmore, L. V., Bonds, D. E., Karter, A. J., et al. (2006). Disparities in HbA1c levels between African-American and non-Hispanic White adults with diabetes: A meta-analysis. *Diabetes Care, 29*(9), 2130–2136.

Kjos, S. L., & Buchanan, T. A. (1999). Gestational diabetes mellitus. *New England Journal of Medicine, 341*(23), 1749–1756.

Knowler, W. C., Barrett-Connor, E., Fowler, S. E., Hamman, R. F., Lachin, J. M., Walker, E. A., et al. (2002). Reduction in the incidence of type 2 diabetes with lifestyle intervention or metformin. *New England Journal of Medicine, 346*(6), 393–403.

Kogan, S. M., Brody, G. H., Crawley, C., Logan, P., & Murry, V. M. (2007). Correlates of elevated depressive symptoms among rural African American adults with type 2 diabetes. *Ethnicity and Disease, 17*(1), 106–112.

Koya, D. L., & Egede, L. E. (2007). Association between length of residence and cardiovascular disease risk factors among an ethnically diverse group of United States immigrants. *Journal of General Internal Medicine, 22*(6), 841–846.

Krentz, A. J., & Bailey, C. J. (2005). Oral antidiabetic agents: Current role in type 2 diabetes mellitus. *Drugs, 65*(3), 385–411.

Krueger, P. M., & Chang, V. W. (2008). Being poor and coping with stress: Health behaviors and the risk of death. *American Journal of Public Health, 98*(5), 889–896.

La Greca, A. M., Swales, T., Klemp, S., Madigan, S., & Skyler, J. (1995). Adolescents with diabetes: Gender differences in psychosocial functioning and glycemic control. *Children's Health Care, 24*(1), 61–78.

Lamberti, J. S., Costea, G. O., Olson, D., Crilly, J. F., Maharaj, K., Tu, X., et al. (2005). Diabetes mellitus among outpatients receiving clozapine: Prevalence and clinical-demographic correlates. *Journal of Clinical Psychiatry, 66*(7), 900–906.

Lamberti, J. S., Crilly, J. F., Maharaj, K., Olson, D., Wiener, K., Dvorin, S., et al. (2004). Prevalence of diabetes mellitus among outpatients with severe mental disorders receiving atypical antipsychotic drugs. *Journal of Clinical Psychiatry, 65*(5), 702–706.

Langer, O., Yogev, Y., Most, O., & Xenakis, E. M. (2005). Gestational diabetes: The consequences of not treating. *American Journal of Obstetrics and Gynecology, 192*(4), 989–997.

Laumann, E. O., West, S., Glasser, D., Carson, C., Rosen, R., & Kang, J. H. (2007). Prevalence and correlates of erectile dysfunction by race and ethnicity among men aged 40 or older in the United States: from the male attitudes regarding sexual health survey. *Journal of Sex and Medicine, 4*(1), 57–65.

Lea, J. P., & Nicholas, S. B. (2002). diabetes mellitus and hypertension: Key risk factors for kidney disease. *Journal of National Medical Association, 94*(8, Suppl.), 7S–15S.

Leahy, J. L. (2005). Pathogenesis of type 2 diabetes mellitus. *Archives of Medical Research, 36*(3), 197–209.

Lett, H. S., Blumenthal, J. A., Babyak, M. A., Sherwood, A., Strauman, T., Robins, C., et al. (2004). Depression as a risk factor for coronary artery disease: Evidence, mechanisms, and treatment. *Psychosomatic Medicine, 66*(3), 305–315.

Liburd, L. C., Namageyo-Funa, A., & Jack, L., Jr. (2007). Understanding "masculinity" and the challenges of managing type-2 diabetes among African-American men. *Journal of National Medical Association, 99*(5), 550–558.

Lin, E., Keaton, W., Korf, V., Reuter, C., Simon, G., Oliver, M., et al. (2004). Relationship of depression and diabetes self-care, medication adherence, and preventive care. *Diabetes Care, 27*, 2154–2160.

Lipman, T. H., Jawad, A. F., Murphy, K. M., Tuttle, A., Thompson, R. L., Ratcliffe, S. J., et al. (2006). Incidence of type 1 diabetes in Philadelphia is higher in Black than White children from 1995 to 1999: Epidemic or misclassification? *Diabetes Care, 29*(11), 2391–2395.

Lipton, R. B., Drum, M., Li, S., & Choi, H. (1999). Social environment and year of birth influence type 1 diabetes risk for African-American and Latino children. *Diabetes Care, 22*(1), 78–85.

Love-Gregory, L., Sherva, R., Sun, L., Wasson, J., Schappe, T., Doria, A., et al. (2008). Variants in the CD36 gene associate with the metabolic syndrome and high-density lipoprotein cholesterol. *Human Molecular Genetics, 17*(11), 1695–1704.

Lustman, P. J., Griffith, L. S., Freedland, K. E., & Clouse, R. E. (1997). The course of major depression in diabetes. *General Hospital Psychiatry, 19*(2), 138–143.

Lustman, P. J., Griffith, L. S., Gavard, J. A., & Clouse, R. E. (1992). Depression in adults with diabetes. *Diabetes Care, 15*(11), 1631–1639.

Luthar, S. S., & Cicchetti, D. (2000). The construct of resilience: Implications for interventions and social policies. *Development and Psychopathology, 12*(4), 857–885.

Matteucci, E., & Giampietro, O. (2007). Building a bridge between clinical and basic research: The phenotypic elements of familial predisposition to type 1 diabetes. *Current Medicinal Chemistry, 14*(5), 555–567.

McMillan, T. (2008, May). Urban farmers' crops go from vacant lot to market. *New York Times.* Retrieved July 1, 2008, from *www.nytimes.com/2008/05/07/dining/07urban.html.*

Meinert, J. A., Blehar, M. C., Peindl, K. S., Neal-Barnett, A., & Wisner, K. L. (2003). Bridging the gap: Recruitment of African-American women into mental health research studies. *Academic Psychiatry, 27*(1), 21–28.

Narayan, K. M., Boyle, J. P., Thompson, T. J., Gregg, E. W., & Williamson, D. F. (2007). Effect of BMI on lifetime risk for diabetes in the U.S. *Diabetes Care, 30*(6), 1562–1566.

Nathan, D. M. (1993). Long-term complications of diabetes mellitus. *New England Journal of Medicine, 328*(23), 1676–1685.

Nathan, D. M. (2002). Clinical practice. Initial management of glycemia in type 2 diabetes mellitus. *New England Journal of Medicine, 347*(17), 1342–1349.

Newcomer, J. W. (2005). Second-generation (atypical) antipsychotics and metabolic effects: A comprehensive literature review. *Central Nervous System Drugs, 19*(Suppl. 1), 1–93.

Nicolucci, A., Cavaliere, D., Scorpiglione, N., Carinci, F., Capani, F., Tognoni, G., et al. (1996). A comprehensive assessment of the avoidability of long-term complications of diabetes. *Diabetes Care, 19*, 927–933.

Norris, S. L., Kansagara, D., Bougatsos, C., & Fu, R. (2008). Screening adults for Type 2 diabetes: A review of the evidence for the U.S. Preventive Services Task Force. *Annals of Internal Medicine, 148*, 855–868.

Ogden, C. L., Carroll, M. D., & Flegal, K. M. (2008). High body mass index for age among US children and adolescents, 2003–2006. *Journal of the American Medical Association, 299*(20), 2401–2405.

O'Malley, A. S., Forrest, C. B., & Miranda, J. (2003). Primary care attributes and care for depression among low-income African American women. *American Journal of Public Health, 93*(8), 1328–1334.

Outlaw, F. H. (1993). Stress and coping: The influence of racism on the cognitive appraisal processing of African Americans. *Issues in Mental Health Nursing, 14*, 399–409.

Paradies, Y. C., Montoya, M. J., & Fullerton, S. M. (2007). Racialized genetics and the study of complex diseases: The thrifty genotype revisited. *Perspectives in Biology and Medicine, 50*(2), 203–227.

Peek, M. E., Cargill, A., & Huang, E. S. (2007). Diabetes health disparities: A systematic review of healthcare interventions. *Medical Care Research and Review, 64*(Suppl. 5), 101S–156S.

Penckofer, S., Ferrans, C. E., Velsor-Friedrich, B., & Savoy, S. (2007). The psychological impact of living with diabetes: Women's day-to-day experiences. *Diabetes Educator, 33*, 680–690.

Pinterova, D., E. J., Kolostova, K., Pruhova, S., Novota, P., Romzova, M., et al. (2007). Six novel mutations in the GCK gene in MODY patients. *Clinical Genetics, 71*(1), 95–96.

Powell, A., & Kahn, A. (1995). Racial differences in women's desire to be thin. *International Journal of Eating Disorders, 17*, 191–195.

Powell, L. H., Hoffman, A., & Shahabi, L. (2001). Socioeconomic differential in health and disease: Let's take the next step. *Psychosomatic Medicine, 63*(5), 722–723.

Preskorn, S., & Irwin, H. (1982). Toxicity of tricyclic antidepressants—Kinetics, mechanism, intervention: A review. *Journal of Clinical Psychiatry, 43*(4), 151–156.

Rana, J. S., Li, T. Y., Manson, J. E., & Hu, F. B. (2007). Adiposity compared with physical inactivity and risk of type 2 diabetes in women. *Diabetes Care, 30*(1), 53–58.

Raphael, S. (2004). *The socioeconomic status of Black males: The increasing importance of incarceration.* Retrieved July 2, 2008, from *gsppi.berkeley.edu/faculty/sraphael/the_socioeconomic_status_of_Black_males_march2004.pdf.*

Reichard, P., Nilsson, B. Y., & Rosenqvist, U. (1993). The effect of long-term intensified insulin treatment on the development of microvascular complications of diabetes mellitus. *New England Journal of Medicine, 329*(5), 304–309.

Rhee, M. K., Cook, C. B., Dunbar, V. G., Panayioto, R. M., Berkowitz, K. J., Boyd, B., et al. (2005). Limited health care access impairs glycemic control in low income urban African Americans with type 2 diabetes. *Journal of Health Care for the Poor and Underserved, 16*(4), 734–746.

Roy, M. S. (2004). Proteinuria in African Americans with type 1 diabetes. *Journal of Diabetes Complications, 8*(1), 69–77.

Roy, M. S., & Skurnick, J. (2007). Six-year incidence of visual loss in African Americans with type 1 diabetes mellitus: The New Jersey 725. *Archives of Ophthalmology, 125*(8), 1061–1067.

Sale, M. M., Smith, S. G., Mychaleckyj, J. C., Keene, K. L., Langefeld, C. D., Leak, T. S., et al. (2007). Variants of the transcription factor 7-like 2 (TCF7L2) gene are associated with type 2 diabetes in an African-American population enriched for nephropathy. *Diabetes, 56*(10), 2638–2642.

Salmon, J., Booth, M. L., Phongsavan, P., Murphy, N., & Timperio, A. (2007). Promoting physical activity participation among children and adolescents. *Epidemiologic Reviews, 29*, 144–159.

Sambamoorthi, U., Olfson, M., Wei, W., & Crystal, S. (2006). Diabetes and depression care among Medicaid beneficiaries. *Journal of Health Care for the Poor and Underserved, 17*, 141–161.

Sanders-Thompson, V. L. (2002). Racism: Perceptions of distress among African-Americans. *Community Mental Health Journal, 38*(2), 111–118.

Saydah, S. H., Brancati, F. L., Golden, S. H., Fradkin, J., & Harris, M. I. (2003). Depressive symptoms and the risk of type 2 diabetes mellitus in a US sample. *Diabetes Metabolism Research and Review, 19*(3), 202–208.

Schneider, E., Zaslavsky, A., & Epstein, A. (2002). Racial disparities in the quality of care for enrollees in Medicare managed care. *Journal of the American Medical Association, 287*(10), 1288–1294.

Schoen, C., Doty, M. M., Collins, S. R., & Holmgren, A. L. (2005). Insured but not protected: How many adults are underinsured? *Health Affairs.* Retrieved June 15, 2008, from *content.healthaffairs.org/cgi/content/abstract/hlthaff.w5.289.*

Schulze, M. B., Manson, J. E., Ludwig, D. S., Colditz, G. A., Stampfer, M. J., Willett, W. C., et al. (2004). Sugar-sweetened beverages, weight gain, and incidence of type 2 diabetes in young and middle-aged women. *Journal of American Medical Association, 292*(8), 927–934.

SEARCH for Diabetes in Youth Study Group. (2006). The burden of diabetes mellitus among US youth: Prevalence estimates. *Pediatrics, 118*, 1510–1518.

Sequist, T. D., Fitzmaurice, G. M., Marshall, R., Shaykevich, S., Safran, D. G., & Ayanian, J. Z. (2008). Physician performance and racial disparities in diabetes mellitus care. *Archives of Internal Medicine, 168*, 1145–1151.

Sernyak, M. J., Gulanski, B., Leslie, D. L., & Rosenheck, R. (2003). Undiagnosed hyperglycemia in clozapine-treated patients with schizophrenia. *Journal of Clinical Psychiatry, 64*(5), 605–608.

Silliman, R. A., Bhatti, S., & Khan, A. (1996). The care of older persons with diabetes mellitus: Families and primary care physicians. *Journal of American Geriatric Society, 44*(11), 1314–1321.

Simon, G. E., Katon, W., Lin, E. H., Rutter, C., Manning, W. G., Von Korff, M., et al. (2007). Cost-effectiveness of systematic depression treatment among people with diabetes mellitus. *Archives of General Psychiatry, 64*, 65–72.

Skinner, T. C., Davies, M. J., Farooqi, A. M., Jarvis, J., Tringham, J. R., & Khunti, K. (2005). Diabetes screening anxiety and belief. *Diabetic Medicine, 22*(11), 1497–1502.

Stein, C. J., & Colditz, G. A. (2004). The epidemic of obesity. *Journal of Clinical Endocrinology and Metabolism, 89*(6), 2522–2525.

Stratton, I. M., Adler, A. I., Neil, H. A., Matthews, D. R., Manley, S. E., Cull, C. A., et al. (2000). Association of glycaemia with macrovascular and microvascular complications of type 2 diabetes (UKPDS 35): Prospective observational study. *British Medical Journal, 321,* 405–412.

Tolle, T., Xu, X., & Sadosky, A. B. (2006). Painful diabetic neuropathy: A cross-sectional survey of health state impairment and treatment patterns. *Journal of Diabetes Complications, 20*(1), 26–33.

U.S. Census Bureau. (2003). *Health insurance coverage in the United States: 2002.* Washington, DC: Author. Retrieved July 2, 2008, from *www.census.gov/prod/2003pubs/p60-223.pdf.*

U.S. Department of Health and Human Services. (2001). *Mental health: Culture, race, and ethnicity—A supplement to mental health: A report of the surgeon general.* Rockville, MD: U.S. Department of Health and Human Services, Substance Abuse and Mental Health Services Administration, Center for Mental Health Services.

U.S. Department of Health and Human Services. (2006). *Depression.* Rockville, MD: Author. Retrieved June 15, 2008, from *www.nimh.nih.gov/publicat/depression.cfm.*

Wagner, J., Tsimikas, J., Abbott, G., de Groot, M., & Heapy, A. (2007). Racial and ethnic differences in diabetic patient-reported depression symptoms, diagnosis, and treatment. *Diabetes Research and Clinical Practice, 75*(1), 119–22.

Watve, M. G., & Yajnik, C. S. (2007). Evolutionary origins of insulin resistance: A behavioral switch hypothesis. *Biomed Central, 7,* 61.

West, D. S., DiLillo, V., Bursac, Z., Gore, S. A., & Greene, P. G. (2007). Motivational interviewing improves weight loss in women with type 2 diabetes. *Diabetes Care, 30,* 1081–1087.

Whooley, M. A. (2006). Depression and cardiovascular disease—Healing the brokenhearted. *Journal of American Medical Association, 295*(24), 2874–2881.

Williams, D. R., & Collins, C. (1995). US socioeconomic and racial differences in health: Patterns and explanations. *Annual Reviews in Sociology, 21,* 349–386.

Williams, D. R., & Collins, C. (2001). Racial residential segregation: A fundamental cause of racial disparities in health. *Public Health Report, 116,* 404–416.

Williams, M. M., Clouse, R. E., & Lustman, P. J. (2006). Treating depression to prevent diabetes and its complications: Understanding depression as a medical risk factor. *Clinical Diabetes, 24,* 79–86.

Williams, R. A., Gavin, J. R., Phillips, R. A., Sumner, A. E., Duncan, A. K., Hollar, D., et al. (2006). High-risk African Americans with multiple risk factors for cardiovascular disease: challenges in prevention, diagnosis, and treatment. *Ethnicity and Disease, 16*(3), 633–639.

Wolford, J. K., & Vozarova de Courten, B. (2004). Genetic basis of type 2 diabetes mellitus: Implications for therapy. *Treatments in Endocrinology, 3*(4), 257–267.

Yoon, J. W., & Jun, H. S. (2001). Cellular and molecular pathogenic mechanisms of insulin-dependent diabetes mellitus. *Annals of the New York Academy of Science, 928,* 200–211.

# 12

# Cardiovascular Disease

Charles H. Hennekens
Wendy R. Schneider
Robert S. Levine

## CONTRIBUTIONS OF DIFFERENT TYPES OF EVIDENCE

Improvements in both individual health and the health of the general public result from advances in medical knowledge that proceed on several fronts, ideally simultaneously. Basic research offers insights into the most plausible biological mechanisms to explain why an exposure or intervention reduces premature death and disability. Although basic research has the unique advantage of precision, its immediate relevance to free-living humans is not always clear. Clinicians provide enormous benefits to affected patients as well as apparently healthy individuals by their applications of advances in diagnosis and treatment, and they formulate hypotheses from their own clinical experiences (namely, their case reports and case series).

Epidemiologists and biostatisticians formulate hypotheses from descriptive studies and—optimally, in collaboration with clinicians—test hypotheses in analytic studies. These include observational (i.e., case–control or cohort) studies, as well as randomized trials. For small to moderate benefits or risks of exposures or interventions, large-scale randomized evidence is crucial: The amount of uncontrolled and uncontrollable confounding inherent in all observational studies, no matter how large and well designed, can be as big as the effect sizes. Analytic epidemiological studies answer the equally crucial and complementary question of whether an exposure or intervention reduces premature death and disability.

271

Although the domain of epidemiology is free-living humans, this discipline is crude and inexact. Observations on free-living humans can never take place under the rigidly controlled conditions possible in a laboratory. Thus each of these disciplines and strategies provides importantly relevant and complementary contributions. Rational clinical decisions for individual patients and apparently healthy individuals, as well as policy decisions for the health of the general public, can safely be based on this totality of evidence (Hennekens & Buring, 1987).

In this chapter, we review the evidence on African Americans and cardiovascular disease (CVD) and discuss interventions that do and do not work, with the goal of decreasing this major and avoidable contributor to disparities in mortality between African Americans and Caucasians.

## WORLDWIDE TRENDS

CVD includes morbidity and mortality from myocardial infarction (MI), stroke, and peripheral vascular disease (PVD). Worldwide, CVD has been the fifth leading cause of mortality, accounting for more than one in four total deaths. In 2004 17.1 million people died from CVD, but by 2030 the World Health Organization (2008) projects that this figure will rise to 23.4 million. Worldwide, CVD is predicted by the World Health Organization to be the leading cause of mortality, accounting for more than one in three deaths. The causes for these increases in mortality from CVD are multifactorial. They include the reassuring decreases in deaths due to malnutrition and infection, as well as the alarming increases in two major risk factors for CVD: cigarette smoking and obesity (Hennekens, 1998; Mackay & Mensah, 2004).

As a specific example of the alarming trends contributing to the emerging pandemic of CVD, 58% of men in Beijing, China, smoke cigarettes—a figure comparable to that in the United States in the 1950s (Liu et al., 1998; Niu et al., 1998). Body mass index (BMI), defined as weight in kilograms divided by height in meters squared, is a reasonably good measure of adiposity (Prospective Studies Collaboration [PSC], 2009). The current average BMI figure of 24.8 for Beijing is comparable to that for the United States in the early 1990s (Z. Chen, personal communication, 2004). In addition, the percentage of Beijing children under the age of 5 who are overweight for their age increased from 4.6% in 1990–1999 to 6.3% in 2000–2007 (World Health Organization, 2009).

## U.S. TRENDS

CVD is the leading cause of death in the United States and most developed Western countries, and will remain so during the 21st century (Hennekens, 1998). Specifically, in 2002 total mentions of CVD constituted about 58% of all deaths. In 2004 CVD was the underlying cause of death for 36.3% (871,517) of all 2,398,000 deaths, or 1 of every 2.8. Finally, as illustrated in Figure 12.1 (Hennekens & Schneider, 2008), with respect to proportional mortality from CVD, coronary heart disease (CHD) accounted for 52% and stroke for 17% (Rosamond et al., 2007).

During the latter part of the 20th century, the United States experienced remarkable declines in mortality from CHD, declines in stroke, and consequent decreases in mortality from CVD. As a result, U.S. life expectancy increased. During the last decade, however, these remarkable trends have been greatly influenced by earlier diagnosis and more aggressive treatment by health care providers, as well as by primary prevention efforts. Ironically, at present the United States is experiencing its greatest life expectancy ever, despite the fact that virtually all untreated risk factors for CVD are worse except for cigarette smoking. It is projected that CVD will remain far and away the leading killer in the United States during the 21st century. It is likely that mortality from CVD will increase in the future because of the increased frequency among U.S. adolescents of cigarette smoking and physical inactivity, as well as obesity and its consequences, which include hypertension, dyslipidemia, and diabetes mellitus (DM) (Flegal, Carroll, Ogden, & Johnson, 2002).

## TRENDS FOR AFRICAN AMERICANS

In the United States, CVD and CHD, its major contributor, are leading causes of death for both men and women from all racial and ethnic backgrounds. However,

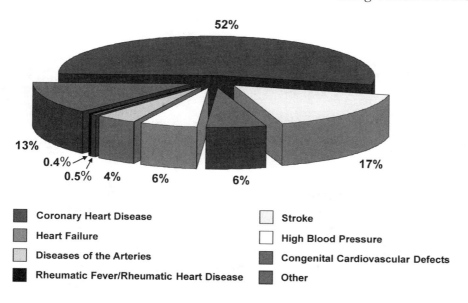

**FIGURE 12.1.** Proportional mortality from cardiovascular diseases in the United States, 2004. Data from the National Center for Health Statistics and the National Heart, Lung, and Blood Institute.

African Americans have the highest overall as well as out-of-hospital CHD death rates of any U.S. ethnic group, particularly at younger ages (Clark et al., 2001). In addition, African Americans have earlier onsets and higher risks of first MI at all ages than their Caucasian counterparts do (Clark et al., 2006). The reasons for the earlier onset and excess deaths from CHD among African Americans are complex and multifactorial. These include a higher prevalence of several major risk factors, patients' delays in seeking medical attention, delays in diagnosis, and less aggressive treatment of patients at higher risk (especially those with evidence of end-organ damage).

Table 12.1 demonstrates that in the United States from 1979 to 2006, age-adjusted mortality from CVD, including MI, PVD, and stroke, declined among African American women and men (Centers for Disease Control and Prevention [CDC], 2000, 2003, 2009). Nevertheless, African Americans have higher absolute rates of acute MI, PVD, and stroke than their Caucasian counterparts. Since the declines in mortality for all three conditions are proportionally smaller among African Americans, Figure 12.2 shows that, not surprisingly, there have been net increases in the mortality rate ratios for both male and female African Americans versus Caucasians (CDC, 2000, 2003, 2009; Levine, Briggs, Husaini, & Hennekens, 2006). Figure 12.3 shows that differences in mortality rates between male and female African Americans and Caucasians have increased for MI and PVD but have remained relatively stable for CVD (CDC, 2000, 2003, 2009).

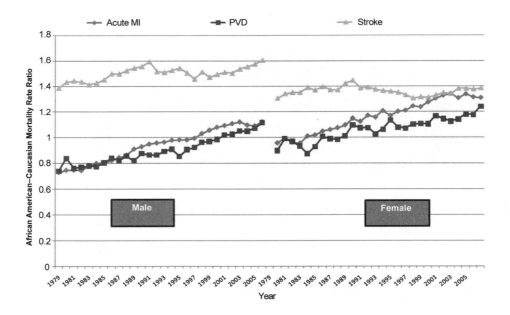

**FIGURE 12.2.** Age-adjusted, male and female, African American–Caucasian mortality rate ratios for acute myocardial infarction (MI), peripheral vascular disease (PVD), and stroke in the United States, 1979–2006. Data from CDC (2000, 2003, 2009).

**TABLE 12.1. Age-Adjusted Mortality per 100,000 among African American Women and Men from Acute Myocardial Infarction (MI), Peripheral Vascular Disease (PVD), and Stroke in the United States, 1979–2006**

| Year | African American women | | | African American men | | |
|------|----------|------|--------|----------|------|--------|
| | Acute MI | PVD | Stroke | Acute MI | PVD | Stroke |
| 1979 | 104.4 | 21.1 | 119.1 | 172.6 | 27.5 | 141.4 |
| 1980 | 107.7 | 23.3 | 121.4 | 173.0 | 31.2 | 144.0 |
| 1981 | 100.4 | 21.3 | 114.2 | 164.8 | 27.1 | 134.1 |
| 1982 | 98.1 | 19.4 | 107.3 | 159.4 | 26.1 | 125.7 |
| 1983 | 100.9 | 18.0 | 105.8 | 160.7 | 25.9 | 119.9 |
| 1984 | 98.4 | 18.1 | 101.6 | 156.8 | 24.6 | 116.5 |
| 1985 | 98.3 | 18.8 | 100.6 | 152.2 | 24.7 | 114.1 |
| 1986 | 94.7 | 17.9 | 94.7 | 142.9 | 24.5 | 112.2 |
| 1987 | 92.5 | 17.4 | 92.8 | 139.4 | 23.7 | 109.6 |
| 1988 | 91.4 | 17.6 | 93.8 | 136.8 | 24.2 | 110.8 |
| 1989 | 93.9 | 17.5 | 90.7 | 140.4 | 22.2 | 105.4 |
| 1990 | 88.4 | 16.4 | 85.1 | 137.2 | 23.0 | 103.8 |
| 1991 | 88.7 | 15.9 | 81.8 | 132.7 | 21.7 | 102.4 |
| 1992 | 83.5 | 14.9 | 79.2 | 128.1 | 20.8 | 96.0 |
| 1993 | 84.5 | 15.4 | 80.1 | 124.7 | 21.5 | 97.5 |
| 1994 | 79.3 | 16.2 | 79.9 | 120.7 | 21.1 | 97.8 |
| 1995 | 78.4 | 15.2 | 80.5 | 116.3 | 19.6 | 98.5 |
| 1996 | 76.3 | 15.1 | 78.5 | 110.8 | 20.2 | 95.7 |
| 1997 | 74.0 | 15.2 | 75.4 | 106.3 | 20.1 | 90.9 |
| 1998 | 71.7 | 14.7 | 74.7 | 105.6 | 20.0 | 89.3 |
| 1999 | 71.5 | 13.9 | 77.2 | 103.5 | 18.4 | 90.8 |
| 2000 | 70.1 | 14.1 | 77.2 | 100.3 | 18.6 | 90.8 |
| 2001 | 67.0 | 13.6 | 74.7 | 94.4 | 17.7 | 86.5 |
| 2002 | 64.1 | 12.7 | 72.8 | 90.7 | 17.2 | 82.7 |
| 2003 | 58.4 | 12.3 | 70.7 | 85.4 | 16.8 | 80.6 |
| 2004 | 53.5 | 11.9 | 66.3 | 75.8 | 15.3 | 75.8 |
| 2005 | 49.5 | 11.5 | 61.5 | 70.7 | 15.2 | 71.4 |
| 2006 | 44.6 | 10.3 | 57.7 | 67.1 | 13.8 | 67.9 |

*Note.* Data from CDC (2000, 2003, 2009).

Thus, while African Americans have experienced absolute improvements in mortality from CVD as well as total mortality, the improvements relative to those of Caucasians are smaller. As a result, the average life expectancy of African Americans remains about 6 years shorter than that of Caucasians. The leading causes of death accounting for the overall 6-year difference are CHD (1.7 years), cancer (1.2 years), homicide (0.6 years), stroke (0.5 years), and perinatal disease (0.5 years). Thus CVD accounts for about 36.7% (2.2/6 years) of the overall reduced life expectancy for African Americans (CDC, 2001).

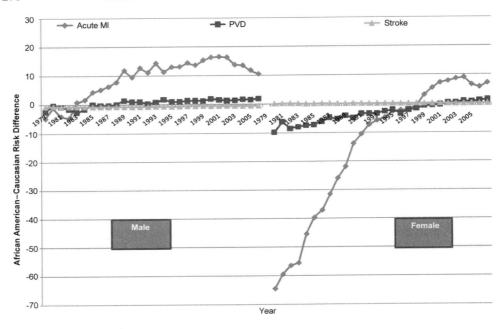

**FIGURE 12.3.** Sex differences in mortality rates between male and female African Americans and Caucasians in age-adjusted mortality from acute MI, PVD, and stroke in the United States, 1979–2006. Data from CDC (2000, 2003, 2009).

# RISK FACTORS: GENERAL CONSIDERATIONS
# FOR CAUCASIANS AND AFRICAN AMERICANS

## Cigarette Smoking

Cigarette smoking is a leading cause of premature total death, especially CVD and cancer (Hennekens & Buring, 1985; Hennekens, Mayrent, & Buring, 1984). In regard to CVD, the risks of cigarettes are proportional chiefly to the amount of current smoking. Upon cessation, CVD risks begin to decrease rapidly and perhaps reach those of persons who have never smoked in 3–5 years. With respect to cancer, the risks of cigarettes are proportional chiefly to the duration of smoking. Upon cessation of smoking, cancer risks do not begin to decrease for several years, and perhaps after a decade reach a level midway between those of persons who continue to smoke and those who have never smoked. Thus for CVD it is never too late to quit smoking, and for cancer it is never too early to quit. Even with respect to CVD in older adults, beneficial changes of smoking cessation begin within a few months (LaCroix et al., 1991).

Among men, African Americans are more likely to smoke cigarettes than Caucasians. Among women, African Americans and Caucasians smoke at about equal rates (Fiore et al., 1989).

## Obesity

The average BMI in the United States is above 27, so about 97 million adults are obese or overweight (National Institutes of Health [NIH], 1998). Thus U.S. society is the fattest in the world, and is likely to be the fattest in the history of the world.

Obesity leads to hypertension, dyslipidemia, and DM. Abdominal (central) obesity is particularly associated with insulin resistance and is more atherogenic than gluteofemoral obesity. In the PSC (2009), BMI is strongly associated with overall and CVD mortality. BMI is also an established risk factor for several causes of death, including CHD (Manson et al., 1990); stroke (Song, Sung, Davey Smith, & Ebrahim, 2004); and cancers of the large intestine, kidney, endometrium, and postmenopausal breast (Calle, Rodriguez, Walker-Thurmond, & Thun, 2003; Reeves et al., 2007). In many populations the average BMI has been rising (typically by a few percent per decade), fueling concern about the effects of greater adiposity on health (World Health Organization Global InfoBase Team, 2005).

Some uncertainties persist, however, about the relationship between BMI and mortality. These include (1) whether some of the reported positive or inverse associations have been distorted by weight loss due to preexisting disease (reverse causality) or by inadequate control for the effects of smoking; (2) whether the shape and strength of BMI's associations with specific diseases differ between smokers and nonsmokers; (3) how the relative and absolute risks for BMI compare with, and also combine with, those for smoking; (4) whether the relative risks differ much by sex or age, and indeed whether any substantial association persists into old age (Janssen & Mark, 2007); (5) how the absolute excess risks for CVD compare with those for neoplastic or respiratory disease; and (6) the extent to which certain less common causes of death, such as kidney (Wang, Chen, Song, Caballero, & Cheskin, 2008) or liver (Gaemers & Groen, 2006) disease, are associated with BMI.

Some of these uncertainties were addressed by the PSC (2009). In this collaborative analysis of data on some 900,000 adults in 57 prospective observational cohort studies, overall mortality was lowest at about 22.5–25 kg/m² in both sexes and at all ages, after the researchers adjusted for smoking status and excluded early follow-up. Above this range, each 5 kg/m² higher BMI was associated with about 30% higher all-cause mortality (40% for CVD; 60–120% for diabetic, renal, and hepatic; 10% for neoplastic; and 20% for respiratory and for all other mortality), and no specific cause of death was inversely associated with BMI. Below 22.5–25 kg/m², the overall inverse association with BMI was predominantly due to strong inverse associations for smoking-related respiratory disease (including cancer), and the only positive association was for CHD. The positive relationships of BMI with risk factors for CVD—such as blood pressure, DM, and (up to about 30 kg/m2) the ratio of non-high-density-lipoprotein cholesterol (non-HDL-C) to high-density-lipoprotein cholesterol (HDL-C)—may well be largely causal, and may in turn account for the excess CVD mortality above 20–22.5 kg/m².

Randomized trials of weight loss interventions have shown that reduced adiposity lowers blood pressure (NIH, 1998), increases insulin sensitivity (Blood Pressure Lowering Treatment Trialists' Collaboration, 2003), and beneficially alters lipoprotein particles (Cholesterol Treatment Trialists' [CTT] Collaborators, 2005). Mendelian randomized evidence indicates that observational associations between BMI and such variables are about as strong as would be expected if the associations were causal (PSC, 2002, 2007). In addition, the deleterious effects of higher blood pressures as well as low-density-lipoprotein cholesterol (LDL-C) on CVD are known from randomized drug trials to be reversible (Blood Pressure Lowering Treatment Trialists' Collaboration, 2003; CTT Collaborators, 2005), so effects of BMI on CVD should also be reversible (NIH, 1998).

In the PSC, the positive association between BMI and CHD can be largely accounted for by blood pressure, lipoproteins, and DM. The relationships of baseline BMI with baseline levels of systolic blood pressure and the non-HDL-C/HDL-C ratio can be taken as associations with usual levels of those variables over the next few years, and predict at least a doubling of CHD mortality between 20 and 30 kg/m$^2$ if the combined effects of systolic blood pressure and the ratio are additive (PSC, 2002, 2007). Indeed, an approximate doubling was what was observed. Merely adjusting for single measurements of blood pressure and total cholesterol would have underestimated the mediating effects of blood pressure and especially lipoproteins (Bogers et al., 2007; Jee et al., 2006). Above 30 kg/m$^2$, the non-HDL-C/HDL-C ratio becomes less relevant, but there may be further adverse changes in lipoprotein particles that cannot be inferred from cholesterol fractions (e.g., an increase in the number of small, dense LDL-C particles). DM becomes particularly relevant above 30 kg/m$^2$.

The consistency of these findings supports the judgment that the observed association between BMI and CHD is causal. Nonetheless, the magnitude of the observed associations could have been confounded to some extent by such factors as physical activity or socioeconomic status. Physical activity is cardioprotective, partly because of its effects on BMI. Physical activity may also be protective at different BMI levels (Li et al., 2006), implying independent effects on CHD. Any such effects could cause the independent effects of BMI on CHD to be overestimated. Confounding by socioeconomic status could have caused the effects of BMI to be either over- or underestimated, but only for all-cause mortality in the upper BMI range, as there were too few deaths to subdivide by cause. This association was much the same for the three large prospective cohort studies of health professionals, in which there would have been relatively little confounding by socioeconomic status. The slight weakening of the association between BMI and CHD mortality at older ages may be due to (1) selective early mortality and/or (2) the slight weakening of the association of BMI with usual levels of blood pressure and the non-HDL-C/HDL-C ratio, and of the usual levels of these intermediate variables with CHD mortality (PSC, 2002, 2007). The weaker associations between BMI and these intermediate variables may in turn reflect a weaker relationship with adiposity in old age, resulting from muscle loss and waist gain (Micozzi &

Harris, 1990). Nonetheless, the PSC shows that higher BMI is associated with definite increases in CHD mortality (and also all-cause mortality), up to 80–89 years at least.

For stroke, the findings in the upper and lower BMI ranges were quite different from each other. In the upper range, BMI was associated positively with ischemic, hemorrhagic, and total stroke. These associations can be largely accounted for by the effect of BMI on blood pressure. In the lower BMI range, however, there was no evidence of a positive relationship with ischemic, hemorrhagic, or total stroke, despite the strong positive association between BMI and blood pressure. Thus, for a given blood pressure, the association between BMI and stroke in this lower range would actually have been inverse. These findings in the lower range were not materially affected by excluding further follow-up or, in contrast with the findings of a large Chinese study (Zhou et al., 2008), by excluding those who had ever smoked. After both exclusions were imposed, there was limited statistical power to detect any association in the lower BMI range.

The evidence from previous large studies of BMI and stroke subtype is not as consistent as might be expected (Asia–Pacific Cohort Studies Collaboration, 2004; Hu, 2008; Kurth et al., 2005; Rexrode et al., 1998; Song et al., 2004). This research suggests that the association of BMI above 25 kg/m² with stroke risk is strongly positive for both ischemic and hemorrhagic stroke. BMI below 25 kg/m² is still positive for ischemic but not for hemorrhagic stroke. In the lower BMI range, the PSC found no evidence of an association for ischemic stroke (although the possibility of a weak positive association was not excluded), and slight evidence of an inverse association for hemorrhagic stroke (PSC, 2009).

African American women have significantly higher rates of overweight and obesity as measured by BMI than their Caucasian counterparts. In contrast, African American men have rates similar to those of their Caucasian counterparts (see Figure 12.4) (Flegal, Carroll, Kuczmarski, & Johnson, 1998). In African American women, randomized trials of short duration show physiological benefits on weight loss as well as psychological benefits, which include improved quality of life, feeling better, looking better, and having more energy (Williams, Flack, Gavin, Schneider, & Hennekens, 2007).

## Physical Inactivity

Physical inactivity is an independent risk factor for CVD. In prospective data from a large prospective cohort study, women who increased their level of physical activity to modest frequency and low intensity experienced significant reductions in risks of CHD (see Table 12.2) (Manson et al., 1999). Furthermore, walking and vigorous exercise were associated with substantial reductions in risks of CHD (Hakim et al., 1998). Finally, the magnitudes of risk reduction associated with brisk walking and vigorous exercise were similar when total energy expenditures were similar. These findings lend further support to current U.S. federal exercise guidelines, which endorse moderate-intensity exercise for at least 30 minutes on

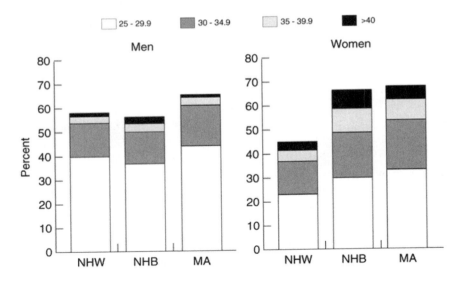

**FIGURE 12.4.** Prevalence of overweight BMI (kg/m²) in U.S. adults by sex and ethnicity, 1988–1994. MA, Mexican American; NHB, non-Hispanic Black; NHW, non-Hispanic White. Three levels of obesity: Class I BMI = 30–34.9; Class II BMI = 35–39.9; Class III BMI = > 40. Data from Flegal, Carroll, Kuczmarski, and Johnson (1998, Table 6, p. 44).

most (preferably all) days of the week (Pate et al., 1995; U.S. Department of Health and Human Services, 1996). Such a regimen (e.g., brisk walking daily for a total of 3 or more hours per week) could reduce the risk of coronary events in women by 30–40%. Increasing walking time or combining walking with more vigorous exercise appears to be associated with even greater risk reductions. Given the high prevalence in the United States of a sedentary lifestyle (78% of adults engage in less physical activity than currently recommended) (U.S. Department of Health and Human Services, 1996), perhaps one-third of CHD among middle-aged U.S. women can be attributed to physical inactivity. Since a brisk walk of at least 20 minutes for at least every other day is associated with a 35–55% reduction in risk of CHD, this strategy could be implemented even among the oldest old persons who are ambulatory (Manson et al., 1999).

## Type 2 Diabetes Mellitus

DM affects 17.9 million Americans. It has been estimated that an additional 5.7 million have it but are undiagnosed. DM is the seventh leading cause of death in the general population, but the fourth leading cause of death among African Americans. The American Diabetes Association (2008) estimates that 3.7 million African Americans (14.7%) have DM, predominantly Type 2. African Americans have a 51% higher prevalence of Type 2 DM than Caucasians. Age-adjusted death

**TABLE 12.2. Relative Risk of Coronary Events According to Quintile Group for Total Physical Activity Score**

| Variable | Quintile group for total activity | | | | | *p* for trend |
|---|---|---|---|---|---|---|
| | 1 | 2 | 3 | 4 | 5 | |
| MET-hr/wk | | | | | | |
| Median | 0.8 | 3.2 | 7.7 | 15.4 | 35.4 | |
| Range | 0–2.0 | 2.1–4.6 | 4.7–10.4 | 10.5–21.7 | > 21.7 | |
| No. of coronary events | 178 | 153 | 124 | 101 | 89 | |
| Person-yr of follow-up | 106,252 | 116,175 | 112,703 | 110,886 | 113,419 | |
| | Relative risk (95% CI) | | | | | |
| Type of analysis | | | | | | |
| Age-adjusted | 1.0 | 0.77 (0.62–0.96) | 0.65 (0.52–0.82) | 0.54 (0.42–0.69) | 0.46 (0.36–0.60) | < .001 |
| Multivariate[a] | 1.0 | 0.88 (0.71–1.10) | 0.81 (0.64–1.02) | 0.74 (0.58–0.95) | 0.66 (0.51–0.86) | .002 |
| Mulitvariate, excluding first 2 yr[a,b] | 1.0 | 0.91 (0.71–1.16) | 0.79 (0.61–1.03) | 0.69 (0.52–0.92) | 0.66 (0.49–0.88) | .004 |
| Mulitvariate, excluding biological intermediate[a,c] | 1.0 | 0.85 (0.69–1.06) | 0.78 (0.62–0.99) | 0.69 (0.54–0.88) | 0.60 (0.46–0.77) | < .001 |

*Note.* The total physical activity score was computed as the cumulative updated average number of MET-hours per week for 1986, 1988, and 1992. The primary endpoint, events due to CHD, included nonfatal MI and death due to coronary causes. In each type of analysis, the women in the lowest quintile group served as the reference group. CI denotes confident interval. From Manson et al. (1999). Copyright 1999 by the Massachusetts Medical Society. Reprinted by permission.

[a]The model included variables for age (in 5-year categories), period during the study (four 2-year periods); smoking status (never smoked, previously smoked, or currently smokes 1 to 14, 15 to 24, or ≥ 25 cigarettes per day); BMI (in five categories); menopausal status (premenopausal, postmenopausal without hormone replacement therapy, postmenopausal with previous hormone replacement therapy, or postmenopausal with current hormone replacement therapy); parental history with respect to MI before the age of 60 years; multivitamin supplement use; vitamin E supplement use; alcohol consumption (0, 1–4, 5–14, ≥ 15 g per day); history of hypertension; history of diabetes; history of hypercholesterolernia; and aspirin use (none, one to six doses per week, or seven or more doses per week).

[b]In this analysis, data from the first 2 years of follow-up after the completion of the physical activity questionnaire were excluded in order to minimize potential bias due to subclinical disease.

[c]In this analysis, biological intermediary covariates that may have had a role in mediating the effect of exercise (BMI, hypertension, high cholesterol level, and diabetes) were excluded from the model.

rates in DM were higher for African American men (117%) and women (167%) than for their Caucasian counterparts.

Although triglycerides (TG) may be an earlier marker, impaired fasting glucose is a precursor to DM, characterized by levels between 110 and 126 mg/dl (6.1 to 7.0 mmol/L). About 50–60% of individuals with impaired fasting glucose also have impaired glucose tolerance (Williams et al., 2007).

## Lipids

In observational studies over decades, a 10% increase in cholesterol is associated with a 20–30% increase in risk of CVD. In randomized trials of statins, decreases in cholesterol are associated with statistically significant and clinically important reductions in risks of CVD, including MI, stroke, and CVD deaths as well as total mortality (CTT Collaborators, 2005).

Specifically, the CTT collaboration included 90,056 patients who were randomized and treated for 5 years in 14 trials of statins. In a meta-analysis, there were 8,086 deaths; 14,348 had major CVD events; and 5,103 developed cancer. At 1 year the mean LDL-C difference ranged from 0.35 mmol/L (13.3 mg/dl) to 1.77 mmol/L (67.3 mg/dl). There were statistically significant proportional reductions in all-cause mortality (12%) and CHD mortality (19%) per mmol/L reduction in LDL-C. There were corresponding statistically significant reductions in MI or CHD deaths (23%), coronary revascularization (24%), fatal or nonfatal stroke (17%), and major CVD events (21%). There were possible but nonsignificant reductions in noncoronary CVD mortality (7%) and non-CVD mortality (5%). The proportional reduction in major CVD events differed significantly according to the absolute reduction in LDL-C achieved. An overall reduction of only about 0.2 mmol/L (7.6 mg/dl) LDL-C reduction translated into 48 fewer participants' having major CVD events per 1,000 among those with prior CHD at baseline, compared with 255 among those without a prior history. There was no evidence that statins increased the incidence of cancer overall or at any particular site. The overall relative risk estimate for statins and cancer of 1.01 is far more reassuring than any subgroup data from any individual trial. There were 15 incident cases of rhabdomyolysis, 9 in the statin group and 6 in the control group—a nonsignificant difference. Statins safely reduced the 5-year incidence of major CHD events, coronary revascularizations, and stroke, regardless of the initial lipid profile or other presenting characteristics. The absolute benefit related chiefly to an individual's absolute risk of such events and to the absolute reduction in LDL-C achieved (CTT Collaborators, 2005).

In the early randomized trials with simvastatin, pravastatin, and lovastatin in secondary and primary prevention, clinical benefits were manifest about 2 years after randomization, which was compatible with the primary postulated mechanism of benefit on antiatherogenic effects of statins via reductions in LDL-C. Several recent trials, however, have suggested early benefits, especially with higher doses of atorvastatin (Cannon et al., 2004; LaRosa et al., 2005; Nissen et al., 2004) and rosuvastatin (Crouse et al., 2007; Nissen et al., 2006; Ridker et al., 2008). These data are compatible with the possibility that early benefits are due to pleiotropic effects of the more potent statins—perhaps via anti-inflammatory, antioxidant, and/or antiplatelet mechanisms, as well as the trapping of free radicals (Novela & Hennekens, 2004). The postulated mechanisms for early benefit are all plausible but unproven, and the magnitude of the major benefits of statins on clinical CVD seems to be either directly or indirectly related to the amount of LDL-C lowering.

Several adjunctive therapies are used to treat lipid abnormalities. The totality of evidence for adjunctive therapies in reducing the risks of CVD is far less than that for statins (Hennekens, Hollar, Eidelman, & Agatston, 2006). Niacin (nicotinic acid) produced statistically significant and clinically important benefits in CHD among 2,835 randomized patients (Berge & Canner, 1991). These beneficial effects were present despite the known glycemic effects of this drug. Omega-3 fatty acids also produced a statistically significant and clinically important benefit on total mortality in 11,324 randomized patients (GISSI-Prevenzione Investigators, 1999). Both these findings, however, preceded the use of statins, and it is unclear whether these benefits were additive to those of statins. Among fibrates, gemfibrozil produced clinical benefits in 2,531 patients in the Veterans Affairs HDL Intervention Trial, but in the U.S. Food and Drug Administration database this drug was responsible for 38% of all rhabdomyolysis, either alone or in combination with statins (Robins et al., 2001). As regards fenofibrates, among diabetic patients in the Fenofibrate Intervention and Event Lowering in Diabetes trial, there was no significant overall benefit in the reduction of CVD. Interestingly, with respect to hypothesis formulation in a post hoc nonrandomized subgroup analysis of patients given fenofibrate who were not treated with statins, there was a significant benefit in the primary prespecified endpoint (Keech et al., 2005). Finally, there are no clinical outcome data for the effects of ezetimibe on CVD, either alone or in combination with statins (Hennekens et al., 2006).

Although numerous drug therapies to modify lipids favorably are currently available either by prescription or over the counter, the 3-hydroxy-3-methylglutaryl coenzyme A reductase inhibitors, or statins, are recommended by the National Cholesterol Education Program (NCEP) as the first-line drugs of choice for virtually all patients eligible for lipid modification by drugs (NCEP Expert Panel on Detection, Evaluation, and Treatment of High Blood Cholesterol in Adults (Adult Treatment Panel III [ATP III]), 2002). The NCEP recommends that primary prevention patients whose LDL-C goal is less than 130 mg/dl (3.36 mmol/L) should have drug therapy initiated simultaneously with therapeutic lifestyle changes. Statins lower total cholesterol (TC), LDL-C, and TG levels, and increase HDL-C levels. With regard to HDL-C levels, both major subfractions (namely, 2 and 3) are protective against CHD (Buring et al., 1992).

In an early meta-analysis of secondary and primary prevention trials, those assigned at random to statins had a 22% reduction in cholesterol levels and a 30% reduction in LDL-C levels (Hebert, Gaziano, Chan, & Hennekens, 1997; Hennekens, 2001). Lowering LDL-C to less than 100 mg/dl (< 2.59 mmol/L), with an optimal goal of less than 70 mg/dl, is the target for patients with prior MI, stroke, or PVD; a 10-year CHD risk of 20% or higher; or DM. For patients with a 10-year CHD risk between 10 and 19%, the LDL-C goal is less than 130 mg/dl (< 3.36 mmol/L), with an optional goal of less than 100 mg/dl. For individuals whose

10-year CHD risk is less than 10%, the LDL-C goal is less than 160 mg/dl (< 4.14 mmol/L) (Grundy et al., 2004).

The revision in 2004 (Grundy et al., 2004) of the original NCEP guidelines (NCEP ATP III, 2002) expanded the prior list of cardiovascular events for which statins should be prescribed to include virtually all occlusive vascular diseases of the heart (stable and unstable angina, angioplasty, or bypass), as well as of the brain (i.e., ischemic stroke, transient ischemic attacks, and symptomatic carotid artery stenosis) and peripheral arteries. These revised U.S. federal guidelines also focus on global risk assessment rather than just lipid parameters. Global risk assessment includes quantitation of the 10-year risk of developing CHD. Such quantitation is based on the novel and important concept of a CHD risk equivalent. In the 2004 updated guidelines, DM is elevated from a major risk factor to a CHD risk equivalent. Thus all diabetic patients should be treated as aggressively as patients who have survived a prior occlusive event of the heart, brain, or peripheral arteries. In addition, based on this concept, a primary prevention patient with a CHD risk equivalent may have an absolute risk for developing a first event equal to or greater than that of a secondary prevention patient for developing a recurrent event. Furthermore, primary prevention patients without a CHD risk equivalent but with multiple risk factors may also have a 10-year risk equal to or greater than that of a secondary prevention patient (i.e., a survivor of a prior event) without additional risk factors. Thus health care providers are asked to quantitate the 10-year risk of all primary prevention patients with two or more risk factors by using the Framingham risk score (NCEP ATP III, 2002) adopted from the Framingham Risk Assessment System (Wilson et al., 1998).

In addition, the 2004 NCEP updated guidelines create two new lipid goals. First, these guidelines raise the level of HDL-C defined as low to less than 40 mg/dl (1.03 mmol/L) rather than 35 mg/dl (0.90 mmol/L). Second, these guidelines lower the level of TG defined as high to greater than 150 mg/dl (1.69 mmol/L) rather than 200 mg/dl (2.26 mmol/L) (Grundy et al., 2004).

The U.S. federal guidelines recommend initial screening based on fasting TC, LDL-C, HDL-C, and TG levels. For individuals with a TG level greater than 200 mg/dl (2.26 mmol/L), health care providers are advised to treat both HDL-C and non-HDL-C levels; the latter lipid parameter is determined by combining the levels of LDL-C and very-low-density-lipoprotein cholesterol (Eidelman, Lamas, & Hennekens, 2002). The global risk assessment should include sex, age, TC level, smoking status, HDL-C level, and systolic blood pressure. If the absolute risk is 20% or greater, a primary prevention patient should be treated as aggressively as a patient who has experienced a previous event.

The NCEP guidelines also target primary prevention patients at high risk due to multiple metabolic risk factors termed the *metabolic syndrome*. This syndrome is a major clinical and public health problem in the United States. The clinical problem results from the fact that the average 10-year global risk of the high-risk primary prevention patient with multiple metabolic risk factors (about 16–18%) is far greater than the simple arithmetic sum of the patient's individual risks.

The public health problem results from the fact that over 25% of all U.S. adults have the metabolic syndrome; the figure rises to about 40% of those over age 40. The NCEP defines the metabolic syndrome as a constellation of any three of the following five criteria: abdominal obesity (waist > 40 in. in men and > 35 in. in women); low HDL-C levels (< 40 mg/dl) in men and < 50 mg/dl in women); high TG levels (> 150 mg/dl); increased blood pressure (> 130/85 mm Hg); and high fasting blood glucose levels (> 110 mg/dl) (see Table 12.3) (NCEP ATP III, 2002).

We should note that the 10-year risks based on Framingham risk scores have been derived from a primarily middle-class Caucasian population. African Americans have higher absolute risks for any given Framingham risk score (Eidelman et al., 2002).

## Blood Pressure

High blood pressure, or hypertension, is defined by the Seventh Report of the Joint National Committee Report on Prevention, Evaluation, and Treatment of High Blood Pressure (Chobanian et al., 2003) as a systolic pressure equal to or greater than 140 millimeters of mercury (mm Hg), or diastolic pressure equal to or greater than 90 mm Hg. Hypertension as thus defined affects more than 50 million people, or 20% of the U.S. population (Lloyd-Jones et al., 2010). Hypertension is a major risk factor for stroke, MI, and death from CVD. In a comprehensive worldwide meta-analysis of the randomized trials of mild to moderate hypertension, drug therapies reduced blood pressures by 4–5 mm Hg. Over 3–5 years, this magnitude of reduction in blood pressure was associated with statistically significant and clinically important decreases of 42% in stroke, 14% in MI, and 23% in deaths from CVD (Collins et al., 1990). A subsequent meta-analysis involving a larger number of trials with greater numbers of clinical CVD endpoints showed a 17% reduction in risk of MI (Moser, Hebert, & Hennekens, 1991). Of note, observational studies have shown that long-term changes of this magnitude were associated with decreases in risks of about 40–45% for stroke, 25–30% for MI, and 20–25% in death from CVD.

The similarities in the magnitudes of the reductions in risks of stroke and death from CVD, and the differences in the magnitude of the reduction in risk of MI, associated with a decrease of 4–5 mm Hg in blood pressure have led to the formulation of three hypotheses. First, the observed differences in the magnitude of the reduction in MI between the trials (14–17%) and the observational studies (25–30%) are due to the play of chance. Second, the beneficial effects of blood pressure lowering on stroke are more immediate and direct than those on MI. Third, the first-line drugs used in the trials were primarily thiazides, which increase LDL-C by about 5% and may have caused a compensatory increase in risk of MI (Collins et al., 1990).

In the Third National Health and Nutrition Examination Survey (NHANES III), the prevalences of hypertension in African American men and women were 35% and 34.2%, respectively, compared to 24.4% and 19.3% in their Caucasian counterparts (Burt et al., 1995). Death rates from hypertension are more than 350% higher in African Americans than in Caucasians (Williams, 2001). African Americans have earlier onset, higher prevalence, and greater severity of hypertension, with double the risk of heart failure (HF) and CHD, as well as approximately fivefold increased risks of fatal stroke and end-stage renal disease (ESRD) (Klag et al., 1997; Ofili, 1995).

Hypertension also causes left ventricular hypertrophy (LVH) and HF. In the Framingham Heart Study, patients with LVH had a five to six times higher risk of sudden death (Kannel, 1983). LVH is more common in African Americans, and increases risks of arrhythmias and silent but lethal ischemic events (Liao, Cooper, McGhee, Mensah, & Ghali, 1995). HF is the leading cause of hospitalizations in the United States among those age 65 and over, and is increasing in prevalence with the increasing age of the population. HF is also more common in African Americans than in Caucasians, and patients with HF have an annual mortality rate of 10% (Hennekens, Pfeffer, & Swedberg, 2007). Finally, among African Americans treated for hypertension, only about 27% achieve their blood pressure goals (Wong et al., 2007).

With respect to costs, the increases in morbidity and mortality due to hypertension in the United States for 2010 are estimated to be over $76 billion in medicines, health services, and loss of productivity (Lloyd-Jones et al., 2010).

## INTERVENTION AND PREVENTION APPROACHES FOR AFRICAN AMERICANS

### General Considerations

In NHANES III, African American men and women, compared to their Caucasian and Hispanic counterparts, had the highest age-adjusted prevalence of high blood pressure; African American women also had the highest age-adjusted prevalence of abdominal obesity (Flegal et al., 2002; Ford, Giles, & Dietz, 2002; Park et al., 2003). African Americans have higher individual risk factors and multiple risk factors that confer greater-than-additive risk, including hypertension, DM, and glucose intolerance. This is due at least in part to the fact that African Americans tend to be diagnosed later and present more frequently with some target organ damage. All these circumstances contribute to the fact that African Americans experience higher morbidity and mortality from CVD than Caucasians do.

At the time of presentation, many African Americans have at least some degree of hypertension, dyslipidemia, and DM. In African Americans, these risk factors (each alone and in combination) increase risks of MI, stroke, and death from CVD as well as PVD and ESRD (Beckman, Creager, & Libby, 2002). CVD events, especially CHD and stroke, are the most common causes of death in both African American and Caucasian patients with ESRD (U.S. Renal Data Systems, 2009).

In African Americans, microalbuminuria is an indicator of early renal disease and is associated with increased risks of CVD even in patients without DM. In the Heart Outcomes Prevention Evaluation (HOPE) trial, microalbuminuria was found in nearly 15% of patients without DM (Gerstein et al., 2001; Mann, Gerstein, Pogue, Bosch, & Yusuf, 2001). Patients with any degree of microalbuminuria have significantly higher risks of CVD, hospitalizations for HF, and all-cause mortality. For every 0.4-mg/mmol increase in the urine albumin–creatinine ratio in the HOPE trial, the risk of major cardiovascular events increased by 5.9% (Gerstein et al., 2001). In the Hypertension Optimal Treatment study, elevated serum creatinine and a glomerular filtration rate of less than 60 ml/min were associated with increased risks of CVD (Ruilope et al., 2001). Moreover, African Americans with even mild renal insufficiency have high risks of LVH and HF, which contribute to increases in morbidity and mortality from CVD.

Finally, African Americans with any given Framingham risk score should be treated more aggressively than Caucasians with a similar score. The reason, as noted earlier, is that their absolute risks are likely to be higher than those of their Caucasian counterparts, in whom the risk scores were derived.

## Interventions That Work

In African Americans, both therapeutic lifestyle change (TLC) and pharmacological interventions of proven efficacy can reduce premature morbidity and mortality from CVD (NCEP ATP III, 2002; Tuomilehto et al., 2001).

### Therapeutic Lifestyle Change

Unfortunately, most individuals in the United States prefer prescription of pills to proscription of harmful lifestyles. TLC, however, will confer large and usually more-than-additive benefits in terms of risk reduction. The emphasis of TLC should be on smoking cessation, weight control, and increased physical activity (Hennekens, 1998, 2000).

#### SMOKING CESSATION

African Americans generally have higher rates of cigarette smoking and lower rates of cessation than their Caucasian counterparts. In the National Health Interview Survey (King, Bendel, & Delaronde, 1998), African American men between 35 and 44 years of age had the highest rates of cigarette smoking. Smoking cessation produces statistically significant and clinically important reductions in risk of CVD, including CHD and stroke. The CDC Task Force on Community Preventive Services recommends provider reminder systems (either alone or in combination with education), as well as reduction of out-of-pocket costs, to achieve smoking cessation (CDC, 2010).

In secondary prevention of CVD, smoking cessation has a 50–70% success rate for patients hospitalized with CHD. In 20 prospective cohort studies, smokers with CHD who quit had a 36% reduction in all-cause mortality (Critchley &

Capewell, 2003). African Americans have lower rates of quitting than their Caucasian counterparts (Royce et al., 1993). Further research with African Americans is needed to determine whether nicotine intake, biological factors, or possibly the preference for mentholated cigarettes affects nicotine dependence and ability to abstain (Mazas & Wetter, 2003).

Cigarette smoking in African Americans should be considered an addictive behavior, and younger men and women (especially pregnant women) should be targeted. Outreach through community or church-based programs offering individual counseling and culturally appropriate self-help materials may be effective.

WEIGHT CONTROL

Weight control and management are critical for all adults and especially for African American women. BMIs in African American women are much higher than in Caucasian women (Ambrosius, Newman, & Pratt, 2001; Dundas, Morgan, Redfern, Lemic-Stojcevic, & Wolfe, 2001). In addition, African American women gain weight at a faster rate than their Caucasian counterparts (Ambrosius et al., 2001). Obesity, defined as BMI > 30 kg/m², is increasing rapidly among both African American men and women (Freedman, Khan, Serdula, Galuska, & Dietz, 2002).

Physical activity (20 minutes of moderate activity several times per week; see below) is an adjunct to diet in weight control and confers a 35–55% decrease in risk of CHD, as well as a reduction in development of DM (Hennekens, 1998).

Watching television may be a risk factor for obesity. African Americans watch TV 75 hours per week per household, versus the U.S. average of 52 hours per week per household (Tirodkar & Jain, 2003). Furthermore, African Americans may be viewing nearly three times as many advertisements for low-nutrition foods (e.g., candy and soda) and more portrayal of overweight characters (Tirodkar & Jain, 2003).

The U.S. National Heart, Lung, and Blood Institute guidelines for ways clinicians can aid their patients with weight control include dietary therapy, physical activity, drug therapy, and (if needed) obesity surgery for those who are grossly overweight (NIH, 1998). All individuals should have BMI and obesity-related disease risks assessed and routinely monitored. For overweight patients, weight maintenance may suffice, if the patients have no additional risk factors and are resistant to weight reduction. Weight reduction is indicated for all obese individuals, and especially for those with other risk factors and increasing severity (BMI > 30 kg/m²). Recommended dietary changes for all patients whose BMI is higher than 25 kg/m2 include caloric restriction and adherence to the U.S. Department of Agriculture's food pyramid guidelines, which include increased intake of fruits, vegetables, and grains. Sound dietary advice should include distribution of meals evenly throughout the day, avoidance of "unconscious" eating, and reduction of daily intake by 200–500 calories to achieve modest weight loss.

With regard to dietary changes to lower LDL-C levels, health care providers are advised to recommend saturated fat less than 7% of total calories and cholesterol less than 200 mg/day, as well as plant stanols and sterols, foods with viscous (soluble) fiber, and soy products. Stanols and sterols are present in certain margarine products and salad dressings. Sources of soluble fiber include legumes, cereal grains, beans, and many fruits and vegetables. Such dietary TLC is likely to have beneficial effects, not just on CHD but also possibly on certain forms of cancer (especially colon and uterus, and possibly breast). Finally, dietary TLC increases the efficacy of drug therapy with statins.

With respect to TV watching, the U.S. Task Force on Community Preventive Services (CDC, 2010) recommends the following behavioral interventions to reduce total screen time (this includes time spent watching TV, videotapes, or DVDs; playing video or computer games; and surfing the Internet):

- Skills building, tips, goal setting, and reinforcement techniques.
- Parent or family support through provision of information on environmental strategies to reduce access to television, video games, and computers.
- A "TV turnoff challenge," in which participants are encouraged not to watch TV for a specified number of days.

Health care providers need to be aware of the effectiveness of community-based, collaborative interventions directed at other obesity-promoting environmental components that disproportionately affect African American communities.

## PHYSICAL ACTIVITY

As noted earlier, low to moderate physical activity, defined as a 20-minute walk every other day, is associated with a 35–55% decrease in CVD (Manson et al., 1999). Regular physical activity well into old age can be achieved if focused on an enjoyable activity, such as dancing, gardening, or dog walking, performed for a sufficient duration on a regular basis (Douglas et al., 2003).

## *Pharmacological Interventions*

### LIPIDS

African Americans at moderate or high risk of a first CHD event, or those with CHD or its equivalent (such as DM), should receive evidence-based doses of statins to achieve the U.S. federal guidelines for LDL-C as the primary goal. Statins will also produce beneficial changes in triglycerides and HDL-C (Jones, 2003).

### BLOOD PRESSURE

African Americans with hypertension should be treated with pharmacological therapy. Drug selection(s) should be governed by compelling indications, contraindications, and clinical judgment. Nonpharmacological treatment (e.g., weight loss, salt restriction) and drug therapy of patients with high-normal elevated diastolic blood pressure (85–89 mm Hg) reduce the rate of development of hypertension (Trials of Hypertension Prevention Collaborative Research Group, 1992).

Lowering blood pressure requires multiple pharmacological agents, including thiazide-type diuretics and possibly other antihypertensive drugs, such as angiotensin-converting enzyme (ACE) inhibitors and calcium channel blockers. Aggressive management of blood pressure with multiple pharmacological agents leads to significant reductions in MI, stroke, death from CVD, and HF (ALLHAT Officers and Coordinators for the ALLHAT Collaborative Research Group, 2002). In hypertensive patients with DM, lowering diastolic blood pressures to 80–85 mm Hg reduces CVD events (Bakris, 2001; Hansson et al., 1998; U.K. Prospective Diabetes Study [UKPDS] Group, 1998). In African Americans, because baseline blood pressures tend to be high, multiple-drug therapy is likely to be needed; inclusion of an ACE inhibitor at an appropriate dose may provide simultaneous benefits on diabetes and renal function (Wright et al., 2002).

Despite a large number of safe and effective antihypertensive agents, substantial numbers of African Americans with elevated blood pressure are not receiving treatment. A survey of Midwest primary care physicians showed that those who were not treating hypertension aggressively were satisfied with elevated systolic blood pressure readings. In 93% of visits, systolic blood pressure readings were ≥ 140 mm Hg, which is above the currently recommended cutoff point (Chobanian et al., 2003; Oliveria et al., 2002). Interestingly, blood pressure was not addressed in 29% of visits, because the visits were not initially set up as blood pressure checks or there were competing medical problems.

Guidelines for treatment of African Americans with hypertension (Douglas et al., 2003) include the following:

- Combination therapy.
- Target of 130/80 mm Hg for those with CHD, DM, or renal insufficiency.
- Inclusion of renin–angiotensin system blocking agents, ACE inhibitors, or angiotensin receptor blockers (ARBs) in the combination therapy for patients with diabetes or renal disease.

Racial differences practically disappear when the combination therapies that most patients need to achieve blood pressure control are used (Williams et al., 2007). ACE inhibitors are the first choice in patients with metabolic syndrome or DM (Bakris et al., 2000). Indeed, ACE inhibitors and ARBs affect the renin–angiotensin system and provide target organ protection superior to that of other agents, even when blood pressure lowering is similar (Agodoa et al., 2001; Fogo, 2001; HOPE Study Investigators, 2000; Lewis, Hunsicker, Bain, & Rohde, 1993; UKPDS Group, 1998). Some data suggest that African Americans may have a less beneficial response to ACE inhibition. Nonetheless, ACE inhibitors have beneficial effects on kidney function and HF. In multidrug regimens, there is virtually no difference in blood pressure lowering between initial therapy with an ACE inhibitor or calcium blocker (Agodoa et al., 2001). In the African American Study of Kidney Disease and Hypertension, ramipril produced a 36% slower mean decline in glomerular filtration rates over 3 years, and a 38% reduction in the risk of renal clinical endpoints among African Americans with hypertensive renal disease (Agodoa et al., 2001).

## GLUCOSE

Glycemic control decreases microvascular complications of Type 2 DM, including renal and ocular. In addition, a recent meta-analysis of randomized trials suggests statistically significant and clinically important reductions in macrovascular complications, including CHD and stroke (Ray et al., 2009).

The American Diabetes Association (2008) outlines management of glucose intolerance and addresses criteria for screening obese African Americans. Randomized trials in patients with Type 1 (Diabetes Control and Complications Trial Research Group, 1995) or Type 2 (UKPDS Group, 1998) DM indicate beneficial effects of lifestyle modifications, such as weight loss and exercise, as well as aspirin, ACE inhibitors, and a variety of hypoglycemic agents. In patients with Type 2 DM, sulfonylurea or insulin therapy significantly reduced the risk of microvascular complications (e.g., retinopathy, nephropathy) by 25% (UKPDS Group, 1998).

## ADJUNCTIVE DRUG THERAPIES

In African Americans, adjunctive drug therapies to TLC should be used aggressively and early to reach treatment goals. In diabetics, use of an ACE inhibitor is associated with statistically significant and clinically important reductions in CVD, including MI, stroke, and CVD death (HOPE Study Investigators, 2000). In addition, ACE inhibitors and ARBs reduce the risks of developing Type 2 DM (Yusuf et al., 2001, 2005). It is possible, although unproven, that African Americans will need higher doses of ACE inhibitors than their Caucasian counterparts to achieve similar benefits.

Daily aspirin (75–325 mg) should be considered for all patients who have suffered a prior occlusive event and may be considered in primary prevention in those whose 10-year risk of CHD is 10% or greater (Hennekens & Schneider, 2008). Aspirin should be used as an adjunct, not an alternative, to management of other risk factors for CVD; in primary prevention, its use should be based on individual clinical judgment until a sufficient totality of randomized evidence emerges for those with a 10-year risk of 10–19% (Antithrombotic Trialists' Collaboration, 2009).

## Interventions That Do Not Work

### Therapeutic Lifestyle Changes

CIGARETTE SMOKING

Switching to a safer cigarette will not work for any population because there is no demonstrated "safer" cigarette.

OBESITY

Fad diets will not work in the long run for any population although many diets show promise over weeks to months in some populations.

### Pharmacological Interventions

LIPIDS

Some nutraceuticals—such as polycosanol and garlic, as well as psyllium as an adjunct to a low-fat diet—will lower LDL-C. Nonetheless, for African Americans at moderate to high risk, the magnitude of the reduction is wholly insufficient to confer any meaningful decreases in risks of MI, stroke, or death from CVD. Such decreases are easily achievable with evidence-based doses of statins.

BLOOD PRESSURE

Although some nutraceuticals lower blood pressure, there are no randomized data for African Americans at moderate to high risk to demonstrate whether any nutraceutical confers statistically significant or clinically important reductions in MI, stroke, or death from CVD.

ADJUNCTIVE DRUG THERAPIES

In observational studies, individuals with high homocysteine levels have consistently been shown to have higher risks of CVD. In addition, in observational studies and randomized trials, folic acid supplementation has been consistently shown to lower levels of homocysteine. At present, however, sufficient data from large-scale randomized trials with clinical endpoints are now available that demonstrate neither statistically significant nor net clinically important reductions in MI, stroke, or CVD death after folic acid supplementation (Lonn et al., 2006).

Basic research demonstrates plausible mechanisms of benefit for antioxidant vitamins on CVD. In observational studies, individuals who self-select for higher intakes of antioxidant vitamins have lower risks of CVD, but this is likely to be due to confounding by indication. Specifically, individuals who self-select for antioxidant vitamins by either diet or supplements also tend to make other beneficial TLC of proven benefit. Large-scale randomized trials of antioxidants, including both beta-carotene and vitamin E, demonstrate no consistent statistically significant or clinically important reduction in MI, stroke, or CVD death (Williams et al., 2006).

## CONCLUSIONS

CVD remains far and away the leading cause of death in African Americans, despite downward trends. African American men clearly have a lower prevalence of the metabolic syndrome (Park et al., 2003)—the constellation of obesity, hypertension, dyslipidemia, and insulin resistance leading to DM (see Table 12.3)—than their Caucasian counterparts. Nonetheless, African American men and women are more insulin-resistant at similar degrees of adiposity, and have higher blood pressures, than Caucasians; African American women also have more obesity. Furthermore, African Americans are diagnosed later; they have higher individual risk factor levels, as well as more risk factors; and multiple risk factors confer greater-than-additive risks. In short, CVD in African Americans poses significant clinical and public health challenges for health care providers (Williams et al., 2006). However, most risk factors are identifiable and modifiable even in early life, and preventive efforts need to be focused on these.

Innovative approaches are necessary to improve adherence with TLC of proven benefit (Haynes, McKibbon, & Kanani, 1996). For the general population, dropout rates for most physical activity programs are 50% within 3–6 months. Even cardiac rehabilitation patients, regardless of the severity of their illness, drop out at a rate of 50% within a year. Group cohesion and social support are important to decrease dropout rates (Fraser & Spink, 2002).

Informal care incorporating nontraditional settings, as well as alternative and complementary medicine, may be more culturally acceptable and cost-effective means of maintaining and promoting health for African American than "treatment as usual" may be. Effective ways of overcoming barriers to accessing traditional care (including financial, transportation, organizational, and linguistic barriers), as well as of offering ongoing education and support, must be found.

Cultural differences between patients and care providers may affect adherence and outcomes. Cultural competence requires providers to be sensitive to

---

**TABLE 12.3. National Cholesterol Education Program (NCEP) Criteria for the Metabolic Syndrome**

- Abdominal obesity (waist circumference > 40 in. [men], 35 in. [women])
- Hypertriglyceridemia (TG ≥ 150 mg/dl)
- Low HDL-C (< 40 mg/dl [men], < 50 mg/dl [women])
- Hypertension (blood pressure ≥ 130/85 mm Hg)
- High fasting plasma glucose (≥ 110 mg/dl)

*Note.* Data from NCEP ATP III (2002). Patients meeting any three of these criteria are deemed to have the syndrome.

African Americans' communication methods and belief systems, as well as to the impact of their culture on health care relationships (National Center for Primary Care at the Morehouse School of Medicine, 2004). African American providers and those who appreciate and understand the diversity of African American communities are most likely to exhibit cultural competence and support informal care practices that help empower these communities for health improvement. If empowerment—the right for individuals to determine their own destinies—can be conveyed to African Americans through informal care delivery systems, this may be an effective, approach to improve health status (Chen, 1999).

Efforts are needed to increase the number of trained minority health professionals and to improve the cross-cultural interaction skills of all health care providers. The majority of African Americans are not treated by African American health care professionals. The following four steps can and should be taken to make services more ethnically sensitive:

1. Improve access to services (especially by hiring bilingual, bicultural staff).

2. Learn about patients' culture so that interventions can be appropriately tailored to it.

3. Modify services as necessary/appropriate (e.g., integrate traditional medicine with formal Westernized medicine).

4. Initiate an appropriate organization development model/specialized program model (e.g., a faith-based health care delivery model).

In addition to TLC, drug therapies of proven benefit should be utilized. For both dyslipidemia and hypertension, "lower is better"; thus aggressive management strategies for high-risk African Americans with multiple risk factors will be beneficial. Whereas for dyslipidemia statins alone will generally enable patients to reach their goals, for hypertension multiple-drug therapies are necessary.

Finally, the current reimbursement environment impedes diagnosis, treatment, and overall access to health care for many African Americans. This is likely to be a factor in the disparities between African Americans and Caucasians in CVD and total mortality, as well as morbidity. The magnitude and duration of these disparities, as well as the major impact of CVD on African Americans, make it urgently necessary for health care providers to use the best clinical information available to diagnose and aggressively treat this population. Further research is needed to acquire sufficient data to achieve evidence-based changes in public health policy. Meanwhile, we must not "let the perfect be the enemy of the possible," because the immediate clinical and public health challenges in the secondary and primary prevention of CVD among African Americans are clear. The achievement of these goals would produce statistically significant and clinically important reductions in the higher total and CVD mortality and morbidity rates experienced by African Americans versus with their Caucasian counterparts.

These, in turn, would produce statistically significant and clinically important reductions in disparities in total mortality between African Americans and Caucasians.

# REFERENCES

Agodoa, L. Y., Appel, L., Bakris, G. L., Beck, G., Bourgoignie, J., Briggs, J. P., et al. (2001). Effect of ramipril vs. amlodipine on renal outcomes in hypertensive nephrosclerosis. *Journal of the American Medical Association, 285,* 2719–2728.

ALLHAT Officers and Coordinators for the ALLHAT Collaborative Research Group. (2002). Major outcomes in high-risk hypertensive patients randomized to angiotensin-converting enzyme inhibitor or calcium channel blocker vs diuretic. The Antihypertensive and Lipid-Lowering Treatment to Prevent Heart Attack Trial (ALLHAT). *Journal of the American Medical Association, 288,* 2981–2997.

Ambrosius, W. T., Newman, S. A., & Pratt, J. H. (2001). Rates of change in measures of body size vary by ethnicity and gender. *Ethnicity and Disease, 11,* 303–310.

American Diabetes Association (2008). Standards of medical care in diabetes—2008. *Diabetes Care, 31*(Suppl. 1), S12–S54.

Antithrombotic Trialists' Collaboration. (2009). Aspirin in the primary and secondary prevention of vascular disease: collaborative meta-analysis of individual participant data from randomized trials. *Lancet, 373,* 1849–1860.

Asia–Pacific Cohort Studies Collaboration. (2004). Body mass index and cardiovascular disease in the Asia–Pacific Region: An overview of 33 cohorts involving 310,000 participants. *International Journal of Epidemiology, 33,* 751–758.

Bakris, G. L. (2001). A practical approach to achieving recommended blood pressure goals in diabetic patients. *Archives of Internal Medicine, 161,* 2661–2667.

Bakris, G. L., Williams, M., Dworkin, L., Elliott, W. J., Epstein, M., Toto, R., et al. (2000). Preserving renal function in adults with hypertension and diabetes: A consensus approach. *American Journal of Kidney Disease, 36,* 646–661.

Beckman, J. A., Creager, M. A., & Libby, P. (2002). Diabetes and atherosclerosis: Epidemiology, pathophysiology, and management. *Journal of the American Medical Association, 287,* 2570–2581.

Berge, K. G., & Canner, P. L. (1991). Coronary drug project: Experience with niacin. Coronary Drug Project Research Group. *European Journal of Clinical Pharmacology, 40*(Suppl. 1), S49–S51.

Blood Pressure Lowering Treatment Trialists' Collaboration. (2003). Effects of different blood-pressure-lowering regimens on major cardiovascular events: Results of prospectively-designed overviews of randomised trials. *Lancet, 362,* 1527–1535.

Bogers, R. P., Bemelmans, W. J., Hoogenveen, R. T., Boshuizen, H. C., Woodward, M., Knekt, P., et al. (2007). Association of overweight with increased risk of coronary heart disease partly independent of blood pressure and cholesterol levels: A meta-analysis of 21 cohort studies including more than 300,000 persons. *Archives of Internal Medicine, 167,* 1720–1728.

Buring, J. E., O'Connor, G. T., Goldhaber, S. Z., Rosner, B., Herbert, P. N., Blum, C. B., et al. (1992). Decreased HDL2 and HDL3 cholesterol, ApoA-I and ApoA-II, and increased risk of myocardial infarction. *Circulation, 85,* 22–29.

Burt, V. L., Whelton, P., Roccella, E. J., Brown, C., Cutler, J. A., Higgins, M., et al. (1995). Prevalence of hypertension in the US adult. *Hypertension, 25*, 305–313.

Calle, E. E., Rodriguez, C., Walker-Thurmond, K., & Thun, M. J. (2003). Overweight, obesity, and mortality from cancer in a prospectively studied cohort of U.S. adults. *New England Journal of Medicine, 348*, 1625–1638.

Cannon, C. P., Braunwald, E., McCabe, C. H., Rader, D. J., Rouleau, J. L., Belder, R., et al. (2004). Intensive versus moderate lipid lowering with statins after acute coronary syndromes. *New England Journal of Medicine, 350*, 1495–1504.

Centers for Disease Control and Prevention (CDC). (2000). Compressed Mortality File 1979–1998: CDC WONDER Online Database, compiled from Compressed Mortality File CMF 1968–1988, Series 20, No. 2A, 2000. Retrieved February 18, 2010, from *wonder.cdc.gov/cmf-icd9.html*

Centers for Disease Control and Prevention (CDC). (2001). Influence of homicide on racial disparity in life expectancy—United States, 1998. *Morbidity and Mortality Weekly Report, 50*, 780–783.

Centers for Disease Control and Prevention (CDC). (2003). CDC WONDER Online Database, compiled from Compressed Mortality File CMF CMF 1989–1998, Series 20, No. 2E, 2003. Retrieved February 18, 2010, from *wonder.cdc.gov/cmf-icd9.html*

Centers for Disease Control and Prevention (CDC). (2009). Compressed Mortality File 1999–2006. CDC WONDER Online Database, compiled from Compressed Mortality File 1999–2006 Series 20 No. 2L, 2009. Retrieved February 18, 2010, from *wonder. cdc.gov/cmf-icd10.html*

Centers for Disease Control and Prevention (CDC). (2010). *Increasing tobacco use cessation and obesity prevention: Interventions in community settings.* Atlanta, GA: Author. Retrieved January 9, 2010, from *www.thecommunityguide.org*

Chen, M. S., Jr. (1999). Informal care and the empowerment of minority communities: Comparisons between the USA and the UK. *Ethnicity and Health, 4*, 139–151.

Chobanian, A. V., Bakris, G. L., Black, H. R., Cushman, W. C., Green, L. A., Izzo, J. L., Jr., et al. (2003, May 21). The seventh report of the Joint National Committee on Prevention, Detection, Evaluation, and Treatment of High Blood Pressure: The JNC 7 report. *Journal of the American Medical Association, 289*, 2560–2572.

Cholesterol Treatment Trialists' (CTT) Collaborators. (2005). Efficacy and safety of cholesterol-lowering treatment: Prospective meta-analysis of data from 90,056 participants in 14 randomised trials of statins. *Lancet, 366*, 1267–1278.

Clark, L. T., Ferdinand K. C., Flack, J. M., Gavin, J. R., 3rd, Hall, W. D., & Kumanyika, S. K. (2001). Coronary heart disease in African Americans. *Heart Disease, 3*, 97–108.

Clark, L. T., Maki, K. C., Galant, R., Maron, D. J., Pearson, T. A., & Davidson, M. H. (2006). Ethnic differences in achievement of cholesterol treatment goals: Results from the National Cholesterol Education Program evaluation project utilizing novel e-technology II. *Journal of General Internal Medicine, 21*, 320–326.

Collins, R., Peto, R., MacMahon, S., Hebert, P., Fiebach, N. H., Eberlein, K. A., et al. (1990). Blood pressure, stroke, and coronary heart disease: Part 2. Short-term reductions in blood pressure: Overview of randomised drug trials in their epidemiological context. *Lancet, 335*, 827–838.

Critchley, J. A., & Capewell, S. (2003). Mortality risk reduction associated with smoking cessation in patients with coronary heart disease: A systematic review. *Journal of the American Medical Association, 290*, 86–97.

Crouse, J. R., III, Raichlen, J. S., Riley, W. A., Evans, G. W., Palmer, M. K., O'Leary, D. H., et al. (2007). Effect of rosuvastatin on progression of carotid intima-media thickness in low-risk individuals with subclinical atherosclerosis: The METEOR Trial. *Journal of the American Medical Association, 297*, 1344–1353.

Diabetes Control and Complications Trial Research Group. (1995). Effect of intensive therapy on the development and progression of diabetic nephropathy in the Diabetes Control and Complications Trial (DCCT). *Kidney International, 47*, 1703–1720.

Douglas, J. G., Bakris, G. L., Epstein, M., Ferdinand, K. C., Ferrario, C., Flack, J. M., et al. (2003). Management of high blood pressure in African Americans: Consensus statement of the Hypertension in African Americans Working Group of the International Society on Hypertension in Blacks. *Archives of Internal Medicine, 163*, 525–541.

Dundas, R., Morgan, M., Redfern, L., Lemic-Stojcevic, N., & Wolfe, C. (2001). Ethnic differences in behavioural risk factors for stroke: Implications for health promotion. *Ethnicity and Health, 6*, 95–103.

Eidelman, R. S., Lamas, G. A., & Hennekens, C. H. (2002). The new National Cholesterol Education Program guidelines. *Archives of Internal Medicine, 162*, 2033–2036.

Fiore, M. C., Novotney, T. E., Pierce, J. P., Hatziandreu, E. J., Patel, K. M., & Davis, R. M. (1989). Trends in cigarette smoking in the United States: The changing influence of gender and race. *Journal of the American Medical Association, 261*, 49–55.

Flegal, K. M., Carroll, M. D., Kuczmarski, R. J., & Johnson, C. L. (1998). Overweight and obesity in the United States: Prevalence and trends, 1960–1994. *International Journal of Obesity, 22*, 39–47.

Flegal, K. M., Carroll, M. D., Ogden, C. L., & Johnson, C. L. (2002). Prevalence and trends in obesity among US adults, 1999–2000. *Journal of the American Medical Association, 288*, 1723–1727.

Fogo, A. B. (2001). Progression and potential regression of glomerulosclerosis. *Kidney International, 59*, 804–819.

Ford, E. S., Giles, W. H., & Dietz, W. H. (2002). Prevalence of the metabolic syndrome among US adults: Findings from the Third National Health and Nutrition Examination Survey. *Journal of the American Medical Association, 287*, 356–372.

Fraser, S. N., & Spink, K. S. (2002). Examining the role of social support and group cohesion in exercise compliance. *Journal of Behavioral Medicine, 25*, 233–249.

Freedman, D. S., Khan, L. K., Serdula, M. K., Galuska, D. A., & Dietz, W. H. (2002). Trends and correlates of class 3 obesity in the United States from 1990 through 2000. *Journal of the American Medical Association, 288*, 1758–1761.

Gaemers, I. C., & Groen, A. K. (2006). New insights in the pathogenesis of non-alcoholic fatty liver disease. *Current Opinions in Lipidology, 17*, 268–273.

Gerstein, H. C., Mann, J. F., Yi, Q., Zinman, B., Dinneen, S. F., Hoogwerf, B., et al. (2001). Albuminuria and risk of cardiovascular events, death, and heart failure in diabetic and nondiabetic individuals. *Journal of the American Medical Association, 286*, 421–426.

GISSI-Prevenzione Investigators. (1999). Dietary supplementation with n-3 polyunsaturated fatty acids and vitamin E after myocardial infarction: Results of the GISSI-Prevenzione trial. *Lancet, 354*, 447–455.

Grundy, S. M., Cleeman, J. I., Bairey Merz, C. N., Brewer, H. B., Jr., Clark, L. T., Hunninghake, D. B., et al. (2004). Implications of recent clinical trials for the National

Cholesterol Education Program Adult Treatment Panel III guidelines. *Circulation,* *110,* 227–239.

Hakim, A. A., Petrovitch, H., Burchfiel, C. M., Ross, G. W., Rodriguez, B. L., White, L. R., et al. (1998). Effects of walking on mortality among nonsmoking retired men. *New England Journal of Medicine, 338,* 94–99.

Hansson, L., Zanchetti, A., Carruthers, S. G., Dahlof, B., Elmfeldt, D., Julius, S., et al. (1998). Effects of intensive blood-pressure lowering and low-dose aspirin in patients with hypertension: Principal results of the Hypertension Optimal Treatment (HOT) randomized trial. *Lancet, 351,* 1755–1762.

Haynes, R. B., McKibbon, K. A., & Kanani, R. (1996). Systematic review of randomised trials of interventions to assist patients to follow prescriptions for medications. *Lancet, 348,* 383.

Heart Outcome Prevention Evaluation (HOPE) Study Investigators. (2000). Effects of ramipril on cardiovascular and microvascular outcomes in people with diabetes mellitus: Results of the HOPE study and MICRO-HOPE study. *Lancet, 355,* 253–259.

Hebert, P. R., Gaziano, J. M., Chan, K. S., & Hennekens, C. H. (1997). Cholesterol lowering with statin drugs, risk of stroke and total mortality: An overview of randomized trials. *Journal of the American Medical Association, 278,* 313–321.

Hennekens, C. H. (1998). Increasing burden of cardiovascular disease: Current knowledge and future directions for research on risk factors. *Circulation, 97,* 1095–1102.

Hennekens, C. H. (2000). Clinical and research challenges in risk factors for cardiovascular diseases. *European Heart Journal, 21,* 1917–1921.

Hennekens, C. H. (2001). Current perspectives on lipid lowering with statins to decrease risk of cardiovascular disease. *Clinical Cardiology, 24*(Suppl. 7), II2–II5.

Hennekens, C. H., & Buring, J. E. (1985). Smoking and coronary heart disease in women. *Journal of the American Medical Association, 253,* 3003–3004.

Hennekens, C. H., & Buring, J. E. (1987). *Epidemiology in medicine.* Boston: Little, Brown.

Hennekens, C. H., Hollar, D., Eidelman, R. S., & Agatston, A. S. (2006). Update for primary healthcare providers: Recent statin trials and revised National Cholesterol Education Program III guidelines. *Medscape General Medicine, 8*(1), 54. Retrieved February 18, 2010, from *www.medscape.com/viewarticle/523079*

Hennekens, C. H., Mayrent, S. L., & Buring, J. (1984). Epidemiologic aspects of aging, mortality and smoking. In R. Bosse & C. Rose (Eds.), *Smoking and aging* (pp. 117–129). Lexington, MA: Heath.

Hennekens, C. H., Pfeffer, M. A., & Swedberg, K. (2007). The CHARM Program: Study design leads to findings of clinical and public health importance. *Journal of Cardiovascular Pharmacology and Therapeutics, 12,* 124–126.

Hennekens, C. H., & Schneider, W. R. (2008). The need for wider and appropriate utilization of aspirin and statins in the treatment and prevention of cardiovascular disease. *Expert Review of Cardiovascular Therapy, 6,* 95–107.

Hu, F. (2008). *Obesity epidemiology.* Oxford, UK: Oxford University Press.

Janssen, I., & Mark, A. E. (2007). Elevated body mass index and mortality risk in the elderly. *Obesity Review, 8,* 41–59.

Jee, S. H., Sull, J. W., Park, J., Lee, S. Y., Ohrr, H., Guallar, E., et al. (2006). Body-mass index and mortality in Korean men and women. *New England Journal of Medicine, 355,* 779–787.

Jones, P. H. (2003). Cholesterol and coronary events. The current thinking. *Postgraduate Medicine, 113*(4, Suppl.), 5–14.

Kannel, W. B. (1983). Prevalence and natural history of electrocardiographic left ventricular hypertrophy. *American Journal of Medicine, 75*(Suppl. 3A), 4–11.

Keech, A., Simes, R. J., Barter, P., Best, J., Scott, R., Taskinen, M. R., et al. (2005). Effects of long-term fenofibrate therapy on cardiovascular events in 9795 people with Type 2 diabetes mellitus (the FIELD study): Randomised controlled trial. *Lancet, 366,* 1849–1861.

King, G., Bendel, R., & Delaronde, S. R. (1998). Social heterogeneity in smoking among African Americans. *American Journal of Public Health, 88,* 1081–1085.

Klag, M. J., Whelton, P. K., Randall, B. L., Neaton, J. D., Brancati, F. L., & Stamler, J. (1997). End-stage renal disease in African-American and White men: 16-year MRFIT findings. *Journal of the American Medical Association, 277,* 1293–1298.

Kurth, T., Gaziano, M., Rexrode, K. M., Kase, C. S., Cook, N. R., Manson, J. E., et al. (2005). Prospective study of body mass index and risk of stroke in apparently healthy women. *Circulation, 111,* 1992–191998.

LaCroix, A. Z., Lang, J., Scherr, P., Wallace, R. B., Cornoni-Huntley, J., Berkman, L., et al. (1991). Smoking and mortality among older men and women in three communities. *New England Journal of Medicine, 324,* 1619–1625.

LaRosa, J. C., Grundy, S. M., Waters, D. D., Shear, C., Barter, P., Fruchart, J. C., et al. (2005). Intensive lipid lowering with atorvastatin in patients with stable coronary disease. *New England Journal of Medicine, 352,* 1425–1435.

Levine, R. S., Briggs, N. C., Husaini, B. A., & Hennekens, C. H. (2006). Geographic studies of Black–White mortality. In D. Satcher & R. J. Pamies (Eds.), *Multicultural medicine and health disparities* (pp. 33–104). New York: McGraw-Hill.

Lewis, E. J., Hunsicker, I. G., Bain, R. P., & Rohde, R. D. (1993). The effect of angiotensin-converting enzyme inhibition on diabetic nephropathy: The Collaborative Study Group. *New England Journal of Medicine, 329,* 1456–1462.

Li, T. Y., Rana, J. S., Manson, J. E., Willett, W. C., Stampfer, M. J., Colditz, G. A., et al. (2006). Obesity as compared with physical activity in predicting risk of coronary heart disease in women. *Circulation, 113*(4), 499–506.

Liao, Y., Cooper, R. S., McGhee, D. L., Mensah, G. A., & Ghali, J. K. (1995). The relative effects of left ventricular hypertrophy, coronary artery disease, and ventricular dysfunction on survival among Black adults. *Journal of the American Medical Association, 273,* 1592–1597.

Liu, B. Q., Peto, R., Chen, Z. M., Boreham, J., Wu, Y. P., Li, J. Y., et al. (1998). Emerging tobacco hazards in China: 1. Retrospective proportional mortality study of one million deaths. *British Medical Journal, 317,* 1411–1422.

Lloyd-Jones, D., Adams, R. J., Brown, T. M., Carnethon, M., Dai, S., De Simone, G., et al. (2010). Heart disease and stroke statistics 2010 update: A Report from the American Heart Association. *Circulation, 121,* e1–e170.

Lonn, E., Yusef, S., Arnold, M. J., Sheridan, P., Poque, J., Micks, M., et al. (2006). Homocysteine lowering with folic acid and B vitamins in vascular disease. *New England Journal of Medicine, 355,* 746.

Mackay, J., & Mensah, G. (2004). *The atlas of heart disease and stroke.* Geneva: World Health Organization. Retrieved February 18, 2010, from *www.who.int/cardiovascular_diseases/resources/atlas/en*

Mann, J. F., Gerstein, H. C., Pogue, J., Bosch, H., & Yusuf, S. (2001). Renal insufficiency as a predictor of cardiovascular outcomes and the impact of ramipril: The HOPE randomized trial. *Annals of Internal Medicine, 134,* 629–636.

Manson, J. E., Colditz, G. A., Stampfer, M. J., Willett, W. C., Rosner, B., Monson, R. R., et al. (1990). A prospective study of obesity and risk of coronary heart disease in women. *New England Journal of Medicine, 322,* 882–889.

Manson, J. E., Hu, F. B., Rich-Edwards, J. W., Colditz, G. A., Stampfer, M. J., Willett, W. C., et al. (1999). A prospective study of walking as compared with vigorous exercise in the prevention of coronary heart disease in women. *New England Journal of Medicine, 341,* 650–658.

Mazas, C. A., & Wetter, D. W. (2003). Smoking cessation interventions among African Americans: Research needs. *Cancer Control, 10*(5), 87–89.

Micozzi, M. S., & Harris, T. M. (1990). Age variations in the relation of body mass indices to estimates of body fat and muscle mass. *American Journal of Physical Anthropology, 881,* 375–379.

Moser, M., Hebert, P., & Hennekens, C. H. (1991). An overview of the meta-analyses of the hypertension treatment trials. *Archives of Internal Medicine, 151,* 1277–1279.

National Center for Primary Care at the Morehouse School of Medicine. (2004). *CRASH course in cultural competency skill* [PowerPoint presentation]. Retrieved from *web. msm.edu/NCPC/crash/cultural_competency_pp.pdf*

National Cholesterol Education Program (NCEP) Expert Panel on Detection, Evaluation, and Treatment of High Blood Cholesterol in Adults (Adult Treatment Panel III [ATPIII]). (2002). Third Report of the National Cholesterol Education Program (NCEP) Expert Panel on Detection, Evaluation, and Treatment of High Blood Cholesterol in Adults (Adult Treatment Panel III) final report. *Circulation, 106,* 3143–3421.

National Institutes of Health (NIH). (1998). Clinical guidelines on the identification, evaluation, and treatment of overweight and obesity in adults: The evidence report. *Obesity Research, 6*(Suppl. 2), 51S–209S.

Nissen, S. E., Nicholls, S. J., Sipahi, I., Libby, P., Raichlen, J. S., Ballantyne, C. M., et al. (2006). Effect of very high-intensity statin therapy on regression of coronary atherosclerosis: The ASTEROID Trial. *Journal of the American Medical Association, 295,* 1556–1565.

Nissen, S. E., Tuzcu, E. M., Schoenhagen, P., Brown, B. G., Ganz, P., Vogel, R. A., et al. (2004). Effect of intensive compared with moderate lipid-lowering therapy on progression of coronary atherosclerosis: A randomized controlled trial. *Journal of the American Medical Association, 291,* 1071–1080.

Niu, S. R., Yang, G. H., Chen, Z. M., Wang, J. L., Wang, G. H., He, X. Z., et al. (1998). Emerging tobacco hazards in China: 2. Early mortality results from a prospective study. *British Medical Journal, 317,* 1423–1424.

Novela, C., & Hennekens, C. H. (2004). Hypothesis: Atorvastatin has unique pleiotropic effects leading to early clinical benefits. *Journal of Cardiovascular Pharmacology and Therapeutics, 9,* 61–63.

Ofili, E. O. (1995). Managing high blood pressure and cardiovascular disease in Blacks. *Association of Black Cardiologists Digest of Urban Cardiology, 2,* 220–225.

Oliveria, S. A., Lapuerta, P., McCarthy, B. D., L'Italien, G. J., Berlowitz, D. R., & Asch, S. M. (2002). Physician-related barriers to the effective management of uncontrolled hypertension. *Archives of Internal Medicine, 162,* 413–420.

Park, Y. W., Zhu, S., Palaniappan, L., Heshka, S., Carnethon, M. R., & Heymsfield, S. B. (2003). The metabolic syndrome: Prevalence and associated risk factor findings in the US population from the Third National Health and Nutrition Examination Survey, 1988–1994. *Archives of Internal Medicine, 163,* 427–436.

Pate, R. R., Pratt, M., Blair, S. N., Haskell, W. L., Macera, C. A., Bouchard, C., et al. (1995). Physical activity and public health: A recommendation from the Centers for Disease Control and Prevention and the American College of Sports Medicine. *Journal of the American Medical Association, 273,* 402–7.

Prospective Studies Collaboration (PSC). (2002). Age-specific relevance of usual blood pressure to vascular mortality: A meta-analysis of individual data for one million adults in 61 prospective studies. *Lancet, 360,* 1903–1913.

Prospective Studies Collaboration (PSC). (2007). Blood cholesterol and vascular mortality by age, sex, and blood pressure: A meta-analysis of individual data from 61 prospective studies with 55,000 vascular deaths. *Lancet, 370,* 1829–1839.

Prospective Studies Collaboration (PSC). (2009). Body-mass index and cause-specific mortality in 900,000 adults: Collaborative analyses of 57 prospective studies. *Lancet, 373,* 1083–1096.

Ray, K. K., Seshasai, S. R. K., Wijesuria, S., Sivakumaran, R., Nethercott, S., Preiss, D., et al. (2009). Effect of intensive control of glucose on cardiovascular outcomes and death in patients with diabetes mellitus: A meta-analysis of randomised controlled trials. *Lancet, 373,* 1765–1772.

Reeves, G. K., Pirie, K., Beral, V., Green, J., Spencer, E., Bull, D. (2007). Cancer incidence and mortality in relation to body mass index in the Million Women Study: Cohort study. *British Medical Journal, 335,* 1134–1139.

Rexrode, K. M., Carey, V. J., Hennekens, C. H., Walters, E. E., Colditz, G. A., Stampfer, M. J., et al. (1998). Abdominal adiposity and coronary heart disease in women. *Journal of the American Medical Association, 280,* 1843–1848.

Ridker, P. M., Danielson, E., Fonseca, F. A., Genest, J., Gotto, A. M., Jr., Kastelein, J. J., et al. (2008). Rosuvastatin to prevent vascular events in men and women with elevated C-reactive protein. *New England Journal of Medicine, 359,* 2195–2207.

Robins, S. J., Collins, D., Wittes, J. T., Papademetriou, V., Deedwania, P. C., Schaefer, E. J., et al. (2001). Insulin resistance and cardiovascular events with low HDL cholesterol: The Veterans Affairs HDL Intervention Trial (VA-HIT). *Journal of the American Medical Association, 285,* 1585–1591.

Rosamond, W., Flegal, K., Friday, G., Furie, K., Go, A., Greenlund, K., et al. (2007). Heart disease and stroke statistics—2007 update: A report from the American Heart Association Statistics Committee and Stroke Statistics Subcommittee. *Circulation, 115,* e69–e171.

Royce, J. M., Hymowitz, N., Corbett, K., Hartwell, T. D., & Orlandi, M. A. (1993). Smoking cessation factors among African Americans and Whites: COMMIT Research Group. *American Journal of Public Health, 83,* 220–226.

Ruilope, L. M., Salvetti, A., Jamerson, K., Hansson, L., Warnold, I., Wedel, H., et al. (2001). Renal function and intensive lowering of blood pressure in hypertensive participants of the Hypertension Optimal Treatment (HOT) study. *Journal of the American Society of Nephrology, 12,* 218–225.

Song, Y.-M., Sung, J., Davey Smith, G., & Ebrahim, S. (2004). Body mass index and ischemic and hemorrhagic stroke: A prospective study in Korean men. *Stroke, 35,* 831–836.

Tirodkar, M. A., & Jain, A. (2003). Food messages on African American television shows. *American Journal of Public Health, 93,* 439–441.

Trials of Hypertension Prevention Collaborative Research Group. (1992). The effects of nonpharmacologic interventions on blood pressure of persons with high normal levels. Results of the Trials of Hypertension Prevention, Phase I. *Journal of the American Medical Association, 267,* 1213–1220.

Tuomilehto, J., Lindström, J., Eriksson, J. G., Valle, T. T., Hämäläinen, H., Ilanne-Parikka, P., et al. (2001). Prevention of Type 2 diabetes mellitus by changes in lifestyle among subjects with impaired glucose tolerance. *New England Journal of Medicine, 344,* 1343–1350.

U.K. Prospective Diabetes Study (UKPDS) Group. (1998). Tight blood pressure control and risk of macrovascular and microvascular complications of type 2 diabetes: UKPDS 38. *British Medical Journal, 317,* 703–713.

U.S. Department of Health and Human Services. (1996). A report of the Surgeon General, physical activity and health, at-a-glance 1996. Retrieved February 18, 2010, from *www.cdc.gov/nccdphp/sgr/pdf/sgraag.pdf*

U.S. Renal Data Systems. (2009). *Annual data report* [Slides]. Retrieved January 11, 2010, from *www.usrds.org/slides.htm*

Wang, Y., Chen, X., Song, Y., Caballero, B., & Cheskin, L. J. (2008). Association between obesity and kidney disease: A systematic review and meta-analysis. *Kidney International, 73,* 19–33.

Williams, R. A. (2001). Cultural diversity in medicine. In R. A. Williams (Ed.), *Humane medicine: A new paradigm in medical education and health care delivery* (Vol. 2, p. 13). Philadelphia: Lippincott Williams & Wilkins.

Williams, R. A., Flack, J. M., Gavin, J. R., III, Schneider, W. R., & Hennekens, C. H. (2007). Guidelines for management of high-risk African Americans with multiple cardiovascular risk factors: Recommendations of an expert consensus panel. *Ethnicity and Disease, 17,* 214–220.

Williams, R. A., Gavin, J. R., III, Phillips, R. A., Sumner, A. E., Duncan, A. K., Hollar, D., et al. (2006). High-risk African Americans with multiple risk factors for cardiovascular disease: Challenges in prevention, diagnosis, and treatment. *Ethnicity and Disease, 16,* 633–639.

Wilson, P. W., D'Agostino, R. B., Levy, D., Belanger, A. M., Silbershatz, H., & Kannel, W. B. (1998). Prediction of coronary heart disease risk factor categories. *Circulation, 97,* 1837–1847.

Wong, N. D., Lopez, V. A., L'Italien, G., Chen, R., Kline, S. E., & Franklin, S. S. (2007). Inadequate control of hypertension in US adults with cardiovascular disease comorbidities in 2003–2004. *Archives of Internal Medicine, 167,* 2431–2436.

World Health Organization. (2008). *World health statistics 2008.* Geneva: Author. Retrieved February 18, 2010, from *www.who.int/whosis/whostat/2008/en*

World Health Organization. (2009). *World health statistics 2009.* Geneva: Author. Retrieved February 18, 2010, from *www.who.int/whosis/whostat/2009/en*

World Health Organization Global InfoBase Team. (2005). *The SuRF Report 2. Surveillance of chronic disease risk factors: Country-level data and comparable estimates.* Geneva: Author. Retrieved January 11, 2010, from *apps.who.int/infobase/surf2/start.html*

Wright, J. T., Jr., Bakris, G., Greene, T., Agodoa, L. Y., Appel, L. J., Charleston, J., et al. (2002). Effect of blood pressure lowering and antihypertensive drug class on progression of hypertensive kidney disease: Results from the AASK trial. *Journal of the American Medical Association, 288,* 2421–2431.

Yusuf, S., Gerstein, H., Hoogwerf, B., Pogue, J., Bosch, J., Wolffenbuttel, B. H., et al. (2001). Ramipril and the development of diabetes. *Journal of the American Medical Association, 286,* 1882–1885.

Yusuf, S., Östergren, J., Gerstein, H., Pfeffer, M. A., Swedberg, K., Granger, C. B., et al. (2005). Effects of candesartan on the development of a new diagnosis of diabetes mellitus in patients with heart failure. *Circulation, 112,* 48–53.

Zhou, M., Offer, A., Yang, G., Smith, M., Hui, G., Whitlock, G., et al. (2008). Body mass index, blood pressure, and mortality from stroke: A nationally representative prospective study of 212,000 Chinese men. *Stroke, 39,* 753–759.

# 13

# Cancer

DERRICK J. BEECH

**N**early 1.5 million people will be newly diagnosed with cancer in 2007 (American Cancer Society, 2007). Despite significant advances in the treatment of many types of cancer, patients diagnosed with a malignancy face clinical psychological and economic challenges directly or indirectly related to their cancer. These challenges are not limited to the person diagnosed with cancer. The diagnosis of cancer in a patient extends beyond the individual to involve family members, friends, and associates. Thus, for every new cancer diagnosis, multiple people are directly or indirectly affected. Although there are numerous forms of cancer, the social, psychological, and emotional impact of the initial diagnosis and ultimate therapy is universally the same. Differences exist with regard to patients' response to cancer based on aspects of their culture, religious beliefs, and social support system.

The goal of helping patients adjust to a cancer diagnosis has led to a field of study focused on the behavioral, social, and psychological aspects of cancer. Psycho-oncology has emerged as a subspecialty of psychology exploring the unique issues inherent in cancer patients' lives. Within the field of psycho-oncology, issues emerge during difference phases of the illness. These unique phases—the initial diagnosis, treatment, survivorship, and aspects of psychosocial adjustments experienced by patients who have advanced disease—affect not only the patients themselves but also those involved in their lives and care.

Derogatis and associates (1983) reported that reaction to a new cancer diagnosis represented nearly 90% of observed psychoactive disorders. This new and typically unexpected health information represents a life-altering event that requires successful coping mechanisms. People's coping mechanisms are highly dependent on their cultural beliefs, thus creating an arena to evaluate ethical aspects of handling the initial diagnosis phase. Numerous factors play a role in the initial response to being informed of a new diagnosis of cancer. Spiritual, social, and environmental factors frame the individuals' coping mechanism. These socioenviromental factors can shape patients and their family's adjustment to the diagnosis of cancer irrespective of ethnicity. However, there are unique social and environmental factors that shape African American patients' response to initial diagnosis.

Unique to the African American community is the component of mistrust of the medical establishment as a result of societal biases and discrimination along with unethical medical experimentation. Patients often reference the Tuskegee syphilis study conducted by the Public Health Service from 1932 to 1972 (Jones, 1991). This investigation involved 400 sharecroppers with untreated syphilis and was designed as an observational study to evaluate the course of the disease and clinical manifestation of syphilis in Blacks compared with Whites. The tragic part of this often-cited medical misadventure is that penicillin was known to be curative treatment for syphilis but was intentionally withheld from the African American study participants. The news of this unethical, government-sponsored study broke in 1972, forcing the study to terminate. The Tuskegee syphilis study represents one glaring example of the breech of trust between African Americans and health care agencies (Jones, 1991).

Inherent in the issue of the psychology of cancer diagnosis is the relevant topic of delayed presentation for patients with symptomatic malignancies. Why do African Americans avoid accessing the health care system when clinical signs and symptoms explicitly support the diagnosis of cancer? There are numerous factors associated with this delay, not least among them financial issues, which also prevail with regard to ethnic differences in timely cancer diagnosis and access to the health care system. However, economic factors alone do not explain the many instances of delayed presentation and late-stage diagnosis, which occur among noninsured and insured patients alike. Even in managed-care environments, there are disparities in rates of early diagnosis and survival based on race. Analysis of screening practices shows lower levels of compliance with recommended cancer screening guidelines among minority populations. The psychological platform from which African Americans view society permeates decisions regarding health care even when there is convincing evidence of the possibility of cancer threatening their survival.

Numerous studies have explored the reasons for delayed cancer diagnosis in African Americans. Many define patient and systems factors contributing to delayed presentations. With regard to breast cancer, Kerr-Cresswell and associates (2005) reported that nearly 30% of women with symptomatic breast cancer delay seeking medical attention for at least 3 months. This study is particularly relevant because it evaluated treatment behavior in an environment where insurance and economic status should have had very little influence on medical care access. Factors associated with delayed presentation included attributing the self-discovered clinical finding as a benign event, fear of cancer, use of nontraditional therapies, fatalism, concern regarding their significant other's ability to cope with a cancer diagnosis, and absence of a family history of cancer. This Canadian study provides some insight into attributes and beliefs that drive noncompliant behavior and ultimately impact cancer survival. However, Black patients comprised only 13% of the study sample (compared with 62% Caucasian and 16% Asian). The unique sociopolitical environment of the United States and the associated psychological impact of past slavery and current racism and discrimination require an expanded analysis of delayed cancer diagnosis within the confines of the U.S. borders.

Farmer, Reddick, D'Agostino, and Jackson (2007), in a cross-sectional survey, evaluated the relevant psychosocial variables involved in the decision making of older African American women regarding whether to undergo screening mammograms. These authors unmasked similar findings as those reported in the Canadian study; cancer knowledge (risk factors, fatalism) and absence of social support (not having a family member or friend to encourage them) played a role in noncompliance with screening guidelines.

Following the psychological adjustment after diagnosis, cancer patients, spouses, parents, friends, and professional associates are presented with the challenges associated with the treatment and posttreatment phases of cancer. Each phase relies on continued social and emotional support. Dunkel-Schetter (1984) noted that the overwhelming majority of cancer patients (81%) viewed emotional support as much more important than informational or instrumental aid. The foundation to successful psychological adjustment during the treatment phase of cancer relies heavily on the stability of the social and financial environments. Anchored by a loving support network, patients undergoing treatment for malignancy have a greater likelihood of successfully adjusting to toxic treatments and potential therapeutic setbacks. This circle of support can often shield the cancer patient in stressful times. Furthermore, financial constraint of the ongoing treatment cycle can layer additional obstacles to the seemingly insurmountable challenges inherent in the daily battle against cancer.

## BIOLOGICAL/GENETIC FACTORS

There have been significant advances in unmasking key genetic and molecular factors that influence the development and progression of malignancy. Many of the novel developments in cancer biology parallel the recent discoveries associated with the Human Genome Project. These technological advancements have improved assessment of risk evaluation of heredity link prognostic markers for specific malignancies and finally targeted molecular therapies for specific cancers. This section briefly explores new technologies that expand the current understanding of malignant disease. However, the focus is on genetic and familiar factors associated with cancer and the impact of these factors on the psychological status of patients and their family members.

Regarding the biological basis of cancer development and genetics, several terms are often used: heredity, familial, and sporadic. Familial cancers are those that occur in families at a greater frequency than expected simply by chance. They may be associated with known genetic mutations or the result of a shared environmental experience. Heredity cancers are malignancies with associated genes that are transmitted from one or both parents to their offspring. Heredity and cancer are usually linked by identifiable syndromes that represent cancers that occur in family members as a result of specific genes transmitted through the lineage. Although frequently referred to interchangeably, heredity (genetic) and familial cancers are very different and confer unique sets of psychological and emotional stresses to patients and their family members.

The expansion of our knowledge of molecular techniques has enabled investigators to explore trends and patterns in families with actual genetic mutations. The use of assays to evaluate DNA and RNA along with traditional protein analysis has expanded the understanding of heredity or genetic cancer syndromes. Mutated genes can now be evaluated by amplification techniques that permit small samples of tissue to be used for the evaluation of multiple possible genetic mutations. A major molecular technique used is polymerase chain reaction (PCR). Various forms of PCR analysis are currently in use to allow the targeted analysis of specific genetic defects that might drive the development and progression of cancer. PCR analysis allows small samples of tissue or body fluids to be used to generate huge results with regard to the genetic factors involved in cancer. A new era in molecular cancer biology evolved with the advancement of technologies that allows the analysis of thousands of human genes at one time. The use of DNA microarray technology was a direct result of the Human Genome Project (National Human Genome Institute, 2003). Microarray technology permits the profiling of specific tumors to determine genetic trends and subclassify cancers for targeted therapies. For example, BRCA1 and BRCA2 genes are associated with hereditary breast cancer. These can be further subcategorized as a result of identifiable subgroups using microarray analysis. At present, no genetic factor has been identified that places African Americans at higher risk for a specific form of cancer.

## INDIVIDUAL FACTORS
## INFLUENCING RISK AND RESILIENCY

The psychology of cancer has a different dimension when associated with the sociopolitical construct of race. To unmask key factors associated with cancer in African Americans, it is essential to understand the social and economic climate surrounding cultural attitudes and beliefs. Individual community and large-scale population behavior directly relates to fundamental cultural beliefs.

Individual factors like exposure to environmental carcinogens can promote specific cancer development. Furthermore, patients' access to the health care sector and ultimately decisions of cancer therapy directly impact outcome. Notable toxins that have been shown to negatively impact health and, more specifically, to promote the development of certain cancers include tobacco exposure, sedentary lifestyle, and poor nutrition. Exposure to human papillomavirus, associated with sexual behavior, increases the risk of cervical cancer.

The estimated 39 million African Americans living in the United States represent a heterogeneous group, with more than 2 million foreign born. African Americans compromise approximately 13% of the U.S. population. An unequal burden of cancer-related morbidity and mortality is shouldered by African Americans. Racial disparities appear to underly the fact that African Americans are more likely than any other ethnic group to die from cancer (American Cancer Society, 2007). The incidence of the more common cancers (lung, prostate, colon, and rectal) is higher among African Americans.

Lung cancer is directly associated with tobacco use. It is the second most common cancer in African Americans in 2007, comprising nearly 22,000 cases of the estimated U.S. total of 229,000 per year. These figures translate to 112 African American men compared with 81.7 Caucasian men per 100,000 population (National Cancer Institutes Division of Cancer Control and Population Science, 2006). The annual incidence in 2003 was 40% higher per capita for African American men compared with their Caucasian counterparts. The ethnic differences in the incidence of lung cancer in women was less dramatic (53.1 African American vs. 54.7 Caucasian).

The harmful effects of tobacco are evident from numerous studies. Smoking accounts for 87% of all lung cancer–related deaths and 30% of all cancer deaths (Doll & Peto, 1981). The risk of developing lung cancer is more than 13 times higher in smokers (U.S. Department of Health and Human Services, 2004). However, the negative health impact of tobacco use goes well beyond lung and bronchial cancer development. Tobacco use is directly associated with the development of many other malignant and benign conditions. Cancers of the upper aerodigestive region (nasopharynx, oral cavity, pharynx, and larynx) are associated with tobacco use. Furthermore, a positive association has been demonstrated between tobacco use and esophageal, pancreatic, renal, bladder, and stomach cancers. Nonmalignant diseases associated with cigarette smoking include cardiovascular disease, bronchitis, emphysema, and stomach ulcers (U.S. Department of Health and Human Services, 2004).

The economic impact of tobacco use parallels the dramatic negative health consequences. Smoking reduces life expectancy by approximately 14 years (Centers for Disease Control and Prevention [CDC], 2002). Premature death of a wage earner results in the greater dependence of family members on government-supported welfare programs; thus, in essence, cigarette use results in an annual expense of approximately $167 billion. This figure is even greater when other forms of smokeless tobacco and secondhand smoke exposure are included.

Critical analysis of smoking initiative and race is paramount to understanding the social components of racial differences in tobacco use. Numerous investigations have demonstrated substantially lower rates of cigarette smoking among African American adolescents compared with Caucasians. In fact, African American youth have the lowest rate of tobacco use compared with all other ethnic groups (CDC, 2006b). Among high school students, 14% of African Americans boys and 11.8% of African American girls reported cigarette use compared with the much higher national statistics—30% and 25%, respectively—for all ethnics groups (CDC, 2006a).

Unfortunately, however, this positive trend changes in young adulthood, where the rate of tobacco use among African Americans surpasses that of their Caucasian counterparts: 26.7% versus 24% for African Americans and Caucasians, respectively.

Tobacco use is strongly associated with many cancers and is included in the subcategory of individual factors that contribute to malignancy. However, the sociopolitical forces and context must be taken into consideration when this behavior-based factor is evaluated. Similar to tobacco use, poor nutrition, obesity, and physical inactivity may be viewed as individual factors that contribute to cancer development and the associated psychological aspects of diagnosis and treatment. Obesity and obesity-related health consequences have reached epidemic levels, threatening the overall health and well-being of Americans. Obesity and metabolic syndrome have moved to the forefront of U.S. health problems.

The health consequences of obesity are extensive, including cerebrovascular disease, cardiovascular disease, and diabetes. Numerous cancers are associated with obesity, including breast, colorectal, endometrial, renal, gastric, and esophageal cancers (Cole, Rodriquez, Walker-Thurmond, & Thun, 2003). More than two-thirds of African Americans are considered to be overweight, and nearly one-half are classified as obese (Ogden et al., 2006).

A variety of factors are involved in the increasing rates of obesity among African Americans. Generally, obesity is related to energy imbalance. The psychosocial aspects that create this energy imbalance in African Americans can be explained from individual and social perspectives. Weight gain, and obesity, occurs when the calories consumed exceed the calories expended. Typically, this imbalance is associated with individual behavior; however, there are numerous social factors, such as higher cost for foods with favorable glycemic index, a paucity of health food stores in economically deprived areas, availability of less expensive prepackaged food, and desire for heavily promoted sweetened beverages and soft drinks. Other contributing factors include increased food portions available in restaurants and prevalence of fast-food kitchens specializing in high-fat meals.

One-third of African Americans report no leisure time physical activity overall, and African American women are more likely to report being physically inactive (36.3%). The current environment and lifestyle trends create and maintain the obesity-promoting imbalance just discussed: Decreased physical activity leads to a reduction in the amount of calories burned. Physical activity has been noted to decrease the risk for colon and breast cancers (Doyle et al., 2006).

## EVIDENCE-BASED TREATMENT INTERVENTIONS

*What Works*

- Religious-based or spiritually anchored support programs
- Small-group sessions delivered with a culturally sensitive approach
- Involvement of African American physicians, nurses, and social workers in planning and implementing treatment

*What Might Work*

- Direct psychotherapy with a culturally sensitive approach
- Cognitive-behavioral therapy techniques
- Behavioral intervention
- Treatment of underlying health causes of distress
- Involvement of current social network in counseling

*What Does Not Work*

- Pharmacological therapies alone
- Internet-based communications
- Traditional disease-specific support groups

Successful interventions address the majority of factors that contribute to individual- and community-based disparities in African Americans. These interventions rely on the unique sociocultural characteristics of African American communities and span the complete spectrum, addressing issues of delayed cancer screening to low participation rates in innovative clinical trials.

Farmer and associates (2007) evaluated the psychosocial factors that correlated with adherence to annual mammography screening in a cohort of older African American women. This cross-sectional survey included 198 African American women between the ages of 50 and 98 years. Dispositional optimism and presence of social support correlated with improved adherence to screening guidelines.

Spurlock and Cullins (2006) attribute current negative trends in breast cancer detection and control among African Americans to the pervasive issue of cancer fatalism, an attitude that undermines their participation in breast cancer screening programs.

Fowler (2007) expanded the current knowledge of psychosocial factors associated with improved breast cancer screening by emphasizing the importance of social support networks. In addition, further light is cast on relevant issues involved in the decision to develop proactive, positive health practices. Fowler's earlier work (2006) suggested that there are five social processes associated with a women's decision to have a screening mammogram: acknowledging prior experiences with health care providers and systems; reporting fears and fatalistic beliefs of breast cancer and its associated treatment; valuing the opinion of significant others; relying on religious beliefs and support networks; and being able to rely on the caregiving responsibilities of the significant other. Caregiving responsibility heavily influenced adherence to mammography screening.

Unlike breast cancer screening, cancer fatalism plays a very minor role in prostate cancer screening among African American men. Sanchez, Bowen, Hart, and Spigner (2007) explored factors associated with prostate cancer screening among African American men ages 40–70 years. Participants indicated many sociocultural reasons for avoiding screening, among them a lack of knowledge of prostate cancer and clinical services; the perception of prostate cancer and the screening technique as threats to manhood; and distrust of the medical community.

Of particular importance is that the most commonly used screening approach naturally used is the least effective technique among African American men with regard to prostate cancer screening. Weinrich, Boyd, Bradford, Mossa, and Weinrich (1988) suggest that effective screening must change from a provider/health site orientation to a consumer/community mindset. Engagement of community organizations and community leaders will significantly enhance screening rates among African American men.

Anxiety is a ubiquitous component of nearly all cancer patients' initial diagnosis, treatment, and follow-up. It is only considered to be pathological if the level of anxiety significantly impairs day-to-day function or quality of life. Dysfunctional anxiety may become clinically evident manifesting in heightened levels of fear, hypervigilance, heart palpitations, muscle tension, and jitteriness. The somatic manifestations of anxiety are the result of the physiological fight-or-flight response. This typically protective response can result in poor compliance with therapy and maladjustment (Noyes, Holt, & Mossic, 1998). The treating physician faces the difficult task of determining whether symptoms associated with anxiety are psychological in nature or a direct result of the cancer. Side effects from any of the medications can present with similar symptoms as those manifested by anxiety (Shuster & James, 1998). Typical symptoms of anxiety can mimic those seen in posttraumatic stress disorder (PTSD). Successful approaches in the management of dysfunctional anxiety or PTSD in the cancer patient include focused intervention to help the patient address and minimize fears and regain a sense of control. Occasionally, antianxiety medications may be required such as benzodiazepines, buspirone, or other nonbenzodiazepine antidepressants. Again, these pharmacological approaches should be paired with patient counseling by a psychiatrist, psychologist, social worker, or chaplain. Other less proven but potentially beneficial approaches include cognitive-behavioral techniques such as hypnosis, relaxation therapy, medication, and focused diaphoretic breathing.

Many cancer patients experience transient episodes of depressed moods. However, major episodes of depression can cause significant impairment. Typical symptoms include decreased appetite, insomnia, fatigue, excess guilt, sense of worthlessness, poor concentration, and possibly thoughts of suicide. Paramount in the evaluation of depression in cancer patients is a vigilant search for possible drug-related causes. Once a diagnosis of depression is made, patients should be appropriately counseled in addition to receiving antidepression medication such as a selective serotonin reuptake inhibitor (SSRI) or tricyclic antidepressant. As with dysfunctional anxiety, cognitive-behavioral therapy is beneficial in treating patients with depression.

Delirium, unlike anxiety or depression, includes a degree of disturbance in consciousness or cognition (American Psychiatric Association, 1994). Delirium is not unique to cancer patients, but can occur in anyone with serious illness. Metabolic derangement can result in delirium. A search for the underlying cause of delirium should be undertaken along with institution of supportive, nonpharmacological therapy. Creating a pleasant, soothing physical environment and optimizing the degree of emotional stimulation from others can assist in redirecting the delirious patient.

## Pharmacological Therapies

The general categories of medication-based therapies for treating psychiatric disturbances or maladjustment in cancer patients include SSRIs, psychostimulants, tricyclic antidepressants, bupropion, and benzodiazepines. Of these, SSRIs are most commonly used. Although cytochrome P450 drug interactions can occur, the side-effect profile to this class of medications is generally mild (headache, jitteriness, and nausea). The use of SSRIs has been associated with thrombocytopenia and abnormal bleeding.

Tricyclic antidepressants are also used for managing depression in cancer patients. Imipramine, nortriptyline, and desipramine are all inexpensive and effective. However, the toxicity profile is greater than that seen with SSRIs. Useful benefits of tricyclic antidepressants include appetite stimulation, analgesia, and a sedative effect. Bupropion, mirtazapine, and trazodone may also be beneficial in treating cancer patients with psychiatric maladjustment.

## Nonpharmacological Therapies

Nonpharmacological interventions are effective in the management of maladjustment or psychiatric dysfunction in cancer patients. These approaches include cognitive-behavioral therapy, behavioral and relaxation therapies, supportive

(supportive–expressive) therapies, meaning-based psychotherapy, group therapy, and the use of support groups.

## RECOMMENDED BEST PRACTICES

The approach to successful implementation of cancer-preventive practices should emphasize peer-to-peer and small-group influences to provide optimal reinforcement of health behavior. Frequently, these small groups can be centered around the church or social organizations that are relevant to patients' daily lives. These optimal health behaviors should be reinforced using the motivational interview approach by physicians and nurses during periodic clinic visits.

Gender-specific and culturally sensitive seminars are useful in promoting compliance with cancer screening guidelines. Typically, these sessions should be delivered in a comfortable, nonthreatening environment. It is essential to create an interactive session rather than a lecture seminar. Participants must feel unrestricted and unjudged in asking questions. Guidelines for cancer screening should be delivered in an encouraging, not punitive, fashion. Follow-up sessions are essential within a short time interval (2–4 months) to ensure retention of information delivered and compliance. Church-supported programs work best; however, social organizations with active participation can also provide benefit.

Community centers may serve to promote positive health practices and increased compliance with screening guidelines. These venues are especially beneficial if information is delivered in a nonaccusatory manner with peer-specific sessions (i.e., all-male group for prostate cancer or prostate health discussions). The foundation of successful psychological support for patients undergoing treatment for cancer relies on effective communication throughout the diagnosis and treatment phase of the illness. A sense of hope must be imparted to the patients and their families regardless of a potentially guarded or poor prognosis.

The health care professional must maintain an honest, encouraging tone throughout the care process and must encourage patients and their families to be active participants in every aspect of care. Follow-up sessions during active treatment should provide patients and families with updated, easy-to-understand information regarding the disease status. Furthermore, patients must be given an opportunity to express their frustrations, anxieties and fears during these clinic visits. Best-practice approaches include frequent patient consultation with a psychiatrist, psychologist, social worker, or nurse navigator to address these concerns. Regarding survivorship, patients will universally maintain a heightened level of concern regarding the possibility of recurrent or progressive cancer. Allowing cancer survivors to participate in culturally sensitive, typically church-based support groups will assist them in adjusting to life with a history of cancer.

## REFERENCES

American Cancer Society. (2007). *Cancer facts and figures*. Atlanta, GA: Author.

American Psychiatric Association. (1994). *Diagnostic and statistical manual of mental disorders* (4th ed.). Washington, DC: Author.

Centers for Disease Control and Prevention. (2002). Annual smoking-attribual mortality, years of potential life lost, and economic costs—United States, 1995–1999. *Morbidity and Mortality Weekly Report, 51*(14), 300–303.

Centers for Disease Control and Prevention. (2006a). Tobacco use among adults—United States, 2005. *Morbidity and Mortality Weekly Report, 55*(42), 1145–1148.

Centers for Disease Control and Prevention. (2006b). Youth risk behavior surveillance—United States, 2005. *Morbidity and Mortality Weekly Report, 55*, 1–108.

Cole, E. E., Rodriquez, C., Walker-Thurmond, K., & Thun, M. J. (2003). Overweight, obesity and mortality—From cancer in a prospectively studied cohort of U.S. adults. *New England Journal of Medicine, 348*(17), 1625–1638.

Derogatis, L. R., Morrow, G. R., Fetting, J., Penman, D., Piasetsky, S., Schmale, A. M., et al. (1983). The prevalence of psychiatric disorders among cancer patients. *Journal of the American Medical Association, 249*(6), 751–757.

Doll, R., & Peto, R. (1981). *The causes of cancer*. New York: Oxford University Press.

Doyle, C., Kushi, L. H., Byers, T., Courneya, K. S., Demark-Wahnefried, W., Grant, B., et al. (2006). Nutrition and physical activity during and after cancer treatment: An American Cancer Society guide for informed choices. *CA: A Cancer Journal for Clinicians, 56*(6), 323–353.

Dunkel-Schetter, C. (1984). Social support and cancer: Findings based on patient interviews and their implications. *Journal of Social Issues, 40*, 77–98.

Farmer, D., Reddick, B., D'Agostino, R., & Jackson, S. A. (2007). Psychosocial correlates of mammography screening in older African American women. *Oncology Forum, 34*(1), 117–123.

Fowler, B. A. (2006). Social process used by African American women in making decisions about mammography screening. *Journal Nurses Scholarship, 38*(3), 247–254.

Fowler, B. A. (2007). The influence of social support relationships on mammography screening in African American women. *Journal of National Black Nurses Association, 18*(1), 21–29.

Jones, J. H. (1991). *Bad blood: The Tuskegee syphilis experiment*. New York: Free Press.

Kerr-Cresswell, D. M., Fitzgerald, B., Fergus, K., Gould, J., Lenis, M., & Clemons, M. (2005). Why so late?: Presentation delay in locally advanced breast cancer (LABC). *Journal of Clinical Oncology, 23*(16S), 712.

National Cancer Institutes, Division of Cancer Control and Population Science. (2006). *Surveillance, epidemiology, and end results (SEER) program 17 registries, 2000–2003*. Washington, DC: Author.

National Human Genome Institute. (2003). *International consortium completes Human Genome Project*. Washington, DC: National Institutes of Health.

Noyes, R., Jr., Holt, C. S., & Mossic, M. J. (1998). Anxiety disorder. In J. C. Holland (Ed.), *Psycho-oncology* (pp. 548–563). New York: Oxford University Press.

Ogden, C. L., Carrol, M. D., Curfin, L. R., McDowell, M. A., Tabak, L. J., & Flegal, K. M. (2006). Prevalence of overweight and obesity in the United States, 1999–2004. *Journal of the American Medical Association, 295*(13), 1549–1555.

Sanchez, M. A., Bowen, D. J., Hart, A., & Spigner, C. (2007). Factor's influencing prostate cancer screening decisions among African American men. *Ethnicity and Disease, 17*(2), 374–380.

Shuster, J. L., & James, G. R. (1998). Approach to the patient receiving palliative care. In T. A. Stern & J. Herman (Eds.), *The MGH guide to psychiatry in primary care prevention* (pp. 147–165). New York: McGraw-Hill.

Spurlock, W. R., & Cullins, L. S. (2006). Cancer fatalism and breast cancer screening in African American women. *Association of Black Nursing Faculty Journal, 17*(1), 38–43.

U.S. Department of Health and Human Services. (2004). *The health consequence of smoking—A report of the surgeon general.* Rockville, MD: U.S. Department of Health and Human Services, Public Health Service, Centers for Disease Control and Prevention, Center for Chronic Disease Prevention and Health Promotion, Office on Smoking and Health.

Weinrich, S. P., Boyd, M. D., Bradford, D., Mossa, M. S., & Weinrich, M. (1988). Recruitment of African Americans into prostate cancer screening. *Cancer Practice, 6*(1), 23–30.

# 14

# Tobacco Use

Tamika D. Gilreath
Guy-Lucien Whembolua
Gary King

In the 20th century, the use of tobacco was a major topic of interest to public health professionals and researchers globally because of its negative health consequences and resultant social costs. As the most preventable public health problem in the United States, cigarette smoking has had a devastating impact on the health of minority populations, particularly African Americans. It is responsible for a considerable proportion of the health disparities and excess mortality of African Americans in comparison to Caucasian Americans or Whites.

The health of African Americans cannot be separated from the social history of race and racism; thus, the study of African American cigarette smoking behavior necessarily entails sociological, psychosocial, political, economic, and biological perspectives. This chapter presents an important overview of key factors related to the use of tobacco, attempts to quit, and its consequences with respect to African Americans.

From the outset, it is important to note that substantial progress has been made recently in reducing smoking prevalence among African Americans. Since 1985, the rate of smoking among men and women has declined for both Whites and African Americans. The reasons, however, for the respective reductions are different; the reduced prevalence of smoking among Whites is due to higher quitting rates, whereas among African Americans it is due to lower initiation rates (King, Polednak, Bendel, Vilsaint, & Nahata, 2004).

In 2006, 23% of African Americans reported smoking cigarettes, a figure very similar to that for White Americans (21.9%). African American men had a prevalence rate of 27.6% compared with 19.2% of African American women, a substantial difference (Centers for Disease Control and Prevention, 2007). Differences in smoking among African Americans vary considerably by social class, region, and nativity (King, Bendel, & Delaronde, 1998). For example, a much lower percentage of nonnative African Americans smoke cigarettes (especially women) than native-born African Americans (King, Polednak, Bendel, & Hovey, 1999). Also, African Americans who live in the Midwest have the highest smoking prevalence rate compared with those residing in the Northeast, West, or South (King, Polednak, & Bendel, 1999).

This chapter begins with a discussion of research on the biology and genetics of smoking among African Americans. We also address health disparities and the conceptualization of "race." In addition, we review the empirical literature on risk and resiliency with respect to cigarette smoking from the perspectives of the individual, family, and community, suggesting the need to use a multilevel approach to the problem. Structural impediments related to social class or social position are explored in the context of tobacco control research and policies. Last, we provide recommendations to prevent tobacco use and present state-of-the-art smoking cessation strategies.

## BIOLOGICAL/GENETIC FACTORS

Cigarette smoke is known to contain more than 4,000 chemical compounds. Tobacco-related morbidity and mortality have been found to be associated with the toxic and carcinogenic chemicals inhaled in cigarette smoke, such as polycyclic aromatic hydrocarbons and tobacco-specific nitrosamines (Hecht, 2002; Hoffmann, Djordjevic, & Hoffmann, 1997). Exposure to these toxins per cigarette smoked is small but accumulates over a lifetime, thus increasing smokers' cancer risk dramatically (Hecht, 2002).

African Americans smoke fewer cigarettes per day (Clark, Gautam, & Gerson, 1996), take fewer puffs per cigarettes (W. J. McCarthy et al., 1995), and have higher levels of cotinine compared with other ethnic groups (Caraballo et al., 1998; Perez-Stable, Herrera, Jacob, & Benowitz, 1998). Despite less use, the health status of African Americans is disproportionately affected by tobacco use. In particular, African Americans have higher rates of tobacco-related deaths from coronary heart disease, stroke, and lung cancer (Moore, 2006) Rates of heart disease and stroke among Blacks and Whites are presented in Tables 14.1 and 14.2 (National Center for Health Statistics, 2007) with lung cancer rates presented in Tables 14.3 and 14.4 (American Cancer Society, 2007).

Several studies have tried to identify the causes of these differences in the incidence of tobacco-related illnesses. One theory is that the type of cigarette smoked may influence carcinogenic exposure and result in disparate cancer rates.

**TABLE 14.1. Age–Adjusted Heart Disease Death Rates per 100,000 (2005)**

| Sex | African American | Non-Hispanic White | African American/non-Hispanic White ratio |
|-----|------------------|--------------------|-------------------------------------------|
| Men | 329.8 | 262.2 | 1.3 |
| Women | 228.3 | 170.3 | 1.3 |

*Note.* From CDC (2008). *Health United States, 2008,* Table 35.

In this respect, menthol has been postulated as an important factor to consider. Gardiner (2004) observed that 70% of African Americans prefer mentholated cigarettes, and that the 25-year period of increased use of menthol cigarettes corresponded to the latency period necessary for the jump in lung cancer mortality rates observed in 1990 (Gardiner, 2004).

Two mechanisms may be responsible for the hypothesized relationship between menthol in the increase of lung cancers. First, the anesthetic and cooling effects of menthol permit deeper inhalation and larger puffs, which would lead to greater exposure to the carcinogenic elements in tobacco smoke (Hebert & Kabat, 1988; Sidney, Tekawa, Friedman, Sadler, & Tashkin, 1995). Second, the combustion of menthol itself may have a carcinogenic effect on lung tissue (Schmeltz & Schlotzhauer, 1968; Sidney et al., 1995). Nonetheless, the association between mentholated cigarettes and cancer is still being debated. Research from Brooks, Palmer, Strom, and Rosenberg (2003) and Werley, Coggins, and Lee (2007) suggests that mentholated cigarettes may not be associated with any greater risk for lung cancers (Brooks et al., 2003; Werley et al., 2007).

## Genetics and Tobacco Use

The use of a biomarker is essential for quantifying human exposure to nicotine for predicting potential health risks for exposed individuals. At present, cotinine, the major metabolite of nicotine, measured in blood, saliva, or urine, appears to be one of the most specific and sensitive biomarkers. It outlasts the presence of nicotine in the human body with a half-life of 14 to 20 hours (Buccafusco, Shuster, & Terry, 2007). Cotinine levels in nonsmokers are primarily the consequence of tobacco smoke under conditions of sustained exposure to environmental tobacco

**TABLE 14.2. Age–Adjusted Stroke Death Rates per 100,000 (2005)**

| Sex | African American | Non-Hispanic White | African American/non-Hispanic White ratio |
|-----|------------------|--------------------|-------------------------------------------|
| Men | 70.5 | 44.8 | 1.6 |
| Women | 60.7 | 44.4 | 1.4 |

*Note.* From CDC (2008). *Health United States, 2008,* Table 36.

**TABLE 14.3. Lung Cancer Death Rates per 100,000 for Men (2002–2006)**

| African American | Non-Hispanic White | African American/non-Hispanic White ratio |
|---|---|---|
| 90.1 | 69.9 | 1.3 |

*Note.* Data from Horner et al. (2009).

smoke (i.e., over hours or days) (Centers for Disease Control and Prevention, 2006).

The association between racially classified social groups (RCSGs) and cotinine has been the subject of several studies (Ahijevych, Tyndale, Dhatt, Weed, & Browning, 2002; Caraballo et al., 1998; Perez-Stable et al., 1998). Cotinine levels were found to be higher in African Americans smokers than in their White counterparts (Perez-Stable et al., 1998; Wagenknecht, Burke, Perkins, Haley, & Friedman, 1992). These differences are hypothesized to be the product of differences in metabolic variations among adult smokers (Caraballo et al., 1998; Perez-Stable et al., 1998). Berlin, Radzius, Henningfield, and Moolchan (2001) found that saliva cotinine levels are significantly higher in African Americans than in Caucasians for equal numbers of cigarettes smoked, suggesting that cotinine elimination or nicotine metabolism may be slower in African Americans. Moolchan, Franken, and Jaszyna-Gasior (2006) demonstrated that the trans-3'-hydroxycotinine/cotinine metabolite ratio is lower in African American adolescents compared with Caucasian adolescents. Their results suggest that ethnoracially based differences in nicotine metabolism among adolescent smokers could be the result of an association with the phenotypic expression of cytochrome P450 2A6, the primary liver enzyme responsible for the conversion of nicotine into cotinine (Moolchan et al., 2006).

Despite the research focus of race and ethnicity on differences related to biological and genetic factors of tobacco use and nicotine addiction, the term *race* in public health and social sciences requires careful consideration. Sociostructural factors such as education, tobacco industry promotion, institutional racism and discrimination, and health practices play a major role in differences seen in smoking (de Beyer, Lovelace, & Yurekli, 2001; Gardiner, 2004; Gilman, Abrams, & Buka, 2003; Orr, Newton, Tarwater, & Weismiller, 2005). Additionally, race or ethnicity is often used in social sciences to explain differences in smoking, although notable criticisms have raised questions about the significance (Griesler & Kandel, 1998; King, 1997; S. S. Lee, Mountain, & Koenig, 2001).

**TABLE 14.4. Lung Cancer Death Rates per 100,000 for Women (2002–2006)**

| African American | Non-Hispanic White | African American/non-Hispanic White ratio |
|---|---|---|
| 40.0 | 41.9 | 0.9 |

*Note.* Data from Horner et al. (2009).

A conventional school of thought views race as a biological or genetic category, or "racial biology." Adherents to this school of thought view the variable as an entity able to explain presumed differences in disease susceptibility, clinical manifestations, and medical outcomes (Cooper, 1984; King, 1997).

However, several arguments have been made against the use of racial biology and for the use of a more sociological perspective. The addition of elements such as genetic admixture, genetic drift, natural selection, and a lack of cross-national or migration studies seems to indicate that the use of racial categories is more related to sociopolitical conventions than the distribution of a population's genes (King, 1997). Thus, racial biology may explain in some cases the differences between ethnic groups within a nation but cannot be generalized worldwide. Krieger (2005) has illustrated this last point by describing the history of the use of the word *Caucasian* and its ties to an unscientific and subjective ideology (Krieger, 2005). Despite these dubious links, it is still used ostensibly as a scientific category. The fact that Caucasian Americans may not have much in common with their Russian counterparts or that conclusions made regarding African Americans cannot totally explain patterns observed in mainland Africans has not stopped the use of a racial category as a variable that is assumed to have universal application.

Another argument against the use of racial biology is that "biological differences are not by definition the same as genetic differences" (Polednak & Janerich, 1989). Variation in the case of cotinine levels among ethnic groups is influenced by many factors such as overall health status, physical activity level, age, thermic effects of food, caffeine consumption, diet, and physical fitness (Ahijevych & Wewers, 1993; Bauman & Ennett, 1994). When one looks at racial categories from a genetic perspective, a "genetic categorization is probabilistic" with "no absolute criterion for how great the genetic distance between groups must be in order to justify labeling them distinct races" (Whitfield & McClearn, 2005, p. 105).

The emergence of pharmacogenomics research, the study of the genetic basis for differential drug responses among individuals, has increased the understanding of single-nucleotide polymorphisms (SNPs). These SNPs may play a role in how humans respond to chemicals such as nicotine (J. E. Lee et al., 2004). Further research should avoid targeting variations within RCSGs and focus on individuals' differences in order to avoid reinforcing categories based on presumed "inherent differences" (King, 1997). In this respect, ancestry and migration have emerged as important analytic categories.

## INDIVIDUAL FACTORS INFLUENCING RISK AND RESILIENCY

Recent research has indicated that African Americans start smoking later than their majority counterparts (Geronimus, Neidert, & Bound, 1993; Moon-Howard, 2003; Royce, Hymowitz, Corbett, Hartwell, & Orlandi, 1993; Trinidad, Gilpin,

Lee, & Pierce, 2004). According to Trinidad and colleagues (2004), approximately 50% of African Americans reported that they started smoking between the ages of 18 and 25 years. However, a substantial proportion (24.5%) of African Americans ages 12 and older are current smokers (National Center for Health Statistics, 2007).

Risk factors that have been found to be related to adolescent African American smoking behavior include poor academic achievement, depressive symptoms, positive attitudes toward tobacco use, unconventional behaviors, socioeconomic status (SES), lack of social integration, and exposure to stress (Brook, Ning, & Brook, 2006; Gardiner, 2001; Juon, Ensminger, & Sydnor, 2002; Mermelstein, 1999; Payne & Diefenbach, 2003; Repetto, Caldwell, & Zimmerman, 2005; White, Violette, Metzger, & Stouthamer-Loeber, 2007). For example, in a longitudinal study of smoking initiation trajectories among African American adolescents who were monitored from first grade to age 32, Juon and colleagues (2002) found several risk factors for early initiation of smoking. Specifically, early initiators were more likely to leave home at a younger age, reported less familial interaction, and exhibited problem behaviors as early as the first grade.

Multiple protective factors have been found as well. Religiosity and moral beliefs, ethnic identity, and participation in prosocial activities (including sports and academics) have been found to be protective against adolescent tobacco use (Gardiner, 2001; Juon et al., 2002; Taylor et al., 1999; Wallace, Brown, Bachman, & LaVeist, 2003; Wills et al., 2007). It has been hypothesized that these multiple protective factors may explain the lower rates of smoking among African American adolescents compared with other RCSGs.

Rates of smoking among African American and White adults have been found to be similar (Centers for Disease Control and Prevention, 1991; Moon-Howard, 2003). Several key risk factors for initiation of smoking in adulthood have been identified in the literature. Notable among them are stress, depressive symptoms, and unconventional behaviors (Payne & Diefenbach, 2003; Repetto et al., 2005). Nonsmoking among African Americans has been found to be associated with marital status, educational attainment, SES, ethnic identity, religiosity, geographic region of residence, and nativity (King et al., 1998, 2006; King, Polednak, & Bendel, 1999; King, Polednak, Bendel, & Hovey, 1999; Nasim, Corona, Belgrave, Utsey, & Fallah, 2007; Nasim, Utsey, Corona, & Belgrave, 2006). Specifically, King, Polednak, Bendel, and Hovey (1999) found that foreign-born Blacks were less likely to be current smokers. Fewer native-born African Americans reported smoking as education and income increased. King and colleagues (1998) also found that older age, lower education, and male gender were associated with being a smoker.

African American women have a lower prevalence of smoking compared with their male counterparts (King et al., 1998; King, Polednak, Bendel, & Hovey, 1999). Despite their lower smoking rates, it is important to identify correlates of smoking among women. In a study of the heterogeneity of smoking among African American women, King and colleagues (2006) identified marriage, education, geographic region of residence (Black women in the South were significantly less likely to smoke than those in the Northeast), and income as protective factors against ever and current smoking (King et al., 2006).

## Risk and Resiliency for Smoking Cessation

Despite smoking fewer cigarettes per day, African Americans are less likely to quit smoking than their White counterparts (King et al., 2004). Few studies have attempted to assess the correlates of this epidemiological finding. Motivation to quit, positive parental relationship, and social support have been shown to be protective mechanisms for African American adolescents and adults wishing to quit (Boardman, Catley, Mayo, & Ahluwalia, 2005; Marcus, Pahl, Ning, & Brook, 2007). Conversely, levels of concurrent stress have been found to be predictive of smoking relapse (Manning, Catley, Harris, Mayo, & Ahluwalia, 2005). Because African Americans tend to smoke fewer cigarettes per day, the majority are classified as light smokers (Okuyemi et al., 2004; Okuyemi, Ahluwalia, Richter, Mayo, & Resnicow, 2001). This is significant for the fact that light smokers are less likely to receive cessation advice from physicians (Okuyemi et al., 2001), an intervention that has been shown to be predictive of successful smoking cessation (Stead, Bergson, & Lancaster, 2008).

# FAMILY FACTORS INFLUENCING RISK AND RESILIENCY

## Familial Resiliency

Familial characteristics are important factors in initiating smoking during adolescence and smoking cessation in adolescence and young adulthood (Brook, Pahl, & Ning, 2006; Glendinning, Shucksmith, & Hendry, 1997; Tillson, McBride, Lipkus, & Catalano, 2004). African American adolescent smoking has been found to be inversely related to parental smoking status and family closeness (Glendinning et al., 1997). African American adolescents are also more likely than their White counterparts to live in households where (1) smoking is prohibited (Payne & Diefenbach, 2003), (2) there are parental restrictions on tobacco use (Clark, Scarisbrick-Hauser, Gautam, & Wirk, 1999), and (3) there are higher levels of parental supervision and family connectedness (Mermelstein & the Tobacco Control Network Writing Group, 1999). In conjunction with familial tobacco use restriction and supervision, Mermelstein and the Tobacco Control Network Writing Group (1999) found that African American adolescents reported strong family proscription against smoking regardless of parental smoking status.

Qualitative studies of African American adolescent substance use have revealed possible areas for future research (Clark et al., 1999; Mermelstein & the Tobacco Control Network Writing Group, 1999). For example Clark, Scarisbrick-Hauser, Gautam, and Wirk (1999) found that African American youth consistently reported that family members would be disappointed in them if they smoked. In addition, regardless of parental smoking status, they expected to be disciplined if they were caught smoking. In this same study, African American parents reported feeling higher parental self-efficacy in enforcing no-smoking policies among their children (Clark et al., 1999).

## Familial Risk

In general, parental neglect, poor family communication, and the normalization of smoking within families have been found to be risk factors for adolescent smoking (Glendinning et al., 1997). Family substance use has also been consistently related to tobacco use in adolescents. Parental and sibling substance use contribute to adolescent tobacco use in two ways. First, adolescents who reside in homes with smokers tend to have access to cigarettes (Kegler et al., 2002). In addition, despite verbal messages, family behaviors may indicate that smoking is socially acceptable in adulthood (Brook, Pahl, & Ning, 2006). In a study of the interaction between parent–child relationships and parental smoking status, Tillson and colleagues (2004) found that close parental relationships were protective against smoking. However, if parents smoked, this relationship was significantly diminished (Tillson et al., 2004). Their sample consisted of minority respondents, 28% of whom were African American. These results reflect the influence of parental smoking practices on the prevention of tobacco use in some African American adolescents.

Additionally, adolescents residing in single-parent homes have also been found to be at higher risk for smoking (Aguilar & Pampel, 2007). Family SES is predictive of smoking status; high-risk adolescents tend to reside in households with incomes at or below national poverty levels.

## COMMUNITY AND SOCIAL FACTORS INFLUENCING RISK AND RESILIENCY

### Communities as Risk Factors

Several studies have identified the various community traits that serve as risk factors for tobacco use across demographic groups. African Americans disproportionately live in impoverished communities (Polednak, 1997). Studies on tobacco advertisements have shown significantly higher numbers of commercial promotion (e.g., in storefronts, on billboards) in predominantly poor minority communities compared with middle-class minority and White communities (Gardiner, 2004; Primack, Bost, Land, & Fine, 2007; U.S. Department of Health and Human Services [USDHHS], 1998). Related to the proliferation of pro-tobacco advertising in African American communities are the historical ties that tobacco companies purposely developed with several important African American organizations. Particularly, the tobacco industry has sponsored events and supported civic efforts by the National Association for the Advancement of Colored People, National

Urban League, and the United Negro College Fund (Yerger & Malone, 2002). In an examination of tobacco industry documents, Yerger and Malone (2002) discovered three primary reasons for these liaisons: to increase consumption of tobacco products by African Americans, to garner African American support for industry policies, and to ameliorate federal tobacco control.

## Community Resiliency

Despite the overwhelming evidence of the tobacco industries' careful targeting of African Americans as consumers, there are community characteristics that have been found to be protective against tobacco use. Xue, Zimmerman, and Caldwell (2007) found that adolescents who resided in predominantly African American neighborhoods were less likely to smoke than those who lived in communities with a low percentage of African Americans. In addition, adolescent participation in prosocial activities (e.g., church or after-school programs) diminished the influence of community composition on tobacco use (Xue et al., 2007).

## Tobacco Control and Social Class

Control policies implemented to reduce access to tobacco products have not had the desired impact across all groups. For example, laws that prohibit the sale of tobacco products to minors are expected to reduce smoking initiation among youth by limiting access. However, a study by Landrine, Klonoff, Campbell, and Reina-Patton (2000) identified ethnicity as the sole predictor of whether store clerks chose to sell tobacco products to underage purchasers. Hispanic and African American youth were more likely to be able to purchase tobacco products than their White counterparts (Landrine et al., 2000).

In addition, laws have been passed recently to increase tobacco taxes, which was intended to, among other goals, act as a deterrent to smoking. However, this policy has had the unintended effect of popularizing the sale of cigarettes. African American participants in Smith and colleagues' (2007), qualitative study reported that the illegal sale of loose cigarettes served as a convenient means to continue smoking (Smith et al., 2007). Furthermore, a qualitative study of New York City residents regarding the purchase of cigarettes from unlicensed vendors revealed a similar theme. In both instances, "loosies" and "the $5 man" made it easier for African Americans to continue smoking regardless of tobacco taxes (Shelley, Cantrell, Moon-Howard, Ramjohn, & VanDevanter, 2007; Smith et al., 2007; Stillman et al., 2007). In addition, tobacco control policies meant to curtail the use of tobacco may inadvertently increase the availability of tobacco products to adolescents within these communities because illegal street merchants are not likely to limit sales to customers 18 years and older.

Rates of smoking among low-income community-based samples of African Americans adults have surpassed 40 to 60% in some studies (Delva et al., 2005; D. Lee, Turner, Burns, & Lee, 2007; Stillman et al., 2007). This is a cause for concern because African Americans in underserved communities have easier access to these illegal and informal economic exchanges than to cessation services (Shelley et al., 2007).

## Racism and Discrimination

Studies have shown that perceived racism has been associated with myriad poor health outcomes in African Americans (Jackson et al., 1996; Klonoff, Landrine, & Ullman, 1999; Krieger & Sidney, 1996; Kwate, Valdimarsdottir, Guevarra, & Bovbjerg, 2003; Steffen, McNeilly, Anderson, & Sherwood, 2003; Stuber, Galea, Ahern, Blaney, & Fuller, 2003; Wyatt et al., 2003). Combining perceptions of racist events with low SES, low educational attainment, and limited social mobility may increase the likelihood of substance use (Kwate et al., 2003; Landrine & Klonoff, 2000). This topic has not been studied thoroughly as it pertains to tobacco use and African Americans. However, Bennett, Wolin, Robinson, Fowler, and Edwards (2005) found that young African American adults who reported harassment were twice as likely to report daily tobacco use (Bennett et al., 2005).

## EVIDENCE-BASED TREATMENT INTERVENTIONS

As mentioned, African Americans are less likely to successfully quit smoking (abstinence > 1 year) than their White counterparts (King et al., 2004). We now discuss published peer review studies of cessation programs that targeted African Americans or involved a substantial proportion of African Americans as subjects.

## African American Self-Quitters

The majority of successful quitters do so without the aid of treatment. Few studies have attempted to identify the sociodemographic characteristics of successful African American self-quitters (Orleans et al., 1989; Royce et al., 1993). In a study of African American adults, Orleans and colleagues (1989) reported that ex-smokers cited concerns about associated health risks as the major reason for quitting. In general, smokers and ex-smokers reported similar numbers of quit attempts and believed that smoking is socially unacceptable. Ex-smokers were less likely to have used cessation aids and more likely to have relied on willpower. However, these data are nearly 20 years old, and more recent research is warranted.

Smoking cessation for African Americans is not a simple pursuit. Previous studies have shown that African Americans metabolize nicotine and cotinine more slowly, smoke fewer cigarettes per day but inhale more deeply, smoke mentholated cigarettes, and smoke cigarette products that contain more nicotine and tar than their majority counterparts, all factors in strong nicotine addiction (Benowitz,

2002; Royce et al., 1993). Several types of evidence-based treatments are available to aid smokers in cessation efforts.

## Treatment and Interventions That Work

### NICOTINE REPLACEMENT THERAPY

Nicotine, a psychoactive ingredient in cigarettes and other tobacco products, has been shown to be the primary cause of smoking addiction. Nicotine replacement therapy (NRT) has been proven as an effective pharmacotherapy in supporting cessation attempts among smokers (Stead, Perera, Bullen, Mant, & Lancaster, 2008). With NRT, the body's craving for nicotine is sated through another medium, reducing smoking and exposure to its harmful constituents.

Currently, the NRT media available include gum, lozenges, transdermal patches, inhalers, and nasal spray. Presently, only the gum, lozenge, and patch are available over the counter in the United States. There is no conclusive evidence that one particular NRT is more effective than another (Gibson et al., 2005; Lancaster, Stead, & Cahill, 2008). The patch provides continuous nicotine compared with other methods that have to be ingested at specific intervals to diminish nicotine withdrawal symptoms. Overall, NRT therapies have been shown to nearly double the odds of successful cessation in clinical trials (Frishman, Mitta, Kupersmith, & Ky, 2006; Lancaster et al., 2008).

Okuyemi and colleagues (2007), in a randomized trial of nicotine gum and motivational interviewing, found no significant difference between the comparison control (no nicotine gum or motivational interview) and intervention (nicotine gum and motivational interview) groups in a sample of African Americans living in low-income housing (Okuyemi et al., 2007). This nonsignificant finding may be due to the low compliance rate for nicotine gum use (only 26% of the treatment sample reported using most of the nicotine gum) or to the short trial period (8 weeks with follow-up at 26 weeks). Despite this finding, other studies of NRT in African Americans show that it does support cessation (Ahluwalia, McNagny, & Clark, 1998; Frishman et al., 2006).

### BUPROPION HYDROCHLORIDE

As it pertains to pharmacotherapy, antidepressants such as bupropion and nortriptyline have been designated as therapies for smoking cessation. The mechanisms through which antidepressants can impact quit attempts include the alleviation of nicotine withdrawal symptoms by serving as nicotinic receptor agonists (or an exogenous chemical that can illicit a response from a cell or receptor in lieu of an endogenous transmitter) (Hughes, Stead, & Lancaster, 2007; Warner & Shoaib, 2005). As an agonist, bupropion acts on receptors that are normally activated by nicotine to cause the psychosomatic responses normally elicited by nicotine use.

Although bupropion is an accepted aid in smoking cessation, only one study of its efficacy has been conducted exclusively in African American smokers. Ahluwalia, Harris, Catley, Okuyemi, and Mayo (2002) conducted a randomized controlled trial of the efficacy of sustained-release bupropion in African Americans recruited from a community-based health care center. At the end of the 7-week intervention, the cessation rate for the intervention group was 36% compared with 19% for the placebo/comparison group. After 26 weeks these rates were 21% and 13.7%, respectively. These results, in combination with those from other trials with smaller samples of African Americans, indicate that this method is, in fact, an effective cessation tool (Frishman et al., 2006; Lancaster et al., 2008; McCarthy et al., 2008). Recently, McCarthy and colleagues (2008) reported that use of bupropion doubled 7-day abstinence (biochemically validated) and nearly tripled self-report prolonged abstinence.

## *Treatment and Interventions That Might Work*

### COMBINATION INTERVENTIONS

According to the 2006 technical report commissioned by the Agency for Healthcare Research and Quality, combined pharmacotherapy and psychological interventions are highly effective for long-term smoking cessation (Ranney et al., 2006). Andrews, Felton, Wewers, Waller, and Tingen (2007) assessed the effectiveness of a combined cessation intervention for African American women residing in public housing. The intervention consisted of nurse-led counseling on empowerment and self-efficacy to quit, NRT, and individual meetings with community-based health workers to provide social support and enhance self-efficacy. Smoking abstinence was verified by expired air carbon monoxide measures. Six-month continuous smoking abstinence rates were 27.5% and 5.7% for the intervention and control groups, respectively (Andrews et al., 2007).

Other studies of combination interventions did not demonstrate such significant differences in cessation between intervention and control groups (Nollen et al., 2007; Okuyemi et al., 2007). Okuyemi and colleagues (2007) examined the effectiveness of an intervention combining nicotine gum, educational materials, and motivational interviewing in a sample of participants, 70% of whom were women, recruited from 20 low-income housing projects. Unlike the intervention group, who received all three components, the comparison group received only motivational interviews and educational materials regarding fruit and vegetable consumption. After 26 weeks, cessation was higher in the comparison group than the intervention group (9.3% vs. 7.6%, respectively [ns]; Okuyemi et al., 2007). Similarly, Nollen and colleagues (2007) assessed the utility of targeted educational materials combined with nicotine patches. Again, no statistically significant cessation results were obtained.

Although none of these three studies produced significant findings, it is important to note that Andrews and colleagues' (2007) intervention included two components that might prove critical in helping African Americans quit smoking.

The use of community members (who were also former smokers) as liaisons and the provision of additional social support for those seeking to quit should be replicated in a larger sample of African American smokers (Andrews et al., 2007).

## CLINICAL INTERVENTIONS

Data regarding self-quitting indicate that care provider advice regarding the health consequences of smoking is important in increasing the motivation to quit (Fiore et al., 2000). Previous studies have shown that physician advice to quit is associated with attempts among the general population and that African Americans are less likely to receive provider advice (Fiore et al., 2000). Conversely, Pollack, Yarnall, Rimer, Lipkus, and Lyna (2002) assessed the reported cessation advice given to African American patients in a community health clinic and found that a majority of the smokers reported that they had been advised to quit (70%); however, these smokers tended to be older, be in poorer health, and to not smoke menthol cigarettes. Younger patients were significantly less likely to receive cessation advice. Despite the high rate of cessation advice, these results indicate a need for additional provider training, especially because 70% of African American smokers use mentholated products.

## COMMUNITY- AND CHURCH-BASED INTERVENTIONS

Community- and church-based interventions to stop smoking have also been implemented (Darity et al., 2006; Schorling et al., 1997; Voorhees et al., 1996). In Voorhees and colleagues' (1996) church-based smoking cessation program, "Heart, Body, and Soul," 21 churches were randomized to provide either intervention or comparison treatment. The intervention program included baseline and postintervention health fairs, sermons on smoking, testimony regarding the cessation process during church services, individual and group support, spiritual audiotapes, and a spiritual-based smoking cessation guide. Comparison programs included the baseline health fair and a pamphlet from the American Lung Association designed for African Americans. Results indicated that there were no statistically significant differences in biologically validated quit rates between intervention and comparison church-based programs (Voorhees et al., 1996). Similarly, Schorling and colleagues (1997), in a smoking cessation program implemented across counties via a church-based health coalition, also found nonsignificant differences in cessation rates.

Darity and colleagues (2006) assessed the effectiveness of a community-based smoking cessation program utilizing a media-only control group and media plus community organizing as the intervention for several predominantly African American communities. Study results indicated significant reductions in smoking after 18 months in a community sample. However, no biological validation was obtained for these results. These community- and church-based intervention programs appear to be promising but require additional replication and the consistent use of biological verification of smoking abstinence.

## Treatment and Interventions That Do Not Work

A review of the literature for treatment and interventions that do not work did not reveal any cessation/intervention programs or treatments deemed unreliable in aiding tobacco use cessation among African Americans.

## Psychopharmacology and Nicotine/Tobacco

Each year only 3% of smokers are able to quit, far less than the 10% who try to quit (Benowitz, 1999). Many smokers wish to quit but are impeded by the nicotine withdrawal symptoms experienced when one suddenly stops smoking. Nicotine acts as an agonist (Rosenzweig, Breedlove, & Leimnan, 2002), and its psychoactive properties are due to its affinity to a class of receptors called nicotinic acetylcholine receptors, located in the peripheral and central nervous systems (Watkins, Koob, & Markou, 2000). When nicotine binds to these receptors, it causes the increased release of several neurotransmitters. Specifically, acetylcholine, dopamine, serotonin, norepinephrine, and beta-endorphin are released (Benowitz, 2001). These neurotransmitters are involved in several important bodily functions and cognitive functions, such as performance and memory, pleasure and reward (Pomerleau & Pomerleau, 1984), and body weight regulation and mood (e.g., anxiety and tension) (Palfai & Jankiewicz, 1997). Furthermore, nicotine also increases the release of norepinephrine and epinephrine from the adrenal glands, which results in increases in heart rate, blood pressure, and gastrointestinal activity.

Nicotine is rapidly absorbed through the alveoli in the lungs when smokers inhale (Winger, Hofmann, & Woods, 1992) and is quickly distributed (within seconds) to the brain (Russell, 1987). It also has a brief half-life of approximately 2 hours (Tricker, 2003). The rewarding properties of nicotine include mild euphoria (Pomerleau & Pomerleau, 1992), increased energy, heightened arousal, and appetite suppression (Stolerman & Jarvis, 1995). Cigarette smokers have reported that smoking produces arousal (Benowitz, 1988) and relaxation during periods of stress (Parrott, 1999). The rapid absorption, distribution, and short half-life of nicotine require frequent self-administration if a smoker is to maintain nicotine levels and its associated rewarding properties.

The majority of smokers (> 77%) are dependent on nicotine (Douglas, 1997; Stolerman, 1991). Thus, periods of tobacco abstinence produce an aversive withdrawal syndrome. Smokers who attempt to abstain from tobacco use experience somatic and affective withdrawal symptoms, including, but not limited to, increased food intake, anxiety, restlessness, depressed mood, headache, irritability, sleep disturbances, and an inability to concentrate (American Psychiatric Association, 2000; Hughes, Gust, Skoog, Keenan, & Fenwick, 1991; Hughes & Hatsukami, 1986).

Among persons who have been smoking long term, withdrawal symptoms can appear within minutes (Schuh & Stitzer, 1995) of the last cigarette. Furthermore, withdrawal symptoms peak in intensity within 1 to 4 days after cessation (Hatsukami, Hughes, Pickens, & Svikis, 1984). The aversive withdrawal symptoms that accompany a quit attempt contribute to relatively low cessation rates, especially considering that relapse to cigarette use is an effective method for suppressing these symptoms (Skjei & Markou, 2003). Therefore, the suppression of this aversive withdrawal syndrome by continued nicotine self-administration (i.e., cigarette smoking) is thought to perpetuate smoking behavior (USDHHS, 1988; Watkins, Stinus, Koob, & Markou, 2000). Nicotine dependence contributes enormously to smoking-related death and disease because it is difficult to quit.

As noted earlier, African Americans have been shown to have higher levels of cotinine and to metabolize cotinine more slowly compared with other ethnic groups (Caraballo et al., 1998; Perez-Stable et al., 1998). Berlin and colleagues (2001) found that saliva cotinine levels are significantly higher in African Americans than in Caucasians for equal numbers of smoked cigarettes, suggesting that cotinine elimination or nicotine metabolism may be slower in African Americans (Berlin et al., 2001). Slower metabolism of nicotine may indicate a greater level of dependence and more difficulty quitting. Additionally, as mentioned, African Americans are also more likely to smoke mentholated cigarettes. The anesthetic and cooling effects of menthol, which permit deeper inhalation and larger puffs, may also lead to greater nicotine exposure (Hebert & Kabat, 1988; Sidney et al., 1995) and subsequent nicotine dependence.

## Prevention of Tobacco Use

The societal and individual costs of tobacco use are high. African Americans disproportionately experience negative health consequences of tobacco use. Relatively few published prevention programs include substantial numbers of African Americans in their samples (Metz, Fuemmeler, & Brown, 2006; Robinson, Klesges, Levy, & Zbikowski, 1999). Additionally, studies tend to target school-age children, a focus that is largely irrelevant for African Americans because this population tends to start smoking at later ages. There is a paucity of research on preventive interventions for young adult and adult populations not associated with an educational institution. A lack of preventive efforts across developmental periods may be associated with increases in prevalence for African American adults.

### Programs That Work

COMBINATION PROGRAMS

There is evidence that combination tobacco use prevention programs can be highly effective (Pentz, 1999). Such programs usually include media campaigns, tobacco control policies, and implementation of a school-based anti-smoking curriculum. As such, several states adopted comprehensive anti-tobacco programs during the 1990s (Friend & Levy, 2002). These programs and policies specifically included increases in tobacco excise taxes, restrictions on environmental tobacco exposure, school-based tobacco control educational programs, and increases in enforcement of age requirements for purchasing tobacco products (Bauer, Johnson, Hopkins, & Brooks, 2000; Centers for Disease Control and Prevention, 2004; Friend & Levy, 2002). It is important to note that none of these programs solely targeted African Americans.

Research indicates that comprehensive programs implemented in Florida and California lowered youth smoking prevalence, with higher influences on middle school students. In contrast, an assessment of smoking susceptibility after a similar campaign in Minnesota showed increased susceptibility among adolescents (Centers for Disease Control and Prevention, 2004).

## MEDIA AND TOBACCO CONTROL

In 2006, the National Institutes of Health State-of-the-Science Panel indicated that there are three effective means to prevent tobacco use: increasing the price of tobacco products, passing laws that limit youth access to tobacco products, and mass media campaigns. Media campaigns have been touted as a high-impact, low-cost way to increase knowledge about the dangers of smoking among the general population and youth in particular (Glantz & Mandel, 2005b). These campaigns are normally used to supplement other tobacco control activities. Most recently, the American Legacy Foundation's "truth" anti-smoking campaign was found to be associated with an overall decrease in national rates of smoking between 1999 and 2002 (Farrelly, Davis, Haviland, Messeri, & Healton, 2005). Additionally, in their study of the impact of environmental smoking restrictions, Farkas, Gilpin, White, and Pierce (2000) found that workplace and household smoking restrictions decrease the likelihood of smoking and increase the likelihood of smoking cessation among adolescents ages 15 to 17 years.

Presently, Congress is considering legislation that will allow the U.S. Food and Drug Administration (FDA) to regulate tobacco products more strictly (Saul, 2008a). The bill would ban most flavored cigarettes and further restrict advertisements. However, the proposed bill exempts menthol products (Saul, 2008a, 2008b). For African Americans, this is a significant concern because, as mentioned, a majority of Black smokers use mentholated cigarette products (Gardiner, 2004). There is presently no conclusive evidence that menthol increases tobacco-related morbidity/mortality as indicated in the prior discussion of biology and genetics; however, there is some evidence that mentholation may increase the level of nicotine dependence (Pletcher et al., 2006), possibly by influencing smoking behaviors (Garten & Falkner, 2004).

In its present form, the bill does include a provision whereby menthol may be banned from cigarettes if and when it is found to be an additional harmful component. However, it may take years after conclusive evidence is found to enforce such a ban. It is well known that the tobacco industry has been targeting African Americans for the use of mentholated products for more than 30 years. Additionally, Kreslake, Wayne, Alpert, Koh, and Connolly (2008) assert that the tobacco industry also titrated the levels of mentholation in their products to promote early dependence among adolescent and young adult smokers. Thus, the exemption of menthol as a banned additive may result in fewer new smokers among racial/ethnic groups who do not smoke menthol cigarettes but may maintain the higher risk for initiation and dependence of smoking among those African American youth and young adults who prefer mentholated products. Tobacco control policies are an effective means for preventing tobacco use initiation. However, these policies must be developed so that they do not leave vulnerable populations at greater risk for tobacco industry targeting through policy exemptions and loopholes.

### Programs That Might Work

SCHOOL-BASED PREVENTION PROGRAMS

Several school-based programs have targeted tobacco use specifically or as part of a larger program to reduce health-compromising behaviors among adolescents (Bruvold, 1993; Metz et al., 2006; Wiehe, Garrison, Christakis, Ebel, & Rivara, 2005). However, some evidence indicates that these programs are expensive, ineffective methods for preventing tobacco use initiation long term. In a meta-analysis of school-based prevention programs with long-term follow-up (from time of intervention to 12th grade or 18 years of age), Wiehe and colleagues (2005) found only one program that was associated with statistically significant reductions in smoking prevalence.

This program, however, was administered to a predominantly White middle-class population (Botvin, Baker, Dusenbury, Botvin, & Diaz, 1995). Additionally, the Hutchinson Smoking Prevention Project carried out in 40 Washington State school districts adopted a rigorous randomized trial design to assess the long-term effectiveness of its intervention on social influences. The program, administered to students in third to 12th grades, had no significant impact on smoking outcomes compared with a control (Peterson, Kealey, Mann, Marek, & Sarason, 2000).

Of four programs that targeted African Americans, one did not assess behavioral outcomes (Robinson et al., 1999). In a pilot evaluation of the Memphis Smoking Prevention program, which included approximately 1,000 predominantly African American students, Robinson and colleagues (1999) found that the program increased knowledge of health effects of tobacco and decreased the beliefs that smoking has social value, produces relaxation, or is associated with weight reduction. Although promising, these results should be replicated with more diverse samples (data were collected from one southern city) using behavioral outcomes as well as attitudinal and skill assessments (Robinson et al., 1999).

Some tobacco use prevention programs targeted or included substantial numbers of African Americans in their samples and assessed behavioral outcomes. Among them, Storr, Ialongo, Kellam, and Anthony (2002) assessed the influence of two preventive interventions for tobacco use in first grade on smoking initiation 6 years later at the end of seventh grade. The rate of smoking was 33% for the control group and 26% for both intervention groups, and the relative risk of smoking was significantly lower for the intervention groups compared with the control group (Storr et al., 2002). In an evaluation of the Life Skills Training (LST) curriculum, Zollinger and colleagues (2003) assessed the impact of receiving LST zero, one, or two times on current, ever, and never smoking. Overall, fewer participants from LST reported being a current smoker compared with the control sample. However, there were no statistically significant differences in smoking prevalence for African Americans (who comprised 59% of the sample).

### Programs That Do Not Work

A search for prevention programs that do not work did not reveal any that were deemed wholly unreliable in aiding tobacco use prevention among African Americans. There has been some discussion as to the cost-effectiveness of school-based prevention programs (Glantz & Mandel, 2005a, 2005b). However, until consistent results can be identified, it is possible that differences in program implementation and outcome measurement may account for some of the null results.

## RECOMMENDED BEST PRACTICES

Tobacco use prevention and cessation for African Americans are major public health concerns. African Americans disproportionately bear the health burden of tobacco use, as evidenced in this chapter. We now make recommendations for the prevention of tobacco use among African Americans and present state-of-the-art smoking cessation strategies.

## Prevention: Future Research and Recommendations

Research suggests that African Americans tend to start smoking in young adulthood, which indicates it is important to maintain the protective factors found in adolescence across the life span. As such, tobacco use prevention science needs to extend the targeted developmental period beyond adolescence into young adulthood. Specifically, research thus far has shown that the development of family-oriented preventive interventions addressing the health consequences for all family members when one member smokes may be highly effective. However, targeting individuals and families is only the first step in preventing tobacco use.

Tobacco control policies have yielded mixed results in facilitating tobacco use prevention in African American communities. For example, laws have limited the tobacco industry targeting of minors by restricting the use of images that are deemed to be appealing to youth. This policy, however, does less for inner-city African American youth, who are exposed to ubiquitous advertisements portraying young adult African Americans who, because they smoke, appear to be having fun and are popular. In addition, policies to increase taxation of tobacco products have also been found to have contradictory effects (Shelley et al., 2007; Smith et al., 2007). The emergence of an underground economy for cigarette sales reduces the effectiveness of such policies. The current FDA legislation under consideration serves as an opportunity for policymakers to consider the impact of policies on vulnerable populations.

Finally, based on a review of the literature, we recommended that multicomponent prevention programs be developed, implemented, and evaluated long term in African American communities. These programs should include media campaigns, equitable enforcement of current tobacco control policies across communities, and school- and community-based tobacco use prevention curricula.

## Smoking Cessation

Persons residing in low-income communities tend to experience more stressful life situations. Because a disproportionate number of African Americans reside in impoverished communities, it is important to identify healthful coping mechanisms aside from the self-medication that might be the reason behind tobacco use among African Americans. Treatment options should include pharmacotherapy combined with counseling.

Physicians who treat African Americans also need to receive training to address tobacco use among this population. Tobacco use has been associated with myriad chronic diseases that are more prevalent among African Americans than Whites. African Americans who are overweight, diagnosed with heart disease, or diagnosed with diabetes are also likely to be smokers. Through training, physicians must be made aware of the need to address all health concerns, both distal and proximal.

The best-practice recommendation for African American smoking cessation programs is to develop community infrastructure such that the professional services known to be required for successful long-term cessation will be made available to underserved populations. Counseling, physician advice, and pharmacotherapy have been found to be effective tools for smoking cessation. Unfortunately, in many instances, it is easier and less expensive in the short term to continue smoking. The long-term productivity and life losses associated with smoking provide impetus for policymakers and medical professionals to ensure that all persons have the opportunity and means to quit smoking successfully.

# REFERENCES

Aguilar, J., & Pampel, F. (2007). Changing patterns of cigarette use among White and Black youth, US 1976–2003. *Social Science Research, 36*, 1219–1236.

Ahijevych, K., & Wewers, M. E. (1993). Factors associated with nicotine dependence among African American women cigarette smokers. *Research in Nursing and Health, 16*(4), 283–292.

Ahijevych, K. L., Tyndale, R. F., Dhatt, R. K., Weed, H. G., & Browning, K. K. (2002). Factors influencing cotinine half-life during smoking abstinence in African American and Caucasian women. *Nicotine and Tobacco Research, 4*(4), 423–431.

Ahluwalia, J., McNagny, S. E., & Clark, W. S. (1998). Smoking cessation among inner-city African Americans using the nicotine transdermal patch. *Journal of General Internal Medicine, 13*(1), 1–8.

Ahluwalia, J. S., Harris, K. J., Catley, D., Okuyemi, K. S., & Mayo, M. S. (2002). Sustained-release bupropion for smoking cessation in African Americans: A randomized controlled trial. *Journal of the American Medical Association, 288*(4), 468–474.

American Cancer Society. (2007). *Cancer facts & figures 2007*. Atlanta: Author.

American Psychiatric Association. (2000). *Diagnostic and statistical manual of mental disorders* (4th ed., text rev.). Washington, DC: American Psychiatric Association.

Andrews, J. O., Felton, G., Wewers, M. E., Waller, J., & Tingen, M. (2007). The effect of a multi-component smoking cessation intervention in African American women residing in public housing. *Research in Nursing and Health, 30*, 45–60.

Bauer, U. E., Johnson, T. M., Hopkins, R. S., & Brooks, R. G. (2000). Changes in youth cigarette use and intentions following implementation of a tobacco control program: Findings from the Florida Youth Tobacco Survey, 1998–2000. *Journal of the American Medical Association, 284*, 723–728.

Bauman, K. E., & Ennett, S. E. (1994). Tobacco use by Black and White adolescents: The validity of self-reports. *American Journal of Public Health, 84*(3), 394–398.

Bennett, G. G., Wolin, K. Y., Robinson, E. L., Fowler, S., & Edwards, C. L. (2005). Perceived racial/ethnic harassment and tobacco use among African American young adults. *American Journal of Public Health, 95*(2), 238–240.

Benowitz, N. L. (1988). Pharmacologic aspects of cigarette smoking and nicotine addiction. *New England Journal of Medicine, 319*, 1318–1330.

Benowitz, N. L. (1999). Nicotine addiction. *Primary Care, 26*(3), 611–631.

Benowitz, N. L. (2001). The nature of nicotine addiction. In P. Slovic (Ed.), *Smoking: Risk, perception and policy* (pp. 159–187). Thousand Oaks, CA: Sage.

Benowitz, N. L. (2002). Smoking cessation trials targeted to racial and economic minority groups. *Journal of the American Medical Association, 288*(4), 497–499.

Berlin, I., Radzius, A., Henningfield, J. E., & Moolchan, E. T. (2001). Correlates of expired air carbon monoxide: Effect of ethnicity and relationship with saliva cotinine and nicotine. *Nicotine and Tobacco Research, 3*(4), 325–331.

Boardman, T., Catley, D., Mayo, M. S., & Ahluwalia, J. S. (2005). Self-efficacy and motivation to quit during participation in a smoking cessation program. *International Journal of Behavioral Medicine, 12*(4), 266–272.

Botvin, G. J., Baker, E., Dusenbury, L., Botvin, E. M., & Diaz, T. (1995). Long-term follow up results of a randomized drug abuse prevention trial in a White middle-class population. *Journal of the American Medical Association, 273*, 1106–1112.

Brook, J. S., Ning, Y., & Brook, D. W. (2006). Personality risk factors associated with trajectories of tobacco use. *American Journal on Addictions, 15*(6), 426–433.

Brook, J. S., Pahl, K., & Ning, Y. (2006). Peer and parental influences on longitudinal trajectories of smoking among African Americans and Puerto Ricans. *Nicotine and Tobacco Research, 8*(5), 639–651.

Brooks, D. R., Palmer, J. R., Strom, B. L., & Rosenberg, L. (2003). Menthol cigarettes and risk of lung cancer. *American Journal of Epidemiology, 158*(7), 609–616; discussion, 617–620.

Bruvold, W. H. (1993). A meta-analysis of adolescent smoking prevention programs. *American Journal of Public Health, 83*, 872–880.

Buccafusco, J. J., Shuster, L. C., & Terry, A. V. (2007). Disconnection between activation and desensitization of autonomic nicotinic receptors by nicotine and cotinine. *Neuroscience Letters, 413*(1), 68–71.

Caraballo, R. S., Giovino, G. A., Pechacek, T. F., Mowery, P. D., Richter, P. A., Strauss, W. J., et al. (1998). Racial and ethnic differences in serum cotinine levels of cigarette smokers: Third National Health and Nutrition Examination Survey, 1988–1991. *Journal of the American Medical Association, 280*(2), 135–139.

Centers for Disease Control and Prevention. (1991). Current trends and differences in the age of smoking initiation between Blacks and Whites–United States. *Morbidity and Mortality Weekly Report, 40*(44), 754–757.

Centers for Disease Control and Prevention. (2004). Effect of ending an antitobacco youth campaign on adolescent susceptibility to cigarette smoking—Minnesota, 2002–2003. *Morbidity and Mortality Weekly Report, 53*(14), 301–304.

Centers for Disease Control and Prevention. (2007). Cigarette smoking among adults—United States, 2006. *Morbidity and Mortality Weekly Report, 56*(44), 1157–1161.

Centers for Disease Control and Prevention. (2010). *Second-hand smoke.* Atlanta, GA: Author. Retrieved December 20, 2008, from *www.cdc.gov.tobacco/data_statistics/fact_sheets/secondhand_smoke/general_facts/index.htm.*

Clark, P. I., Gautam, S., & Gerson, L. W. (1996). Effect of menthol cigarettes on biochemical markers of smoke exposure among Black and White smokers. *Chest, 110*(5), 1194–1198.

Clark, P. I., Scarisbrick-Hauser, A., Gautam, S. P., & Wirk, S. J. (1999). Anti-tobacco socialization in homes of African-American and White parents, and smoking and nonsmoking parents. *Journal of Adolescent Health, 24*, 329–339.

Cooper, R. S. (1984). A note on the biologic concept of race and its application in epidemiologic research. *American Heart Journal, 108*, 715–723.

Darity, W. A., Chen, T. T., Tuthill, R. W., Buchanan, D. R., Winder, A. E., Stanek, E., III, et al. (2006). A multi-city community based smoking research intervention project in the African-American population. *International Quarterly of Community Health Education, 26*(4), 323–336.

de Beyer, J., Lovelace, C., & Yurekli, A. (2001). Poverty and tobacco. *Tobacco Control, 10*(3), 210–211.

Delva, J., Tellez, M., Finlayson, T. L., Gretebeck, K. A., Siefert, K., Williams, D. R., et al. (2005). Cigarette smoking among low-income African Americans: A serious public health problem. *American Journal of Preventive Medicine, 29*(3), 218–220.

Douglas, C. E. (1997). Manipulation of cigarette production to cause and enhance addiction. *Lung Cancer, 18*(52), 5–6.

Farkas, A. J., Gilpin, E. A., White, M. M., & Pierce, J. P. (2000). Association between household and workplace smoking restrictions and adolescent smoking. *Journal of the American Medical Association, 284,* 717–722.

Farrelly, M. C., Davis, K. C., Haviland, M. L., Messeri, P., & Healton, C. G. (2005). Evidence of a dose-response relationship between "truth" antismoking ads and youth smoking prevalence. *American Journal of Public Health, 95*(3), 425–431.

Fiore, M. C., Bailey, W. C., Cohen, D. J., Dorfman, S. F., Goldstein, M. G., Gritz, E. R., et al. (2000). *Treating tobacco use and dependence. Clinical practice guideline.* Rockville, MD: U.S. Department of Health and Human Services.

Friend, K., & Levy, D. T. (2002). Reductions in smoking prevalence and cigarette consumption associated with mass media campaigns. *Health Education Research, 17,* 85–98.

Frishman, W. H. M. D., Mitta, W. M. D., Kupersmith, A. M. D., & Ky, T. M. D. (2006). Nicotine and non-nicotine smoking cessation Pharmacotherapies. *Cardiology in Review, 14*(2), 57–73.

Gardiner, P. S. (2001). African American teen cigarette smoking: A review. In D. Burns (Ed.), *Changing adolescent smoking prevalence: Where is it and why* (Tobacco Control Monograph No. 14, NIH Publication No. 02-5086) (pp. 213–226). Bethesda, MD: National Cancer Institute.

Gardiner, P. S. (2004). The African Americanization of menthol cigarette use in the United States. *Nicotine and Tobacco Research, 6*(Suppl. 1), S55–S65.

Garten, S., & Falkner, R. V. (2004). Role of mentholated cigarettes in increased nicotine dependence and greater risk of tobacco-attributable disease. *Preventive Medicine, 38*(6), 793–798.

Geronimus, A., Neidert, L., & Bound, J. (1993). Age patterns of smoking in US Black and White women of childbearing age. *American Journal of Public Health, 87*(7), 1131–1135.

Gibson, P., Irving, L., Abramson, M., Wood-Baker, R., Volmink, J., Hensley, M., et al. (Eds.). (2005). *Evidence-based respiratory medicine.* Malden, MA: BMJ Books.

Gilman, S. E., Abrams, D. B., & Buka, S. L. (2003). Socioeconomic status over the life course and stages of cigarette use: Initiation, regular use, and cessation. *Journal of Epidemiology and Community Health, 57*(10), 802–808.

Glantz, S. A., & Mandel, L. L. (2005a). Letters to the editor: The guest editors reply. *Journal of Adolescent Health, 37,* 7–8.

Glantz, S. A., & Mandel, L. L. (2005b). Since school-based tobacco prevention programs do not work, what should we do? *Journal of Adolescent Health, 36*(3), 157–159.

Glendinning, A., Shucksmith, J., & Hendry, L. (1997). Family life and smoking in adolescence. *Social Science and Medicine, 44*(1), 93–101.

Griesler, P. C., & Kandel, D. B. (1998). Ethnic differences in correlates of adolescent cigarette smoking. *Journal of Adolescent Health, 23*(3), 167–180.

Hatsukami, D. K., Hughes, J. R., Pickens, R. W., & Svikis, D. (1984). Tobacco withdrawal symptoms: An experimental analysis. *Psychopharmacology, 84*(2), 231–236.

Hebert, J. R., & Kabat, G. C. (1988). Menthol cigarettes and esophageal cancer. *American Journal of Public Health, 78*(8), 986–987.

Hecht, S. S. (2002). Tobacco smoke carcinogens and breast cancer. *Environmental Molecular Mutagenesis, 39*(2–3), 119–126.

Hoffmann, D., Djordjevic, M. V., & Hoffmann, I. (1997). The changing cigarette. *Preventive Medicine, 26*(4), 427–434.

Horner, M. J., Ries, L. A. G., Krapcho, M., Neyman, N., Aminou, R., Howlader, N., et al. (Eds.). (2009). *SEER Cancer Statistics Review, 1975–2006*. Bethesda, MD: National Cancer Institute. Available at *http://seer.cancer.gov/csr/1975_2006/*.

Hughes, J. R., Gust, S. W., Skoog, K., Keenan, R. M., & Fenwick, J. W. (1991). Symptoms of tobacco withdrawal. *Archives of General Psychiatry, 48,* 52–59.

Hughes, J. R., & Hatsukami, D. K. (1986). Signs and symptoms of tobacco withdrawal. *Archives of General Psychiatry, 43,* 289–294.

Hughes, J. R., Stead, L., & Lancaster, T. (2007). Antidepressants for smoking cessation. *Cochrane Database of Systematic Reviews,* Issue 1 (Article No.: CD000031), DOI: 10.1002/14651858.CD000031.pub3.

Jackson, J. S., Brown, T. N., Williams, D., Torres, M., Sellers, S. L., & Brown, K. (1996). Racism and the physical and mental health status of African Americans: A thirteen year panel study. *Ethnicity and Disease, 6,* 132–147.

Juon, H., Ensminger, M. E., & Sydnor, K. D. (2002). A longitudinal study of developmental trajectories to young adult cigarette smoking. *Drug and Alcohol Dependency, 66,* 303–314.

Kegler, M. C., McCormick, L., Crawford, M., Allen, P., Spigner, C., & Ureda, J. (2002). An exploration of family influences on smoking among ethnically diverse adolescents. *Health Education and Behavior, 29*(4), 473–490.

King, G. (1997). The "race" concept in smoking: A review of the research on African Americans. *Social Science and Medicine, 45*(7), 1075–1087.

King, G., Bendel, R. B., & Delaronde, S. R. (1998). Social heterogeneity in smoking among African Americans. *American Journal of Public Health, 88*(7), 1081–1085.

King, G., Polednak, A., Fagan, P., Gilreath, T., Humphrey, E., Fernander, A., et al. (2006). Heterogeneity in the smoking behavior of African American women. *American Journal of Health Behavior, 30*(3), 237–246.

King, G., Polednak, A. P., & Bendel, R. B. (1999). Regional variation in smoking among African Americans. *Preventive Medicine, 29*(2), 126–132.

King, G., Polednak, A. P., Bendel, R. B., & Hovey, D. (1999). Cigarette smoking among native and foreign-born African Americans. *Annals of Epidemiology, 9*(4), 236–244.

King, G., Polednak, A. P., Bendel, R. B., Vilsaint, M., & Nahata, S. (2004). Disparities in smoking cessation between African Americans and Whites: 1990–2000. *American Journal of Public Health, 94*(11), 1965–1971.

Klonoff, E. A., Landrine, H., & Ullman, J. (1999). Racial discrimination and psychiatric symptoms among Blacks. *Cultural Diversity and Ethnic Minority Psychology, 5*(4), 329–339.

Kreslake, J. M., Wayne, G. F., Alpert, H. R., Koh, H. K., & Connolly, G. N. (2008). Tobacco industry control of menthol in cigarettes and targeting of adolescents and young adults. *American Journal of Public Health, 98,* 1685–1692.

Krieger, N. (2005). Stormy weather: Race, gene expression, and the science of health disparities. *American Journal of Public Health, 95*(12), 2155–2160.

Krieger, N., & Sidney, S. (1996). Racial discrimination and blood pressure: The CARDIA study of young Black and White adults. *American Journal of Public Health, 86*(10), 1370–1378.

Kwate, N. O. A., Valdimarsdottir, H. B., Guevarra, J. S., & Bovbjerg, D. H. (2003). Experiences of racist events have negative health consequences for African American women. *Journal of the National Medical Association, 95*, 450–460.

Lancaster, T., Stead, L., & Cahill, K. (2008). An update on therapeutics for tobacco dependence. *Expert Opinions in Pharmacotherapy, 9*(1), 15–22.

Landrine, H., & Klonoff, E. A. (2000). Racial discrimination and cigarette smoking among Blacks: Findings from two studies. *Ethnicity and Disease, 10*(2), 195–202.

Landrine, H., Klonoff, E. A., Campbell, R., & Reina-Patton, A. (2000). Sociocultural variables in youth access to tobacco: Replication 5 years later. *Preventive Medicine, 30*(5), 433–437.

Lee, D., Turner, N., Burns, J., & Lee, T. (2007). Tobacco use and low-income African Americans: Policy implications. *Addictive Behaviors, 32*(2), 332–341.

Lee, J. E., Lee, S. J., Namkoong, S. E., Um, S. J., Sull, J. W., Jee, S. H., et al. (2004). Gene-gene and gene-environmental interactions of p53, p21, and IRF-1 polymorphisms in Korean women with cervix cancer. *International Journal of Gynecological Cancer, 14*(1), 118–125.

Lee, S. S., Mountain, J., & Koenig, B. A. (2001). The meanings of "race" in the new genomics: Implications for health disparities research. *Yale Journal of Health Policy, Law, and Ethics, 1*, 33–75.

Manning, B. K., Catley, D., Harris, K. J., Mayo, M. S., & Ahluwalia, J. (2005). Stress and quitting among African American smokers. *Journal of Behavioral Medicine, 28*(4), 325–333.

Marcus, S. E., Pahl, K., Ning, Y., & Brook, J. S. (2007). Pathways to smoking cessation among African American and Puerto Rican young adults. *American Journal of Public Health, 97*(8), 1444–1448.

McCarthy, D. E., Piasecki, T. M., Lawrence, D. L., Jorenby, D. E., Shiffman, S., Fiore, M. C., et al. (2008). A randomized controlled clinical trial of bupropion SR and individual smoking cessation counseling. *Nicotine and Tobacco Research, 10*(4), 717–729.

McCarthy, W. J., Caskey, N. H., Jarvik, M. E., Gross, T. M., Rosenblatt, M. R., & Carpenter, C. (1995). Menthol vs nonmenthol cigarettes: Effects on smoking behavior. *American Journal of Public Health, 85*(1), 67–72.

Mermelstein, R. (1999). Ethnicity, gender and risk factors for smoking initiation: An overview. *Nicotine and Tobacco Research, 1*(Suppl. 2), S39–S43.

Mermelstein, R., & the Tobacco Control Network Writing Group. (1999). Explanations of ethnic and gender differences in youth smoking: A multi-site, qualitative investigation. *Nicotine and Tobacco Research, 1*, S91–S98.

Metz, A. E., Fuemmeler, B. F., & Brown, R. T. (2006). Implementation and assessment of an empirically validated intervention program to prevent tobacco use among African American middle school youth. *Journal of Clinical Psychology in Medical Settings, 13*(3), 229–238.

Moolchan, E. T., Franken, F. H., & Jaszyna-Gasior, M. (2006). Adolescent nicotine metabolism: Ethnoracial differences among dependent smokers. *Ethnicity and Disease, 16*(1), 239–243.

Moon-Howard, J. (2003). African American women and smoking: Starting later. *American Journal of Public Health, 93*(3), 418–420.

Moore, M. A. (2006). Do cross-registry comparisons of Black and White Americans provide support for N-acetylation as an important determinant for urinary bladder and other tobacco-related cancers? *Asian Pacific Journal of Cancer Prevention, 7*(2), 267–273.

Nasim, A., Corona, R., Belgrave, F. Z., Utsey, S. O., & Fallah, N. (2007). Cultural orientation as a protective factor against tobacco and marijuana smoking for African American young women. *Journal of Youth and Adolescence, 36,* 503–516.

Nasim, A., Utsey, S. O., Corona, R., & Belgrade, F. Z. (2006). Religiosity, refusal efficacy, and substance use among African-American adolescents and young adults. *Journal of Ethnicity in Substance Abuse, 5*(3), 29–49.

National Center for Health Statistics. (2007). *Health, United States, 2007 with chartbook on trends in the health of Americans.* Hyattsville, MD: Centers for Disease Control and Prevention.

National Institutes of Health State-of-the-Science Panel. (2006). Tobacco use: Prevention, cessation and control. *Annals of Internal Medicine, 145*(11), 839–844.

Nollen, N., Ahluwalia, J., Mayo, M. S., Richter, K. P., Choi, W. S., Okuyemi, K. S., et al. (2007). A randomized trial of targeted educational materials for smoking cessation in African Americans using transdermal nicotine. *Health Education and Behavior, 34*(6), 911–927.

Okuyemi, K. S., Ahluwalia, J. S., Banks, R., Harris, K. J., Mosier, M. C., Nazir, N., et al. (2004). Differences in smoking and quitting experiences by levels of smoking among African Americans. *Ethnicity and Disease, 14*(1), 127–133.

Okuyemi, K. S., Ahluwalia, J. S., Richter, K. P., Mayo, M. S., & Resnicow, K. (2001). Differences among African American light, moderate, and heavy smokers. *Nicotine and Tobacco Research, 3*(1), 45–50.

Okuyemi, K. S., James, A. S., Mayo, M. S., Nollen, N., Catley, D., Choi, W. S., et al. (2007). Pathways to health: A cluster randomized trial of nicotine gum and motivational interviewing for smoking cessation in low-income housing. *Health Education and Behavior, 34*(1), 43–54.

Orleans, C. T., Schoenbach, V. J., Salmon, M. A., Strecher, V. J., Kalsbeek, W., Quade, D., et al. (1989). A survey of smoking and quitting patterns among Black Americans. *American Journal of Public Health, 79*(2), 176–181.

Orr, S. T., Newton, E., Tarwater, P. M., & Weismiller, D. (2005). Factors associated with prenatal smoking among Black women in eastern North Carolina. *Maternal and Child Health Journal, 9*(3), 245–252.

Palfai, T., & Jankiewicz, H. (1997). *Drugs and human behavior.* New York: Brown & Benchmark.

Parrott, A. C. (1999). Does cigarette smoking cause stress? *American Psychologist, 54*(10), 817–820.

Payne, T. J., & Diefenbach, L. (2003). Characteristics of African American smokers: A brief review. *American Journal of the Medical Sciences, 326*(4), 212–215.

Pentz, M. A. (1999). Effective prevention programs for tobacco use. *Nicotine and Tobacco Research, 1,* S99–S107.

Perez-Stable, E. J., Herrera, B., Jacob, P., III, & Benowitz, N. L. (1998). Nicotine metabolism and intake in Black and White smokers. *Journal of the American Medical Association, 280*(2), 152–156.

Peterson, A. V., Kealey, K. A., Mann, S. L., Marek, P. M., & Sarason, I. G. (2000). Hutchinson Smoking Prevention Project: Long-term randomized trial in school-based tobacco use prevention—Results on smoking. *Journal of the National Cancer Institute,* 92(24), 1979–1991.

Pletcher, M. J., Hulley, B. J., Houston, T., Kiefe, C. I., Benowitz, N. L., & Sidney, S. (2006). Menthol cigarettes, smoking cessation, artherosclerosis, and pulmonary function: The Coronary Artery Risk Development in Young Adults (CARDIA) Study. *Archives of Internal Medicine, 166,* 1915–1922.

Polednak, A. (1997). *Segregation, poverty and mortality in urban African Americans.* New York: Oxford University Press.

Polednak, A. P., & Janerich, D. T. (1989). Lung cancer in relation to residence in census tracts with toxic-waste disposal sites: A case-control study in Niagara County, New York. *Environmental Research, 48*(1), 29–41.

Pollack, K. I., Yarnall, K. S., Rimer, B. K., Lipkus, I., & Lyna, P. R. (2002). Factors associated with patient-recalled smoking cessation advice in a low-income clinic. *Journal of the National Medical Association, 94*(5), 354–363.

Pomerleau, C. S., & Pomerleau, O. F. (1984). Neuroregulators and the reinforcement of smoking: Towards a biobehavioral explanation. *Neuroscience and Biobehavioral Reviews, 8*(4), 503–513.

Pomerleau, C. S., & Pomerleau, O. F. (1992). Euphoriant effects of nicotine in smokers. *Psychopharmacology, 108,* 460–465.

Primack, B. A., Bost, J. E., Land, S. R., & Fine, M. J. (2007). Volume of tobacco advertising in African American markets: Systematic review and meta-analysis. *Public Health Reports, 122*(5), 607–615.

Ranney, L., Melvin, C., Lux, L., McClain, E., Morgan, L., & Lohr, K. (2006). *Tobacco use: Prevention, cessation, and control.* Rockville, MD: Agency for Healthcare Research and Quality.

Repetto, P. B., Caldwell, C. H., & Zimmerman, M. A. (2005). A longitudinal study of the relationship between depressive symptoms and cigarette use among African American adolescents. *Health Psychology, 24*(2), 209–219.

Robinson, L. A., Klesges, R. C., Levy, M. C., & Zbikowski, S. M. (1999). Preventing cigarette use in a bi-ethnic population: Results of the Memphis Smoking Prevention Program. *Cognitive and Behavioral Practice, 6,* 136–143.

Rosenzweig, M. R., Breedlove, S. M., & Leimnan, S. C. (2002). *Biological psychology.* Sunderland, MA: Sinauer.

Royce, J. M., Hymowitz, N., Corbett, K., Hartwell, T. D., & Orlandi, M. A. (1993). Smoking cessation factors among African Americans and Whites. *American Journal of Public Health, 83*(2), 220–226.

Russell, M. A. H. (1987). Nicotine intake and its regulation by smokers. In W. D. Martin, G. R. Van Loon, E. T. Iwamoto, & L. Davis (Eds.), *Tobacco smoking and nicotine* (pp. 25–50). New York: Plenum Press.

Saul, S. (2008a, May 13). Cigarette bill treats menthol with leniency. *New York Times.* Available at *www.nytimes.com/2008/05/13/business/13menthol.htm#.*

Saul, S. (2008b, June 5). Opposition to menthol cigarettes grows. *New York Times.* Available at *www.nytimes.com/2008/06/05/business/05tobacco.html.*

Schmeltz, I., & Schlotzhauer, W. S. (1968). Benzo(a)pyrene, phenols and other products from pyrolysis of the cigarette additive, (d,1)-menthol. *Nature, 219,* 370–371.

Schorling, J. B., Roach, J., Siegel, M., Baturka, N., Hunt, D. E., Guterbock, T. M., et al.

(1997). A trial of church-based smoking cessation interventions for rural African Americans. *Preventive Medicine, 26*(1), 92–101.

Schuh, K. J., & Stitzer, M. L. (1995). Desire to smoke during spaced smoking intervals. *Psychopharmacology, 120*(3), 289–295.

Shelley, D., Cantrell, J., Moon-Howard, J., Ramjohn, D. Q., & VanDevanter, N. (2007). The $5 man: The underground economic response to a large cigarette tax increase in New York City. *American Journal of Public Health, 97*(8), 1483–1488.

Sidney, S., Tekawa, I. S., Friedman, G. D., Sadler, M. C., & Tashkin, D. P. (1995). Mentholated cigarette use and lung cancer. *Archives of Internal Medicine, 155*(7), 727–732.

Skjei, K. L., & Markou, A. (2003). Effects of repeated withdrawal episodes, nicotine dose, and duration of nicotine exposure on the severity and duration of nicotine withdrawal in rats. *Psychopharmacology, 168*, 280–292.

Smith, K. C., Stillman, F., Bone, L., Yancey, N., Price, E., Belin, P., et al. (2007). Buying and selling "loosies" in Baltimore: The informal exchange of cigarettes in the community context. *Journal of Urban Health, 84*(4), 494–507.

Stead, L. F., Bergson, G., & Lancaster, T. (2008). Physician advice for smoking cessation. *Cochrane Database of Systematic Reviews*, Issue 2 (Article No.: CD000165), DOI: 10.1002/14651858.CD000165.pub3.

Stead, L. F., Perera, R., Bullen, C., Mant, D., & Lancaster, T. (2008). Nicotine replacement therapy for smoking cessation. *Cochrane Database of Systematic Reviews*, Issue 1 (Article No.: CD000146), DOI: 10.1002/14651858.CD000146.pub2.

Steffen, P., McNeilly, M., Anderson, N., & Sherwood, A. (2003). Effects of perceived racism and anger inhibition on ambulatory blood pressure in African Americans. *Psychosomatic Medicine, 65*, 746–750.

Stillman, F. A., Bone, L., Avila-Tang, E., Smith, K., Yancey, N., Street, C., et al. (2007). Barriers to smoking cessation in inner-city African American young adults. *American Journal of Public Health, 97*(8), 1405–1408.

Stolerman, I. P. (1991). Behavioral pharmacology of nicotine: Multiple mechanisms. *British Journal of Addiction, 86*, 533–536.

Stolerman, I. P., & Jarvis, M. J. (1995). The scientific case that nicotine is addictive. *Psychopharmacology, 117*, 2–10.

Storr, C. L., Ialongo, N. S., Kellam, S. G., & Anthony, J. C. (2002). A randomized controlled trial of two primary school intervention strategies to prevent early onset tobacco smoking. *Drug and Alcohol Dependence, 66*, 51–60.

Stuber, J., Galea, S., Ahern, J., Blaney, S., & Fuller, C. (2003). The association between multiple domains of discrimination and self-assessed health: A multilevel analysis of Latinos and Blacks in four low-income New York City neighborhoods. *Health Services Research, 38*(6, Pt. 2), 1735–1759.

Taylor, W. C., Ayars, C. L., Gladney, A. P., Peters, R. J., Roy, J. R., Prokhorov, A. V., et al. (1999). Beliefs about smoking among adolescents—Gender and ethnic differences. *Journal of Child and Adolescent Substance Abuse, 8*(3), 34–54.

Tillson, E. C., McBride, C. M., Lipkus, I., & Catalano, R. F. (2004). Testing the interaction between parent-child relationship factors and parent smoking to predict youth smoking. *Journal of Adolescent Health, 35*(3), 182–189.

Tricker, A. R. (2003). Nicotine metabolism, human drug metabolism polymorphisms and smoking behavior. *Toxicology, 183*(1–3), 151–173.

Trinidad, D. R., Gilpin, E. A., Lee, L., & Pierce, J. P. (2004). Do the majority of Asian-

American and African-American smokers start as adults? *American Journal of Preventive Medicine, 26*(2), 156–158.

U.S. Department of Health and Human Services. (1988). *The health consequences of smoking: Nicotine addiction.* Retrieved December 20, 2008, from *profiles.nlm.nih.gov/NN/B/B/Z/D/_/nnbbzd.pdf.*

U.S. Department of Health and Human Services. (1998). *Tobacco use among U.S. racial/ethnic minority groups—African Americans, American Indians and Alaska Natives, Asian Americans and Pacific Islanders and Hispanics: A report of the Surgeon General.* Atlanta, GA: U.S. Department of Health and Human Services, Centers for Disease Control and Prevention, National Center for Chronic Disease Prevention and Health Promotion, Office on Smoking and Health.

Voorhees, C. C., Stillman, F. A., Swank, R. T., Heagerty, P. J., Levine, D. M., & Becker, D. M. (1996). Heart, body, and soul: Impact of church-based smoking cessation interventions on readiness to quit. *Preventive Medicine, 25*(3), 277–285.

Wagenknecht, L. E., Burke, G. L., Perkins, L. L., Haley, N. J., & Friedman, G. D. (1992). Misclassification of smoking status in the CARDIA study: A comparison of self-report with serum cotinine levels. *American Journal of Public Health, 82*(1), 33–36.

Wallace, J. M., Jr., Brown, T. N., Bachman, J. G., & LaVeist, T. A. (2003). The influence of race and religion on abstinence from alcohol, cigarettes and marijuana among adolescents. *Journal of Studies on Alcohol, 64,* 843–848.

Warner, C., & Shoaib, M. (2005). How does bupropion work as a smoking cessation aid? *Addiction Biology, 10*(3), 219–231.

Watkins, S. S., Koob, G. F., & Markou, A. (2000). Neural mechanisms underlying nicotine addiction: Acute positive reinforcement and withdrawal. *Nicotine and Tobacco Research, 2,* 19–37.

Watkins, S. S., Stinus, L., Koob, G. F., & Markou, A. (2000). Reward and somatic changes during precipitated nicotine withdrawal in the rat: Central and peripheral mechanisms. *Journal of Pharmacology and Experimental Therapeutics, 292,* 1053–1064.

Werley, M. S., Coggins, C. R., & Lee, P. N. (2007). Possible effects on smokers of cigarette mentholation: A review of the evidence relating to key research questions. *Regulatory Toxicology and Pharmacology, 47*(2), 189–203.

White, H. R., Violette, N. M., Metzger, L., & Stouthhamer-Loeber, M. (2007). Adolescent risk factors for late-onset smoking among African American young men. *Nicotine and Tobacco Research, 9*(1), 153–161.

Whitfield, K. E., & McClearn, G. (2005). Genes, environment, and race: Quantitative genetic approaches. *American Psychologist, 60*(1), 104–114.

Wiehe, S. E., Garrison, M. M., Christakis, D. A., Ebel, B. E., & Rivara, F. P. (2005). A systematic review of school-based smoking prevention trials with long-term follow-up. *Journal of Adolescent Health, 36*(3), 162–169.

Wills, T. A., Murry, V. M., Brody, G. H., Gibbons, F. X., Gerrard, M., Walker, C., et al. (2007). Ethnic pride and self-control related to protective and risk factors: Test of the theoretical model for the strong African American families program. *Health Psychology, 26*(1), 50–59.

Winger, G., Hofmann, F. G., & Woods, J. H. (1992). *A handbook on drug and alcohol abuse: The biomedical aspects* (3rd ed.). New York: Oxford University Press.

Wyatt, S. B., Williams, D. R., Calvin, R., Henderson, F. C., Walker, E. R., & Winters, K.

(2003). Racism and cardiovascular disease in African Americans. *American Journal of Medical Science, 325,* 315–331.

Xue, Y., Zimmerman, M. A., & Caldwell, C. H. (2007). Neighborhood residence and cigarette smoking among urban youths: The protective role of prosocial activities. *American Journal of Public Health, 97*(10), 1865–1872.

Yerger, V. B., & Malone, R. E. (2002). African American leadership groups: Smoking with the enemy. *Tobacco Control, 11*(4), 336–345.

Zollinger, T. W., Saywell, R. M., Muegge, C. M., Wooldridge, J. S., Cummings, S. F., & Caine, V. A. (2003). Impact of the life skills training curriculum on middle school students' tobacco use in Marion County, Indiana, 1997–2000. *Journal of School Health, 73*(9), 338–346.

# 15

# Anxiety

ANGELA NEAL-BARNETT
LORI E. CROSBY
BERNADETTE BLOUNT SALLEY

**A**nxiety disorders are the most prevalent mental health problems in this country (Kessler et al., 2004; U.S. Department of Health and Human Services, 2006). Annually, anxiety disorders cost this country more than $42 billion in lost wages, missed workdays, and health benefits (Greenberg et al., 1999). Among African American communities, anxiety disorders commonly are classified as "nerves" or "bad nerves" (Neal-Barnett, 2003). These colloquialisms capture the key components of most anxiety disorders: anxiety and fear. Anxiety is the perception or awareness of a future threat. Often the perceived threat is far worse than anything that actually happens. In some cases, the future threat is unrealistic. However, it feels real to the person who is experiencing it. Fear is brought on by an imminent or immediate threat. Fearful individuals have a physical reaction to the threat.

Recent data from the National Comorbidity Survey (NCS; Kessler et al., 1994) and the National Comorbidity Survey—Replication (NCS-R; Kessler et al., 2004) reveal that African American adults have a lower lifetime prevalence rate for anxiety disorders than their non-Hispanic White counterparts (Breslau, Kendler, Su, Gaxiola-Aguilar, & Kessler, 2005). Between 23.8 and 24.7% of the 12 million African Americans in this country will develop an anxiety disorder compared with 29.1% of non-Hispanic Whites (Breslau et al., 2005; Breslau, Gaxiola-Aguilar, Su, Williams, & Kessler, 2006). Among those African Americans who suffer from anxiety disorders however, the manifestations appear to be more persistent (Breslau et al., 2005). African Americans with anxiety disorders have higher rates of suicide attempts than those with other psychiatric diagnoses (Joe, Baser, Breeden, Neighbors, & Jackson, 2006). Clearly, anxiety disorders can have a devastating impact on the lives of affected African Americans and their families.

Anxiety disorders are also among the most common psychiatric disorders among U.S. youth (Safren et al., 2000), with prevalence rates ranging from 12 to 20% (Mash & Barkley, 2003). Research suggests that African American children likewise experience anxiety and anxiety disorders (Last & Perrin, 1993; Neal & Knisley, 1995). However, determining the prevalence rate for any of the anxiety disorders in African American children is extremely difficult. To date, no studies have assessed the entire range of anxiety disorders in African American youth.

According to the text revision of the fourth edition of the *Diagnostic and Statistical Manual of Mental Disorders* (DSM-IV-TR; American Psychiatric Association, 2000), there are six major anxiety diagnoses: panic disorder (PD), obsessive–compulsive disorder (OCD), posttraumatic stress disorder (PTSD), generalized anxiety disorder (GAD), social anxiety disorder (also known as social phobia [SAP]), and specific phobia (SP). A seventh diagnosis, separation anxiety disorder (SAD), is found under the DSM-IV-TR category "disorders first diagnosed in infancy, childhood, or adolescence." Additional anxiety diagnoses include acute stress disorder, substance-induced anxiety disorder, and anxiety disorder resulting from a general medical condition. This chapter focuses on the major anxiety diagnoses manifested in African American adults and children. In this next section, we provide a general description of each disorder.

## GENERAL DESCRIPTIONS

### Panic Attacks/PD

Panic attacks are a common component of most anxiety disorders. Panic attack symptoms include increased heart rate, heart pounding; sweating; trembling or shaking; body temperature going from hot to cold or cold to hot; chest pain; shortness of breath or choking; fear of losing control or going crazy; feeling like you are going to die; and numbing/tingling sensations (American Psychiatric Association, 2000). Panic attacks can either be cued by the situation, be predisposed by the situation, or appear to come out of the blue. A panic attack that occurs for no apparent reason is known as panic disorder.

With PD, once the individual experiences the uncued panic attack, one begins to worry that it will happen again. This worry is a hallmark of PD and can lead to agoraphobia. Agoraphobia is defined as fear of having a panic attack and not being able to get out or get help. Because of this fear, an individual begins to avoid going places where he or she believes a panic attack may take place or where he or she has previously experienced a panic attack. Agoraphobic avoidance can range from mild to severe. Most individuals who are diagnosed with PD report some form of agoraphobic avoidance.

Unlike their White or Hispanic counterparts, African Americans with PD also experience recurrent isolated sleep paralysis (ISP). ISP occurs just before falling asleep or just before waking up and makes one feel as though he or she cannot move (Bell, Dixie-Bell, & Thompson, 1986; Bell & Jenkins, 1994). During this period, an individual experiences vivid hallucinations or feeling of acute danger. When the paralysis ends, the individual sits up and experiences panic-like symptoms, including tachycardia, hyperventilation, and fear (Bell et al., 1986; Neal, Nagle, Smith, & Smucker, 1994). Among African Americans with southern roots, the phenomenon is often referred to as "witch riding" (Bell et al., 1986; Walker, 2003). Current research suggests that recurrent ISP may either be a precursor to or a different manifestation of panic (Bell & Jenkins, 1994; Carter, Sbrocco, & Carter, 1996; Friedman & Paradis, 2002; Neal et al., 1994). Numerous African Americans with essential hypertension also experience recurrent ISP, suggesting a mind–body connection (Bell, Hildreth, Jenkins, & Carter, 1988; Neal et al., 1994). Untreated, recurrent isolated sleep paralysis and PD may affect an individual's blood pressure and be a contributing factor in the development of hypertension (Bell et al., 1988; Neal et al., 1994; Neal-Barnett, 2003).

## Obsessive–Compulsive Disorder

OCD is characterized by unwanted, unreasonable, and intrusive repetitive thoughts, images, or ideas (obsessions) that create a high level of anxiety and are relieved by repetitive and excessive behaviors (compulsions). The most widespread obsessions center on contamination/germs, behavior affecting well-being, and inappropriate sexual thoughts and sin. Common compulsions include washing, cleaning, checking, counting, and praying (American Psychiatric Association, 2000).

Clinical evidence suggests that rates of OCD may be higher among African Americans (Williams, Chambless, & Steketee, 1998; Williams & Turkheimer 2007). A review of the literature finds that, based on OCD measurement scale scores, African Americans endorse clinically significant higher levels of anxiety related to contamination and washing (Williams & Turkheimer, 2007). In-depth analysis has found that these higher scores are directly related to African Americans' attitudes about cleanliness; when statistically controlled, the higher levels of reported anxiety disappear (Williams & Turkheimer, 2007).

## Generalized Anxiety Disorder

GAD is a chronic, debilitating form of anxiety involving excessive worry and physical tension (American Psychiatric Association, 2000). Individuals with GAD constantly engage in "what if" thinking. The excessive worry associated with GAD may literally "make one sick." Illnesses associated with GAD include irritable bowel syndrome and ulcers (Neal-Barnett, 2003). Worry and the negativity associated with it breed depression. Many people with GAD experience some form of clinical depression (U.S. Department of Health and Human Services, 2006). Little published research is available about the manifestation of GAD among African Americans.

## Social Anxiety Disorder/Social Phobia

SAP is an excessive fear of being criticized or evaluated in social or performance situations. The disorder may be confined to one type of social/performance situation (i.e., giving a speech) or may generalize to almost all social situations (American Psychiatric Association, 2000). Research suggests that for African American adolescents and emerging adults issues such as racial socialization, racial identity, and the accusation of "acting White" may play a role in the manifestation of this disorder (Breslau et al., 2006; Neal-Barnett, 2003, 2004).

## Specific Phobias

SPs involve excessive fear in the presence of objects, animals, and nonevaluative nonperformance situations that pose little or no threat. Common SPs include animals, blood, and injury (American Psychiatric Association, 2000). Whereas it is true that everyone is afraid of something, for individuals with SPs the fear is excessive and interferes with their lives. Many people with SPs experience panic attacks in the presence of the feared stimulus. Early epidemiological data suggested that SPs were more prevalent among African Americans (Neal & Turner, 1991). Subsequent epidemiological studies have indicated the opposite (Kessler et al., 1994, 2004).

## Posttraumatic Stress Disorder

PTSD develops after experiencing or witnessing a terrifying event that involved physical harm or the threat of physical harm. An import caveat is that not everyone who experiences or witnesses a traumatic event develops PTSD. Indeed, the available data indicate that after a traumatic event only 8% of men and 20% of women develop the disorder. PTSD is characterized by emotional numbness, avoidance of remindful situations and people, reexperiencing of the event via flashbacks, quick startle response, and extreme hypervigilance (American Psychiatric Association, 2000).

African American women are three to five times more likely than White women to experience trauma through victimization and violence (Neal-Barnett & Crowther, 2000; Wyatt, 1998), leading some to hypothesize that PTSD may be higher among this group. The available data from the NCS and NCS-R studies (Breslau et al., 2005, 2006) do not bear this out.

## African American Children and Anxiety Disorder Diagnoses

All children occasionally feel fearful, anxious, or worried; therefore, it is important to distinguish normal fears and worries from pathological anxiety. Pathological anxiety is defined as fears or worries that are experienced frequently, cause subjective discomfort, have been present for some time, and result in some interference/impairment in functioning at home, at school, or with peers (Christophersen & Mortweet, 2001).

Although children can develop any of the aforementioned DSM-IV-TR-identified anxiety disorders, some tend to be more common. For example, SAD, the experiencing of extreme anxiety when separated from one's parents or primary caregiver, and SP tend to be more common in school-age children (i.e., 6–9 years old), whereas GAD and SAP may be more common in later childhood and adolescence. PD may be more common in adolescence (Anxiety Disorders Association of America, 2008). As for African American adults, little information is available about the manifestation of anxiety disorders in African American youth.

## RISK AND RESILIENCE FACTORS

One's risk and resilience to the development of an anxiety disorder is biopsychosocial in nature. Several factors, not just one, combine to influence the development and maintenance of an anxiety disorder. Given the lower prevalence of anxiety disorders in African Americans and the higher persistence rates among those who develop the disorders, Breslau and colleagues (2006) have hypothesized that resiliencies developed in childhood and adolescence serve as proactive factors for African Americans. In these next sections, we explore a variety of anxiety risk and resilience factors for African American adults and children.

## Biological/Genetic Factors

A single gene does not account for the development of anxiety disorders in African Americans. However, some individuals appear to have a genetic predisposition for anxiety. Technical advances in genetics have allowed researchers to learn more about the role of genes in anxiety development. Using these advances, as reported in Neal-Barnett (2003), Canadian researchers found that individuals who suffer from panic attacks had a gene that increased the level of the chemical cholecystokinin in their brain. Research with German women (Montag et al., 2008) found that individuals with a common variation of the catechol-O-methyltransferase gene have an exaggerated startle reflex when viewing unpleasant pictures. The researchers hypothesize that this sensitivity, in combination with other biopsychosocial risk factors, may place women with this gene variation at higher risk for anxiety disorders (Montag et al., 2008).

Hormonal changes also appear to place women at risk for the development of anxiety. Lower levels of the female hormones estrogen and progesterone are associated with panic attacks. For this reason, it is not unusual to find women experiencing their first panic attack when pregnant or to find an increase in panic attacks among pregnant panic patients (Neal-Barnett, 2003).

The advances in brain imaging and neurochemical research provide a better understanding of the role that various parts of the brain play in the development of anxiety. Brain scans have identified the amygdala, an almond-shaped structure deep in the brain, as the section that alerts the rest of the brain that a threat is present and triggers a fear or anxiety response (U.S. Department of Health and Human Services, 2006). Emotional memories appear to be stored in the amygdala, and these memories may play a role in the development of certain specific phobias (U.S. Department of Health and Human Services, 2006).

The hippocampus, located within the left temporal lobe, is the part of the brain that affects our short-term memory. This region also encodes threatening events into memories. Research reveals that the hippocampus of individuals who were victims of child abuse or who served in military combat is smaller than those who have not experienced these traumatic events (U.S. Department of Health and Human Services, 2006). This finding has implications for PTSD, and more research is being conducted to ascertain the role of the hippocampus in the development of PTSD (U.S. Department of Health and Human Services, 2006).

The periaqueductal gray region of the brain is associated with flight–fright–freeze response to threat (Mobbs et al., 2007). Research has found that this response is activated more quickly in women and remains activated longer. Although African Americans participate in genetic studies, to the best of our knowledge, no evidence currently exists that indicates racial differences in genetic risk or resilience for anxiety disorders.

Several studies with children lend support for a genetic component to the development of anxiety. For example, twin studies of children with anxiety have found that genetics account for a significant amount of the variance (up to half in some studies) in self-reported and parent-reported anxiety (Eaves et al., 1997; Topolski et al., 1997). In addition, studies have shown that the rate for first-degree biological relatives of youth with anxiety disorders is higher than in the general population (Last, Hersen, Kazdin, Orvaschel, & Perrin, 1991; S. M. Turner, Beidel, & Costello, 1987). Data from these studies, however, have not provided proof of a direct link between a specific gene or genetic pathway and anxiety. Rather, they suggest that children inherit a "general vulnerability" (i.e., general risk factor) for anxiety disorders (Barlow, 2002; S. M. Turner et al., 1987).

It should be noted that African American children are included in the sample for some of the heritability studies (e.g., S. M. Turner et al., 1987), but there is not enough evidence to support or refute the heritability of a genetic risk factor for African American children. The same is true for biological factors. Researchers at the National Institute of Mental Health have reported that there appears to be a relationship between OCD and group A beta-hemolytic streptococcal infection, or strep throat (da Rocha, Correa, & Teixeira, 2008); however, there has been very little research on this relationship in African American children.

## Individual Factors Influencing Risk and Resiliency

### Gender

Being female places one at higher risk for the development of anxiety disorders (U.S. Department of Health and Human Services, 2006). Based on the published research, African American females appear more at risk than African American males. Little research exists overall on adult gender differences in anxiety, and there is a paucity of research on African American adult males and anxiety disorders (Neal & Turner, 1991; Neal-Barnett, 2003).

Research is available, however, to suggest that female gender may be a risk factor for the development of anxiety in African American children. Douglas and Rice (1979) studied anxiety symptoms using standardized self-report measures for 80 fifth and sixth graders and found that girls had higher general anxiety scores than boys. Similarly, a study of somatic symptoms and anxiety in African American adolescents revealed that girls reported significantly more somatic symptoms than boys (Kingery, Ginsburg, & Alfano, 2007). Results suggest that African American girls may be slightly more at risk than their male counterparts for developing anxiety, although this may not be true for all. McLaughlin, Hilt, and Nolen-Hoeksema (2007) found that African American males reported significantly higher levels of physiological anxiety than other males of other races and higher levels, but not significantly so, than African American females.

### Age

Older and younger African Americans appear to be at higher risk for the development of certain anxiety disorders. According to data from the African American subsample of the National Survey of American Life (Jackson et al., 2004), older African Americans are at higher risk for development of PTSD and social phobia (Ford et al., 2007).

Pubertal maturation research has shown that children who experience early puberty are at risk for emotional distress. Ge, Brody, Conger, and Simons (2006) examined the relationship between pubertal maturation and internalizing and externalizing symptoms in 867 10- to 12-year-old African American children. Pubertal status and timing (i.e., early maturity) were associated with symptoms of GAD for African American girls and boys. It is notable that the same relationship was not found for adolescents who matured late (Ge et al., 2006).

### Anxiety Sensitivity

"Anxiety sensitivity is the belief that anxiety-related symptoms have negative physical, social, and psychological consequences" (Neal-Barnett, 2004, p. 277).

This construct has received support in the larger literature as a risk factor for anxiety, especially PD (Schmidt, Lerew, & Jackson, 1997). Little research has been conducted on anxiety sensitivity in African American adult samples. In a factor analysis of the Anxiety Sensitivity Index, M. M. Carter, Miller, Sbrocco, Suchday, and Lewis (1999) found that, rather than the often-reported three-factor solution, a fourth factor emerged: mental incapacitation. It should be noted that Carter and colleagues' sample was composed of college students.

Some research studies suggest that anxiety sensitivity may be elevated in African American children (Lambert, Cooley, Campbell, Benoit, & Stansbury, 2004), but this has not been true for all samples (Ginsburg & Drake, 2002a). Lambert, Cooley, and colleagues (2004) administered an anxiety sensitivity measure, the Childhood Anxiety Sensitivity Index (Silverman, Fleisig, Rabian, & Peterson, 1991), to 140 inner-city fourth- and fifth-grade African American children. Results revealed that the proposed factor structure (three factors) did not fit the data. Exploratory factor analysis revealed two factors: physical concerns and mental incapacitation concerns. Mental incapacitation also emerged in the Carter and colleagues (1999) college student study, suggesting a possible unique factor for anxiety sensitivity among African Americans.

In a follow-up study, Lambert, McCreary, Joiner, Schmidt, and Ialongo (2004) found that fear of cardiovascular sensations and fear of unsteadiness were uniquely related to anxiety in African American adolescents. Thus, African American children with high levels of anxiety sensitivity to physical symptoms and feelings of unsteadiness may be at an increased risk for developing anxiety disorders.

### Racial Identity

Racial identity is defined as that part of a person's self-concept that is related to membership within a specific race (African American Racial Identity Research Lab, 2008; Sellers & Shelton, 2003; Sellers, Smith, Shelton, Rowley, & Chavous, 1998; Yip, Seaton, & Sellers, 2006). Some researchers use the terms *racial identity* and *ethnic identity* synonymously, whereas others argue that the two are different. Within the anxiety disorders literature, the former approach appears to have been adopted. Several researchers have highlighted the importance of considering racial identity when examining mental health and well-being among African Americans (Banks & Kohn-Wood, 2007; Carter, 1995; Franklin-Jackson & Carter, 2007; Marks, Settles, Cooke, Morgan, & Sellers, 2004). Carter and colleagues (1996) have theorized that various levels of racial identity would impact not only one's vulnerability to anxiety but also how one chooses to cope with anxiety. Despite Carter and colleagues' development of a testable theoretical framework, few researchers have examined racial identity and anxiety disorders. Carter and coauthors (2005) reported an inverse relationship between ethnic identity and state–trait anxiety, with greater levels of ethnic identity associated with lower levels of anxiety in a college student sample (Carter et al., 2005). Neal-Barnett,

Statom, and Stadulis (2003) examined the impact of racial identity on the manifestation and perception of trichotillomania, an anxiety-related disorder, among middle-class African American women. Results indicated that the racial identity dimensions of public and private regard directly influenced women's perceptions of the disorder and how it interfered in their lives (Neal-Barnett et al., 2003). The regard dimensions tap into socioevaluative perceptions of being African American by the outside world and by one's self (African American Racial Identity Research Lab, 2008).

Among adolescents, higher levels of racial identity serve as a buffer for psychological distress, including anxiety. In particular, racial identity is found to have a buffering effect against discrimination, a societal stressor (Caldwell, Zimmerman, Hilkene, Sellers, & Notaro, 2002; Sellers, Caldwell, Schmeelk-Cone, & Zimmerman, 2003).

Racial socialization may also play an influential role in the development of anxiety. A study by Silverman, La Greca, and Wasserstein (1995) found that African American boys reported more performance worries than African American girls. One explanation for this finding is that it actually reflects the differences in socialization of African American boys and girls (Safren et al., 2000). Although African American boys may be reinforced for performing both at school and in extracurricular activities, African American girls may be reinforced for succeeding more in relational or social areas. Thus, it would follow that boys would develop more performance-related fears and girls more social fears.

### *Spirituality*

Spirituality is an essential part of the African American personality and appears to serve as a protective factor against anxiety disorders (Brown & Keith, 2003; Chatters & Taylor, 1989; Cook & Wiley, 2000; Lawson & Thomas, 2007). An analysis of several national data sets (Taylor, Chatters, Jayakody, & Levin, 1996) found that eight of 10 African Americans reported that religious beliefs are very important to them, and 43.6% said they "almost always" sought spiritual comfort through religion.

Older adults use spirituality and spiritual activities to cope with negative life events (Koenig, George, & Seigler, 1988; Krause & Van Tran, 1989; Lawson & Thomas, 2007). Prayer is a daily component of older African Americans' lives, as revealed by approximately 78% of Chatters and Taylor's (1989) sample, and is an important source of emotional support and coping for African American adults (Cook & Wiley, 2000; McAdoo, 1995).

Directly related to anxiety disorders, qualitative research with older African American Katrina survivors reveals that spirituality, prayer, belief in a higher power, daily Bible reading, and service facilitated coping with the traumatic events of the storm (Lawson & Thomas, 2007). McLeish and Del Ben (2008) found that prayer was effective in decreasing PTSD symptoms among Katrina survivors receiving services from an outpatient clinic. In our own work with middle-class African

American women, spiritual affirmations are used as a form of self-talk to alleviate anxiety associated with panic attacks (Neal-Barnett, 2003, 2008). Research with African American children living in urban poverty has suggested that spirituality serves as a buffer in the development of anxiety (Breslau et al., 2006).

## Temperament

Evidence exists for a relationship between temperament (i.e., behavioral inhibition) and anxiety disorders in children. Longitudinal research studies have corroborated the link between behavioral inhibition and the development of anxiety disorders (Biederman et al., 2001), and research has supported a predictive relationship between behavioral inhibition and anxiety disorders such as social anxiety disorder. This link is suspected to exist for African American children, although the available research is extremely limited. African American children, have been included in the samples of studies of behavioral inhibition and anxiety, but we were unable to find one study examining behavioral inhibition in a predominantly African American sample.

## Other Individual Risk Factors in Children

The presence of test anxiety in African American children may increase their risk of developing an anxiety disorder. One study found a higher rate of test anxiety in urban lower socioeconomic status (SES) African American children, and these children were more likely to have symptoms of social anxiety disorder (B. G. Turner, Beidel, Hughes, & Turner, 1993). These children were also more likely to score lower on academic achievement tests and on measures of perceived social competencies, cognitive competencies, and general self-concept. The presence of anxiety symptoms at an early age may be an additional risk factor. Grover, Ginsburg, and Ialongo (2005) found that African American children who showed anxiety symptoms in first grade were more likely to demonstrate anxiety symptoms in eighth grade (Grover, Ginsburg, & Ialongo, 2007).

## Family Factors Influencing Risk and Resiliency

Little information is available regarding the role of family factors in the development of anxiety among African American adults (Neal-Barnett, 2003). A naturalistic study of Black and White women with PD and agoraphobia found that, significantly more so than Whites, Black women had experienced the early loss of a parent via death, divorce, or estrangement (Friedman, Paradis, & Hatch, 1994).

Assessment and treatment outcome studies point toward the central role of familial factors in the development of anxiety disorders in children (Barrett, Dadds, & Rapee, 1996; S. M. Turner, Beidel, Roberson-Nay, & Tervo, 2003). S. M. Turner and colleagues (2003) examined the role of familial factors in African

American families by assessing and comparing the parenting behaviors of African American and White parents diagnosed with an anxiety disorder with behaviors of their counterparts with no diagnosis. Results suggested that the role of transmission from parents to children is complex. Anxiety may be transmitted via social learning and information transfer.

In addition, the emotional climate of the family may also influence the development of anxiety in children. Families of anxious parents rated the family environment lower on expressiveness. Anxious parents also reported feelings of distress when their children engaged in risk-taking behaviors. An unexpected finding was that anxious parents remained physically distant and were more likely to engage in play with their child through conversation rather than physical proximity (S. M. Turner et al., 2003). Other studies have reported similar characteristics of anxious parents. Barrett and colleagues (1996) found that anxious parents spend a significant amount of time discussing threatening situations, misinterpret ambiguous cues, and reinforce avoidance.

Grover and colleagues' (2005) study provides further support for the role of family factors in the development of anxiety symptoms in African American children. They examined childhood predictors of anxiety symptoms in a predominantly African American sample of 149 children. Results indicated that children who experienced a negative family environment, grief-related losses, and academic failures by first grade had higher levels of anxiety in sixth grade.

Dulmus and Wodarski (2000) examined the relationship between parental victimization and distress symptoms in 30 6- to 12-year-old African American children. Results showed that parents of children who were victimized exhibited higher levels of distress, lending support to the role of family victimization in the development of anxiety symptoms.

Family composition may also be a risk factor for developing anxiety. Results from a study by Barbarin and Soler (1993) indicate that children with single mothers reported higher levels of anxiety than children with multiple caregivers. Additional research is needed to better understand the role of the family in the development of anxiety disorders for African American children.

## Social and Community Factors Influencing Risk and Resiliency

### Socioeconomic Status

Among the many social and community factors that can serve as risk factors for African American adults, SES, racism, and discrimination appear to stand out. Much has been written about poverty's role in mental health. It is not necessarily being poor that places one at risk but rather the associated consequences of poverty (e.g., inadequate housing, lack of access to resources, education). Recent epidemiological research, however, suggests that resilience factors that are present early in one's life, such as spirituality, racial identity, and cultural values/ethnic socialization, may negate poverty's impact on anxiety development (Breslau et al., 2006).

The bulk of the research on African American adults and anxiety has focused on low-income samples. Information on how middle-income status affects anxiety is sparse. Neal-Barnett (2003) and Neal-Barnett and Crowther (2000) suggest that middle-income women are often seen as "strong Black women." The pressure and stress of being all things to all segments of the Black community may increase anxiety. In a diary study examining blood pressure and panic attacks, middle-class Black women recorded their activities and emotions while wearing an ambulatory blood pressure machine (Neal-Barnett, 2003). Based on their dairies, anxiety was not experienced; however, the blood pressure and heart rate data revealed a different story. When questioned about the discrepancies, many women replied, "Baby, if I thought about that, I'd have to think about everything" (Neal-Barnett & Crowther, 2000).

Children from families with lower SES levels tend to be at higher risk for mental health problems, including anxiety disorders. Minority youth are disproportionately represented in the lower SES strata (American Psychological Association Task Force on Resilience and Strength in Black Children and Adolescents, 2008). The contribution of SES to the development of anxiety cannot be underestimated. In fact, SES is a significant confound in studies that examine racial differences in anxiety (Papay & Hedl, 1978).

### Racism

Racism is a societal stressor that has been hypothesized to place African Americans at risk for anxiety (Carter et al., 1996; Neal & Turner, 1991; Neal-Barnett, 2003). To date, research specifically examining racism as a variable in the development of anxiety disorders appears nonexistent. A small body of literature exists, however, that demonstrates race-related stress, which includes racism, to be a powerful risk factor for psychological distress (Utsey, 1999; Utsey, Giesbrecht, Hook, & Stanard, 2008). Psychological factors such as optimism and ego resilience serve as protective factors against racism.

### Peer Victimization

Storch and Esposito (2003) examined the relationship between peer victimization and PTSD symptoms in Hispanic and African American children. Consistent with available research on White adolescents, victimization, both overt and relational, was associated with PTSD, indicating that children who are bullied are at increased risk for developing an anxiety disorder.

### Cultural Values

Cultural values may also play a role in the development of anxiety in African American children. It is hypothesized that children will show less anxiety about things that are not consistent with their cultural, familial, or community values. Support from this hypothesis comes from the work of Silverman and colleagues (1995), who interviewed 141 boys and 132 girls in the second through seventh grades at a public school and also had the children complete self-report measures of anxiety. Their results indicated that African American children (33% of the sample) reported more worries related to war, personal harm, family, and health than White children. These results have been discussed in light of differences in cultural values. That is, worries related to school may not be as prominent for African American children who live in a community that values communalism, harmony, and a present time orientation rather than competition, individualism, and a future time orientation. In fact, these children may experience more social fears.

Similarly, fears/anxiety may develop related to contextual or situational factors. This is supported by early research that examined fears of African American children in community samples. A study by Lapouse and Monk (1959) found that Black children had greater fear regarding the use of other people's property. Given the racial and social climate of the 1950s, when the research was conducted, this is not surprising. At that time, it was reasonable, and some would argue healthy, for Black children to develop a fear of the use of other people's property given the consequences for using a White person's property (Safren et al., 2000).

Another example of the contribution of contextual factors to the development in anxiety in children comes from the research on community violence and anxiety. That there is an association between community violence and anxiety in urban youth has been well documented (Garbarino, Kostelny, & Dubrow, 1991). Exposure to violence has an adverse affect on children's functioning and has been associated with increased psychological distress, including anxiety disorders (Cooley-Quille, Boyd, Frantz, & Walsh, 2001). Although the association between community violence and anxiety disorders is complex, it is clear that exposure to community violence is a risk factor for anxiety disorders in children. Given that African American youth are more likely to experience community violence, some boys and girls may be especially vulnerable to developing anxious symptoms.

Kliewer and colleagues (2004) has examined resiliency factors for African American children that may mediate the relationship between internalizing disorders/adjustment problems and community violence. The study identified the following factors as mediating this relationship: internal locus of control, high self-efficacy, optimism, and goal orientation (Kliewer et al., 2004).

## EVIDENCE-BASED TREATMENT INTERVENTIONS

### What Works

Treatment studies conducted primarily with Whites have found various forms of cognitive-behavioral therapy (CBT) to be most effective in the treatment of adult anxiety disorders (U.S. Department of Health and Human Services, 2006).

As it relates to anxiety, CBT consists of three major components: understanding the relationship among thoughts, emotions, and behaviors; alleviating physical symptoms of anxiety; and eliminating avoidance or agoraphobic behavior (Neal-Barnett, 2003). Common techniques of CBT include progressive relaxation, self-monitoring, self-talk, and exposure. As with almost all aspects of research on African American adults and anxiety, open and randomized controlled intervention studies are extremely limited. The glaring absence of intervention research was highlighted during the 2008 conference, "Culturally Informed Evidence Based Practices: Translating Research and Policy for the Real World," where anxiety interventions were not part of the agenda.

The Society of Clinical Child and Adolescent Psychology, Committee on Evidence-Based Practice, developed a list of empirically validated treatments for children and adolescents with anxiety disorders, depression, attention-deficit/hyperactivity disorder, and conduct/oppositional problems (Society of Clinical Child and Adolescent Psychology, n.d.). The list provides information about well-established and promising treatments for childhood anxiety disorders. Well-established treatments are those for which at least two studies have shown the treatment to be efficacious compared with another treatment, placebo or medication, or in a large number of single-case design trials. Studies of well-established treatments involve the use of a treatment manual, provide specifics about the sample and randomization procedures, and have been replicated by at least one other set of researchers. Promising or probably efficacious treatments are those for which at least one study shows the treatment is more effective than a medication, another treatment or placebo, two studies show the treatment is more effective than a waiting-list control or a small number of single-case design studies.

The only childhood anxiety disorder with well-established treatments (Participant Modeling and Reinforced Practice) listed on the Society of Clinical Child and Adolescent Psychology evidence-based website is specific phobia. Participant modeling is a combination of modeling and in vivo exposure. This treatment involves a therapist or peer modeling positive coping responses in a fearful situation and then having the therapist or peer coach the child through the situation. Treatment begins with easier situations and moves toward more difficult/fearful situations. Reinforced practice builds on this treatment and involves providing rewards to the child for practicing engaging in and coping with feared situations (Society of Clinical Child and Adolescent Psychology, n.d.).

A recent systematic review of efficacy of CBT for childhood anxiety disorders indicated that CBT is beneficial for children older than 6 years (Cartwright-Hatton, Roberts, Chitsabesan, Fothergill, & Harrington, 2004). Most studies report that children who receive CBT have a reduction in symptoms and that these gains are maintained for at least 1 year (Cartwright-Hatton et al., 2004). CBT involves teaching children to alter their thoughts and learn new behaviors in anxiety-provoking situations. Children learn to identify anxiety triggers, decrease anxiety-laden thoughts, and practice effective coping strategies. CBT has been provided to children individually, as a family-based intervention, and via groups (Virginia

Commission on Youth, 2003). CBT-based family interventions typically entail teaching parents to reward coping behaviors and to redirect or ignore fear-laden behaviors (e.g., complaining). Parents are also instructed in communication and problem-solving skills. CBT-based family interventions have been found to be effective for children with anxiety disorders, particularly separation anxiety, but may not be as beneficial for adolescents. Group CBT treatments have been found to be effective in reducing anxiety symptoms for children in clinical and school-based settings (Virginia Commission on Youth, 2003). A modular approach to CBT has also been proposed (Friedberg & Gorman, 2007).

The existing data suggest that CBT is equally effective across racial and gender groups (Beidel et al., 2007; Treadwell, Flannery-Schroeder, & Kendall, 1995). These studies have not conceptualized race outside of racial group membership. Neal-Barnett (2004) has suggested that, in order to fully understand whether CBT is effective, researchers must incorporate psychological aspects of race (i.e., racial identity, racial socialization, accusation of acting White) into the treatment design.

## What Might Work

To date, only one randomized control study has been published on PD treatment for African American women. Using Barlow's panic control therapy, Carter, Sbrocco, Gore, Marin, and Lewis (2003) provided group treatment for 14 African American women. Group treatment was chosen because it meshed with sense of community observed among many African Americans. Women in the group treatment reported significant improvement compared with the 15 women assigned to a waiting-list control (Carter et al., 2003).

Carter and colleagues (2003) did not discuss what aspects of the treatment worked best. They noted, however, that they found it important to incorporate into the group treatment discussions regarding African Americans' beliefs about emotion, the role of the workplace in exacerbation of symptoms for African Americans, and the role of ethnicity in completing homework assignments. Although not empirically evaluated, the authors felt that inclusion of this culturally specific information made the treatment more effective (Carter et al., 2003).

Carter and colleagues' research (2003) suggests that a culture-infused group approach to panic treatment may be effective. Sister circles are groups that build on existing friendships, fictive kin networks, and the sense of community found among African Americans. The curriculum is embedded within a Black female cultural framework. Gaston, Porter, and Thomas (2007) have reported on the success of Prime Time Sister Circles to reduce health risk for middle-age African American women. The possibility exists that this intervention can be successful with certain anxiety diagnoses. Within out research lab, we have undertaken an exploratory open-trial study to determine the efficacy of sister circles in the treatment of panic attacks. Funded by the National Institute of Mental Health, data from the project's first phase confirm African American women's belief that a group approach that takes into account issues of race and gender would be beneficial in addressing panic (Neal-Barnett, 2008).

In addition to PD, some information is available regarding evidence-based treatment of PTSD in African American populations. In a clinical trial study of CBT for female sexual assault victims, Zoellner, Feeny, Fitzgibbons, and Foa (1999) found no difference between African American and Caucasian women's response to CBT. An ongoing clinical trial conducted with African American and White HIV-positive women with PTSD has found CBT in the form of brief prolonged exposure therapy to be effective (Lambert, 2007). At this point, what is unknown is whether, similar to panic, cultural issues need to be incorporated into PTSD interventions with African Americans.

Given the importance of spirituality in African Americans' lives and its perceived role as a buffer against the development of an anxiety disorder, alternative therapies might be considered. A link exists between spirituality and music (Lane, 1994). For generations, songs filled with messages of hope, encouragement, spirituality, and empowerment have permeated the hearts and minds of African Americans, often giving them the strength to persevere in the face of great odds. From a cognitive-behavioral standpoint, positive affirmations set to music could potentially be integrated into existing treatment for anxiety. In a therapeutic sense, music can be an excellent resource for teaching anxious people how to calm themselves, redirect their thoughts, and envision themselves free of fear and anxiety. Music has also been shown to relieve the physical symptoms of performance anxiety, a form of social phobia.

South Korean researchers have explored music's effect on psychiatric patients with anxiety and depressive disorder (Choi, Lee, & Lim, 2008). Patients who received a 15-session music intervention showed a significant decrease in anxiety symptoms, as measured by the state–trait anxiety scales, and depressive symptoms, as measured on the Beck Depression Scale, compared with patients who received treatment as usual (Choi et al., 2008).

CBT has been designated as a promising treatment for SAD, GAD, and SP in children (Society of Clinical Child and Adolescent Psychology, n.d.). Recent research suggests that CBT is also a promising treatment for SAP and OCD (Barrett, Farrell, Pina, Peris, & Piacentini, 2008). In addition, trauma-based CBT may be an effective treatment for children (Cohen, Deblinger, Mannarino, & Steer, 2004); however, more studies are needed before it can be labeled as promising.

Relaxation training is another form of treatment that has been designated as promising for GAD and SAD in children (Society of Clinical Child and Adolescent Psychology, n.d.). This treatment involves instructing children in exercises (e.g., diaphragmatic breathing) that help them achieve a state of physical relaxation. The goal is to provide them with skills to achieve a state of physical relaxation in anxiety-provoking situations.

With all promising treatments, it is essential that the therapist providing the intervention be sensitive to cultural issues. This is particularly true for youth because the therapist–child relationship appears to be a crucial component of treatment. Interventions with African Americans are less likely to be effective if the therapist is unfamiliar with various aspects of African American culture.

## What Does Not Work

Eye movement desensitization reprocessing (EMDR; Shapiro, 1989) has been touted as a viable treatment of PTSD. EMDR combines rapid eye movements with the visualization of the traumatic event (Shapiro, 1989). Research has found that the effective aspects of EMDR are its cognitive-behavioral components. The rapid eye movement aspect does not appear effective (Lilienfeld, 1996). A search of the literature does not reveal treatment studies specifically focused on African Americans and EMDR.

Some professional and lay experts have suggested that certain herbs or over-the-counter medications may be helpful in treating youth anxiety. It has also been suggested that medications used for more severe psychiatric difficulties may be helpful (Virginia Commission on Youth, 2003). There is no evidence for the effectiveness of antihistamines, neuroleptics (e.g., haloperidol), herbs, or over-the-counter medications (Virginia Commission on Youth, 2003) in treating childhood anxiety disorders.

Overall, the existing research speaks to the need for more evidence-based treatment research on African Americans and anxiety interventions. A combination of qualitative and quantitative research methods would appear necessary to facilitate this work. As discussed earlier in this chapter, certain cultural factors such as spirituality and racial identity appear to serve as buffers against anxiety. Community stakeholders might best inform research on how these factors promote resilience and whether and how they should be incorporated into existing evidence-based interventions. A hallmark of community-based participatory research is qualitative research including focus groups.

## PREVENTION

### What Works

Ideally, anxiety prevention begins in childhood. Too often, however, this is not the case. Most programs aimed at preventing the development of anxiety disorders in children target anxiety symptoms (e.g., anxiety sensitivity). These programs may take the form of primary/universal prevention programs (e.g., FRIENDS; Lowry-Webster, Barrett, & Dadds, 2001) with the goal of reducing anxiety symptoms in normal children or secondary/targeted prevention programs (e.g., Cool Teens; Cunningham & Wuthrich, 2007) that target children who screen positive on anxiety measures. Although prevention programs may not be effective for all youth, several have been shown to decrease anxiety symptoms in primary and high school children (Donovan & Spence, 2000). To date, there are not enough studies of any treatment to meet criteria for a well-established anxiety prevention program.

As indicated earlier, few African American adults are aware of the various forms of anxiety and their causes. As a result, anxiety symptoms go untreated, increasing the risk for development of a full-blown anxiety disorder. Education raises awareness, and often awareness leads to behavior that reduces the likelihood of symptoms turning into a disorder. For example, when an individual is feeling anxious, caffeine increases those feelings (Neal-Barnett, 2003). Simply raising awareness about caffeine's role in anxiety may make a marked difference. A review of the literature did not reveal studies on awareness education and anxiety prevention among African Americans.

Individuals who experience panic attack often misinterpret their bodily sensations. For example, an individual who has just walked up three flights of stairs may mistake difficulty catching her breath as the same sensation experienced with a panic attack. This erroneous belief can lead the individual to incorrectly believe she is having a panic attack when, in actuality, she is simply winded. Neal-Barnett (2003) reports that teaching African American women to correctly interpret and label physical sensations can be an effective form of prevention.

Biofeedback may serve as another form of prevention. Biofeedback encourages awareness of anxiety symptoms. The most common form of biofeedback, electromyography provides feedback on muscle tension (Mayo Clinic Staff, 2008). Muscle tension is a common symptom in GAD and in panic attacks. From a prevention standpoint, individuals can use biofeedback as a cue to begin to tense or relax their muscles. Biofeedback is also covered by most health insurance plans (Mayo Clinic Staff, 2008).

## What Might Work

Music may be an effective form of secondary prevention for African American adults with anxiety symptoms. Research has shown that music can affect one's muscle activity, heart rate, and skin temperature, all of which are associated with anxiety (Lane, 1994; Levitin, 2006; Walworth, 2003). Numerous studies have demonstrated music's impact on test and performance anxiety. Currently, the need exists for well-controlled prevention studies on music and anxiety prevention among African Americans.

CBT appears to be a promising treatment for both the secondary and tertiary prevention of anxiety disorders in children. Dadds, Spence, Holland, Barrett, and Laurens (1997) compared a family-based CBT group intervention with a monitoring group. This 10-week study included 128 7- to 14-year-old Australian children and their families. The intervention group showed a reduction in existing anxiety diagnosis and decreased onset of new anxiety diagnoses 6 months and 2 years after the intervention (Dadds et al., 1999). In a second study, 489 10- to 12-year-old children were enrolled in a 12-session, school-based CBT program (Barrett & Turner, 2001). The children were assigned to either an intervention group led by a psychologist, an intervention group led by a teacher, or a monitoring group. At the end of treatment, children in the intervention groups had fewer anxiety symptoms than those in the monitoring group. A later study by the same research group found similar results when classrooms were randomly assigned to the intervention or monitoring group (Lowry-Webster et al., 2001). This intervention was also found to be effective for primary and high school students from diverse backgrounds (Chinese, Yugoslavian, and mixed-ethnicity) (Barrett, Sonderegger, & Sonderegger, 2002).

Studies have demonstrated that CBT is a promising prevention treatment for African American youth. Cooley, Boyd, and Grades (2004) developed a preventive school-based intervention specifically for African American children exposed to community violence. Analyses revealed decreases in anxiety symptoms, including physiological symptoms, concentration problems, and environmental worries. Likewise, Ginsburg and Drake (2002b) adapted a group CBT intervention for African American adolescents. Despite the small sample size ($n = 12$), Ginsburg and Drake found that adapted intervention was superior to an attention control group.

## What Does Not Work

Exercise interventions have been proposed as a preventive treatment for childhood anxiety disorders. To date, the evidence does not support the effectiveness of these types of interventions (Lauren, Nordheim, Ekeland, Hagen, & Heian, 2006).

Some African American adolescents and adults use alcohol or marijuana to relieve their anxiety symptoms (Neal-Barnett, 2003). Neither has been proven as an effective means of prevention. Both forms of self-medication simply mask symptoms; when the effects of the substances abate, the anxiety still remains.

## PSYCHOPHARMACOLOGY AND ANXIETY

Anxiety medication is an issue that creates division among African Americans, particularly women. Many are reluctant to use medication because they believe it is a sign of weakness. The negative beliefs about medication may stem from a historical mistrust of medication. This stigma appears associated with the inability to manage one's mental health and beliefs about being a strong Black woman (Neal-Barnett, 2003; Neal-Barnett & Crowther, 2000; Wagner et al., 2005). Spiritual beliefs and reliance on a higher power may also influence medication decisions for anxious African Americans (Neal-Barnett, 2003).

For those African Americans who do look to medication as a cure for their anxiety, unfortunately there is no medication that alone will accomplish this task. Anxiety medication reduces the intensity and, in some cases, the amount of anxiety a person experiences. This reduction in anxiety, combined with behavioral or cognitive-behavioral intervention, facilitates the ability to overcome and manage anxiety.

The most widely prescribed medications for relieving anxiety can be divided into six categories: selective serotonin reuptake inhibiters (SSRIs), benzodiazepines, tricyclic antidepressants (TCAs), beta-blockers, azaspirones, and monoamine oxidase inhibitors (MAOIs).

## Selective Serotonin Reuptake Inhibitors

Fluvoxamine (Luvox), fluoxetine (Prozac), sertraline (Zoloft), paroxetine (Paxil), citalopram (Celexa), and escitalopram (Lexapro) are all SSRIs. These medications work by increasing the amount of serotonin, a hormone and neurotransmitter that is found between the nerves endings in the brain. Paroxetine is effective in reducing generalized anxiety and social anxiety symptoms. Both paroxetine and citalopram have been shown to alleviate panic attack symptoms. Research has found fluoxetine and fluvoxamine to be helpful in reducing obsessions (Neal-Barnett, 2003). Escitalopram is effective in the treatment of GAD. SSRIs are also the medication of choice for treatment of childhood anxiety disorders. Pediatric OCD is the only disorder for which medications have received an U.S. Food and Drug Administration (FDA) indication. The following SSRIs have been approved for use in childhood OCD: fluoxetine, sertraline, citalopram, and fluvoxamine (Seidel & Walkup, 2006). Care should be taken when prescribing SSRIs for anxious youth, particularly if the anxiety is accompanied by depression. The FDA has issued a Black box warning regarding a tendency for an increase in suicidal thoughts in depressed adolescents and children (U.S. FDA, 2007).

## Benzodiazepines

Benzodiazepines are the earliest forms of antianxiety medication. This class of medication acts as a sedative and produces a calming affect on the body. Among some African Americans, benzodiazepines are known as "nerve pills." The mostly commonly prescribed benzodiazepines are alprazolam (Xanax), clonazepam (Klonopin), and lorazepam (Ativan). Unlike the SSRIs, which are taken on a daily basis, benzodiazepines are taken only as needed. Two major drawbacks exist to their use. First, when an individual discontinues the medication, a rebound effect occurs: the anxious symptomatology returns with greater frequency and intensity. Second, more so than other anxiety medications, benzodiazepines have an addictive quality, particularly when combined with alcohol. Benzodiazepines are contraindicated for children.

## Tricyclic Antidepressants

Although this class of medication is often used to treat depression, two TCAs, clomipramine (Anafranil) and impramine (Tofranil), are also used to treat anxiety. TCAs work by blocking the passage of natural neural chemical stimulants to the nerve endings of the brain, producing a calming effect. Clomipramine is prescribed to reduce obsessive thoughts associated with OCD; it has also been approved for use in childhood OCD (Seidel & Walkup, 2006). Imipramine is used to control panic attacks (Neal-Barnett, 2003)

## Beta-Blockers

Many African Americans are familiar with beta-blockers because they are used to control blood pressure. Beta-blockers reduce anxiety by lowering one's heart rate and blood pressure, thereby reducing symptoms such as sweating, rapid heartbeat, and rapid body temperature changes. Specifically, two beta-blockers, atenolol (Tenormin) and propranolol (Inderal), help reduce social anxiety that is confined to one or two social situations. For anxiety difficulties, beta-blockers are taken on an as-needed basis. Once again, some African Americans eschew beta-blockers because they do not want to become overly dependent on medication to solve their anxiety problem. Beta-blockers are nonaddictive and have few side effects. Beta-blockers are not used in the treatment of childhood anxiety.

## Azaspirones

Buspirone (BuSpar) is the only medication in this category and is prescribed for adults. Although it is unclear how it works inside the body and the brain, buspirone works fairly quickly to reduce symptoms associated with generalized anxiety.

## Monoamine Oxidase Inhibitors

For adults whose anxiety has not been reduced using the other categories of medication, MAOIs are prescribed. These medications work by breaking down certain hormones in the brain. Commonly prescribed MAOIs for anxiety include phenelzine (Nardil) and tranylcypromine sulfate (Parnate).

The greatest drawback for MAOIs is that patients prescribed these must eliminate certain foods and beverages from their diet, including cheese, caffeine, chocolate, and cured and processed meats. These foods contain tyramine and when combined with a MAO inhibitor produce an adverse reaction. An MAOI patch has been approved by the FDA, which eliminates the need for food restrictions when using the medications (U.S. Food and Drug Administration, 2006).

## RECOMMENDED BEST PRACTICES

Simply stated, the empirical evidence needed to make a definitive statement regarding best practices for treating anxiety disorders in African American adults is lacking. CBT is effective in treating anxiety among predominantly Caucasian adult populations, and there is little reason to doubt it would be effective in African American populations. The broader question, however, is, will CBT be enough or is it, as at least one study has suggested, important to infuse cultural aspects into the treatment? Within the year, we anticipate research emerging from our own work (Neal-Barnett, 2008) to shed light on this issue.

What is apparent from research is that a need exists to educate African Americans about anxiety disorders. Many within the African American community are unaware of the diagnoses. Raising awareness is an important preventive step. For example, research has shown that among hypertensives panic attacks are erroneously viewed as symptoms of hypertension, an idiopathic disorder (Neal et al., 1994). Our own research with sister circles has highlighted the importance of psychoeducation (Neal-Barnett, 2008); many women are simple unaware that anxiety disorders have another name other than "bad nerves."

Despite the small number of evidence-based treatment studies with African American youth, the available research suggests that evidence-based treatments, particularly those incorporating CBT, are probably effective for this population and should be the first line of treatment, particularly given that many alternate treatments have not been tested. CBT has also been shown to be promising for anxiety prevention in youth (Cooley et al., 2004; Ginsburg & Drake, 2002a).

Ho (1992) has argued that ethnic minorities might respond best to treatments that are time limited, practical, goal oriented, and structured. In an effort to apply the treatment in a culturally responsive manner, the clinician should consider any culturally relevant issues and how they may impact treatment. The clinician should then make adaptations to meet each client's needs. Individualizing treatment provides greater flexibility and allows the clinician to take into account all relevant dimensions of culture (e.g., gender, developmental level). Adaptations are important, but additional research is needed to demonstrate the impact of cultural adaptations on treatment outcomes (Huey & Polo, 2008).

Research is needed to address gaps in the literature in understanding the prevalence of anxiety disorders in community and clinical samples, how anxiety is expressed, differences in the conceptualization of anxiety, best practices for the assessment of anxiety in African American adults and youth, and treatment outcomes. Studies need to better document the inclusion of African Americans and control for socioeconomic factors. Recruitment issues will also need to be addressed given concerns about participant bias. Studies across groups and within the African American population will help us better understand the correlates and predictors of anxiety. Studies would also be strengthened if they were conducted with adequate sample sizes. In addition, it will be important to use a variety of assessment methods and, when possible, cross-culturally valid instruments (Huey & Polo 2008).

## ACKNOWLEDGMENT

Work on this chapter was supported in part by Grant No. 5R21MH076722-02 awarded by the National Institute of Mental Health to Angela Neal-Barnett.

## REFERENCES

African American Racial Identity Research Lab. (2008, June). *The Multidimensional Inventory of Black Identity*. Retrieved June 30, 2008, from *http://sitemaher.umich.edu/aaril/home*.

American Psychiatric Association. (2000). *Diagnostic and statistical manual of mental disorders* (4th ed., text rev.). Washington, DC: Author.

American Psychological Association Task Force on Resilience and Strength in Black Children and Adolescents. (2008). *Resilience in African American children and adolescents: A vision for optimal development*. Washington, DC: Author.

Anxiety Disorders Association of America. (2008). *Anxiety disorders in children and teens*. Silver Spring, MD: Author. Retrieved August 1, 2008, from *www.adaa.org/GettingHelp/FocusOn/Children&Adolescents.asp*.

Banks, K. H., & Kohn-Wood, L. P. (2007). The influence of racial identity profiles on the relationship between racial discrimination and depressive symptoms. *Journal of Black Psychology, 33*, 331–354.

Barbarin, O. A., & Soler, R. E. (1993). Behavioral, emotional, and academic adjustment in a national probability sample of African American children: Effects of age, gender, and family structure. *Emotional Development of African American Children, 19*(4), 423–446.

Barlow, D. H. (2002). *Anxiety and its disorders: The nature and treatment of anxiety and panic* (2nd ed.). New York: Guilford Press.

Barrett, P., & Turner, C. (2001). Prevention of anxiety symptoms in primary school children: Preliminary results from a universal school-based trial. *British Journal of Clinical Psychology, 40*(4), 399–401.

Barrett, P. M., Dadds, M. R., & Rapee, R. M. (1996). Family treatment of childhood anxiety: A controlled trial. *Journal of Consulting and Clinical Psychology, 64*(2), 333–342.

Barrett, P. M., Farrell, L., Pina, A. A., Peris, T. S., & Piacentini, J. (2008). Evidence-based psychosocial treatments for child and adolescent obsessive–compulsive disorder. *Journal of Clinical Child and Adolescent Psychology, 37*(1), 131–155.

Barrett, P. M., Sonderegger, R., & Sonderegger, N. L. (2002). Assessment of child and adolescent migrants to Australia: A crosscultural comparison. *Behaviour Change, 19*(4), 220–235.

Beidel, D. C., Turner, S. M., Sallee, F. R., Ammerman, R. T., Crosby, L. A., & Pathak, S. (2007). SET-C versus fluoxetine in the treatment of childhood social phobia. *Journal of the American Academy of Child and Adolescent Psychiatry, 46*(12), 1622–1632.

Bell, C. C., Dixie-Bell, D. D., & Thompson, B. (1986). Further studies on the prevalence of isolated sleep paralysis in Black subjects. *Journal of the National Medical Association, 72*, 331–334.

Bell, C. C., Hildreth, C. J., Jenkins, E. J., & Carter, C. (1988). The relationship of isolated sleep paralysis and panic disorder to hypertension. *Journal of the National Medical Association, 80,* 289–294.

Bell, C. C., & Jenkins, E. J. (1994). Isolated sleep paralysis and anxiety disorders. In S. Friedman (Ed.), *Anxiety disorders in African Americans* (pp. 117–127). New York: Springer.

Biederman, J., Hirshfeld-Becker, D. R., Rosenbaum, J. F., Herot, C., Friedman, D., Snidman, N., et al. (2001). Further evidence of association between behavioral inhibition and social anxiety in children. *American Journal of Psychiatry, 158*(10), 1673–1679.

Breslau, J., Gaxiola-Aguilar, S., Su, M., Williams, D., & Kessler, R. (2006). Specifying race-ethnic differences in risk for psychiatric disorder in USA national sample. *Psychological Medicine, 36,* 57–68.

Breslau, J., Kendler, K. S., Su, M., Gaxiola-Aguilar, S., & Kessler, R. (2005). Lifetime risk and persistence of psychiatric disorders across ethnic groups in the United States. *Psychological Medicine, 35,* 317–327.

Brown, D. R., & Keith, V. (2003). *In and out of our right minds: The mental health of African American women.* New York: Columbia University Press.

Caldwell, C. H., Zimmerman, M. A., Hilkene, D., Sellers, R. M., & Notaro, P. (2002). Racial identity, maternal support and psychological distress among African American adolescents. *Child Development, 73,* 1322–1336.

Carter, M. M., Miller, O., Sbrocco, T., Suchday, S., & Lewis, E. L. (1999). Factor structure of the Anxiety Sensitivity Index among African-American college students. *Psychological Assessment, 11,* 525–533.

Carter, M. M., Sbrocco, T., & Carter, C. (1996). African Americans and anxiety disorders research: Development of a testable theoretical framework. *Psychotherapy, 33,* 449–463.

Carter, M. M., Sbrocco, T., Gore, K. L., Marin, N. W., & Lewis, E. L. (2003). Cognitive behavior therapy versus a wait list control in the treatment of African American women with panic disorder. *Cognitive Therapy and Research, 27*(5), 505–518.

Carter, M. M., Sbrocco, T., Miller, O., Suchday, S., Lewis, E., L., & Freedman, R. E. K. (2005). Factor structure, reliability, and validity of the Penn State Worry Questionnaire: Differences between African-American and White-American college students. *Journal of Anxiety Disorders, 19*(8), 827–843.

Carter, R. T. (1995). *The influence of race and racial identity in psychotherapy: Towards a racially inclusive model* (pp. 139–156). San Francisco: Wiley.

Cartwright-Hatton, S., Roberts, C., Chitsabesan, P., Fothergill, C., & Harrington, R. (2004). Systematic review of the efficacy of cognitive behaviour therapies for childhood and adolescent anxiety disorders. *British Journal of Clinical Psychology, 43*(2), 421–436.

Chatters L. M., & Taylor R. J. (1989). Life problems and coping strategies of older Black adults. *Social Work, 34,* 313–319.

Choi, A. N., Lee, M. S., & Lim, H. J. (2008). Effects of group music intervention on depression, anxiety, and relationships in a psychiatric population: A pilot study. *Journal of Alternative Complementary Medicine, 14*(5), 567–570.

Christophersen, E. R., & Mortweet, S. L. (2001). Diagnosis and management of anxiety disorders. In E. R. Christophersen & S. L. Mortweet (Eds.), *Treatments that work with children: Empirically supported strategies for managing childhood problems* (pp. 49–78). Washington, DC: American Psychological Association.

Cohen, J. A., Deblinger, E., Mannarino, A. P., & Steer, R. A. (2004). A multisite, randomized controlled trial for children with sexual abuse-related PTSD symptoms. *Journal of the American Academy of Child and Adolescent Psychiatry, 43*(4), 393–402.

Cook, D. A., & Wiley, C. Y. (2000). Psychotherapy with members of African American churches and spiritual traditions. In S. P. Richards & A. E. Bergin (Eds.), *Handbook of psychotherapy and religious diversity* (pp. 369–396) Washington, DC: American Psychological Association.

Cooley, M. R., Boyd, R. C., & Grades, J. J. (2004). Feasibility of an anxiety preventive intervention for community violence exposed African-American children. *Multiculturalism and Primary Prevention: Toward a New Primary Prevention Culture, 25*(1), 105–123.

Cooley-Quille, M., Boyd, R. C., Frantz, E., & Walsh, J. (2001). Emotional and behavioral impact of exposure to community violence in inner-city adolescents. *Journal of Clinical Child Psychology, 30*(2), 199–206.

Cunningham, M., & Wuthrich, V. (2007). Review of the Cool Teens CD-ROM: An anxiety management program for young people. *Journal of Family Studies, 13*(1), 104–108.

da Rocha, F. F., Correa, H., & Teixeira, A. L. (2008). Obsessive-compulsive disorder and immunology: A review. *Progress in Neuro-Psychopharmacology and Biological Psychiatry, 32*(5), 1139–1146.

Dadds, M. R., Holland, D. E., Laurens, K. R., Mullins, M., Barrett, P. M., & Spence, S. H. (1999). Early intervention and prevention of anxiety disorders in children: Results at 2-year follow-up. *Journal of Consulting and Clinical Psychology, 67*(1), 145–150.

Dadds, M. R., Spence, S. H., Holland, D. E., Barrett, P. M., & Laurens, K. R. (1997). Prevention and early intervention for anxiety disorders: A controlled trial. *Journal of Consulting and Clinical Psychology, 65*(4), 627–635.

Donovan, C. L., & Spence, S. H. (2000). Prevention of childhood anxiety disorders. *Clinical Psychology Review, 20*(4), 509–531.

Douglas, J. D., & Rice, K. M. (1979). Sex differences in children's anxiety and defensiveness measures. *Developmental Psychology, 15*(2), 223–224.

Dulmus, C. N., & Wodarski, J. S. (2000). Trauma-related symptomatology among children of parents victimized by urban community violence. *American Journal of Orthopsychiatry, 70*(2), 272–277.

Eaves, L. J., Silberg, J. L., Maes, H. H., Simonoff, E., Pickles, A., Rutter, M., et al. (1997). Genetics and developmental psychopathology: 2. The main effects of genes and environment on behavioral problems in the Virginia twin study of adolescent behavioral development. *Journal of Child Psychology and Psychiatry, 38*(8), 965–980.

Ford, B. C., Bullard, K., McKeever, K. M., Taylor, R. J., Toler, A. K., Neighbors, H. W., et al. (2007). Lifetime and 12-month prevalence of *Diagnostic and Statistical Manual of Mental Disorders*, fourth edition disorders among older African Americans: Findings from the National Survey of American life. *American Journal of Geriatric Psychiatry, 15*, 652–659.

Franklin-Jackson, D., & Carter, R. T. (2007). The relationship between race-related stress, racial identity, and mental health for Black Americans. *Journal of Black Psychology, 33*, 5–26.

Friedberg, R. D., & Gorman, A. A. (2007). Integrating psychotherapeutic processes with cognitive behavioral procedures. *Journal of Contemporary Psychotherapy, 37*(3), 185–193.

Friedman, S., & Paradis, C. (2002). Panic disorder in African-Americans: Symptomatology and isolated sleep paralysis. *Culture, Medicine, and Psychiatry, 26*, 179–198.

Friedman, S., Paradis, C., & Hatch, M. (1994). Characteristics of African American and White patients with panic disorder and agoraphobia. *Hospital and Community Psychiatry, 45*, 798–803.

Garbarino, J., Kostelny, K., & Dubrow, N. (1991). What children can tell us about living in danger. *American Psychologist, 46*(4), 376–383.

Gaston, M. H., Porter, G. K., & Thomas, V. G. (2007). Prime Time™ Sister Circles: Evaluating a gender-specific, culturally relevant health intervention to decrease major risk factors in mid-life African-American women. *Journal of the National Medical Association, 99*(4), 428–438.

Ge, X., Brody, G. H., Conger, R. D., & Simons, R. L. (2006). Pubertal maturation and African American children's internalizing and externalizing symptoms. *Journal of Youth and Adolescence, 35*(4), 528–537.

Ginsburg, G. S., & Drake, K. L. (2002a). Anxiety sensitivity and panic attack symptomatology among low-income African American adolescents. *Journal of Anxiety Disorders, 16*(1), 83–96.

Ginsburg, G. S., & Drake, K. L. (2002b). School-based treatment for anxious African-American adolescents: A controlled pilot study. *Journal of the American Academy of Child and Adolescent Psychiatry, 41*(7), 768–775.

Greenberg, P. E., Sisitsky, T., Kessler, R. C., Finklestein, S. N., Berndt, E. R., Davidson, J. R., et al. (1999). The economic burden of anxiety disorders in the 1990s. *Journal of Clinical Psychiatry, 60*, 427–435.

Grover, R. L., Ginsburg, G. S., & Ialongo, N. (2005). Childhood predictors of anxiety symptoms: A longitudinal study. *Child Psychiatry and Human Development, 36*(2), 133–153.

Grover, R. L., Ginsburg, G. S., & Ialongo, N. (2007). Psychosocial outcomes of anxious first graders: A seven-year follow-up. *Depression and Anxiety, 24*(6), 410–420.

Ho, M. K. (1992). Differential application of treatment modalities with Asian American youth. In L. Vargas & J. D. Koss-Chioino (Eds.), *Working with culture: Psychotherapeutic interventions with ethnic minority children and adolescents* (pp. 182–203). San Francisco: Jossey-Bass.

Huey, S. J., & Polo, A. J. (2008). Evidence-based psychosocial treatments for ethnic minority youth. *Journal of Clinical Child and Adolescent Psychology, 37*(1), 262–301.

Jackson, J. J., Torres, M., Caldwell, C. H., Neighbors, H. W., Nesse, R. M., Taylor, R. J., et al. (2004). The National Survey of American Life: A study of racial, ethnic, and cultural influences on mental disorders and mental health. *International Journal of Methods in Psychiatric Research, 13*(4), 196–207.

Joe, S., Baser, R. E., Breeden, G., Neighbors, H. W., & Jackson, J. S. (2006). Prevalence of and risk factor for lifetime suicide attempts among Blacks in the United States. *Journal of the American Medical Association, 296*, 2112–2123.

Kessler, R. C., Berglund, P., Chiu, W. T., Demler, O., Heeringa, S., Hiripi, E., et al. (2004). The USA National Comorbidity Survey Replication (NCS-R): Design and field procedures. *International Journal of Methods in Psychiatric Research, 13*, 69–92.

Kessler, R. C., McGonagle, K. A., Zhao, S., Nelson, C. B., Hughes, M., Eshleman, S., et al. (1994). Lifetime and 12-month prevalence of DSM-III-R psychiatric disorder in the United States. *Archives of General Psychiatry, 51*, 8–19.

Kingery, J. N., Ginsburg, G. S., & Alfano, C. A. (2007). Somatic symptoms and anxiety among African American adolescents. *Journal of Black Psychology, 33*(4), 363–378.

Kliewer, W., Cunningham, J. N., Diehl, R., Parrish, K. A., Walker, J. M., Atiyeh, C., et al. (2004). Violence exposure and adjustment in inner-city youth: Child and caregiver emotion regulation skill caregiver-child relationship quality, and neighborhood cohesion as protective factors. *Journal of Clinical Child and Adolescent Psychology, 33*(3), 477–487.

Koenig, H. G., George, L. K., & Seigler, I. C. (1988, June). The use of religion and other emotion-regulating coping strategies among older adults. *Gerontologist, 28*(3), 303–310.

Krause, N., & Van Tran, T. (1989). Stress and religious involvement among older Blacks. *Journal of Gerontology, 44*(1), S4–S13.

Lambert, L. (2007, Fall). Facing AIDS. *Kent State Magazine*. Retrieved September 1, 2008, from *www.glpdigitaleditions.com/publication*.

Lambert, S. F., Cooley, M. R., Campbell, K. D. M., Benoit, M. Z., & Stansbury, R. (2004). Assessing anxiety sensitivity in inner-city African American children: Psychometric properties of the Childhood Anxiety Sensitivity Index. *Journal of Clinical Child and Adolescent Psychology, 33*(2), 248–259.

Lambert, S. F., McCreary, B. T., Joiner, T. E., Schmidt, N. B., & Ialongo, N. S. (2004). Structure of anxiety and depression in urban youth: An examination of the tripartite model. *Journal of Consulting and Clinical Psychology, 72*(5), 904–908.

Lane, D. (1994). *Music as medicine: Deforia Lane's life of music, healing and faith*. Grand Rapids, MI: Zondervan.

Lapouse, R., & Monk, M. (1959). Fears and worries in a representative sample of children. *American Journal of Orthopsychiatry, 209*, 803–818.

Last, C. G., Hersen, M., Kazdin, A., Orvaschel, H., & Perrin S. (1991). Anxiety disorders in children and their families. *Archives of General Psychiatry, 48*(10), 928–934.

Last, C. G., & Perrin, S. (1993). Anxiety disorders in African-American and White children. *Journal of Abnormal Child Psychology, 21*(2), 153–164.

Lauren, L., Nordheim, L. V., Ekeland, E., Hagen, K. B., & Heian, F. (2006). Exercise for preventing and treating anxiety and depression in children and young people. *Cochrane Database of Systematic Reviews*, Issue 3 (Article No. CD004-691), DOI: 10.1002/14651858.CD0040691.pub2.

Lawson, E. J., & Thomas, C. (2007). Wading in the waters: Spirituality and older Black Katrina survivors. *Journal of Healthcare for the Poor and Underserved, 18*, 341–345.

Levitin, D. (2006). *This is your brain on music*. New York: Dutton.

Lilienfeld, S. O. (1996). EMDR: Less than meets the eye? *Skeptical Inquirer, 20*(1), 25–31. Retrieved September 1, 2008, from *findarticles.com/p/articles/mi_m2843/is_n1_v20/ai_17849139/print?tag=artBody;col1*.

Lowry-Webster, H. M., Barrett, P. M., & Dadds, M. R. (2001). A universal prevention trial of anxiety and depressive symptomatology in childhood: Preliminary data from an Australian study. *Behaviour Change, 18*(1), 36–50.

Marks, B., Settles, I. H., Cooke, D. Y., Morgan, L., & Sellers, R. M. (2004). African American racial identity: A review of contemporary models and measures. In R. L. Jones (Ed.), *Black psychology* (4th ed., pp. 383–404). Hampton, VA: Cobb & Henry.

Mash, E. J., & Barkley, R. A. (Eds.). (2003). *Child psychopathology* (2nd ed.). New York: Guilford Press.

Mayo Clinic Staff. (2008). *Biofeedback: Using your mind to improve your health.* Rochester, MN: Mayo Clinic. Retrieved October 8, 2008, from *www.mayoclinic.com/health/biofeedback/SA00083.*

McAdoo, H. (1995). Stress levels, family help patterns, and religiosity in middle- and working class African American single mothers. *Journal of Black Psychology, 21*(4), 424–449.

McLaughlin, K. A., Hilt, L. M., & Nolen-Hoeksema, S. (2007). Racial/ethnic differences in internalizing and externalizing symptoms in adolescents. *Journal of Abnormal Child Psychology, 35*(5), 801–816.

McLeish, A. C., & Del Ben, K. S. (2008). Symptoms of depression and posttraumatic stress disorder in an outpatient population before and after Hurricane Katrina. *Depression and Anxiety, 25,* 406–421.

Mobbs, D., Petrovic, P., Marchant, J. L., Hassabis, D., Weiskopf, N., Seymour, B., et al. (2007). When fear is near: Threat imminence elicits prefrontal–periaqueductal gray shifts in humans. *Science, 24,* 1079–1083.

Montag, C., Buckholtz, J. W., Hartman, P., Merz, M., Burk, C., Hennig, J., et al. (2008). COMT genetic variation affects fear processing: Psychophysiological evidence. *Behavioral Neuroscience, 122*(4), 901–909.

Neal, A. M., & Knisley, H. (1995). What are African-American children afraid of?: Part II. A twelve month follow-up. *Journal of Anxiety Disorders, 9,* 151–161.

Neal, A. M., Nagle, L., Smith, J., & Smucker, W. (1994). The presence of panic disorder among African American hypertensives: A pilot study. *Journal of Black Psychology, 20*(1), 29–35.

Neal, A. M., & Turner, S. M. (1991). Anxiety disorders research with African Americans: Current status. *Psychological Bulletin, 109,* 400–410.

Neal, A. M., & Ward-Brown, B. J. (1994). Fears and anxiety disorders in African American children. In S. Friedman (Ed.), *Anxiety disorders in African Americans* (pp. 65–75). New York: Springer.

Neal-Barnett, A. (2004). Orphans no more: A commentary on anxiety and African American youth. *Journal of Clinical Child and Adolescent Psychology, 33*(2), 276–278.

Neal-Barnett, A. M. (2003). *Soothe your nerves: The Black women's guide to understanding and overcoming anxiety, panic, and fear.* New York: Fireside/Simon & Schuster.

Neal-Barnett, A. M. (2008). *Sister circles for professional African American women with panic attacks.* Unpublished manuscript.

Neal-Barnett, A. M., & Crowther, J. H. (2000). To be female, anxious, middle class, and Black. *Psychology of Women Quarterly, 24*(2), 132–140.

Neal-Barnett, A. M., Statom, D., & Stadulis, R. (2003, September). *Tenderheaded: The experience of trichotillomania in African American women.* Paper presented at the 2nd International Symposium of the L'Oreal Ethnic Hair and Skin Institute, Chicago.

Papay, J. P., & Hedl, J. J. (1978). Psychometric characteristics and norms for disadvantaged third and fourth grade children on the State–Trait Anxiety Inventory for Children. *Journal of Abnormal Child Psychology, 6*(1), 115–120.

Safren, S. A., Gonzalez, R. E., Horner, K. J., Leung, A. W., Heimberg, R. G., & Juster, H. R. (2000). Anxiety in ethnic minority youth: Methodological and conceptual issues and review of the literature. *Behavior Modification, 24*(2), 147–183.

Schmidt, N. B., Lerew, D. R., & Jackson, R. J. (1997). The role of anxiety sensitivity in the pathogenesis of panic: Prospective evaluation of spontaneous panic attacks during acute stress. *Journal of Abnormal Psychology, 106*(3), 355–364.

Seidel, L., & Walkup, J. T. (2006). Selective serotonin reuptake inhibitor use in the treatment of the pediatric non-obsessive–compulsive disorder anxiety disorders. *Journal of Child and Adolescent Psychopharmacology, 16*(1–2), 171–179.

Sellers, R. M., Caldwell, C. H., Schmeelk-Cone, K. H., & Zimmerman, M. A. (2003). The role of racial identity and racial discrimination in the mental health of African American young adults. *Journal of Health and Social Behavior, 44*, 302–317.

Sellers, R. M., & Shelton, J. N. (2003). The role of racial identity in perceived racial discrimination. *Journal of Personality and Social Psychology, 84*, 1079–1092.

Sellers, R. M., Smith, M. A., Shelton, J. N., Rowley, S. A. J., & Chavous, T. M. (1998). Multidimensional model of racial identity: A reconceptualization. *Personality and Social Psychology Review, 2*, 18–39.

Shapiro, F. (1989). Eye movement desensitization: A new treatment for post-traumatic stress disorder. *Journal of Behavior Therapy and Experimental Psychiatry, 20*, 211–217.

Silverman, W. K., Fleisig, W., Rabian, B., & Peterson, R. A. (1991). Child Anxiety Sensitivity Index. *Journal of Clinical Child Psychology, 20*(2), 162–168.

Silverman, W. K., La Greca, A. M., & Wasserstein, S. (1995). What do children worry about?: Worries and their relation to anxiety. *Child Development, 66*(3), 671–686.

Society of Clinical Child and Adolescent Psychology. (n.d.). *Evidence-based treatment for children and adolescents*. Retrieved September 25, 2008, from *www.abct.org/sccap*.

Storch, E. A., & Esposito, L. E. (2003). Peer victimization and posttraumatic stress among children. *Child Study Journal, 33*(2), 91–98.

Taylor, R. J., Chatters, L. M., Jayakody, R., & Levin, J. S. (1996). Black and White differences in religious participation: A multisample comparison. *Journal for the Scientific Study of Religion, 35*(4), 403–410.

Topolski, T. D., Hewitt, J. K., Eaves, L. J., Silberg, J. L., Meyer, J. M., Rutter, M., et al. (1997). Genetic and environmental influences on child reports of manifest anxiety and symptoms of separation anxiety and overanxious disorders: A community-based twin study. *Behavior Genetics, 27*(1), 15–28.

Treadwell, K. R. H., Flannery-Schroeder, E. C., & Kendall, P. C. (1995). Ethnicity and gender in relation to adaptive functioning, diagnostic status, and treatment outcome in children from an anxiety clinic. *Journal of Anxiety Disorders, 9*(5), 373–384.

Turner, B. G., Beidel, D. C., Hughes, S., & Turner, M. W. (1993). Test anxiety in African American school children. *School Psychology Quarterly, 8*(2), 140–152.

Turner, S. M., Beidel, D. C., & Costello, A. (1987). Psychopathology in the offspring of anxiety disorders patients. *Journal of Consulting and Clinical Psychology, 55*(2), 229–235.

Turner, S. M., Beidel, D. C., Roberson-Nay, R., & Tervo, K. (2003). Parenting behaviors in parents with anxiety disorders. *Behaviour Research and Therapy, 41*(5), 541–554.

U.S. Department of Health and Human Services. (2006). *Anxiety disorders* (NIH Publication No. 06-3879). Rockville, MD: Author.

U.S. Food and Drug Administration. (2006). *FDA approves Emsam (Selegiline) as first drug patch for depression*. Washington, DC: Author. Retrieved September 1, 2008, from *www.fda.gov/bbs/topics/NEWS/2006/NEW01326.html*.

U.S. Food and Drug Administration. (2007). *Antidepressant use in children, adolescents, and adults.* Washington, DC: Author. Retrieved September 1, 2008, from *www.fda. gov/cder/drug/antidepressants/default.htm.*

Utsey, S. O. (1999). Development and validation of a short form of the Index of Race-Related Stress—Brief version. *Measurement and Evaluation in Counseling and Development, 32,* 149–166.

Utsey, S. O., Giesbrecht, N., Hook, J., & Stanard, P. M. (2008). Resources that inhibit psychological distress in African Americans exposed to stressful life vents and race-related stress. *Journal of Counseling Psychology, 55,* 49–62.

Virginia Commission on Youth. (2003). *Anxiety disorders.* Retrieved August 30, 2008, from *coy.state.va.us/Modalities/anxiety.htm.*

Wagner, A. W., Bystritsky, A., Russo, J. E., Craske, M. G., Sherbourne, C. D., Stein, M. B., et al. (2005). Beliefs about psychotropic medication and psychotherapy among primary care patients with anxiety disorders. *Depression and Anxiety, 21,* 99–105.

Walker, A. (2003). *The third life of Grange Copeland.* New York: Harcourt Books.

Walworth, D. D. (2003). The effect of preferred music genre selection versus preferred song selection on experimentally induced anxiety levels. *Journal of Music Therapy, XL*(1), 2–14.

Williams, K. E., Chambless, D. L., & Steketee, G. (1998). Behavioral treatment of obsessive-compulsive disorder in African Americans: Clinical issues. *Journal of Behavior Therapy and Experimental Psychiatry, 23,* 161–170.

Williams, M., & Turkheimer, E. (2007). Identification and explanation of racial differences on contamination measures. *Behaviour Research and Therapy, 45,* 3041–3050.

Wyatt, G. (1998). *Stolen women.* New York: Wiley.

Yip, T., Seaton, E. K., & Sellers, R. M. (2006). African American racial identity across the lifespan: Identity status, identity content, and depressive symptoms. *Child Development, 7,* 1504–1517.

Zoellner, L. A., Feeny, N. G., Fitzgibbons, L. A., & Foa, E. B. (1999). Response of African American and Caucasian women to cognitive behavior therapy for PTSD. *Behaviour Research and Therapy, 30,* 581–595.

# 16

# Attention-Deficit/ Hyperactivity Disorder

JACQUELYN DUVAL–HARVEY
KENNETH M. ROGERS

Attention-deficit/hyperactivity disorder (ADHD) is one of the most common reasons for psychiatric and educational referral for school-age children, with a prevalence rate of 3–7% of the childhood population (American Psychiatric Association, 2000). The current clinical profile of ADHD includes two highly correlated but psychometrically distinct symptom domains: inattention–disorganization and hyperactivity–impulsivity. These two domains are the basis of the three subtypes in the *Diagnostic and Statistical Manual of Mental Disorders* (fourth edition, text revision [DSM-IV-TR]; American Psychological Association, 2000): predominantly inattentive (ADHD-PI), predominantly hyperactive–impulsive (ADHD-PHI), and combined (ADHD-C). It is well documented that children with ADHD are at significant risk for negative outcomes in a variety of important life domains. Our understanding of this disorder is the result of more than a century of clinical and scientific investigation aided by technological advances in neuroimaging and genetics research.

Despite the prevalence, effect, and extensive study of ADHD, there is a lack of research on the disorder as it relates to African Americans. Given the impact of ADHD, the existence of treatments with substantial evidence of effectiveness with the general population of children with ADHD, as well as some empirical ADHD research suggesting race/ethnicity effects, it is important that efforts be made to better understand any unique features of etiology, symptomology, outcomes, and treatment relative to African Americans. This chapter contributes to this effort by summarizing the important findings and issues related to ADHD that may be helpful to African Americans with ADHD, their families, health professionals, and researchers. We place particular emphasis on (1) discussing findings from the limited amount of research that specifically addresses race effects, (2) summarizing the findings and evidence-based practices that have grown out of the extensive body of research on ADHD conducted with primarily White samples, and (3) providing a context in which the responsible parties (e.g., parents, health professionals) might utilize these two areas of research in making decisions regarding ADHD among African Americans.

## OVERVIEW OF ADHD RESEARCH AND ISSUES

Early clinical descriptions of children with significant difficulties sustaining attention were detailed by Still (1902) more than a century ago. Since then, there has been considerable effort exploring specific symptoms and associated theoretical frameworks to identify the precise nature of the impairment and its etiology. At present, ADHD is one of the best researched disorders in medicine as well as the most researched psychiatric disorder affecting children. A considerable amount of research continues to be generated, the complexity of which has increased considerably owing to the greater focus on the neuroscience and genetic components resulting from advances in neuron-imaging techniques. (See Barkley, 2006, for a comprehensive review.) Use of this technology is already producing significant gains in understanding the neurological aspects of the disorder.

Despite this abundance of knowledge, there are some prevailing controversies about ADHD and shortcomings associated with the existing research. At the core of the controversy is the issue of whether ADHD is a "true" illness, because restlessness, inattention, and impulsive behavior are seen as common characteristics of children. Concern has also been raised about whether it may be overdiagnosed to mask poor educational environment or teacher intolerance. Finally, the use of psychotropic medications in the treatment of ADHD is perceived by some to be an attempt at financial gain by pharmaceutical companies and physicians.

The research on ADHD is discussed in more detail in subsequent sections; however, it is important to point out that the prevalence of the disorder can vary considerably depending on several factors, perhaps chief among these being the methodology used for defining and measuring ADHD (Lambert, Sandoval, & Sassone, 1978). Barkley (2006) has shown that changes in the DSM-based diagnostic criteria result in increased prevalence, with the adoption of the DSM-IV and its addition of new subtypes ADHD-PI and ADHD-PHI nearly doubling the prevalence rate.

The use of prevalence rates is necessary, but not sufficient, to classify any behavior as a disorder. Establishing an appropriate standard for cutoff scores on rating scales or structured interviews is important to prevent both underidentification of children in need of treatment to prevent negative outcomes and overidentification, which results in more children with behaviors inappropriately labeled as deviant. Ultimately, utilizing a scientific process to identify children whose symptoms are severe enough to result in impairment in one or more major life domains is the primary goal and the focus of continuing research. Research has identified negative outcomes, including school dropout, poor social relationships, and engaging in antisocial activities, and other high-risk behaviors in association with ADHD symptoms.

## OVERVIEW OF RESEARCH AND ISSUES REGARDING ADHD IN AFRICAN AMERICANS

One of the limitations of the research on ADHD is that, despite both national and international investigations, few studies have focused on the racial or ethnic issues related to ADHD (Miller, Nigg, & Miller 2009). Attention in this area is warranted because of several factors that have been summarized by Miller and colleagues (2009). First, different racial groups may have varying behavioral expectations and tolerances for acceptable child and adolescent behavior and mental health care (Livingston, 1999), which may function as moderators of developmental processes.

Second, there is a history of differential misdiagnosis of African Americans in the psychiatric assessment of adults, wherein clinicians using nonstandard assessment practices tend to judge the same clinical presentation differently by race, obscuring any objective differences in rates of disorder (Friedman, Paradis, & Hatch, 1994; Whaley & Geller, 2007). Third, African Americans have the highest poverty rate among all racial and ethnic groups in the United States (Kendall & Hatton, 2002). Low socioeconomic status (SES) is associated with less access to health care, increased psychological and physiological stress, and general health problems. There may also be some specific race-related effects separate from SES that may account for differences in health outcome among African Americans. For example, racial health disparities exist between African Americans and Caucasians even when SES is controlled, including higher rates of morbidity and mortality and a higher incidence of HIV/AIDS and many forms of cancer (Centers for Disease Control and Prevention [CDC], 2006).

An initial review by Samuel and colleagues (1997) of the available literature from 1965 to 1997 identified only 16 research articles relevant to ADHD in African American youth. A more recent analysis (Miller et al., 2009) of all peer-reviewed journal articles written in English and published from 1990 to 2007 yielded 73 of 462 articles with ADHD in African American children as the major topic of investigation. These reviewers found discrepancies in the prevalence of ADHD behaviors and diagnosis in African American children, the role of ethnicity in treatment response to ADHD, and differences in parental perceptions/attitudes regarding ADHD and the treatment implications thereof.

Emblematic of the importance and lack of clarity regarding ADHD issues of concern for the African American community was the decision to draft the following consensus statement by the National Medical Association, the oldest and largest organization representing African American physicians and their patients, in collaboration with leading experts convened by Children and Adults with Attention Deficit Hyperactivity Disorder (2005), the nation's leading advocacy organization serving families and individuals affected by ADHD:

- ADHD exists, it occurs in African American children and adults, and it can be detrimental to African Americans.
- There is evidence-based medicine to support the contention that ADHD is an actual disorder.
- African American children and adults directly and indirectly may suffer a disproportionate burden because of ADHD.
- African American children deserve the highest quality of psychiatric medical care, including optimal assessment, evaluation, and diagnosis, and full, unrestricted, open access to the best available medication for the treatment of ADHD and depression.

Clearly, the African American community, as well as researchers and practitioners interested in how best to understand and treat ADHD, could benefit from additional efforts to broaden and disseminate our knowledge of ADHD. The following sections provide a brief summary of issues and research regarding various aspects of the ADHD discussion (e.g., risk factors, evidence-based treatment/approaches) as well as our practice recommendations.

## BIOLOGICAL AND GENETIC FACTORS

The initial investigation of ADHD-related behaviors began in the United States as a result of the encephalitis epidemic of 1918, with much of the focus on the presumed causal relationship between brain damage and its subsequent behavioral impacts (Barkley, 2006). This early work gave rise to a long history of investigations on the biological factors thought to underlie ADHD as well as other disorders. In the mid-20th century, some of these relationships were found to lack support. However, as for ADHD, there is now substantial evidence and agreement that neurological factors play a principal role in its development (Barkley, 2006).

### Genetic Factors

Across multiple studies and countries, ADHD and its symptoms have been consistently found to be among the most genetically influenced psychiatric conditions (Levy & Hay, 2001). The research supporting a genetic linkage to ADHD has included studies of thousands of identical and fraternal twin pairs, studies involving comparisons of siblings reared together and those reared apart, and comparisons of biological versus adoptive families of ADHD children (Barkley, 2006). All of these different methods supported a strong level of heritability of the disorder and its defining symptoms. Consistent with this association, Faraone and colleagues (2005), in their review of twin studies, concluded that the estimated heritability of ADHD was 76%.

Many of the studies investigating a genetic link to ADHD examined the prevalence of ADHD among family members. Several of these early studies estimated that about 5% of mothers and 15% of fathers of children with ADHD reported having similar problems (Morrison & Stewart, 1973), whereas later investigations pointed to rates as high as 20% for mothers and 80% for fathers (Nigg & Hinshaw, 1998). Among biological siblings, the risk of having ADHD is in the range of 17–37%, with an average risk of 25–37% for first-degree biological relatives of children with ADHD.

In addition to research examining the heritability of ADHD, there have also been efforts to identify the genetic mechanisms by which the transmission of ADHD might occur. Two prominent examples of this are the work of Faraone and colleagues (2005) and Congdon and Canli (2008). Faraone and colleagues identified seven genes that showed statistically significant associations with ADHD. In their review of the current state of research on the neural and genetic basis of trait impulsivity, Congdon and Canli identified three gene polymorphisms that may influence impulsivity: the D4 dopamine receptor (DRD4), the dopamine transporter, and the catechol-$O$-methyltransferase enzyme. Although the focus of their study was not strictly ADHD but impulsivity as a broad, multidimensional construct, each of the three potential genetic influences identified in their research has support linking it to ADHD. Barkley (2006) concluded that a review of existing molecular genetic research suggests that the greatest research support for a specific genetic association with ADHD exists for the DRD4 receptor.

## Neurological Factors

Early researchers hypothesized that specific regions and dysfunctions within the brain were likely associated with ADHD. For example, Hastings and Barkley (1978) and Klorman (1992) suggested that brain underactivity in the frontal lobe was a contributing factor in ADHD. Similarly, several studies in the 1990s found that children with ADHD did less well on tests designed to assess frontal lobe functions (Barkley, 1997; Goodyear & Hynd, 1992). The utilization of neuroimaging to detect states of brain activity contributed to greater specificity related to brain functioning (e.g., Semrud-Clikeman et al., 1994), activity levels (e.g., Zametkin et al., 1990), and regional demarcations (Hynd, Semrud-Clikeman, Lorys, Novey, & Eliopulos, 1990) associated with ADHD. These findings and others like them provide strong support that impaired brain development is an important factor in ADHD.

A review by Willcutt, Doyle, Nigg, Faraone, and Pennington (2005), which involved a meta-analysis of 83 studies and several thousand subjects, found that patients with ADHD tended to exhibit impairments in executive functioning domains, specifically response inhibition, vigilance, working memory, and some measures of planning. Barkley (2006) summarizes the research on the neuropsychology of ADHD by noting that neuroimaging to evaluate brain activity and structures has contributed to a substantial increase in the research in this area. Consistent with the findings of Willcutt and colleagues, Barkley further suggests that the results of this research support the view that ADHD involves a problem with behavioral (executive) inhibition (Nigg, 2001), and that the attention problems found in ADHD likely represent deficits in the broader domain of executive functioning, especially working memory.

## African Americans and Genetic and Biological Factors in ADHD

There has been little research regarding the genetic etiology of ADHD in African Americans and whether the relationships found in this area in other groups (generally Caucasian males) hold true among African Americans (Miller et al., 2009). The concern is based on the limited participation of African Americans in twin studies of ADHD (Mazei-Robison, Couch, Shelton, Stein, & Blakely, 2005) and the existence of only one study, Samuel and colleagues (1999), examining heredity of ADHD among African Americans. Samuel and colleagues found a heightened prevalence of ADHD among family members of African American participants who had been diagnosed with the disorder than that among families of participants with no ADHD. These findings are consistent with those of studies investigating familial patterns with Caucasian samples. Miller and colleagues (2009) also note that there is a similar absence of research investigating the molecular genetic linkages to ADHD within African American populations. So, as it relates to the biological and genetic factors specific to ADHD in African Americans, the available research does not indicate any racial difference on these factors, but given the dearth of empirical study of this population, it is likely premature to form definitive conclusions.

## INDIVIDUAL FACTORS

The research evidence for individual difference factors in ADHD is most established regarding the relationships of gender and age to ADHD prevalence, but with significantly less research and clarity on the role of other individual characteristics such as SES, race, and ethnicity.

## Gender

A consistent finding in the literature is that more boys than girls are referred and consequently diagnosed with ADHD, despite some variability among studies related to prevalence rates. Barkley's (2006) summary of epidemiological studies of ADHD prevalence found an average ratio of boys to girls of approximately 3.4:1 among community samples; whereas Ross and Ross (1982) reported an average ratio of 6:1 among clinic-referred samples.

Several factors have been suggested to account for the differences in prevalence. There may be actual gender differences in the presentation of symptoms among children with ADHD as well as differences in how specific behaviors are interpreted by adults (parents, teachers, mental health professionals) in terms of gender role and culture. There may also be a true underlying difference in the expression of the disorder.

Studies of gender differences in the presentation of symptoms among children with ADHD suggest that, although there is general commonality on the symptoms expressed, girls tend to manifest somewhat lower symptom levels, particularly as they relate to aggressive behavior (Gaub & Carlson, 1997; Gershon, 2002; Newcorn et al., 2001). Barkley (2006) suggested that this heightened manifestation of aggressive behavior among boys may explain, at least in part, the larger gender gap in ADHD prevalence among clinic-referred samples. In essence, parents, teachers, and other authority/professional figures may be more likely to refer children for treatment who exhibit aggressive or antisocial behavior. To the extent that ADHD is more likely to be manifested through these behaviors in boys than girls, these factors would contribute to a higher proportion of boys in clinic-referred samples.

Gaub and Carlson (1997) and Gershon (2002) both found that girls had lower levels of inattentive, hyperactive, and impulsive symptoms as well as lower levels of other externalizing symptoms, such as aggression and delinquency. These two meta-analytic studies also found that girls tended to experience greater intellectual impairment.

## Socioeconomic Status

Research on the relationship of SES to ADHD is somewhat mixed. When summarizing the state of research on the relationship between SES and ADHD, Barkley (2006) make three general points. First, there is abundant evidence that ADHD occurs across all socioeconomic levels. Second, several studies have found a negative relationship between SES and measures of ADHD or some element of ADHD symptoms (Boyle & Lipman, 2002; Lambert et al., 1978; Szatmari, 1992; Szatmari, Offord, & Boyle, 1989).

In addition to the two points just presented, Barkley (2006) suggests that when differences in ADHD have been found across SES levels, the finding may have been an artifact of other disorders known to be related to SES or a methodological factor such as the means used to determine ADHD. He notes that the SES–ADHD relationship reported in Szatmari and colleagues (1989) was no longer observed when the effects of other disorders known to be associated with SES (e.g., conduct disorder [CD]) were taken into account. Likewise, the relationship between SES and ADHD in the Lambert and colleagues (1978) study also appeared to be influenced by other factors, in that the finding of a relationship between SES and ADHD differed depending on the methodology used to diagnosis ADHD. A negative relationship was observed when only two of three parties (parent, teacher, or physician) had to agree on the diagnosis; however, no relationship was observed when agreement among all three parties was required. Given these findings, the strength, or existence, of a meaningful relationship between SES and prevalence is still to be determined.

## Age

Age differences in ADHD are well documented, with higher precedence levels among younger age groups. Nolan, Gadow, and Sprafkin (2001) reported prevalence rates for ADHD of 18.2% among preschool children, 15.9% among elementary school-age children, and 14.8% for secondary school-age children. Given the relatively high prevalence levels found in this study, it is important to note that ADHD prevalence was determined by teacher ratings, which tend to be higher than when ADHD is determined by more rigorous processes (e.g., determination by clinical diagnostic criteria or even multiple raters). Kashani, Orvaschel, Ronsenberg, and Reid (1989) utilized clinical diagnostic criteria to determine ADHD prevalence levels in a sample of 8-, 12-, and 17-year-olds and reported lower prevalence levels, but a similar pattern of prevalence across age groups, than those found by Nolan and colleagues: 8-year-olds, 7.2%; 12-year-olds, 2.9%; and 17-year-olds, 0%.

Research also supports a general trend of symptom improvement as children with ADHD grow older, although there are many instances where individuals suffer with ADHD into their adult years. In fact, one of the significant developments in the study and treatment of ADHD over the past 20 years has been the increased acknowledgment, study, and treatment of adult ADHD (Barkley, 2006).

Barkley (2006) provides a thorough and informative summary of the developmental course and adult outcomes of children with ADHD, which can provide a useful framework for the consideration and understanding of ADHD across different developmental stages. Elements of Barkley's summary are briefly outlined next.

### Preschool Children

Significantly inattentive and overactive behavior is commonly seen among children by age 3 and generally does not represent any cause for concern. The longer these behaviors persist, however, the greater the likelihood that they will begin to have a negative impact on functioning, with evidence of behavior and academic achievement problems occurring in about 10% of such children by second grade (Palfrey, Levine, Walker, & Sullivan, 1985). However, it is not uncommon for the more active and aggressive preschoolers to show early adjustment problems that ultimately may contribute to frequent change in day care and preschool settings.

### School-Age Children

A traditional educational setting presents a major challenge for children with ADHD and is thought to be the greatest source of stress for them and their parents (Barkley, Fischer, Edelbrock, & Smallish, 1990; Biederman, 1997). During this elementary and middle school–age phase, children and parents face the combined challenges of academic and social demands at school as well as behavioral challenges at home. The academic and social demands of school often trigger referrals for evaluation by first grade, and the traditional academic grade progression process may have parents facing decisions about whether to retain their children in their current grade as a result of "immature" behavior or slow academic development.

### Adolescence

Research suggests a decline in levels of hyperactivity and improvement in attention span and impulse control for youth with ADHD-PHI and ADHD-C (Fischer, Barkley, Smallish, & Fletcher, 2004; Hart, Lahey, Loeber, Applegate, & Frick, 1995) during the adolescent years. However, the increasing demands for independent responsible conduct as well as changes resulting from puberty and social relations (e.g., issues of identity, peer group acceptance) have led some to suggest that this developmental age may well be the most difficult for individuals with ADHD.

### Adults

Researchers note the importance of distinguishing between findings from studies of adults with ADHD who had a prior diagnosis of ADHD as children and clinic-referred adults who are seeking help in dealing with ADHD. Among the differences in the two populations are differences in the extent to which individuals qualify fully for an ADHD diagnosis. Many adults monitored to adulthood from childhood may not fully meet the criteria for a diagnosis of ADHD, while this is not likely the case for individuals who have sought treatment for their behavioral issues at clinics as adults and have subsequently been diagnosed as having ADHD.

Only a few studies have followed samples of hyperactive children into adulthood. Summary of this research can be found in Barkley (2006), Weiss and Hechtman (1993), and Klein and Mannuzza (1991). Barkley summarizes some of the key findings of his and others' empirical findings on ADHD among adults as follows:

- Adults who have been diagnosed with ADHD since childhood are more likely to be less educated, underachieving in their occupational settings, and experiencing difficulty working without supervision.
- Clinic-referred adults appear to have somewhat lower educational and social risks than children with ADHD monitored into adulthood (e.g., conduct problems, antisocial personality disorder, depression).
- Adults with ADHD also tend to experience impairments in social, occupational, and educational functioning.
- Differences between the two populations lie chiefly in lower levels of oppositional, conduct, or antisocial problems/disorders and higher levels of intellectual and academic functioning among self-referred adults with ADHD.

## Race

As indicated previously, there is still relatively little information on ADHD risk and resiliency factors in African Americans. Miller and colleagues (2009) represents the most comprehensive and up-to date summary of ADHD research addressing ADHD in African Americans. Their review updates the efforts of Samuel and colleagues (1997), who documented the scarcity of research in this area. Studies identified by Miller and colleagues were classified into three general categories: syndromal characteristics (34 articles), treatment (17 articles), and parent perceptions of ADHD (22 articles). These researchers note that, although the 73 articles that they reviewed represent an increase over the level of research found by Samuel, there are nonetheless many issues related to ADHD and African Americans that still require more research.

Among the key findings in Miller and colleagues' (2009) review were the discrepancies in prevalence of ADHD behaviors and diagnosis in African American children, the role of ethnicity in treatment response to ADHD, and differences in parental perceptions/attitudes regarding ADHD. Treatment response and differences in parental perceptions are discussed in a subsequent section; here we focus on the discrepancies in prevalence.

Miller and colleagues' (2009) review included a mini meta-analysis of five studies of ADHD symptoms and five studies of ADHD diagnosis to determine whether there were racial differences in ADHD prevalence. They found that, although African American youth had more ADHD symptoms on parent and teacher ratings and classroom observations, they received a diagnosis of ADHD by a health professional using International Classification of Diseases or DSM criteria only two-thirds as often as Caucasian youth. Potentially confounding variables such as teacher rating bias, income, insurance coverage, and comorbid learning disability did not account for this finding. One proposed explanation for these results is that access to or utilization of services does not occur until symptoms are relatively severe.

Miller and colleagues (2009) also found some studies that suggested that African Americans may experience higher levels of exposure to factors associated with higher risk of ADHD. These included lower SES (see prior discussion) and exposure to environmental toxins such as lead. Lead exposure has been linked to impaired attention, hyperactivity, and aggression (Stein, Schettler, Wallinga, & Valenti, 2002), and the CDC reports that levels of lead exposure are dramatically higher among inner-city African Americans (36%) than American children overall (CDC, 2000).

In addition, Miller and colleagues (2009) note that there is a relatively small amount of research on the question of whether current ADHD assessment instruments and approaches appropriately measure the disorder in African Americans, and that the findings do not suggest a definitive answer. They cite one effort to develop a culturally specific measure of ADHD, The Terry, an African American version of the Dominic-R (Valla, Bergeron, Bidaut-Russell, St-Georges, & Gaudet, 1997).

In one of the first studies to use ethically sensitive methods to study ADHD in African American children, Samuel and colleagues (1998) suggests that ADHD may be characterized by a narrower pattern of psychiatric comorbidity and dysfunction than has been observed among Whites. However, they acknowledge several methodological limitations of their study (e.g., small sample size) that might limit the generalizability of their findings.

## FAMILY FACTORS INFLUENCING RISK AND RESILIENCY

Family factors influencing risk and resiliency can be generally organized around three categories:

- Family functioning, which refers to the dynamics and impact of having a child with ADHD.
- Family care-seeking attitudes and behavior, which address how the family's beliefs about ADHD influence their care-seeking behavior for their child with ADHD.
- Family characteristics, which relate to the family's contribution to the child's ADHD.

### Family Functioning

Caring for a child with ADHD is a potential stressor for parents and caregivers, as is the case with any other illness. However, unlike other childhood illnesses, it is not unusual for parents to be blamed or seen as contributing to the behavior problems. Children with ADHD tend to exhibit less compliance to parental requests, show poor sustained compliance, and make greater requests for assistance, while parents appear to make more commands, reprimands, and punishment. It is unclear whether the parental behaviors are the cause or consequence of the noncompliance. Parents are faced not only with the demands of caring for their children but are often involved in mediating difficulties in school with peers and other siblings that may likely occur throughout childhood and into adolescence. Given these multiple demands, it is not surprising that parents often view themselves as less skilled and less knowledgeable in their parenting roles. In families with children with comorbid oppositional defiant disorder (ODD) or CD, conflict is even greater and poor disciplinary styles are highest.

## Family Care-Seeking Attitudes and Behavior

Although it is very likely that the prevalence of ADHD in African Americans is similar to that of the general population (3–5%), fewer African Americans are diagnosed and treated for ADHD (Bailey & Owens, 2005), and there is evidence of higher rates of unmet ADHD treatment needs among minority than White children (Bussing, Perwien, & Belin, 1996).

Racial disparities in access to care have been well documented (Bussing, Schoenberg, & Perwien, 1998; Bussing, Zima, & Belin, 1997; dosReis et al., 2003; dosReis, Owens, Puccia, & Leaf, 2004). However, there may be some issues particular to ADHD that may be contributing to challenges in access to care. For example, studies indicate that among families living in the inner city, only one-third will follow up with a mental health referral for their children (Harrison, McKay, & Bannon, 2004). Discontinuation of treatment following initial visits is also common (Kazdin, Stolar, & Marciano, 1995).

The first step in the process of seeking and participating in services is the individual's identification, understanding, and acceptance of a problem. This is followed by the knowledge that treatment is available, determination of access to treatment, and ultimately the willingness to engage fully in the treatment process. Social and cultural norms as well as attitudes and beliefs about the illness can influence this process (Kleinman, Eisenberg, & Good, 1978; McKay, Pennington, Lynn, & McCadam, 2001; Zwaanswijk, Verhaak, Bensing, van der Ende, & Verhulst, 2003).

There have been some earlier studies on the knowledge and attitudes of African American families with children diagnosed with ADHD (Bussing, Schoenberg, & Perwien, 1998; Bussing, Schoenberg, Rogers, Zima, & Angus, 1998; Bussing, Zima, Gary, & Garvan, 2003), but a recent series of studies (dosReis et al., 2006; dosReis & Myers, 2008; Mychailyszyn, dosReis, & Myers, 2008) provide an opportunity to examine whether there has been any shift over time.

In terms of general ADHD knowledge, earlier studies (e.g., Bussing, Schoenberg, & Perwien, 1998) found that fewer African American parents were familiar and knowledgeable about ADHD compared with Whites. The more recent studies indicate that although there has been an increase in familiarity with ADHD among African American parents, the majority continue to see the symptoms of ADHD as related to poor parenting styles in terms of lack of appropriate discipline and poor role modeling. Diet, particularly excess sugar intake, continues to be seen as a cause of ADHD-related hyperactivity despite evidence to the contrary.

Initial reluctance concerning the use of psychotropic medication is consistent among African American parents and Caucasian parents irrespective of SES, but concerns about potential addiction to medications and harmful side effects are more prevalent among African Americans. There are trends that suggest a greater willingness to use medication despite these concerns, but they appear to be largely based on interest in improving academic functioning, particularly when recommended by a physician. The willingness to use medication does not seem to indicate a preference for medication overall; in fact, African American families hold very strong beliefs that medication is prescribed too frequently, and some even see it as a function of inadequate educational environments and overwhelmed or impatient teachers. Even among parents who consent to the use of medication for their own children and would recommend it to others, administration is in accordance with school attendance only.

These attitudes are not exclusive to parents but have also been reported among African American professionals. Davison and Ford (2001) found that these professionals were less likely to diagnose ADHD or to prescribe stimulant medication treatment because of perceived stigma with the diagnostic label, concern about addiction to medication, distrust of the educational system, and perceived lack of cultural awareness on the part of Caucasian educators.

Examination of how attitudes and knowledge influence help-seeking behavior for children with ADHD among urban African American families (dosReis, Mychailyszyn, Myers, & Riley, 2007) has suggested four frameworks for understanding parental motivation regarding treatment:

- *Immediate resolution*: Parents' motivation is to find a quick solution to the problematic behavior. In such cases, medication is likely the preferred treatment option.

- *Pragmatic management*: Parents view the behaviors as medical or biological in origin with long-term consequences that need to be managed. These parents are likely to seek help from multiple sources and could be interested in both medication and therapy as treatment choices.

- *Attributional ambivalence*: Parents recognize that their children's ADHD symptoms are atypical but attribute their origin to environmental or nonbiological factors. Such families may consider engaging in therapy and nonmedication approaches to treatment.

- *Coerced conformance*: Parents do not consider their children's behavior to be problematic but are likely to seek care through the instigation of a third party with established authority, such as school officials. In such cases, there may initially be limited openness to either therapy or medication.

Collectively, these studies all point to the fact that, despite some identification of the medical community as the preferred source of information on ADHD, African American parents utilize their social networks, direct experience, and personal beliefs for assistance in understanding ADHD and making help-seeking and treatment decisions. Effective educational strategies need to include those individuals who are the actual transmitters of information, and professionals are encouraged to have open, frank discussions of these issues whenever the opportunity presents itself.

## Parental Characteristics

As mentioned, there is compelling evidence of a strong genetic component for ADHD. Parental ADHD is associated with an increased risk of psychiatric and emotional problems in their children by late adolescence and a 30–54% risk for ADHD specifically. As with children, comorbid factors such as depression, alcoholism, CD, and personality disorder are also present in parents with ADHD and contribute to greater difficulties when their children enter adolescence.

Although there is no indication that the gender of the parent with ADHD is an important consideration, symptom ratings for children with ADHD are consistently lower when rated by fathers than mothers. This may be due to mothers traditionally spending more time with the children in a variety of settings as well as in caretaking roles, including involvement with tasks or placement of demands that may be more difficult for children with ADHD. There may also be differences in parental style relative to communication and disciple wherein fathers are less likely to repeat commands and reason and more likely to discipline more quickly. However, it is unclear whether these findings would be similar for African American families and in single-parent homes headed by a mother or a father.

## SOCIAL AND COMMUNITY FACTORS

In general, children with ADHD who are referred for clinic treatment often experience poor peer relationships (50–70%) and greater social rejection. These problems are highest among those with comorbid ODD/CD, who may also exhibit greater social aggression, higher expressed emotion, lower thresholds for provoked aggression, and more persistent aggression (Barkley, 2006).

Risk factors associated with the development of ADHD and related pathology in the general population include low SES, juvenile detainee status, prenatal marijuana exposure, and exposure to environmental toxins (Arnold et al., 2003; Bazargan et al., 2005; DuPaul, Barkley, & Connor, 1998; Epstein et al., 2005).

Developmentally, ADHD creates some specific challenges for youth as they move through the various stages of life. For example, preschoolers with ADHD place enormous caretaking demands on their parents and frequently display aggressive behavior when interacting with siblings and peers. As children with ADHD move into the elementary school years, academic problems take on increased importance. This, coupled with ongoing family and peer relationship problems, sets the stage for the development of low self-esteem and other emotional concerns.

Similar problems persist into adolescence but on a more intense level. New problems may develop as well, such as experimentation with alcohol or other drugs, stemming from their natural desire/demand for increasing independence, self-regulation, and self-control and their inability to cope with the associated responsibilities. In addition to the primary ADHD symptoms, individuals are at increased risk for secondary or comorbid diagnoses (Jensen, Martin, & Cantwell, 1997). ODD is especially common early on, affecting approximately 40% of preschoolers and elementary school–age children with ADHD. About 20–30% of these children will eventually display secondary features of CD.

When ADHD is accompanied by either ODD or CD, there is also an increased risk for depression and anxiety disorders, especially during adolescence. Antisocial personality disorder, major depressive disorder, and substance abuse are a few of the comorbid problems that adults with ADHD may experience. These comorbid conditions increase the severity of overall psychosocial impairment and indicate a less favorable prognosis.

Despite the availability of efficacious ADHD treatments, analysis of the National Medical Expenditure Survey data indicates that although ADHD treatment rates have increased significantly across all sociodemographic groups in the United States, the rates for racial and ethnic minority children remain low compared with those for White children (Olfson, Gameroff, Marcus, & Jensen, 2003). African American children are only half as likely as White children to take stimulant medication (Zito, Safer, dosReis, & Riddle, 1997, 1998).

In the previous section, the impact of ADHD on the family was discussed. Specific to African American children, the beliefs and attitudes of primary caregivers are more likely to result in delays in accessing evaluation and treatment services and may contribute to greater severity of symptoms. Reluctance to view ADHD as a condition outside of the control of the youth is supported by community values that may validate or even create these perceptions. It is, therefore, important to provide the community with accurate information about this disorder in order to decrease risk and promote resiliency.

In a study by Olaniyan and colleagues (2007), focus groups were held with African American parents to identify their specific beliefs about ADHD and the general attitudes and beliefs among their community social networks, which may influence the perceptions and care-seeking behavior. A total of 31 African American parents, five male (16%) and 26 (84%) female, from jurisdictions in Maryland and Washington, DC, participated. Diverse education and income levels were represented. Each family included an average of two children younger than 17.

Findings from the study were reported for five general areas: cause of behavioral problems, ADHD as a diagnosis, attitudes toward doctors, opinions about medication, and perceptions of school environment. Overall, the responses to these general areas were consistent with the results discussed in the previous section for parents of children with ADHD. Although there was mention of factors such as the child's developmental age, diet, and genetic factors, poor parenting, which included lack of attention and lack of discipline, was by and large the most frequently cited cause of child behavior problems. There were diverse views on what constituted appropriate discipline, with some strongly recommending spanking and others endorsing communication as a more effective approach.

ADHD was considered only a label for behavior and not an illness requiring treatment. Even as a label, there were concerns that this resulted in stigmatization for youth. Medication was seen as a method of controlling behavior that was reminiscent of practices during slavery. Although attitudes toward doctors were mixed, many saw them as an option of last resort when the parents' own attempts had failed and no other alternatives were apparent. Many believed that physicians were too liberal in their prescription of medication and questioned whether this behavior was perhaps motivated by financial reward from pharmaceutical companies.

In terms of medication use, most were negative, although some saw benefits. Concerns about side effects and addiction were common, and for these reasons many did not consider medication to be a permanent solution. Perceptions of the school environment were also mixed. There were concerns that school administrators are quick to endorse ADHD diagnosis and medication to compensate for ineffective teaching styles and classroom structure. However, teachers were also seen as having difficult jobs, with large classroom sizes and insufficient tools, including discipline options, to maintain control.

Although many of these views may not be unique to African American parents, there was a general sense that these perspectives were intertwined with feelings of racial inequality and discriminatory practice, which are not often discussed or addressed by physicians or other clinicians.

## EVIDENCE-BASED TREATMENT INTERVENTIONS

The guidelines of the Task Force of the American Psychological Association classify treatments into three categories: well established, probably efficacious, and possibly efficacious.

- *Well established*: the highest level of empirical support, requires at least two high-quality (e.g., random assignment, adequate sample size) between-groups trials by different investigative teams showing that treatment is superior to placebo or another treatment or equivalent to an already established treatment (Chambless et al., 1996, 1998).

- *Probably efficacious*: requires only one high-quality trial comparing treatment with placebo (or alternative treatment) or two trials comparing treatment with no treatment (Chambless et al., 1996, 1998).
- *Possibly efficacious*: the existence of at least one study showing the treatment to be efficacious but has not yet met the standard for probably efficacious or well established (Chambless & Hollon, 1998).

At the time these criteria were established, there was no psychotherapy treatment research that met the standards for demonstrating treatment efficacy for ethnic minority populations (Chambless et al., 1996).

The hallmark of evidence-based treatment research on ADHD is the National Institute of Mental Health (NIMH) collaborative multisite Multimodal Treatment Study of Children with ADHD (MTA; MTA Cooperative Group, 1999a, 1999b). The MTA is the first major clinical trial by NIMH to focus on a childhood disorder. It is also the largest and most well-controlled study on children's mental health. The intent of the study was to identify which types of youth benefited most from which interventions. Children were randomly assigned to four treatment groups: medication only, behavior modification alone, the combination of medication and behavior modification, and community comparison. Six sites in the United States and one in Canada were selected in order to obtain a significantly large and diverse sample of youth with ADHD and implement the study using a common intervention protocol.

The participants were 579 children (80% males) ages 7 to 9.9 years; approximately 61% were Caucasian, 20% were African American, and 8% were Hispanic. Treatments were delivered over a 14-month period, with comprehensive assessments of functioning in multiple domains conducted at baseline before randomization and again at 3, 9, and 14 months. Treatment protocols were implemented more rigorously than typical clinic interventions. There were 19 measures of six dependent variables: (1) ADHD symptoms, (2) aggressive-ODD, (3) internalizing symptoms, (4) social skills, (5) parent–child relations, and (6) academic achievement.

As a result of the MTA and other research, only two interventions for ADHD have a well-established evidence base: medication, primarily with a central nervous system stimulant (Spencer et al., 1996; Swanson, McBurnett, Christian, & Wigal, 1995), and behavior modification (Pelham, Wheeler, & Chronis, 1998). The combination of these two is also widely recommended by the American Academy of Pediatrics (2001).

## Pharmacological Interventions

Pharmacological agents, particularly stimulants (methylphenidate, amphetamines) are the most effective treatment to date for the management of ADHD symptoms with a wide range of age groups, including preschoolers, school-age children, adolescents, and adults (Barkley, 2006). Approximately 75% of school-age children initially treated with any kind of stimulants show a positive clinical response. However, the majority of studies included youth referred from specialty clinics or university-based medical centers, resulting in samples that are predominantly male and White. More recent inclusion of youth from community-based settings such as clinics and schools has had little impact in changing the gender and ethnic distribution.

There is compelling evidence of the short-term efficacy of stimulant medications (American Academy of Pediatrics, 2001; Farmer, Compton, Burns, & Robertson, 2002; Pelham et al., 2005) for children with ADHD, including African Americans. Unfortunately, these medications achieve peak effectiveness about 2 hours following ingestion, resulting in the need for multiple doses to manage symptoms during and after school. The newer long-acting oral and transdermal formulations, which are described in more detail in the section on pharmacological treatments, have also been found to be effective in managing ADHD symptoms, although not all at the same levels of effectiveness (Pelham et al., 2005).

Trials using nonstimulant medications for ADHD are also underway. One of the major trials using nonstimulant medication is the Formal Observation of Concerta versus Strattera (FOCUS; Kemner, Starr, Brown, Ciccone, & Lynch, 2004), which involved 323 sites in a randomized, open-label investigation of Concerta (OROS methylphenidate [MPH]), a once-daily controlled-release medication, and Strattera (atomoxetine), a selective norepinephrine reuptake inhibitor and the first nonstimulant medication for ADHD. The study sample included 1,323 children ages 6–12 years with a diagnosis of ADHD based on psychiatric history and a review of the DSM-IV diagnostic checklist.

Given the limited data on ethnic minorities, Starr and Kemner (2005) conducted a subgroup analysis of the FOCUS data to determine the effectiveness of and tolerability for ADHD treatments among African American participants. Of the 183 African American children in the sample (14%, of whom 87% were male, with a mean age of 9 years), 125 received OROS MPH and 58 received atomaxetine. The response to the two treatments among the African American sample was similar to that observed in the overall study. Although children in both treatments showed significant improvements from baseline measures, by Week 3 the OROS MPH group demonstrated greater improvement. The two groups reported similar rates of treatment-related adverse effects: 19.2% for OROS MPH and 19% for atomoxetine. However, slightly more patients in the atomoxetine group (1.7% vs. 0.8%) withdrew from the study as a result of these adverse effects, which included somnolence, sedation, and nausea.

Overall, these results and those from the MTA study point to methylphenidate as a well-established treatment for ADHD among African American youth (Brown & Sexson, 1988; Bukstein & Kolko, 1998).

In addition to the pharmacological findings in the MTA study, secondary analysis of the data, which included "systematic explorations of mediators and moderators of treatment effects" (Swanson et al., 2008, p. 5), indicates a greater impact of behavioral interventions in combination with medication for African American children than for the overall sample. The combination treatment is currently classified as probably efficacious for African American children with ADHD and related problems. Although the MTA study found no ethnic differences in most treatment outcomes, intensive behavioral treatment plus medication was more beneficial than either medication alone or community services for both African American and Latino youth. The use of behavior modification has been found to lower the dosage of MPH needed to achieve improvement in symptoms.

## Psychosocial Interventions

The use of behavioral interventions for ADHD is considered effective and is recommended in clinical practice guidelines (American Academy of Child and Adolescent Psychiatry, 2007; American Academy of Pediatrics, 2001). However, according to Pelham and colleagues (2005), there is a lack of consensus among ADHD experts regarding the effectiveness of behavioral treatments as a result of comparative studies that use "non-intensive clinical levels or outpatient behavior therapy such as parent training or faded behavior therapy" (p. 112). In addition to the intensity of the intervention (Fabiano & Pelham, 2002), Pelham and Murphy (1986) strongly promote contingency management-based behavioral interventions as more potent than clinical behavior therapy.

The evidence does indicate that although combination psychosocial/pharmacological treatment has been found to improve functioning in areas such as academic accuracy and productivity for youth with ADHD, among the psychosocial interventions, contingency management methods applied across multiple setting such as school, after-school settings, and at home have the most empirical support (Barkley, 2006). Parent training in these methods is often necessary for utilization in and outside of the home. These behavioral interventions are one of the few scientifically proven alternatives for children (about 10–25%) who do not respond positively to medication. Brief summaries of the components of the specific behavioral interventions and model program, based on the work of Barkley (2006) are provided in subsequent sections, with additional citation recommendations for more comprehensive reviews.

### Parent Training

Parent training (PT) is often included in a multimodal approach to treatment of ADHD in order to provide parents with instruction on specialized child management techniques (Barkley, 2006). Typically, implementation involves 8–16 weekly sessions with psychoeducation about ADHD and instruction in behavior management strategies (Kaiser, Hoza, & Hurt, 2008). Most programs use a variety of contingency management methods aimed at improving the effectiveness of commands, transition planning, and altering tasks and settings to be more conducive

to performance by children with ADHD. The implementation of positive attending, token or point systems, response cost, and time out from reinforcement can
also be useful. Monitoring programs such as daily school behavior report cards
can be included for tracking and responding to child behavior when away from
home.

Recent evidence has emerged about the usefulness of PT in relation to family functioning, particularly when the child's ADHD symptoms are more severe.
Reduction in parent–child conflict, child defiance, and related disruptive behavior appears to benefit family functioning overall. There is also evidence of good
outcomes for children with comorbid anxiety when used as part of psychosocial
treatment in combination with medication. The education and strategies provided
in PT show good results in conjunction with medication for families of low SES.
Evidence suggests that the positive outcomes associated with PT are maintained
after termination of treatment (Barkley, 2006).

Large-group, community-based approaches to parent counseling and training provide an alternative to clinic-based parent training, and facilitate better
compliance and attendance. The Community Parent Education (COPE) program,
as described by Barkley (2006), is one example of a program that addresses the
needs of culturally diverse communities in several ways. Workshops are located
in community settings, such as neighborhood schools, making it convenient to
attend without the stigma of a clinic setting and using facilitators from similar
cultural backgrounds. The COPE model uses a coping-modeling/problem-solving
approach that encourages participants to formulate solutions to common child
management problems. Training discussions encourage parents to formulate
rationales supporting the strategies developed by the group. These explanations
reflect the unique perspectives that different cultures bring to the group. The
reader is referred to Pfiffner and Kaiser (2009) and Chronis, Chacko, Fabiano,
Wymbs, and Pelham (2004) for detailed overviews of behavioral parent training
for ADHD.

### School-Based Interventions Aimed at Teachers

According to Barkley (2006), the objectives of school-based interventions are to
improve basic knowledge among educators about the nature, causes, course, and
treatments for ADHD and to increase home and school collaboration in order to
produce a more uniform, consistent, and effective plan of management incorporating the primary caregivers. These objectives ultimately lead to the main goal,
which is to improve academic performance and social effectiveness among children with ADHD in the school setting. Core interventions for ADHD involve:

- Altering the physical classroom layout as needed.
- Modifying academic tasks to match each child's abilities and deficits.
- Increasing the use of computer-assisted instruction.

- Improving academic skills.

- Altering teacher-delivered consequences (e.g., attention, reprimands, tokens, time-outs) for appropriate and inappropriate conduct while minimizing adverse side effects.

- Intentionally programming for maintenance of treatment gains and generalization outside the treatment setting.

- Using peers to facilitate academic success and behavioral control.

- Developing home-based reinforcement programs (daily behavior cards).

- Striving to enhance self-monitoring and self-management.

- Modifying these approaches for use with teens with ADHD.

For a comprehensive review of the literature on school-based treatment of ADHD, the reader is referred to DuPaul and Eckert (1997).

### Social Skills Training

Social skills training has shown positive results for assisting children with ADHD in their social adjustment, but results are usually limited to settings with active behavioral programs in place to promote these skills (Barkley, 2006). There continues to be a need for better understanding of how to match specific instructional materials and behavioral management techniques to specific child characteristics, how to improve academic performance, and how to improve maintenance and generalization of intervention effects.

### Interventions with Adolescents

Interventions for families with adolescents with ADHD have a focus similar to those for younger children but recognize the opportunity for improvement in cognitive functioning as a result of maturation. Family training must include instruction in behavior management methods to assist with restructuring the physical and social environments, to help teens with ADHD "show what they know," and to give parents greater influence over teen misconduct (Barkley, 2006). Research indicates that a combination of behavior management training and problem-solving communication training does reduce conflict between teens with ADHD and their parents, but the effects are modest, reliably helping about 25% of these families.

In summary, combined treatment is clearly superior in terms of parent- and teacher-rated symptoms of ADHD, social skills, academic performance, and parenting. In addition, it appears to be better than either behavioral treatment alone or medication alone in normalizing children's functioning, as assessed by symptom composites of ADHD and ODD (Swanson et al., 2001); these effects are maintained at 24-month follow-up.

A review of possible moderators of treatment response to combined treatment (Kaiser et al., 2008) identified child comorbidity, child developmental level, family demographics, and parental psychopathology/cognitions as intervening variables. In addition, the authors point to certain areas as needing further attention in the research and clinical literature. Additional specificity is needed on the essential components of multimodal treatment with an examination of the appropriate intensity and ordering of the components. Because ADHD is more prevalent among boys, resulting in their overrepresentation in research samples, the knowledge base about treatment outcomes for girls is limited (Farmer et al., 2002). The same limitations exist for ethnic minorities. No clinical trials, except the MTA study, address the efficacy of psychosocial treatments for African American youth with ADHD (Huey & Polo, 2008). Virtually nothing is known about how to treat these youth with any other clinical syndromes, and much more is needed to encourage participation, to support the need and value of these studies, and to bridge the gap (Miller et al., 2009).

## PSYCHOPHARMACOLOGY AND ADHD

The effectiveness of psychopharmacological agents in the treatment of ADHD is well established. However, despite this evidence, given the limited involvement of African Americans in these studies and the current understanding of the attitudes, knowledge, and practices of African American caregivers in relation to ADHD and medication, decisions concerning treatment of ADHD should involve a great deal of information sharing and communication among client, caregivers, and the treating physician.

Treating clinicians must understand that African American parents' reluctance or refusal to use medication may be rooted in their culture's history of slavery, discrimination, and documented abuse in drug treatment trials. The most well known of these is the Public Health Service's Tuskegee syphilis study, which ran from 1932 to 1972, commissioned to determine the long-term effects of untreated syphilis. In this study, more than 200 African American men who were syphilis positive were denied both knowledge of their diagnosis as well as effective treatment.

Although such research would not be permitted today, born from its legacy are feelings of distrust by African Americans for the medical and broader research communities, which still persist. Distrust leads to avoidance of medical care until the late stages of illness, resulting in a self-fulfilling prophesy of sorts: Effective treatment of late-state illness is either limited in its impact or unavailable, making recovery less likely.

Children with ADHD can demonstrate remarkable improvement with medication. However, in addition to parental or caregiver beliefs about the use of medications, other factors should be considered, such as the severity of the symptoms and the efficacy of prior treatments, both medical and nonmedical. Inasmuch as parental attitudes toward ADHD and psychotropic medication have been discussed in sufficient detail in previous sections, the focus here is on the available medications, their side effects, selection, and other standards of care.

Medications used to treat ADHD can be divided into three classes: stimulant medication (e.g., Ritalin), nonstimulant medications (e.g., Strattera), and other medications (e.g., Wellbutrin). Although the mechanism of action for these medications is not fully understood, they do address several deficits observed in individuals with ADHD:

- The brain waves of individuals with ADHD are often slower than would be expected when performing tasks such as reading or when engaging in demanding activities.

- The brain's prefrontal cortex, which sorts and organizes sensations from the body and the environment, does not work as efficiently in youth with ADHD. As a consequence, the youth are often flooded with sensory information that is unfiltered and not prioritized, resulting in an unfocused, scattered mind.

The overall outcome from these, as well as other changes, is decreased concentration and hyperactive behavior.

## Stimulant Medications

Stimulant medications were first introduced in the 1950s as a treatment for narcolepsy, a condition in which individuals fall asleep suddenly. Its use in the treatment of ADHD began in the 1960s. There are two groups of stimulant medications: short acting and intermediate/long acting. The long-acting stimulants have a mean duration of 8–12 hours, and students avoid having to take medication at school. Newer formulations of the long-acting stimulants include Adderall XR and Concerta. Short-acting stimulants have a duration of action of about 3–6 hours, necessitating a midday dose often provided at school.

All of the stimulant medications, whether long or short term, are generally of two types: methylphenidate and dextroamphetamine. Both types of drugs have been designated as Schedule II controlled drugs by the U.S. Drug Enforcement Agency, meaning that there are special restrictions on their use because they have been found to be addictive in adults; however, this has never been established as an issue in children and adolescents with ADHD. In fact, it has been demonstrated that youth with ADHD who are adequately treated with stimulant medication are at lower risk for substance abuse issues later in life.

### Short-/Intermediate-Acting Stimulant Medications

Although there are a number of newer agents on the market, there is still a role for the older, short-acting stimulant medications. The shorter duration of some of the older medications may be beneficial for youth who experience loss of appetite. For example, because the duration of action may be as short as 3–4 hours, a youth taking medication at 7:00 A.M. may have a trough level by noon, allowing his appetite to grow in time for lunch before receiving an afternoon dose to last the rest of the day. Another advantage to shorter acting medications is that they can be used during select periods in the day, for example, with a younger child or one who only attends school part time and is in a less demanding setting during other times. Finally, many of these medications are now available in generic formulations, making them less expensive but as effective as the longer acting agents. This may be a suitable option for uninsured individuals and those who opt to pay out of pocket for medications. A discussion of specific individual short-/intermediate-acting medications is provided next.

### RITALIN

Ritalin (methylphenidate), first introduced in the 1950s, was among one of the most widely prescribed drugs for ADHD. With a duration of 2–4 hours, it often has to be administered two to three times daily. Ritalin, like most stimulants, is effective in more than 75% of individuals with ADHD. A number of different methylphenidate preparations have been introduced over the years, including Ritalin SR, Methylin, Methylin ER, and Metadate CD. These preparations allow for duration of action of up to 8 hours, in the case of Metadate CD.

### DEXEDRINE

Dexedrine (dextroamphetamine) was initially developed in the 1920s for the treatment of obesity and depression. By the 1930s, drug trials demonstrated that Dexedrine was effective in the treatment of hyperactivity. It was approved by the U.S. Food and Drug Administration (FDA) for the treatment of ADHD in 1958. Despite its effectiveness in treating ADHD and its status as the first drug on the market to treat ADHD, several side effects, including insomnia and appetite suppression, have limited its use. However, dextroamphetamine-based products such as Adderall have seen a resurgence in recent years because of their longer duration of action and a lower risk of insomnia and appetite suppression with the newer preparations.

### FOCALIN

Focalin (dexmethylphenidate) is a stimulant that is very similar to methylphenidate. Dexmethylphenidate is one of the active ingredients in methylphenidate, and it was hoped that because only the active ingredient was available in this preparation, there would be fewer side effects. However, this proved not to be the case, and Focalin use has never matched that of the other short-acting stimulant medications. However, there is increased use of the newer, longer-acting Focalin XR.

## Long-Acting Stimulant Medications

### CONCERTA

Concerta is a sustained-release form of methylphenidate (Ritalin) allowing for a full day of effectiveness, eliminating the need for midday doses. Although there were previous medications such as Ritalin SR that were designed to last an entire day, these medications were less effective than Ritalin. Concerta is as effective as Ritalin. It is designed to work for 12 hours but is only approved for children older than 6.

### RITALIN LA

Ritalin LA, like Concerta, is a methylphenidate derivative and also utilizes a technology that allows it to work for a full day. Ritalin LA capsules, like those of Concerta, can be opened and sprinkled on food if swallowing is trouble-some.

### ADDERALL XR

One of the more recent developments in the treatment of ADHD is Adderall XR. It is approved for use in children older than 6, although regular Adderall can be used in children 3 to 5 years of age. Adderall XR is a sustained-release form of Adderall, a popular stimulant, which contains dextroamphetamine. Like Ritalin LA and Concerta, the capsule can sprinkled onto food.

### DAYTRANA

One of the most recent medications released on the market is methylphenidate-based Daytrana. Unlike other long-acting medications that are administered orally to increase the duration of effectiveness, Daytrana is a patch that can be applied each morning and provides a continuous dose of medication throughout the day while worn. The dose of medication may be adjusted by varying the strength of the patch or by varying the amount of time the patch is worn.

### VYVANSE

The most recent dextroamphetamine-based medication introduced for the treatment of ADHD is Vyvanse (lisdexamfetamine dimesylate). This medication exerts its effect through the same mechanism as Adderall; however, the mechanism for extending its effective time is different and appears to be superior, offering up to

12 hours of effective treatment with fewer side effects. Its limitation is its relative cost, which is significantly higher than that of Adderall XR.

### Side Effects of Stimulants

The most common side effects of stimulants include nervousness, difficulty sleeping, loss of appetite, weight loss, headaches, upset stomach, nausea or dizziness, racing heartbeat, restlessness/agitation, irritability/mood swings, lack of spontaneity, social withdrawal, depression, and tics. Although all stimulant medications potentially cause side effects, long-acting stimulants tend to have fewer side effects that are sensitive to the amount of medication present in the body because the medication builds more gradually in the bloodstream and then wears off slowly. As a result, side effects and the rebound effect—the return of symptoms as the drug wears off—are milder.

In February 2006, the Drug Safety and Risk Management Advisory Committee of the FDA (2006) voted to recommend the addition of a warning label to all ADHD stimulant medications highlighting several safety concerns:

- *Heart-related problems*: ADD/ADHD medications can cause sudden death in children with heart problems. They can also cause strokes, heart attacks, and sudden death in adults with a history of heart disease. ADD/ADHD stimulant drugs should not be used by people with heart defects, high blood pressure, heart rhythm irregularities, or other heart problems. Additionally, anyone taking stimulant medication should have their blood pressure and heart rate checked regularly.

- *Psychiatric problems*: Even in people with no history of psychiatric problems, stimulants for ADD/ADHD can trigger or exacerbate hostility, aggressive behavior, manic or depressive episodes, paranoia, and psychotic symptoms such as hallucinations. Individuals with a personal or family history of suicide, depression, or bipolar disorder are at a particularly high risk and should be carefully monitored.

Parents must be educated about the side effects of stimulant medications to ensure that accurate information is provided as part of the informed consent process during discussions of their risks and benefits. Furthermore, side effects must be effectively evaluated and monitored. At a minimum, the following screening and evaluation measures should be undertaken:

- Physical examination: prior to initiating medication and when indicated based on symptoms.

- Height and weight: at initiation and at least one to two times annually.

- Monitoring of blood pressure: at initiation and at least once annually.

Parents should be alerted to contact their health care provider if any of the following symptoms occur: chest pain, shortness of breath, fainting, auditory or visual hallucinations, delusional thinking, or suspicion or paranoia.

## Long-Term Effects of ADD/ADHD Stimulant Medications

Although stimulants have been in widespread use for more than 40 years and their effectiveness in treating the symptoms of ADHD is well established, relatively few studies have examined their long-term safety. For children and young adults, whose brains are still developing, long-term use may cause permanent neurological changes. Because of the physical and mental health risks, all children being treated for ADHD should have a thorough medical workup to rule out other causes of ADHD symptoms. Once medications are initiated, the youth should see his or her health care provider at least monthly until stabilized. Thereafter, follow-up evaluations should be performed a minimum of once every 3 months.

## Nonstimulant Medications

Many parents may decide not to use stimulant medications because of cultural beliefs or a concern about addiction or other side effects. Some youth may not be able to tolerate stimulants because of related insomnia or increased anxiety, and for others stimulant medications may be ineffective in the treatment of ADHD. For these youth, there are other pharmacological options available, including the nonstimulant medications developed to treat ADHD, such as Strattera, and medications developed to treat other disorders (e.g., antidepressants) that have been found to be effective in managing ADHD.

### Strattera

Strattera (atomoxetine) was developed specifically for the treatment of ADHD. Unlike the stimulant medications, which affect dopamine levels, Strattera increases levels of norepinephrine. Strattera is longer acting than the stimulant drugs (> 24 hours), making it a good option for those who have trouble getting started in the morning. Because it has some antidepressant properties, it is also a good option for individuals with coexisting anxiety or depression. Unlike the stimulants that have a fairly rapid onset of action (< 1 hour in some cases), Strattera levels must build to a therapeutic dose in order to be effective. Therefore, it cannot be discontinued, unlike stimulants, which can be discontinued for periods without negatively impacting effectiveness when use is resumed. Strattera does not exacerbate tics or Tourette's syndrome, as do stimulants. However, it does not appear to be as effective for symptoms of hyperactivity.

Common side effects of Strattera include dry mouth, mild diarrhea or constipation, problems sleeping, sexual side effects, difficulty urinating, agitation/irritability, loss of appetite, drowsiness, headache, stomach upset, nausea/vomiting, and dizziness. According to its warning label, Strattera may also cause an increase in suicidal thoughts and actions in some children and teenagers. This is a particular risk if the youth has a mood disorder such as major depressive disorder or bipolar disorder in addition to ADHD. Warning signs include severe anxiety, agitation, impulsivity, irritability, hostility, panic attacks, insomnia, mania, and depression. An increase in any of these symptoms should be reported to the child's doctor immediately.

### Antidepressants

Youth with ADHD and comorbid depression and anxiety disorders will often benefit from antidepressants such as bupropion (Wellbutrin) and venlafaxine (Effexor). These atypical antidepressants target multiple neurotransmitters in the brain and can help with symptoms of depression, anxiety, inattention, and impulsivity. Although they are not as effective in treating ADHD as the stimulants or Strattera, they can be useful adjuncts in treating youth who cannot tolerate the side effects of other medications or who have these comorbid conditions.

### Other Medications

Although the stimulants, Strattera, and antidepressants are often effective in treating decreased attention and poor focus, they are sometimes only minimally effective in treating the behavioral symptoms, including impulsivity, hyperactivity, and aggression. In these situations, the alpha2-adrenergic agonists, initially developed to treat high blood pressure, can be beneficial adjuncts. Options include clonidine (Catapres) and guanfacine (Tenex). They are especially beneficial in children with Tourette's syndrome because they may suppress tics. However, these medications are not as effective with symptoms of inattention and, therefore, are generally used in combination with the other medications discussed previously rather than as a sole treatment.

In summary, the wide array of pharmacological treatments available for the treatment of ADHD and strong evidence of their effectiveness render them a valuable component in successful treatment plans. Comprehensive and accurate information about medication choices, benefits, and side effects is essential for the patient, family, and caregivers. Careful administration and monitoring can successfully manage risks and negative side effects. The addition of behavior management training is the recommended treatment for African American youth.

## PREVENTION OF ADHD

In 2003, the National Institutes of Health brought together representatives from the public and national and international experts in the research and health care fields to review the scientific evidence on ADHD (Ferguson, 2000). The consensus statement of the expert panel revealed that there was insufficient knowledge about the cause or causes of ADHD. Consequently, it was felt that there were "no strategies for the prevention of ADHD."

Today much more is known about the cause of ADHD, and although there is no research that addresses prevention directly, there are signs of progress in that direction. In the online edition of the *Proceedings of the National Academy of Sciences* during the week of November 12, 2007, researchers at the NIMH revealed that in youth with ADHD, although the brain matures in a normal pattern, some regions demonstrate delayed growth by as much as 3 years (Shaw et al., 2007).

The study involved 223 youth with ADHD and a similar-sized control group. In the control group, sensory processing and motor control areas of the back and top of the brain peaked in thickness earlier in childhood. The frontal areas supported the ability to suppress inappropriate actions and thoughts, remember things from moment to moment, control movement, and focus attention. In youth with ADHD, about half of the cortex sites examined attained peak thickness at an average of 10.5 years compared with 7.5 years in youth without ADHD.

The delays are most prominent in regions at the front of the brain's outer cortex, an area important for the ability to control thinking, attention, and planning. It is believed that this pattern may explain why many youth eventually outgrow ADHD. Previously, the focus of brain imaging had been the size of the lobes of the brain. New image analysis techniques, however, provided for greater precision and enhanced the ability to detect focal regional changes where the delay is most marked.

Although there are limitations in the use of this technology, which does not allow for detection of these findings on an individual basis, it does suggest the opportunity to increase recovery from the disorder, which is the beginning of discoveries related to prevention.

## RECOMMENDED BEST PRACTICES

The previous sections reviewed the clinical and scientific knowledge base on ADHD, with emphasis on African American children and their families. The recommendations offered here integrate and expand this information to address the existing gaps in engaging African American families in the evaluation and treatment of ADHD.

A comprehensive evaluation is routinely the first step in the clinical process. This may present a challenge because many African American families do not typically consider hyperactivity and inattentiveness as behaviors that warrant assessment and treatment. Therefore, intervention at an earlier stage is required and should optimally occur during a pediatric visit. The American Academy of Child and Adolescent Psychiatry (AACAP, 2007) provides recommended best-practice guidelines, which are primarily directed toward psychiatrists but can be useful for others in the medical community, particularly pediatricians.

The practice guidelines were first published as the practice parameter for the assessment and treatment of children and adolescents with ADHD in 1997. This was followed in 2002 by specific guidelines related to treatment with stimulant medications (AACAP, 2002). The most current edition, published in 2007, continues the tradition of providing evidence-based guidelines for the effective diagnosis and treatment of ADHD based on the current scientific evidence and clinical consensus of experts in the field. The strength of the underlying empirical and clinical support is identified at the end of each of the recommendations, with coding as follows:

- MS: Minimal standard is applied to recommendations that are based on rigorous empirical evidence and/or overwhelming clinical consensus. Minimal standards apply more than 95% of the time.

- CG: Clinical guidelines are applied to recommendations that are based on strong empirical evidence and/or strong clinical consensus. Clinical guidelines apply about 75% of the time.

- OP: Option is applied to recommendations that are acceptable based on emerging empirical evidence or clinical opinion but lack strong empirical evidence and/or strong clinical consensus.

- NE: Not endorsed is applied to practices that are known to be ineffective or contraindicated.

The parameters are organized in three categories, screening, evaluation, and treatment, with specific recommendations in each category. Reporting of the best-practice recommendations for African American youth with ADHD will be incorporated into the parameters of the AACAP with notation where there is additional or different information for this ethnic minority group. The following summary of the AACAP recommendations comes specifically from the published article (AACAP, 2007).

## Screening

*Recommendation 1*: Screening for ADHD should be part of every patient's mental health assessment (MS).

It is the expectation of the AACAP that specific questions related to the major symptom domains of ADHD (inattention, impulsivity, and hyperactivity) are asked regardless of presenting problem. Reporting symptoms that induce impairment should result in a full evaluation for ADHD if the physician, which is most likely to be the child's pediatrician, has the necessary training. Otherwise, a referral to a competent mental health professional is advised. Although it is suggested that rating scales or questionnaires be included as part of the registration process, no specific screening tools are recommended, information on common behavior rating scales used in the assessment of ADHD is provided in Table 16.1.

## Evaluation

*Recommendation 2*: Evaluation of a preschooler (age 3–5 years), child (6–12 years), or adolescent (13–17 years) for ADHD should consist of clinical interviews with the parent and patient, obtaining information about the patient's school or day care functioning, evaluation of comorbid psychiatric disorders, and review of the patient's medical, social, and family histories (MS). A comprehensive assessment by a health professional with specific training in the evaluation and treatment of ADHD should involve a detailed interview of the parent/caregiver and subsequently teachers. The primary goal of the assessment is to determine whether or not the child has ADHD and to differentiate diagnoses of ADHD from other childhood psychiatric disorders or medical problems. The assessment also serves to identify interventions that

**TABLE 16.1. Common Concerns and Suggested Methods in Assessment of ADHD**

| | |
|---|---|
| Current concerns about the child | • Unstructured interview |
| History of those concerns (onset, course, periodicity) | • Semistructured interview |
| Differentiation among other disorders | • Structured interview based on the DSM<br>• Well-normed behavior rating scales<br>• Semistructured interview of developmental domains (motor, language, social, educational, etc.) |
| Developmental inappropriateness of symptoms or concerns | • DSM diagnostic thresholds<br>• Well-normed behavior rating scales<br>• Psychological testing |
| Comorbidity | • Structured, DSM-based interview<br>• Screen for intelligence (testing)<br>• Screen for achievement skills (testing) |
| Impairments | • Interviews with parent and teachers<br>• Review of prior school and medical records<br>• Adaptive functioning interviews/scales |
| Psychological adjustment of parents | • Symptom Checklist 90—Revised<br>• Marital/couple functioning screen<br>• Parental stress screen<br>• Parental screen for ADHD (or other disorders as appropriate |
| Child and parent strengths | • Semistructured interview |
| Community resources | • Semistructured interview and search for available professional services |

*Note.* From Barkley (2006). Copyright 2006 by The Guilford Press. Reprinted by permission.

may be needed to address specific concerns. Barkley (2006) identifies issues that should be included in the assessment process to ensure a comprehensive review, with suggestions of specific measures for each component. It is also highly recommended that instruments normed for the child's specific ethnic background (if available) be used to preclude problems of overdiagnosis. This list is provided in Table 16.1.

Interviewing the patient along with the parent is recommended for preschool-age or young children, separately from the parents if the patient is an older child or adolescent in order to encourage sharing of sensitive information such as depression, alcohol, and other drug use or abuse. The patient interview also includes a mental status examination and allows the clinician to assess intellectual/cognitive processes as well as thought content and process.

*Recommendation 3*: If the patient's medical history is unremarkable, laboratory or neurological testing is not indicated (NE).

Although there are a few medical conditions with symptoms similar to ADHD (e.g., hyperthyroidism and encephalopathies), these conditions are not common among the vast majority of patients, and symptoms other than those shared with ADHD are also present. Exposure to lead paint or plumbing is a consideration in patients raised in older, inner-city environments and warrant measurement serum lead levels. *In utero* exposure to alcohol and other toxins contributes to a higher incidence of ADHD than for the general population and should be assessed.

*Recommendation 4*: Psychological and neuropsychological tests are not mandatory for the diagnosis of ADHD, but should be performed if the patient's history suggests low general cognitive ability or low achievement in language or mathematics relative to his or her intellectual ability (OP).

The importance of this recommendation relates to the common association between low standardized test scores and ADHD. The clinician will need to determine from the assessment whether the patient has ADHD, with academic difficulties as a consequence of the symptoms, whether there are two separate diagnoses; ADHD and a learning disorder; or whether there is a learning disorder with secondary inattentive symptoms.

Children who are primarily learning disabled often manifest difficulties in the academic subject specific to the disability and less frequently outside of that setting. There are also symptoms of learning/language disorders that are not part of the ADHD spectrum, such as expressive or receptive language difficulties. In such cases, both the learning disability and the ADHD would be diagnosed. Students with ADHD and academic difficulties that are more situational or can be ameliorated with one-on-one assistance or with rewards are more likely to show improved academic performance when the ADHD symptoms are managed.

*Recommendation 5*: The clinician must evaluate the patient with ADHD for the presence of comorbid psychiatric disorders (MS).

As with learning or academic difficulties, comorbid conditions can exist as a function of ADHD symptoms and as a separate diagnosis in addition to the ADHD. Anxiety disorders tend to have an early onset concurrent with ADHD (Kovacs & Devlin, 1998), whereas depressive disorders seem to occur several years after the onset of ADHD (Spencer, Biederman, & Wilens, 1999).

## Treatment

*Recommendation 6*: A well-thought-out, comprehensive treatment plan should be developed for the patient with ADHD (MS).

A plan of care should involve interventions such as psychopharmacological treatments and behavior therapy, which address the chronic nature of the illness. Psychoeducation for the parent and patient about ADHD and the treatment options is necessary. Referrals to community supports as well as school resources may be appropriate. The treatment plan should be reviewed regularly and modified as needed based on needs. In the event that pharmacological treatments will be part of the care plan, this treatment is best provided by a psychiatrist, the specialist best equipped to prescribe, evaluate, and manage its course.

Recommendations 7–10, which follow, directly address the use of these medications by treating physicians. Given the extensive information provided on the use of medication to manage ADHD symptoms, this information is not repeated in this section.

*Recommendation 7*: The initial psychopharmacological treatment of ADHD should be a trial with an agent approved by the FDA for the treatment of ADHD (MS).

*Recommendation 8*: If none of the agents approved for ADHD result in satisfactory treatment, the clinician should undertake a careful review of the diagnosis and then consider behavior therapy or the use of medications not approved by the FDA for the treatment of ADHD.

*Recommendation 9*: During a psychopharmacological intervention for ADHD, the patient should be monitored for treatment-emergent side effects (MS).

Strategies for managing side effects from medication include monitoring, adjustment of dosage, switch to another medication, and use of an adjunctive pharmacotherapy to treat the side effects. The risk of suicidal thoughts associated with atomoxetine use resulted in the addition of a boxed warning to its label. Although the risk is small, it is important to alert parents to the possibility so that symptoms can be monitored, particularly in the first few months of treatment.

> *Recommendation 10*: If a patient with ADHD has a robust response to psychopharmacological treatment and subsequently shows normative functioning in academic, family, and social functioning, then psychopharmacological treatment of the ADHD alone is satisfactory (OP).

The perspective of the AACAP (2007) is that for children without comorbid symptoms, the MTA study does not show significant additional benefit of the psychosocial intervention.

> *Recommendation 11*: If a patient with ADHD has a less-than-optimal response to medication, has a comorbid disorder, or experiences stressors in family life, then psychosocial treatment in conjunction with medication treatment is often beneficial (CG).

Analysis of the MTA study for children with comorbid disorders and psychosocial stressors shows that there are clear benefits to adjunctive psychosocial interventions. Children receiving public assistance as well as African Americans and other ethnic minorities also showed a better outcome with combined treatment. This points to the importance of individualization in treatment decision making for children with psychosocial stressors in addition to ADHD symptoms.

> *Recommendation 12*: Patients should be assessed periodically to determine whether there is continued need for treatment or whether symptoms have remitted. Treatment of ADHD should continue as long as symptoms remain and cause impairment (MS).

This recommendation speaks to the importance of regular follow-up for children with ADHD who are being treated with medication. The AACAP recommends that follow-up should occur at least several times a year to ensure that the medication is still active, the dose is optimal, and side effects are managed. As patients with ADHD enter adolescence, questions about continuation of medication often arise. The academy suggests that decisions to discontinue medication are appropriate if the patient has been symptom free for at least 1 year. Signs that the ADHD is in remission include lack of need to adjust dose despite robust growth, lack of deterioration when a dose of stimulant medication is missed, or new competencies arising during periods of abstinence from medication (drug holidays).

> *Recommendation 13*: Patients treated with medication for ADHD should have their height and weight monitored throughout treatment (MS).

The impact of stimulant medication on growth is at the core of this recommendation. Although the research is inconclusive, with some evidence of risk of small reductions in height gain in some studies, serial plotting of height and weight on growth charts is recommended to monitor changes that may be due to medication.

In summary, although comprehensive and grounded in strong empirical and clinical research, the practice parameters just described reflect the perspective of a specific group of treatment professionals and, with this focus, cannot be expected to provide guidance to all mental health professionals or specialty arenas.

Guidelines on recommendations for best practice related to behavioral interventions for individuals with ADHD, their families, and communities should also stem from the knowledge of efficacious practices such as have been described in the section on evidence-based interventions. However, because there is little to no available evidence-based research on engaging African Americans in the identification, assessment, and treatment of ADHD, recommendations that have been gleaned from the studies and clinical experiences involving African Americans are used as the basis for recommendations for parental engagement.

The previously cited studies involving African American caregivers and youth with ADHD consistently point to one pivotal issue: the disbelief that ADHD is an illness. This misperception results in underutilization of existing services, reluctance to actively and fully engage in the assessment and treatment process, and a tendency to discontinue services more frequently. The challenge, therefore, is bridging the gap between what African Americans, or anyone, believe about ADHD and what is known based on scientific and clinical research.

One recommendation is to provide better education to the African American community rather than exclusively to parents or caregivers of children at risk for or with ADHD (Miller et al., 2009). There is evidence that when ADHD arises as a concern, caregivers seek out information and advice from individuals within their social network. Although this network may include African American health professionals, it is important to note that these individuals may also share the same beliefs (Davison & Ford, 2001). It is important then to educate both professional and lay communities, disseminated by individuals who are likely to be seen as trustworthy. Although targeted outreach by peers with the same training background or discipline may be effective in educating health professional, community residents may benefit more from a diverse group that can address various perspectives (e.g., individuals with direct care experience; various professional groups such as nutritionists, social workers, psychologists, and psychiatrists; a parent of a child with ADHD and a child who is able to share his or her own experience with ADHD). This diverse team could engage community members and groups in order to increase awareness and education about ADHD, decrease stigmatization, and promote the benefits of ADHD treatment (Bailey & Owens, 2005). CHADD has utilized this team concept and sponsored events in partnership with local African American advocacy groups with good success.

Another suggestion is to structure the assessment and treatment process in a manner that addresses the concerns of the African American community. Reports concerning distrust of the educational system and the perceived lack of cultural awareness on the part of White educators indicate that teacher ratings of ADHD would be insufficient in convincing parents that a problem exists. What may be more effective is to review the child's social and academic history: A pattern of behaviors or concerns is more compelling and less easily dismissed as biased or insensitive reporting.

It is also possible that, for African American families of limited means, exposure to toxins and dietary concerns may be a factor. Although excess sugar intake may not cause ADHD, obtaining serum lead levels or referring the family for follow-up assessments related to alcohol exposure as part of an initial assessment would help identify affected children and result in greater engagement by parents because they feel that they have been listened to and taken seriously by the professional. In addition, if the family is treated as partners in care, it results in a cooperative relationship that facilitates open communication and information sharing. A clinician who actively facilitates this type of relationship allows the family to expand their perspective of the medical or scientific community beyond a narrow, more stereotypic view.

There has been some effort to develop culturally sensitive assessment instruments. The value of such measures has been validated by a variety of sources, including the American Psychological Association (2003). It is generally felt that neglecting cultural variables can lead to miscommunication and value conflicts, which increase the level of client discomfort, resulting in poor therapeutic engagement and ultimately failure of treatment (Huey & Polo, 2008. Although culture-responsive methods have been developed and are gaining in popularity, their formal application in controlled trials is rare. Given the reluctance of ethnic minorities to participate in research protocols, it is not surprising that only correlation data are available to assess these methods. Ethnic match between client and therapist (e.g., Genshaft & Hirt, 1979), specialized training (Lochman, Curry, Dane, & Ellis, 2001), and modifications in treatment format (Szapocznik, Hervis, & Schwartz, 2003) are some of the strategies that have been used.

Because little evidence exists that culture-responsive treatment is more beneficial than standard treatment for ethnic minority groups, there is clearly a need for additional experimental work to test the potential of these adaptations (Huey & Polo, 2008). It may also be useful to reframe the research questions to address issues that are more meaningful at this exploratory stage, such as whether more ethnic clients are engaged and retained, until there is a sufficient pool of clients to assess efficacy.

In conclusion, although the evidence base on ADHD is limited for African American children, there are strong data to support the use of stimulant medications in combination with behavioral interventions. Contrary to the perceptions of overdiagnosing and inappropriate use of stimulant medications, the studies suggest delays in accessing care and reluctance to engage in treatment. It is very likely that the prevalence of ADHD among African American children is similar to that of the general population; however, there is some evidence that treatment delays contribute to a more severe symptom presentation when initially referred to psychiatric settings. It is therefore imperative to provide accurate information to African Americans in general and parents of children at risk for ADHD in particular. Once parents do present for assessment, it is important to listen to and address their concerns and to rule out other factors that may contribute to the symptom picture. A comprehensive assessment by a competent professional is essential to forge a therapeutic alliance with the family.

## REFERENCES

American Academy of Child and Adolescent Psychiatry. (2002). Practice parameter for the use of stimulant medications in the treatment of children, adolescents and adults. *Journal of the American Academy of Child and Adolescent Psychiatry, 41*(92), 26S–29S.

American Academy of Child and Adolescent Psychiatry. (2007). Practice parameter for the assessment and treatment of children and adolescents with attention-deficit/ hyperactivity disorder. *Journal of the American Academy of Child and Adolescent Psychiatry, 46*(7), 894–921.

American Academy of Pediatrics. (2001). Clinical practice guideline: Treatment of school-aged children with attention-deficit/hyperactivity disorder. *Pediatrics, 108*, 1033–1044.

American Psychiatric Association. (2000). *Diagnostic and statistical manual of mental disorders* (4th ed., text rev.). Washington, DC: Author.

American Psychological Association. (2003). Guidelines on multicultural education, training, research, practice and organizational change for psychologists. *American Psychologist, 58*, 377–402.

Arnold, L. E., Elliot, M., Sachs, L., Bird, H., Kraemer, H. C., Wells, K. C., et al. (2003). Effects of ethnicity on treatment attendance, stimulant response/dose, and 14-month outcome in ADHD. *Journal of Consulting and Clinical Psychology, 71*(4), 713–727.

Bailey, R. K., & Owens, D. L. (2005). Overcoming challenges in the diagnosis and treatment of attention deficit/hyperactivity disorder in African Americans. *Journal of the National Medical Association, 97*(10, Suppl.), 5S–10S.

Barkley, R. A. (1997). Inhibition, sustained attention, and executive function: Constructing a unifying theory of ADHD. *Psychological Bulletin, 121*, 65–94.

Barkley, R. A. (2006). *Attention-deficit hyperactivity disorder: A handbook for diagnosis and treatment* (3rd ed.). New York: Guilford Press.

Barkley, R. A., Fischer, M., Edelbrock, C. S., & Smallish, L. (1990). The adolescent outcome of hyperactive children diagnosed by research criteria: I. An 8-year prospective follow-up study. *Journal of the American Academy of Child and Adolescent Psychiatry, 29*, 546–557.

Bazargan, M., Calderón, J. L., Heslin, K. C., Mentes, C., Shaheen, M. A., Ahdout, J., et al. (2005). A profile of chronic mental and physical conditions among African-American and Latino children in urban public housing. *Ethnicity and Disease, 15*(4, Suppl. 5) S5–3-9.

Biederman, J. (1997, October). *Comorbidity in girls with ADHD.* Paper presented at the annual conference of the American Academy of Child and Adolescent Psychiatry, Toronto.

Boyle, M. H., & Lipman, E. L. (2002). Do places matter?: Socioeconomic disadvantage and behavioral problems of children in Canada. *Journal of Consulting and Clinical Psychology, 70*(2), 378–389.

Brown, R. T., & Sexson, S. B. (1988) A controlled trial of methylphenidate in Black adolescents. Attentional, behavioral and physiological effects. *Clinical Pediatrics, 27*(2), 74–81.

Bukstein, O. G., & Kolko, D. J. (1998). Effects of methylphenidate on aggressive urban children with attention deficit hyperactivity disorder. *Journal of Clinical Child Psychology, 27*, 340–351.

Bussing, R., Perwien, A. R., & Belin, T. (1996). *Predicting unmet service needs for ADHD among children in special education: Who is at risk?* Poster presented at the annual meeting of the American Psychiatric Association, New York.

Bussing, R., Schoenberg, N. E., & Perwien, A. R. (1998). Knowledge and information about ADHD: Evidence of cultural differences among African-American and White parents. *Social Science and Medicine, 46*(7), 919–928.

Bussing, R., Schoenberg, N. E., Rogers, K. M., Zima, B. T., & Angus, S. (1998). Explanatory models of ADHD: Do they differ by ethnicity, child gender, or treatment status? *Journal of Emotional and Behavioral Disorders, 6*(4), 233–242.

Bussing, R., Zima, B. T., & Belin, T. R. (1997, October). *Mental health service use for ADHD across multiple sectors.* Paper presented at the 44th annual meeting of the American Academy of Child and Adolescent Psychiatry, Toronto.

Bussing, R., Zima, B. T., Gary, F. A., & Garvan, C. W. (2003). Barriers to detection, help-seeking, and service use for children with ADHD symptoms. *Journal of Behavioral Health Services and Research, 30*(2), 176–189.

Centers for Disease Control and Prevention. (2000). *Revised final FY1999 performance plan and FY2000 performance plan XIII.* Atlanta, GA: Author. Retrieved March 13, 2009 *www.cdc.gov/hiv/topics/surveillance/resources/reports/2005report/default.htm.*

Centers for Disease Control and Prevention. (2006). Racial/ethnic disparities in diagnosis of HIV/AIDS—33 states, 2001–2004. *Morbidity and Mortality Weekly Report, 55*, 121–125.

Chambless, D. L., Baker, M. J., Baucom, D. H., Beutler, L. E., Calhoun, K. S., Crits-Christoph, P., et al. (1998). Update on empirically validated therapies: II. *Clinical Psychologist, 51*, 3–16.

Chambless, D. L., & Hollon, S. D. (1998). Defining empirically supported therapies. *Journal of Consulting and Clinical Psychology, 66*, 7–18.

Chambless, D. L., Sanderson, W. C., Shoham, V., Bennett Johnson, S., Pope, K. S., Crits-Christoph, P., et al. (1996). An update on empirically validated therapies. *Clinical Psychologist, 49*, 5–18.

Children and Adults with Attention-Deficit/Hyperactivity Disorder. (2005, August 15). *CHADD applauds National Medical Association for acknowledging AD/HD's impact on African Americans.* Washington, DC: Author.

Chronis, A. M., Chacko, A., Fabiano, G. A., Wymbs, B. T., & Pelham, W. E. (2004). Enhancements to the behavioral parent training paradigm for families of children with ADHD: Review and future directions. *Clinical Child Family Psychology Review, 7*(1), 1–27.

Congdon, E., & Canli, T. (2008). A neurogenetic approach to impulsivity. *Journal of Personality, 76*(6) 1448–1483.

Davison, J. C., & Ford, D. Y. (2001). Perceptions of attention deficit hyperactivity disorder in one African American community. *Journal of Negro Education, 70*(4), 264–274.

dosReis, S., Butz, A., Lipkin, P., Anixt, J., Weiner, C. L., & Chernoff, R. (2006). Attitudes about stimulant medication for attention-deficit/hyperactivity disorder among African-American families in an inner city community. *Journal of Behavioral Health Services and Research, 33*, 423–430.

dosReis, S., Mychailyszyn, M. P., Myers, M. A., & Riley, A. W. (2007). Coming to terms with ADHD: How urban African-American families come to seek care for their children. *Psychiatric Services, 58*, 636–641.

dosReis, S., & Myers, M. A. (2008). Parental attitudes and involvement in psychopharmacological treatment for ADHD: A conceptual model. *International Journal of Psychiatry, 20*(2), 135–141.

dosReis, S., Owens, P. L., Puccia, K. B., & Leaf, P. (2004). Multimodal treatment for ADHD among youths in three Medicaid subgroups: Disabled, foster care and low income. *Psychiatric Services, 55*, 1041–1048.

dosReis, S., Zito, J. M., Safer, D. J., Soeken, K. L., Mitchell, J. W., & Ellwood, L. C. (2003). Parental perceptions and satisfaction with stimulant medication for attention-deficit/hyperactivity disorder. *Journal of Developmental and Behavioral Pediatrics, 24*, 155–152.

DuPaul, G. J., Barkley, R. A., & Connor, D. F. (1998). Stimulants. In R. A. Barkley (Ed.), *Attention-deficit/hyperactivity disorder: A handbook for diagnosis and treatment* (pp. 510–551). New York: Guilford Press.

DuPaul, G. J., & Eckert, T. L. (1997). The effects of school-based interventions for attention deficit hyperactivity disorder: A meta-analysis. *School Psychology Review, 26*(1), 5–28.

Epstein, J. N., Willoughby, M., Valencia, E. Y., Tonev, S. T., Abikoff, H. B., Arnold, L. E., et al. (2005). The role of children's ethnicity in the relationship between teacher ratings of attention-deficit/hyperactivity disorder and observed classroom behavior. *Journal of Consulting and Clinical Psychology, 73*(3), 424–434.

Fabiano, G. A., & Pelham, W. E. (2002). Evidence-based treatment for mental disorders in children and adolescents. *Current Psychiatry Reports, 4*, 93–100.

Faraone, S. V., Perlis, R. H., Doyle, A. E., Smoller, J. W., Goralnick, J. J., Holmgren, M. A., et al. (2005). Molecular genetics of attention-deficit/hyperactivity disorder. *Biological Psychiatry, 57*, 1313–1323.

Farmer, E. M. Z., Compton, S. N., Burns, B. J., & Robertson, E. (2002). Review of the evidence base for treatment of childhood psychopathology: Externalizing disorders. *Journal of Consulting and Clinical Psychology, 70*(6), 1267–1302.

Ferguson, J. H. (2000). National Institutes of Health consensus development conference statement: Diagnosis and treatment of attention deficit/hyperactivity disorder. *Journal of the American Academy of Child and Adolescent Psychiatry, 39*(2) 182–193.

Fischer, M., Barkley, R. A., Smallish, L., & Fletcher, K. (2004). Hyperactive children as young adults: Deficits in inhibition, attention, and response perseveration and their relationship to severity of childhood and current ADHD and conduct disorder. *Developmental Neuropsychology, 27*, 107–133.

Friedman, S., Paradis, C., & Hatch, M. (1994). Characteristics of African-American and White patients with panic disorder and agoraphobia. *Hospital and Community Psychiatry, 45*, 798–803.

Gaub, M., & Carlson, C. L. (1997). Gender differences in ADHD: A meta-analysis and critical review. *Journal of the American Academy of Child and Adolescent Psychiatry, 36*, 1036–1045.

Genshaft, J. L., & Hirt, M. (1979). Race effects in modifying cognitive impulsivity through self-instruction and modeling. *Journal of Experimental Child Psychology, 27*, 185–194.

Gershon, J. (2002). A meta-analytic review of gender differences in ADHD. *Journal of Attentional Disorders, 5*, 143–154.

Goodyear, P., & Hynd, G. (1992). Attention deficit disorder with (ADD/H) and without (ADD/WO) hyperactivity: Behavioral and neuropsychological differentiation. *Journal of Clinical Child Psychology, 21*, 273–304.

Harrison, M., McKay, M. M., & Bannon, W. M. (2004). Inner-city child mental health service use: The real question is why youth and families do not use services. *Community Mental Health Journal, 40*, 119–131.

Hart, E. L., Lahey, B. B., Loeber, R., Applegate, B., & Frick, P. J. (1995). Developmental changes in attention-deficit hyperactivity disorder in boys: A four year longitudinal study. *Journal of Abnormal Child Psychology, 23*, 729–750.

Hastings, J., & Barkley, R. A. (1978). A review of psychophysicological research with hyperactive children. *Journal of Abnormal Child Psychology, 7*, 413–437.

Huey, S. J., & Polo, A. J. (2008). Evidence-based psychosocial treatments for ethnic minority youth. *Journal of Clinical Child and Adolescent Psychiatry, 37*(1), 262–301.

Hynd, G. W., Semrud-Clikeman, M., Lorys, A. R., Novey, E. S., & Eliopulos, D. (1990). Brain morphology in developmental dyslexia and attention deficit disorder/hyperactivity. *Archives of Neurology, 47*, 919–926.

Jensen, P. S., Martin, D., & Cantwell, D. P. (1997). Comorbidity in ADHD: Implications for research, practice and DSM-V. *Journal of the American Academy of Child and Adolescent Psychiatry, 36*, 1065–1079.

Kaiser, N. M., Hoza, B., & Hurt, E. A. (2008). Multimodal treatment for childhood attention-deficit/hyperactivity disorder. *Expert Review of Neurotherapeutics, 8*(10), 1573–1583.

Kazdin, A., Stolar, M., & Marciano, P. (1995). Risk factors in dropping out of treatment among White and Black families. *Journal of Family Psychology, 9*, 402–417.

Kemner, J. E., Starr, H. L., Brown, D. L., Ciccone, P. L., & Lynch, J. M. (2004). Greater symptom improvement and response rates with OROS MPH versus atomoxetine in children with ADHD. XXIVth CINP Congress: Paris, France, 20–24 June 2004. *International Journal of Neuropsychopharmacology, 7*, S273–S274.

Kendall, J., & Hatton, D. (2002). Racism as a source of health disparity in families with children with attention deficit hyperactivity disorder. *Advances in Nursing Science, 25*(2), 22–39.

Kashani, J. H., Orvaschel, H., Ronsenberg, T. K., & Reid, J. C. (1989). Psychopathology in a community sample of children and adolescents: A developmental perspective. *Journal of the American Academy of Child and Adolescent Psychiatry, 28*, 701–706.

Klein, R. G., & Mannuzza, S. (1991). Long-term outcome of hyperactive children: A review. *Journal of the American Academy of Child and Adolescent Psychiatry, 30*, 383–387.

Kleinman, A., Eisenberg, L., & Good, B. (1978). Culture, illness, and care: Clinical lessons from anthropologic and cross-cultural research. *Annals of Internal Medicine, 88*, 251–258.

Klorman, R. (1992). Cognitive event-related potentials in attention deficit disorder. In S. E. Shaywitz & B. A. Shaywitz (Eds.), *Attention deficit comes of age: Toward the twenty-first century* (pp. 221–244). Austin, TX: Pro-Ed.

Kovacs, M., & Devlin, B. (1998). Internalizing disorders in children. *Journal of Abnormal Child Psychology, 29*, 513–528.

Lambert, N. M., Sandoval, J., & Sassone, D. (1978). Prevalence of hyperactivity in elementary school children as a function of social systems definers. *American Journal of Orthopsychiatry, 48*, 446–463.

Levy, F., & Hay, D. A., (2001). *Attention, genes and attention deficit hyperactivity disorder.* Philadelphia: Psychology Press.

Livingston, R. (1999). Cultural issues in diagnosis and treatment of ADHD. *Journal of the American Academy of Child and Adolescent Psychiatry, 38*(12), 1591–1594.

Lochman, J. E., Curry, J. F., Dane, H., & Ellis, M. (2001). The Anger Coping Program: An empirically-supported treatment for aggressive children. *Residential Treatment for Children and Youth, 18*, 63–73.

Mazei-Robison, M. S., Couch, R. S., Shelton, R. C., Stein, M. A., & Blakely, R. D. (2005). Sequence variations in the human dopamine transporter gene in children with attention deficit hyperactivity disorder. *Neuropharmacology, 49*(6), 724–736.

McKay, M. M., Pennington, J., Lynn, C. J., & McCadam, K. (2001). Understanding urban child mental health service use: Two studies of child, family, and environmental correlates. *Journal of Behavioral Health Services and Research, 28*, 475–483.

Miller, T. W., Nigg, J. T., & Miller, R. L. (2009). Attention deficit hyperactivity disorder in African American children: What can be concluded from the past ten years? *Clinical Psychology Review, 29*, 77–86.

Morrison, J. R., & Stewart, M. (1973). The psychiatric status of the legal families of adopted hyperactive children. *Archives of General Psychiatry, 28*, 888–891.

MTA Cooperative Group. (1999a). A 14-month randomized clinical trial of treatment strategies for attention-deficit/hyperactivity disorder. *Archives of General Psychiatry, 56*, 1008–1096.

MTA Cooperative Group. (1999). Moderators and mediators of treatment response for children with attention deficit hyperactivity disorder. *Archives of General Psychiatry, 56*, 1073–1086.

Mychailyszyn, M. P., dosReis, S., & Myers, M. (2008). African American caretakers' views of ADHD and use of outpatient mental health care services for children. *Family Systems and Health, 26*(4), 447–458.

Newcorn, J. H., Halperin, J. M., Jensen, P., Abikoff, H. B., Arnold, E., Cantwell, D. P., et al. (2001). Symptoms profiles I children with ADHD: Effects of comorbidity and gender. *Journal of the American Academy of Child and Adolescent Psychiatry, 40*, 137–146.

Nigg, J. T. (2001). Is ADHD an inhibitory disorder? *Psychological Bulletin, 125*, 571–596.

Nigg, J. T., & Hinshaw, S. P. (1998). Parent personality traits and psychopathology associated with antisocial behaviors in childhood attention-deficit hyperactivity disorder. *Journal of Child Psychology and Psychiatry, 39*, 143–159.

Nolan, E. E., Gadow, K. D., & Sprafkin, J. (2001). Teacher reports of DSM-IV ADHD, ODD, and CD symptoms in school children. *Journal of the American Academy of Child and Adolescent Psychiatry, 40*, 241–249.

Olaniyan, O., dosReis, S., Garriett, V., Mychailyszyn, M. P., Anixt, J., Rowe, P. C., et al.

(2007). Community perspectives of childhood behavioral problems and ADHD among African American parents. *Ambulatory Pediatrics, 7,* 226–231.

Olfson, M., Gameroff, M. J., Marcus, S. C., & Jensen, P. S. (2003). National trends in the treatment of attention deficit hyperactivity disorder. *American Journal of Psychiatry, 160,* 1071–1077.

Palfrey, J. S., Levine, M. D., Walker, D. K., & Sullivan, M. (1985). The emergence of attention deficits in early childhood: A prospective study. *Journal of Developmental and Behavioral Pediatrics, 6,* 339–348.

Pelham, W. E., Burrows-MacLean, L. B., Gnagy, E. M., Fabiano, G. A., Coles, E. K., Tresco, K. A., et al. (2005). Transdermal methylphenidate, behavioral, and combined treatment for children with ADHD. *Experimental and Clinical Psychopharmacology, 13*(2), 111–126.

Pelham, W. E., & Murphy, H. A. (1986). Attention deficit and conduct disorders. In M. Hersen (Ed.), *Pharmacological and behavioral treatment: An integrative approach* (pp. 108–148). New York: Wiley.

Pelham, W. E., Wheeler, T., & Chronis, A. M. (1998). Empirically supported psychosocial treatments for ADHD. *Journal of Child Clinical Psychology, 27,* 189–204.

Pfiffner, L. J., & Kaiser, N. M. (2009). Behavior therapy. In M. K. Dulcan (Ed.), *Dulcan's textbook of child and adolescent psychiatry* (pp. 845–868). Arlington, VA: American Psychiatric Publishing.

Ross, D. M., & Ross, S. A. (1982). *Hyperactivity: Research, theory and action.* New York: Wiley.

Samuel, V. J., Biederman, J., Faraone, S. V., George, P., Mick, E., Thornell, A., et al. (1998). Clinical characteristics of attention deficit hyperactive disorder in African American children. *American Journal of Psychiatry, 155*(5), 696–698.

Samuel, V. J., Curtis, S., Thornell, A., George, P., Taylor, A., Brome, D. R., et al. (1997). The unexplored void of ADHD and African-American research: A review of the literature. *Journal of Attention Disorders, 1*(4), 197–207.

Samuel, V. J., George, P., Curtis, S., Thornell, A., Taylor, A., Brome, D. R., et al. (1999). A pilot controlled family study of DSM-III-R and DSM-IV ADHD in African-American children. *Journal of the American Academy of Child and Adolescent Psychiatry, 38*(1), 34–39.

Semrud-Clikeman, M., Filipek, P. A., Biederman, J., Steingard, R. J., Kennedy, D., Renshaw, P., et al. (1994). Attention-deficit hyperactivity disorder: Magnetic resonance imaging morphometric analysis of the corpus callosum. *Journal of the American Academy of Child and Adolescent Psychiatry, 33,* 875–881.

Shaw, P., Eckstrand, K., Sharp, W., Blumenthal, J., Lerch, J. P., Greenstein, D., et al. (2007). Attention-deficit/hyperactivity disorder is characterized by a delay in cortical maturation. *Proceedings of the National Academy of Sciences, 104*(49), 19649–19654.

Spencer, T., Biederman, J., & Wilens, T. (1999). Attention-deficit/hyperactivity disorder and comorbidity. *Pediatric Clinics of North America, 46,* 915–927.

Spencer, T., Biederman, J., Wilens, T., Harding, M., O'Donnell, D., & Griffin, S. (1996). Pharmacotherapy of ADHD across the life cycle. *Journal of the American Academy of Child and Adolescent Psychiatry, 35,* 409–432.

Starr, H. L., & Kemner, J. (2005). Multi-center, randomized, open-label study of OROS methylphenidate versus atomoxetine: Treatment outcomes in African-American children with ADHD. *Journal of the National Medical Association, 97*(10, Suppl.), 11S–16S.

Stein, J., Schettler, T., Wallinga, D., & Valenti, M. (2002). In harm's way: Toxic threats to child development. *Journal of Developmental and Behavioral Pediatrics, 23*(Suppl. 1), S13–S22.

Still, G. F. (1902). Some abnormal psychical conditions in children. *Lancet, i,* 1008–1012, 1077–1082, 1163–1168.

Swanson, J. M., Arnold, L. E., Kraemer, H., Hechtman, L., Molina, B., Hinshaw, S., et al. (2008). Evidence, interpretation and qualification from multiple reports of long-term outcomes in the multimodal treatment study of children with ADHD (MTA): Part 1. Executive summary. *Journal of Attention Disorders, 12*(1), 4–14.

Swanson, J. M., Kraemer, H. C., Hinshaw, S. P., Arnold, L. E., Conners, C. K., Abikoff, H. B., et al. (2001). Clinical relevance of the primary findings of the MDT: Success rates based on severity of ADHD and ODD symptoms at the end of treatment. *Journal of the American Academy of Child and Adolescent Psychiatry, 40,* 168–170.

Swanson, J. M., McBurnett, K., Christian, D. L., & Wigal, T. (1995). Stimulant medications and the treatment of children with ADHD. In T. H. Ollendick & R. J. Prinz (Eds.), *Advances in clinical child psychology* (Vol. 17, pp. 265–322). New York: Plenum Press.

Szapocznik, J., Hervis, O. E., & Schwartz, S. (2003). *Brief strategic family therapy manual* [NIDA therapy manuals for drug addiction series]. Rockville, MD: National Institute on Drug Abuse.

Szatmari, P. (1992). The epidemiology of attention-deficit hyperactivity disorders. *Child and Adolescent Psychiatric Clinics of North America, 1,* 361–372.

Szatmari, P., Offord, D. R., & Boyle, M. H. (1989). Correlates, associated impairments, and patterns of service utilization of children with attention deficit disorders: Findings from the Ontario Child Health Study. *Journal of Child Psychology and Psychiatry, 30,* 205–217.

U.S. Food and Drug Administration. (2006). *Drug safety and risk management advisory committee meeting, February 9 and 10, 2006.* Washington, DC: Author. Retrieved April 18, 2009, from *www.fda.gov/ohrms/dockets/ac/cder06.html#DrugSafetyRiskMgmt.*

Valla, J. P., Bergeron, L., Bidaut-Russell, M., St-Georges, M., & Gaudet, N. (1997). Reliability of the Dominic-R: A young child mental health questionnaire combining visual and auditory stimuli. *Journal of Child Psychology and Psychiatry, 38*(6), 717–724.

Weiss, G., & Hechtman, L. (1993). *Hyperactive children grown up* (2nd ed.). New York: Guilford Press.

Whaley, A. L., & Geller, P. A. (2007). Towards a cognitive process model of ethnic/racial bias in clinical judgment. *Review of General Psychology, 11*(1), 75–96.

Willcutt, E. G., Doyle, A. E., Nigg, J. T., Faraone, S. V., & Pennington, B. F. (2005). Validity of the executive function theory of attention-deficit/hyperactivity disorder: A meta-analytic review. *Biological Psychiatry, 57,* 1336–1346.

Zametkin, A. J., Nordahl, T. E., Gross, M., King, A. C., Semple, W. E., Rumsey, J., et al. (1990). Cerebral glucose metabolism in adults with hyperactivity of childhood onset. *New England Journal of Medicine, 323,* 1361–1366.

Zito, J. M., Safer, D. J., dosReis, S., & Riddle, M. A. (1997). Methylphenidate patterns among Medicaid youth. *Psychopharmacology Bulletin, 33,* 143–147.

Zito, J. M., Safer, D. J., dosReis, S., & Riddle, M. A. (1998). Racial disparity in psychotropic medications prescribed for youth with Medicaid insurance in Maryland. *Journal of the American Academy of Child and Adolescent Psychiatry, 37,* 179–184.

Zwaanswijk, M., Verhaak, P. F., Bensing, J. M., van der Ende, J., & Verhulst, F. C. (2003). Help seeking for emotional and behavioural problems in children and adolescents: A review of the recent literature. *European Child and Adolescent Psychiatry, 12*(4), 153–161.

# 17

# Major Depressive Disorder

*Meeting the Challenges of Stigma,
Misdiagnosis, and Treatment Disparities*

Rahn Kennedy Bailey
Holly L. Blackmon
Francis L. Stevens

It is estimated that by 2053, nearly half of the entire U.S. population will be composed of ethnically and racially diverse people (Carrington, 2006). With this growing rate of diverse groups, clinicians and researchers will need to understand that the Eurocentric views peculiar to Whites may not be relevant or adequate to address the mental health needs among African Americans and other racially diverse, growing populations (Carrington, 2006). All physicians, those of African American descent and from other groups, are in need of important information related to how best to treat these diverse groups. From enrollment to diagnosis to treatment, all individuals from all backgrounds must be included in the process of the clinical research of affective disorders. This chapter provides an overview of contemporary clinical depression in the African American population. It will address the unique cultural, genetic, and environmental factors that may impact the development and progression of clinical depression and its management. We focus on the many myths and stigmas that adversely impact the diagnosis and treatment of this very debilitating disorder (Ronald et al., 2005). Finally, we outline ways the physician can meet the new challenges of addressing and treating depression in the African American population.

## THE SCOPE AND PREVALENCE OF THE PROBLEM

Major depressive disorder (MDD) is a common and disabling psychiatric disorder in the United States (Demyttenaere et al., 2004; Kessler et al., 2005; Ronald et al., 2005) and occurs across all racial and ethnic groups. The 12-month and lifetime prevalence rates of MDD are estimated at 6.7% and 16.6%, respectively (Kessler, Chiu, Demler, & Walters, 2005; Ronald et al., 2005). MDD is the world's fourth leading cause of disabling disease and the leading cause of nonfatal disease burden, responsible for almost 12% of total years lived with disability (Üstün, Ayuso-Mateos, Chatterji, Mathers, & Murray, 2004). In 2000, the economic burden of MDD in the United States was estimated at $83 billion (Greenberg et al., 2003), which includes costs related to employment, suicide, and medical care.

Kessler and colleagues (2006), using data from the National Comorbidity Survey replication, found that MDD accounts for 27.2 lost workdays per ill worker per year. This estimate includes workdays missed and poor performance on the job. Thus, the data highlights the impact that depression can have on people and society and underscore the need for accurate recognition and management.

The National Study of American Life is the largest study of mental health in the Black population conducted in the United States. In a sample of 6,082 adult patients, of whom 3,570 were African American, Williams and colleagues (2007) reported a 12-month prevalence of depression of 10.4%, highlighting the scope of the problem of MDD among African Americans. This study remains the largest such study including African Americans currently available.

## USUAL SIGNS AND SYMPTOMS AND PERSISTENCE OF MDD

The key diagnostic symptoms of clinical depression are well known and include depressed mood, loss of interest, loss of pleasure, significant weight or appetite change, sleep disturbance, psychomotor disturbance, fatigue/loss of energy, feelings of worthlessness or guilt, impaired concentration, and thoughts of death or suicide. Associated signs and symptoms noted in the fourth edition of the *Diagnostic and Statistical Manual of Mental Disorders* (American Psychiatric Association, 1994) include tearfulness, irritability, anxiety, pain (headaches, joint or abdominal pain), and impaired sexual functioning. Because of the numerous possibilities of the presentation of depression, diagnosis can be difficult.

In terms of severity, Williams and colleagues (2007) showed that, compared with Caucasians, African Americans were more likely to report episodes of depression that were either severe or very severe and more disabling. More than 56.6% of African Americans, compared with 38.6% of Caucasians, described their episodes of depression as disabling. The authors concluded that when African Americans develop MDD, it is likely debilitating and persistent.

## BIOLOGICAL/GENETIC FACTORS

Adding to the challenges health care providers face is that African Americans are more likely to suffer from certain other diseases in addition to MDD. Comorbidities have become a very important consideration in clinical medicine as our understanding grows of the impact of each disease on the whole system. African Americans have been shown to suffer consistently from more episodes of diabetes, obesity, and hypertension. These illnesses, compounded with higher rates of chemical dependency, place patients at greater risk of poor physical health and general disease, all of which increase the likelihood of limited clinical functional outcomes both medically and psychiatrically.

As many as 13.3% of all African Americans age 20 years and older have diabetes (American Diabetes Association 2007) African Americans are 1.8 times more likely to have diabetes than non-Hispanics or Caucasians. Depression can increase the symptoms of diabetes and decrease overall functional well-being (American Diabetes Association 2007) and is a risk factor for the development of Type 2 diabetes (Eaton, Armenian, Gallo, Pratt, & Ford, 1996) African Americans also have higher rates of obesity than Caucasians (American Obesity Society, 2007).

## INDIVIDUAL FACTORS INFLUENCING
## RISK AND RESILIENCY

Although biological issues play a role in the effect of MDD on African Americans, the choices individuals make concerning treatment should also be considered.

In 1996 the National Mental Health Association commissioned a national survey on clinical depression. The survey explored the barriers preventing African Americans from seeking treatment and measured overall knowledge of and attitudes toward depression. Among the major findings are that approximately 63% of African Americans view depression as a "personal weakness," and 31% believed that it is a "health" problem. Nearly 30% of African Americans indicated that if they were depressed they would "handle it" themselves, and almost 20% would seek help for depression from friends and family. Only 25% African Americans recognized changes in eating and sleeping habits as signs of possible depression; 16% identified irritability as a symptom. Only 33% of African Americans said they would accept medication for depression if prescribed by a doctor. Close to 66% indicated that they believe prayer and faith alone will successfully treat depression "almost all of the time" or "some of the time" (Coridan & O'Connell,

2001; Mental Health Association in New Jersey, Inc., 2001; National Mental Health Association, 2000).

## DISPARITIES IN AVAILABILITY OF AND ACCESS TO MENTAL HEALTH CARE

Availability and access to mental health care can play a significant role in the treatment of depression in African Americans. African Americans are less likely to seek psychiatric care than Caucasians, more likely to receive health care in outpatient hospital and emergency departments, and more likely to seek mental health services in emergency care settings. As a result, they are less likely to receive and benefit from the continuity of treatment provided by primary care. The 2000 surgeon general's report on culture, race, and ethnicity in mental health supports the common finding that Blacks are more likely to receive care in the emergency care center (U.S. Department of Health and Human Services, 2001). These facilities are, by definition, not organized to provide good long-term follow-up care or continuity of services. Among clinically trained mental health professionals in the emergency center, 2% are psychiatrists, 2% are psychologists, and 4% are social workers (Holzer, Goldsmith, & Ciarlo, 1998).

More African Americans prefer treatment by African American clinicians, although only a small percentage of medical professionals are African American. African Americans (Allmark, 2004) are more likely to seek treatment for their emotional distress from primary care clinicians than from specialty mental health providers. Yet depression in African Americans may be detected less often in primary care than it is in Whites (Borowsky et al., 2000). In terms of emotional distress, Cooper-Patrick and colleagues (1997) showed that African Americans are still more likely to seek treatment from a primary physician. Another factor complicating treatment involves health insurance. Nearly 25% of African Americans are uninsured, a rate 1.5 times greater than that for Caucasians (Brown, Ojeda, Wyn, & Levan, 2000). In addition, 53% of African Americans have employer-based health insurance versus 73% of Caucasians (Hall, Bromberger, & Matthews, 1999).

Access to health care is a barrier commonly experienced by Blacks. A relatively high proportion of African Americans live in rural areas of the South. However, mental health practices are concentrated in urban areas and are less likely to be found in the most rural counties of the United States (Holzer et al., 1998). Both the Epidemiologic Catchment Area study and the National Comorbidity Survey found that the percentage of African Americans receiving mental health care services from any source was one-half that of Caucasians (Swartz et al., 1988). It was noted that African Americans from counties in San Francisco and Santa Clara, California, were more likely to discontinue treatment and receive care in the emergency room compared with Caucasians (Hu, Snowden, Jerrell, & Nguyen, 1991; Sue, Zane, & Young, 1994).

## SOCIAL AND COMMUNITY FACTORS INFLUENCING RISK AND RESILIENCY

More than any other issue, the stigma associated with depression is a huge obstacle in the assessment and clinical treatment of African Americans. Stigma influences the diagnosis or leads to misdiagnosis; fuels negative attitudes, which deter presentation; and causes African Americans to seek care from a primary care doctor rather than a psychiatrist. Assessment issues to consider include (1) the misdiagnosis of MDD, (2) somatic symptom presentation, (3) attitudes and beliefs regarding depression, and (4) stigma surrounding depression and settings where African Americans typically seek treatment for depression (U.S. Department of Health and Human Services, 2001). Disparities in access to mental health care are another consideration. Some disparities include financial barriers, lack of health care providers, and geographical distribution of African American patients versus the geographical distribution of point-to-care settings (U.S. Department of Health and Human Services, 2001).

## PSYCHIATRIC MISDIAGNOSIS

A very sobering point is that African American patients are incorrectly diagnosed more often than Whites (Borowsky et al., 2000; Strakowski, Hawkins, & Keck, 1997). Race and ethnicity have been shown to be factors in accurate psychiatric diagnosis. One must consider that this is likely due in part to the subjective nature of psychiatric diagnoses. In fact, ongoing research assesses this issue. A variety of reasons exist for such discrepancy in psychiatric diagnostic patterns. Limited resources may prevent some African American patients from receiving a quality initial psychiatric evaluation and assessment (Carrington, 2006). Once an evaluation has been conducted, there is a risk that interpersonal bias can play a role in altering the accuracy of the psychiatric diagnosis (Adebimpe, 1981). Certain strategies/tools can be implemented to address these areas of concern. Critical among them is the high-quality cultural competency training of all clinicians. Such training has the potential to level the playing field and thereby increase the likelihood that all clinicians, regardless of background, will be prepared to make quality and unbiased evaluations of African American patients for clinical depression. Developing an understanding of the role of cultural context in psychiatric diagnoses is critical to the diagnostic process and accurate diagnoses (Quimby, 2006).

## PREVALENCE OF SOMATIC SYMPTOM PRESENTATION

African Americans are more likely to present with somatic symptoms compared with Whites. A possible reason for misdiagnosis among African Americans is that they are most likely to present with complaints of physical discomfort. According to data from Robins and Reiger as cited in Kirp (1992), 15% of African Americans presented with somatic symptoms compared to 9% of Whites.

Data from Brown and colleagues (2000) show that African Americans reported or were seen as having more severe sleep disturbance, appetite and weight loss, and hypochondriasis than Caucasians. Interestingly, these symptoms are in contrast to those of the more common emotional sadness typically addressed. This symptom presentation may account for some of the difficulty in detecting depression in African Americans.

## STIGMA OF DEPRESSION

Again, one of the greatest impediments to the successful treatment of clinical depression is the issue of stigma. Dr. Annelle Primm, Director of Minority and National Affairs for the American Psychiatric Association, expressed that such stigma is worse in African Americans in part because of the social factors specific to their culture (Moran, 2004), which include strongly held religious beliefs, lack of trust in the medical profession, communication barriers, and the long history of suffering in the African American community (Moran, 2004). Clearly, these issues require a more active process in order to satisfactorily screen for this disorder.

## ACCESS TO TREATMENT

Socioeconomic differences in America may play a role in African Americans' ability to access treatment for clinical depression. African Americans, along with other racial ethnic minorities, comprise just over half of the nonelderly uninsured population, partly because they are more likely to be in low-income families whose employers are less likely to offer coverage.

In 2005, 21% of the African American population was uninsured compared with 13% of the Caucasian population (Henry J. Kaiser Family Foundation & Garfield, 2007). African Americans, along with other ethnic groups, are less likely than their Caucasian counterparts to receive standard routine care in one stable setting and are more likely to participate in low-income plans such as Medicaid. African Americans are less likely than Whites to have a regular place to receive care or to have a health care visit. They are most likely to receive health coverage from Medicare or other public providers. Barriers to availability of care and access to clinical services are possible contributors to the severity of disability associated with depression.

## TREATMENT DISPARITIES

African Americans are less likely than Caucasians to receive appropriate care for depression. They are less likely than Caucasians to receive an antidepressant when their depression is first diagnosed (27% vs.44%) and are less likely to receive selective serotonin reuptake inhibitors (SSRIs) for treatment. Melfi, Croghan, Hanna, and Robinson (2000) made this conclusion based on their report on the treatment of 13,065 MDD patients in a state Medicaid study from 1989 through 1994.

## USE OF ANTIDEPRESSANTS

Results of a study by Miranda and Cooper (2004) showed that African Americans are less inclined to use medications prescribed by primary care physicians for treatment. Most African American patients prefer counseling to medications (Brody, Khaliq, & Thompson, 1997; Dwight-Johnson, Sherbourne, Liao, & Wells, 2000), are less likely to find antidepressant medications acceptable for treatment, and are less likely to believe that antidepressant medications are effective. In addition, they are more likely than Caucasians to believe that antidepressants are addictive Cooper et al., 2003).

## EVIDENCE-BASED TREATMENT INTERVENTIONS

The field of psychiatric medicine has worked for years to improve the clinical treatment of depression, and among African Americans, there seem to be specific strategies that are particularly helpful in this regard. As clinicians, we look for ways to improve diagnosis and understand the role of cultural context in psychiatric diagnoses. This is critical to the accuracy of the diagnostic process in particular. Physicians should also consider the stigma associated with mental health illness and treatment when caring for patients suspected to have depression. This factor alone can derail treatment: some patients have become noncompliant because of the stigma of having a "brain illness."

Physicians should assess their patients regarding depression, life stressors, and social conflicts and their relation to any somatic symptoms. Many patients will often focus on somatic concerns significantly. In soliciting their patients' concerns, physicians empower patients to know that their concerns are important. The ability of patients to describe their social stressors, life conflicts, and individual style of coping can be a helpful strategy in successful treatment. Maintaining a respectful, open approach in understanding patients' style of coping with depressive symptoms, including religious beliefs, will facilitate an environment where patients can feel comfortable discussing their concerns.

## RECOMMENDATIONS FOR EFFECTIVE
## MANAGEMENT OF MDD

In order to provide the most effective treatment for clinical depression in their African American patients, physicians must determine their treatment preference, for example, medications or talk therapy (Das, Olfson, McCurtis, & Weissman,

2006). One should ask the patients first if they have a preference. Talk therapy, if desired, should be pursued.

Physicians should educate patients about available treatments, including antidepressant medications, along with their onset of action and side effects (Das et al., 2006). Patients need to be educated about the illness, treatment, and clinical depression as a disorder. Treatment adherence should be regularly checked. Clinicians should assist patients in finding strategies to overcome social or financial barriers (Das et al., 2006). Compliance should be assiduously assessed, and the clinicians should take the lead and work actively to assist patients in overcoming the common social and financial barriers that abort the treatment process.

## PSYCHOPHARMACOLOGY AND MDD

African Americans may avoid or cease antidepressant treatment because of poor tolerance of certain classes of psychotropic medications (Das et al., 2006). Among African American medical circles, there has been frequent discussion of the differences in medication response among patients.

African Americans tend to respond more quickly to antipsychotic medications and tricyclic antidepressants than Caucasians because of differences in drug metabolism in the cytochrome enzyme (specifically CYP2D6) (Bradford, 2002). The hepatic CYP2D6 microenzyme system plays a readily identifiable role in this matter, partially explaining these observed differences. African Americans treated with tricyclic antidepressants, will, therefore, experience higher plasma levels per dose and an earlier onset of action than Whites.

It is estimated that 47–70% of African Americans and Asian Americans may be slow metabolizers of tricyclic antidepressants, which accounts for the higher incidence of side effects in these populations (Ruiz, 2000). Using agents with less effect on the hepatic CYP450 system, such as SSRIs and selective norepinephrine reuptake inhibitors, may reduce the risk of toxicity and overdose among ethnic minorities, making it more likely they will seek psychiatric treatment for depression (Ruiz, 2000). A review by Bradford (2002) found that, for African Americans, nonfunctional and reduced-function alleles for CYP2D6 account for nearly half (48.7%) of alleles observed in African Americans compared with 26% in Caucasians. Functional CYP2D6 alleles represent a median frequency of 71% of alleles among Whites (Bradford, 2002). Although it is unclear whether these differences lead to a higher number of poor metabolizers among African Americans, it is important that clinicians be aware of potential CYP2D6 allele differences. More research is needed in this area to understand the clinical implications of these findings.

## RESEARCH PARTICIPATION

The low research participation rates of ethnic-minority patients in clinical research has long been a point of significant concern. To generalize research results, it is important that all groups be active participants in health research (Allmark, 2004; Freedman et al., 1995). Because of their reluctance to participate, persons of all race and ethnicity minorities must be aggressively pursued for clinical trials if the data results are to be effective. Studies that show a positive endpoint are most useful if the endpoint pertains to all groups who might receive that treatment.

Factors that contribute to lower African American participation in research are medical eligibility, child care demands, job flexibility, and geographic proximity to the research site. There are a number of reasons for the dearth of African Americans in clinical research projects, both as investigators and participants. Perhaps the most significant reason is the well-documented history of research abuse, the Tuskegee syphilis study (Bonner & Miles, 1997; El-Sadr & Capps, 1992; Kirp, 1992; Thomas, Pinto, Roach, & Vaughn, 1994; Wendler et al., 2006). These factors conspire to discourage many African Americans from clinical research participation. Yet there are data suggesting that certain segments of the community are actually willing to participate when invited.

Efforts to increase minority access to clinical research studies should focus on a range of considerations, including invitations to participate, using sites that are accessible to minority groups, and identification of factors that may undermine minority participation, such as lack of trust. Efforts should also focus on overcoming the readily identifiable barriers, and solutions to address them, for example, provision of child care and reimbursement of travel expense (Bonner & Miles, 1997; Wendler et al., 2006). The resolution of job conflicts and the use of nontraditional sites that are more comfortable and convenient for the African American patients would promote greater research participation.

## CONCLUSION

Clinical depression presents a formidable burden for the African American community. Cultural and socioeconomic factors present barriers to accurate diagnosis and treatment. Metabolic differences may play a role in optimal treatment response. Medical comorbidities may present challenges to effective treatment. Last, greater participation in clinical research trials is essential to ensure improved means of accurate diagnosis and to identify successful MDD treatments that may be specific to African Americans.

## REFERENCES

Adebimpe, V. R. (1981). Overview: White norms in psychiatric diagnosis of Black American patients. *American Journal of Psychiatry, 138,* 279–285.

Allmark, P. (2004). Should research samples reflect the diversity of the population? *Journal of Medical Ethics, 30,* 185–189.

American Diabetes Association. (2007). *African American and diabetes facts.* Alexandria, VA: Author. Retrieved May 22, 2007, from *diabetes.org/communityprograms-and-localevents/africanamerican/facts.jsp.*

American Obesity Society. (2007). *AOA fact sheet.* Silver Spring, MD: Author. Retrieved May 22, 200,7 from *www.obesityusa.org/subs/fastfacts/Obesity_Minority_Pop.shtml.*

American Psychiatric Association. (1994). *Diagnostic and statistical manual of mental disorders* (4th ed.). Washington, DC: Author.

Bonner, G. J., & Miles, T. P. (1997). Participation of African Americans in clinical research. *Neuroepidemiology, 16,* 281–284.

Borowsky, S., Rubenstein, L., Meredith, L., Camp, P., Jackson-Triche, M., & Wells, K. (2000). Who is at risk of nondetection of mental health problems in primary care? *Jounal of General Internal Medicine, 15*(6), 381–388.

Bradford, L. D. (2002). CYP2D6 allele frequency in European Caucasians, Asians, Africans and their descendents. *Pharmacogenomics, 3,* 229–243.

Brody, D. S., Khaliq, A., & Thompson T. (1997). Patients' perspectives on the management of emotional distress in primary care settings. *Journal of General Internal Medicine, 12*(7), 403–406.

Brown, E. R., Ojeda, V. D., Wyn, R., & Levan, R. (2000). *Racial and ethnic disparities in access to health insurance and health care.* Los Angeles: University of California at Los Angeles Center for Health Policy Research and the Henry J Kaiser Family Foundation.

Carrington, C. H. (2006). Clinical depression in African American women: Diagnoses, treatment, and research. *Journal of Clinical Psychology, 62*(7), 779–791.

Cooper, L. A., Gonzales, J. J., Gallo, J. J., Rost, K. M., Meredith, L. S., Rubenstein, L. V., et al. (2003). The acceptability of treatment for depression among African-American, Hispanic, and White primary care patients. *Medical Care, 41,* 479–489.

Cooper-Patrick, L., Gallo, J. J., Powe, N. R., Steinwachs, D. M., Eaton, W. W., & Ford, D. E. (1997). Mental health service utilization by African Americans and Whites: The Baltimore epidemiologic catchment area follow-up. *Medical Care, 37,* 1034–1045.

Coridan, C., & O'Connell, C. (2001). *Meeting the challenge: ending treatment disparities for women of color.* Alexandria, VA: National Mental Health Association.

Das, A. K., Olfson, M., McCurtis, H. L., & Weissman, M. M. (2006). Depression in African Americans: Breaking barriers to detection and treatment: Community-based studies tend to ignore high-risk groups of African Americans. *Journal of Family Practice, 55*(1), 30–39.

Demyttenaere, K., Bruffaerts, R., Posada-Villa, J., Gasquet, I., Kovess, V., Lepine, J. P., et al. (2004). Prevalence, severity, and unmet need for treatment of mental disorders in the World Health Organization World Mental Health Surveys. *Journal of the American Medical Association, 291*(21), 2581–2590.

Dwight-Johnson, M., Sherbourne, C., Liao, D., & Wells, K. (2000). Treatment preferences among depressed primary care patients. *Journal of General Internal Medicine, 15*(8), 527–534.

Eaton, W. W., Armenian, H., Gallo, J., Pratt, L., & Ford, D. E. (1996). Depression and risk for onset of Type II diabetes: A prospective population-based study. *Diabetes Care, 19*(10), 1097–1102.

El-Sadr, W., & Capps, L. (1992). The challenge of minority recruitment in clinical trials for AIDS. *Journal of the American Medical Association, 267,* 954–957.

Freedman, L. S., Simon, R., Foulkes, M. A., Friedman, L., Geller, N. L., Gordon, D. J., et al. (1995). Inclusion of women and minorities in clinical trials and the NIH Revitalization Act of 1993: The perspective of NIH clinical trialists. *Control Clinical Trials,* *16,* 277–285.

Greenberg, P. E., Kessler, R. C., Birnbaum, H. G., Leong, S. A., Lowe, S. W., Berglund, P. A., et al. (2003). The economic burden of depression in the United States: How did it change between 1990 and 2000? *Journal of Clinical Psychiatry, 64,* 1465–1475.

Hall, M., Bromberger, J., & Matthews, K. A. (1999). Socioeconomic status and health in industrial nations. *Annals of the New York Academy of Sciences, 896,* 427–430.

Henry J. Kaiser Family Foundation, & Garfield, R. (2007). *Key facts: race, ethnicity and medical care* (Publication No. 6069-02). Menlo Park, CA: Henry J. Kaiser Family Foundation. Retrieved May 22, 2007, from *www.kff.org/minorityhealth/upload/6069-02.pdf.*

Holzer, C. E., Goldsmith, H. F., & Ciarlo, J. A. (1998). Effects of rural-urban county type on the availability of health and mental health care professionals. In R. W. Manderscheid & M. J. Henderson (Eds.), *Mental health, United States* (pp. 204–213). Rockville, MD: Center for Mental Health Services.

Hu, T. W., Snowden, L. R., Jerrell, J. M., & Nguyen, T. D. (1991). Ethnic populations in public mental health: Services choice and level of use. *American Journal of Public Health, 81*(11), 1429–1434.

Kessler, R. C., Akiskal, H. S., Ames, M., Birnbaum, H., Greensberg, P., Hirschfeld, R. M., et al. (2006). Prevalence and effects of mood disorders on work performance in a nationally representative sample of U.S. workers. *American Journal of Psychiatry, 163,* 1561–1568.

Kessler, R. C., Chiu, W. T., Demler, O., & Walters, E. E. (2005). Prevalence, severity, and comorbidity of 12-month DSM-IV disorders in the national comorbidity survey replication. *Archives of General Psychiatry, 62,* 617–627.

Kirp, D. L. (1992, November). What school choice really means. *Atlantic Monthly,* pp. 38–42.

Melfi, C. A., Croghan, T. W., Hanna, M. P., & Robinson, R. L. (2000). Racial variation in antidepressant treatment in a Medicaid population. *Journal of Clinical Psychiatry, 61*(1), 16–21.

Mental Health Association in New Jersey, Inc. (2001). *African American outreach (African American factsheet).* Verona, NJ: Author.

Miranda, J., & Cooper, L. (2004). Disparities in care for depression among primary care patients. *Journal of General Internal Medicine, 19,* 120–126.

Moran, M. (2004). Culture, history can keep Blacks from getting depression treatment. *Psychiatry News, 39,* 11–12.

National Mental Health Association. (2000). *Depression and African Americans (factsheet).* Alexandria, VA: Author.

Quimby, E. (2006). Ethnography's role in assisting mental health research and clinical practice. *Journal of Clinical Psychology, 62,* 859–879.

Ronald, C., Kessler, R. C., Berglund, P., Demler, O., Jin, R., Merikangas, K. R., et al. (2005). Lifetime prevalence and age-of-onset distributions of DSM-IV disorders in the national comorbidity survey replication. *Archives of General Psychiatry, 62,* 593–602.

Ruiz, P. (Ed.). (2000). *Ethnicity and psychopharmacology.* Washington, DC: American Psychiatric Press.

Strakowski, S. M., Hawkins, J. M., & Keck, P. E., Jr. (1997). The effects of race and information variance on disagreement between psychiatric emergency service and research diagnoses in first-episode psychosis. *Journal of Clinical Psychiatry, 58*(10), 457–463.

Sue, S., Zane, N., & Young, K. (1994). Research on psychotherapy on culturally diverse populations. In A. Bergin & S. Garfield (Eds.), *Handbook of psychotherapy and behavior change* (4th ed., pp. 783–817). New York: Wiley.

Swartz, M., Wagner, H., Swanson, J., Burns, B., George, L., & Padgett, D. (1988). Comparing use of public and private mental health services: The enduring barriers of race and age. *Community Mental Health Journal, 34,* 133–144.

Thomas, C. R., Pinto, H. A., Roach, M., III, & Vaughn, C. B. (1994). Participation in clinical trials: Is it state-of-the-art treatment for African Americans and other people of color? *Journal of the National Medical Association, 86,* 177–182.

U.S. Department of Health and Human Services. (2001). *Mental health: Culture, race, and ethnicity—A supplement to mental health: A report of the surgeon general.* Rockville, MD. Author.

Üstün, T. B., Ayuso-Mateos, J. L., Chatterji, S., Mathers, C., & Murray C. J. L. (2004). Global burden of depressive disorders in the year 2000. *British Journal of Psychiatry, 184,* 386–392.

Wendler, D., Kington, R., Madans, J., Van Wye, G., Christ-Schmidt, H., Pratt, L. A., et al. (2006). Are racial and ethnic minorities less willing to participate in health research? *Public Library of Science Medicine, 3,* 201–210. Retrieved December 3, 2007, from *www.plosmedicine.org.*

Williams, D. R., González, H. M., Neighbors, H., Nesse, R., Abelson, J. M., Sweetman, J., et al. (2007). Prevalence and distribution of major depressive disorder in African Americans, Caribbean Blacks, and non-Hispanic Whites: Results from the National Survey of American Life. *Archives of General Psychiatry, 64,* 305–315.

# 18

# Schizophrenia

WILLIAM B. LAWSON
SHANA JEANELLE GAGE

**S**chizophrenia is regarded as the most severe of neuropsychiatric disorders, and its prognosis is often poor. Although dementing illnesses can be just as severe, the early onset of schizophrenia, in the late teens and early 20s, and an only slightly reduced life span means years of lost productivity and immeasurable suffering endured by patients and family members (Dixon, 1999; Mueser & McGurk, 2004). Recent advances have led to improved diagnostic accuracy and to a better understanding of genetic risks and psychosocial stressors. Moreover, improved treatment has made recovery an attainable goal (World Health Organization, 1979). Studies have suggested that recovery from schizophrenia has been underestimated, especially in the third world (Jablensky et al., 1992). Race and ethnicity may impact the diagnosis, course, and treatment of this illness through biopsychosocial factors that are only now beginning to be appreciated. We suspect that a lack of consideration of these factors in the diagnosis and treatment plan limits the likelihood of recovery.

## EPIDEMIOLOGY

The literature has historically presented African Americans as being at increased risk for schizophrenia. However, recent findings show no or lower disparity in prevalence by ethnicity. The differences may be a result of misdiagnosis.

Overdiagnosis of schizophrenia is presumed because racial differences have often disappeared with the use of structured interviews, which presumably minimize bias (Lawson, 2002). Large-scale, door-to-door epidemiological surveys have tended to support this interpretation as well. The Epidemiologic Catchment Area study, which sampled five major cities and oversampled ethnic minorities, found no difference between African Americans and other ethnic groups when socioeconomic class was controlled (Robins, Locke, & Regier, 1991). The National Comorbidity Survey and the more recent National Comorbidity Survey Replication found that African Americans were less likely to have nonaffective psychosis, which is primarily schizophrenia (Kessler et al., 1994, 2005). The lower rates may be the result of the National Comorbidity Studies failing to sample institutionalized populations, including jails, where African Americans are overrepresented.

Nevertheless, clinical studies continue to show that African Americans are more likely to be diagnosed with schizophrenia in a variety of settings. The overdiagnosis occurs in juvenile facilities, in VA hospitals, and in public and private facilities (Barnes, 2004; Blow et al., 2004; DelBello, Lopez-Larson, Soutullo, & Strakowski, 2001). We examined psychiatric disorders in treatment settings in the state of Tennessee (Lawson, Hepler, Holladay, & Cuffel, 1994). Because inpatient admissions were for involuntary patients alone, treatment seeking was not a variable. Nevertheless, schizophrenia was diagnosed in African Americans at a proportionally greater rate than their representation in the population (Figure 18.1).

Overdiagnosis can even occur with structured interview instruments. The development of the DSM-III has certainly improved the validity and the diagnosis of psychiatric disorders. However consistent use of the third edition of the *Diagnostic and Statistical Manual of Mental Disorders* (DSM-III; American Psychiatric Association, 1980) and now DSM-IV (American Psychiatric Association, 1994) often does not prevent the misdiagnosing of African Americans. Strakowski's group (2003) showed that the misdiagnosis was the result of a failure to obtain accurate information rather than misapplication of the diagnostic criteria, although both factors contributed.

In addition, African Americans with affective disorders are more likely to have prominent first-rank psychotic symptoms than Caucasians, which uninformed clinicians often interpret as evidence for schizophrenia while overlooking affective symptoms (Arnold et al., 2004). Other related factors include clinician bias based on preconceived notions of the presence of affective disorders in African Americans, lack of familiarity with culture-based idioms of distress, and social distance (Lawson, 2002).

Misdiagnosis may be a result of cultural misinterpretation. The increased likelihood of psychotic symptoms in African Americans may be a result of a misinterpretation of other intrapsychic experiences. African Americans without schizophrenia, for example, are more likely to report dissociative symptoms (Frueh et al., 2002; Seedat, Stein, & Forde, 2003). Paranoia is often reported by African American patients (Lawson, 2002). A cultural reticence to disclose inner feelings to strangers of a different ethnicity is often reported and has been referred to as a "healthy paranoia" (Jones & Gray, 1986). African Americans will often delay or not seek mental health treatment until symptoms are severe, making

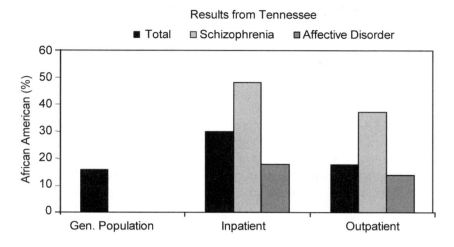

**FIGURE 18.1.** Overdiagnosis of schizophrenia in African Americans. Data from Lawson, Hepler, Holladay, and Cuffel (1994).

diagnosis difficult (Lawson, 2002). Consideration should be given to diagnosing schizophrenia in African Americans only if the diagnostic criteria are fully met and as a diagnosis of exclusion.

In summary, all sources of information should be considered in the diagnostic assessment of schizophrenia in African Americans and other ethnic groups. Family members, caretakers, and medical records should be consulted. Premature closure should be avoided when a patient presents with psychotic symptoms. Hallucinations and delusions may occur in affective and anxiety disorders, especially when treatment has been delayed. Close adherence to the DSM-IV should be encouraged, with the recognition that the DSM does not exclude mood or anxiety disorders when psychotic symptoms are present. Awareness of cultural issues such as specific idioms of distress must be increased. It is difficult for one to know the nuances of every culture, which is why sources other than the patient must be consulted. In any case, the diagnosis of schizophrenia should be presumptive for African Americans until other diagnoses are excluded.

## GENETIC FACTORS

Throughout much of the 20th century, schizophrenia was thought to be the result of family pathology. A stress diathesis model is now prevalent. Schizophrenia clearly has a genetic basis because a heavy loading of biological relatives increases the risk. Other biological factors such as viral infections during the second trimester of pregnancy, perinatal insult, and head injury have all been implicated. A number of putative genes have been identified, and some are now being replicated

(Le-Niculescu et al., 2007). It remains to be seen whether they are rare mutations and whether they can always be confirmed in African Americans because studies involving non-Caucasians are rare (Aliyu et al., 2006).

The Caspi and colleagues (2005) study reminded us that for psychiatric disorders genes should be considered only in the context of environmental factors. In that study, the development of adult psychosis was seen in patients with a risk gene for schizophrenia. Adult psychosis was more likely, however, with adolescent-onset cannabis use. Without the susceptibility gene, cannabis was not associated with increased risk of psychosis. A simple statement of known risk could be misinterpreted. It is also important to educate families that ethnicity probably does not increase risk and that family environment does not cause schizophrenia. Genetics factors are important. However, risk is not conferred by genetic factors alone. Environment in a broad sense is important.

## SOCIOCULTURAL FACTORS

The diagnosis of schizophrenia presents a considerable challenge for the African American family, particularly for those with limited resources and living in a hostile social-cultural environment. The direct costs of schizophrenia often exceed the median family income of African Americans (Lawson, 1986). Moreover, although African Americans are more likely to believe that mentally ill individuals are predisposed to violence (Anglin, Link, & Phelan, 2006), they are more likely to keep family members with schizophrenia in the home despite limited resources. African Americans are more tolerant of the unconventional and often unpredictable behavior associated with schizophrenia. African Americans are less likely than Caucasians to believe that individuals with schizophrenia should be blamed and punished for violent behavior and less likely to feel burdened by and rejecting toward the family member (Rosenfarb, Bellack, & Aziz, 2006a, 2006b). Cultural factors, therefore, may be more important then socioeconomic status in determining whether family will continue to be engaged with a member with schizophrenia.

Although the idea that family dynamics cause schizophrenia has been discredited, family relationships can affect the course of the illness. However, factors that contribute to poor outcome are different for Caucasians than for African Americans. High emotionality and family intrusiveness have been shown consistently to predict poor outcome in Caucasians with schizophrenia. This does not appear to be the case among African Americans. Critical comments by relatives were perceived as expressed criticism by Caucasian and Latino family members with schizophrenia but were not perceived consistently so by their African American counterparts (Weisman, Rosales, Kymalainen, & Armesto, 2006). Moreover, in African Americans, intrusiveness and critical comments, elements considered important in families with high emotionality, showed no association with outcome. Presumably, African American families interpreted such behavior as a greater source of concern (Rosenfarb et al., 2006a, 2006b).

Family factors do play an important role in the lives of African Americans with schizophrenia. African Americans tend to be supportive and to continue family involvement despite being fearful of the mentally ill. Moreover, the relationships between family dynamics and schizophrenia seen in Caucasians do not seem to apply to African Americans. Behavior that may worsen outcome in other cultures may be protective in African Americans.

## TREATMENT AVAILABILITY

Many African Americans lack access to mental health services and often receive suboptimal treatment. In addition, they are more likely to have a lower income, lack health insurance, and be homeless or imprisoned (Folsom et al., 2005; Primm, Ogden, & Gomez, 2005; U.S. Department of Health and Human Services, 2001). Hospitalization is more common and often involuntary (Paul & Menditto, 1992; Strakowski et al., 1995). The disposition after discharge is often medication only, and thereafter emergency room care rather then specialized care such as day treatment or case management is the typical setting for additional treatment (Barrio et al., 2003; Kuno & Rothbard, 2005).

Income differences explain some but not all of these disparities. African Americans have 60% of the income of Caucasians. Because of their cultural history of slavery and job discrimination, the accumulation of wealth has occurred only recently for some African American families (Lawson, 1986). Unfortunately, direct costs for the treatment of schizophrenia exceed the median family income of African Americans. This burden is even greater for African American families with a schizophrenic member because they are more likely to provide care within the home.

African Americans are more likely to delay treatment, often because they view the mental health system as hostile. The greater likelihood of being involuntarily admitted does not help these attitudes.

Moreover, provider attitudes are important. African Americans are viewed as being more hostile then they actually are, a misconception compounded by poor communications and social, economic, and ethnic distance (Lawson, Yesavage, & Werner, 1984; Segal, Bola, & Watson, 1996). Patients become suspicious and hostile to the system and either choose other, often ineffectual, alternatives or are less adherent to treatment (Valenstein et al., 2006; Whaley, 2004).

## PHARMACOTHERAPY

Antipsychotic medications remain essential to reducing acute symptoms, maintaining stable functioning, and achieving possible recovery. Unfortunately, the treatment of ethnic minorities is often inappropriate. African Americans often receive excessive doses of medication, whereas Hispanics and Asians receive lower doses when treated by ethnic providers (USDHHS, 2001). African Americans are more likely to receive first-generation rather then second-generation or atypical antipsychotics, higher doses of all medication, more different types of medications, and more depot or injectable long-term medication (Lawson, 1986; Segal et al., 1996; see Table 18.1). These studies involved Medicaid or VA hospital patients, and presumably income should not have affected the difference.

The biological evidence tends to support lower dosing for ethnic minorities. Ethnic differences have been found in the way many psychotropic agents are metabolized. Most psychotropic agents are metabolized through the CYP450 family of liver isoenzymes. The CYP2D6 isoenzyme, in particular, shows ethnic variation. Relative to the majority of Caucasians, Asian, Hispanic, and African American populations show reduced activity in this enzyme, and many Ethiopians show increased activity. Reduced activity means that a drug is metabolized more slowly, leading, therefore, to higher plasma levels (Bradford, 2002). Individuals with CYP2D6 alleles associated with reduced or no activity and given standard medication doses are more likely to have extrapyramidal side effects with antipsychotics and to discontinue treatment, and those with increased activity may not show any response at all (de Leon et al., 2005). Thus, there is no biological reason for the excessive dosing of African Americans.

Pharmacological studies show some advantage for prescribing atypical antipsychotics to African Americans. Second-generation or atypical antipsychotics are less likely to cause extrapyramidal side effects and are believed to cause less tardive dyskinesia (Tollefson et al., 1997). Moreover, some of the newer antipsychotic agents are not predominantly metabolized through the CYP2D6 system but rather through CYP1A2, with CYP2D6 a minor pathway (Bradford, 2002). African Americans are twice as likely as Caucasians to develop tardive dyskinesia with typical antipsychotics (Glazer, Morgenstern, & Doucette, 1994; Jeste, Caligiuri, & Paulsen, 1995; Morgenstern & Glazer, 1993). African Americans are also more likely to experience acute extrapyramidal symptoms than Caucasians with typical antipsychotics, but these differences disappear with atypical agents (Tran, Lawson, Andersen, & Shavers, 1999).

For ethnic minorities, especially African Americans, atypical medications appear to offer an advantage when movement side effects are considered. However, atypical medications have been associated with unacceptable metabolic consequences such as diabetes and the metabolic syndrome (Fenton & Chavez, 2006). African Americans may be at increased vulnerability because of excessive obesity or risk of diabetes mellitus (Ananth, Kolli, Gunatilake, & Brown, 2005). The CATIE (Clinical Antipsychotic Trials of Intervention Effectiveness) study, a naturalistic, federally funded investigation comparing atypical medications with each other and with a typical agent, showed that the atypical agents did not have

**TABLE 18.1. Summary of Studies on the Use of Antipsychotic Pharmacotherapy in African Americans with Schizophrenia**

| Authors (year) | Population | Findings |
| --- | --- | --- |
| Daumit et al. (2003) | Sample culled from national outpatient database | African Americans are less likely to receive atypical antipsychotics. |
| Mark, Palmer, Russo, & Vasey (2003) | Schizophrenia care and assessment program | African Americans are more likely to receive depot medication and less likely to receive second-generation antipsychotics, even after controlling for the use of depot. |
| Herbeck et al. (2004) | American Psychiatric Institute practice research network sample | African Americans are less likely to receive second-generation antipsychotics when clinic, socioeconomic status, and health system are controlled. |
| Opolka, Rascati, Brown, & Gibson (2004) | Medicaid population | African Americans are less likely to receive olanzapine or risperidone. |
| Yang et al. (2008) | Veterans Administration hospital patients | African Americans are less likely to receive second-generation antipsychotics. |

a great advantage (Lieberman et al., 2005). The CATIE study population included 40% African Americans, so insufficient numbers of minorities cannot be used as an argument against it. Moreover, no genetic variants were found that predicted any racial or ethnic risk (Grossman et al., 2008). Nevertheless, the study excluded those with tardive dyskinesia, limited the dosing range, and involved a limited time period.

The atypical agent clozapine has shown consistently superior efficacy and less movement-disordered side effects compared with other antipsychotics. It is also less available to African Americans but for different reasons than other atypical medications (Kelly et al., 2006; Moeller, Chen, & Steinberg, 1995). Its side effects include those of a metabolic nature seen with atypical medications, but that is not the limiting factor. The difficulty is its greater risk for agranulocytosis, which has led to a requirement for regular blood monitoring. Minimal leukocyte counts are recommended before clozapine can be started despite the lack of evidence that preexisting white cell counts predict agranulocytosis. However, African Americans are known to have a normal leukocyte count whose range can extend well below normal values (i.e., "benign leukopenia"). As a result, the overly cautious clinician may choose not to start otherwise healthy African American patients on clozapine.

The solution appears to be straightforward. No biological reason discovered thus far supports the current treatment protocol for African Americans. Indeed, African Americans must be made to feel welcome in the mental health system. When physicians are more willing to become involved with the patient, ethnic differences and excessive dosing disappears (Segal et al., 1996).

## TREATMENT AND RECOVERY

The concept of recovery from mental illness has gained momentum in recent decades as consumer empowerment has generated interest first among peer support groups and then among many mental health providers (Bellack, 2006). Recovery was once thought to be rare in schizophrenia. Indeed, a patient who became symptom free was thought to have received the wrong diagnosis. Recent long-term studies have now shown that more than 60% of patients become symptom free and are able to function successfully in society (Bellack, 2006; Lieberman et al., 2008). The Vermont study (Harding, Brooks, Ashikaga, Strauss, & Breier, 1987) showed that large numbers of patients with a chronic long-standing history of severe mental illness were able to recover and function successfully in society with adequate community resources and rehabilitation. The criteria for recovery in this study included having a social life indistinguishable from neighbors, employment or volunteer work, being symptom free, and off medication. Recovery formerly meant being restored to health and strength after illness. The empowerment model of recovery emphasizes basic principles of recovery, which are universal in the mental health realm: hope, support, responsibility, education, empowerment, medication, strength, employment, spirituality, and self-help. It recognizes that recovery, and not simply the absence of symptoms, was possible.

Studies have shown that recovery rates of schizophrenia in third-world countries are higher. The World Health Organization cohort outcomes at 15 and 25 years showed that recovery rates in developing nations were roughly twice as high as their developed counterparts (Harrison et al., 2001; Jablensky et al., 1992; World Health Organization, 1979). The old African proverb "I am because we are and because we are I am" parallels the attitude taken by members of society in developing countries regarding those with mental illness. In these cultures, every family member is valued, appreciated, and given a specific role to the play in the family. Family members diagnosed with mental illness are celebrated and reintegrated into the community, in contrast to the dissociation and isolation that are common in developed countries. The nurturing, care, and support characteristic of cultures in underdeveloped countries are in stark contrast to stigma, criticism, and shame demonstrated by society in developed countries.

Culture is a determinant factor in the tolerance shown to those with schizophrenia abroad. Culture forgives the abnormal deviations and allows them to be explained by beliefs in supernatural forces or physical illness. Belief in the possibility of a cure is also common, even for those with long-standing, severe illness. The concept of inborn versus acquired diseases seems to give hope that those diseases that developed after childhood have a greater chance of cure. These beliefs foster feelings of hope and faith for recovery not only by the family but also by the afflicted family member.

A review of recovery shows that the functional realm must also be defined by domains rather then simply globally (Lieberman et al., 2008). When looking at specific domains, evidence for recovery is far more common. Most importantly, improvement in a specific domain can be linked to recent advances in pharmaco-therapy. Such outcomes, although limited in scope at present, provide hope that treatments can be developed that may have a more global impact on functioning.

African Americans with schizophrenia face a double dilemma. They often do not have a positive supportive environment associated with recovery in the United States as in third-world countries. Ironically, such supportive environments are still being provided in Africa, the ancestral home of African Americans. Also, they are less likely to receive the benefits of recent pharmacological advances. More needs to be done to validate the positive values of African culture and to utilize them with peers and families. Similarly, more needs to be done to improve access to new treatments.

## CONCLUSION

Schizophrenia is a devastating disorder for anyone, but especially for ethnic minorities. Recent developments have shown that recovery is common. How-ever, limited access to treatment increases the illness burden for economically depressed families and may inhibit individual recovery. When treatment is avail-able, misdiagnosis is common. Other disorders are mislabeled as schizophrenia and treated inappropriately. Examination of cultural factors indicates that find-ings about family environment for Caucasians may not apply to ethnic minorities. Treatment of schizophrenia is suboptimal for African Americans and not sim-ply because of socioeconomic factors. Excessive dosing with older medications is common and cannot be supported by biological factors. Moreover, there is less access to nonmedication treatments and a lack of appreciation of cultural needs. Race and ethnicity, their cultural determinants, and their interaction with socio-economic and biological factors must be considered in the diagnosis and treat-ment of schizophrenia. Optimizing treatment in the context of a culture-relevant positive perspective can lead to meaningful recovery. Failure to do so increasingly will result in health and mental health disparities.

## REFERENCES

Aliyu, M. H., Calkins, M. E., Swanson, C. L., Jr., Lyons, P. D., Savage, R. M., May, R., et al. (2006). Project among African-Americans to explore risks for schizophrenia (PAART-NERS): Recruitment and assessment methods. *Schizophrenia Research*, 87, 32–44.

American Psychiatric Association. (1980). *Diagnostic and statistical manual of mental dis-orders* (3rd ed.). Washington, DC: Author.

American Psychiatric Association. (1994). *Diagnostic and statistical manual of mental dis-orders* (4th ed.). Washington, DC: Author.

Ananth, J., Kolli, S., Gunatilake, S., & Brown, S. (2005). Equally increased risk for meta-bolic syndrome in patients with bipolar disorder and schizophrenia treated with second-generation antipsychotics. *Expert Opinion on Drug Safety*, 4, 1111–1124.

Anglin, D. M., Link, B. G., & Phelan, J. C. (2006). Racial differences in stigmatizing attitudes toward people with mental illness. *Psychiatry Services, 57*, 857–862.

Arnold, L. M., Keck, P. E., Jr., Collins, J., Wilson, R., Fleck, D. E., Corey, K. B., et al. (2004). Ethnicity and first-rank symptoms in patients with psychosis. *Schizophrenia Research, 67*, 207–212.

Barnes, A. (2004). Race, schizophrenia, and admission to state psychiatric hospitals. *Administration Policy and Mental Health, 31*, 241–252.

Barrio, C., Yamada, A. M., Hough, R. L., Hawthorne, W., Garcia, P., & Jeste, D. V. (2003). Ethnic disparities in use of public mental health case management services among patients with schizophrenia. *Psychiatry Services, 54*, 1264–1270.

Bellack, A. S. (2006). Scientific and consumer models of recovery in schizophrenia: Concordance, contrasts, and implications. *Schizophrenia Bulletin, 32*, 432–442.

Blow, F. C., Zeber, J. E., McCarthy, J. F., Valenstein, M., Gillon, L., & Bingham, C. R. (2004). Ethnicity and diagnostic patterns in veterans with psychoses. *Social Psychiatry and Psychiatric Epidemiology, 39*, 841–851.

Bradford, L. D. (2002). CYP2D6 allele frequency in European Caucasians, Asians, Africans and their descendants. *Pharmacogenomics, 3*, 229–243.

Caspi, A., Moffitt, T. E., Cannon, M., McClay, J., Murray, R., Harrington, H., et al. (2005). Moderation of the effect of adolescent-onset cannabis use on adult psychosis by a functional polymorphism in the catechol-O-methyltransferase gene: Longitudinal evidence of a gene × environment interaction. *Biological Psychiatry, 57*, 1117–1127.

Daumit, G. L., Crum, R. M., Guallar, E., Powe, N. R., Primm, A. B., Steinwachs, D. M., et al. (2003). Outpatient prescriptions for atypical antipsychotics for African Americans, Hispanics, and Whites in the United States. *Archives of General Psychiatry, 60*, 121–128.

de Leon, J., Susce, M. T., Pan, R. M., Fairchild, M., Koch, W. H., & Wedlund, P. J. (2005). The CYP2D6 poor metabolizer phenotype may be associated with risperidone adverse drug reactions and discontinuation. *Journal of Clinical Psychiatry, 66*, 15–27.

DelBello, M. P., Lopez-Larson, M. P., Soutullo, C. A., & Strakowski, S. M. (2001). Effects of race on psychiatric diagnosis of hospitalized adolescents: A retrospective chart review. *Journal of Child and Adolescent Psychopharmacoology, 11*, 95–103.

Dixon, L. (1999). Providing services to families of persons with schizophrenia: Present and future. *Journal of Mental Health Policy and Economics, 2*, 3–8.

Fenton, W. S., & Chavez, M. R. (2006). Medication-induced weight gain and dyslipidemia in patients with schizophrenia. *American Journal of Psychiatry, 163*, 1697–1704.

Folsom, D. P., Hawthorne, W., Lindamer, L., Gilmer, T., Bailey, A., Golshan, S., et al. (2005). Prevalence and risk factors for homelessness and utilization of mental health services among 10,340 patients with serious mental illness in a large public mental health system. *American Journal of Psychiatry, 162*, 370–376.

Frueh, B. C., Hamner, M. B., Bernat, J. A., Turner, S. M., Keane, T. M., & Arana, G. W. (2002). Racial differences in psychotic symptoms among combat veterans with PTSD. *Depression and Anxiety, 16*, 157–161.

Glazer, W. M., Morgenstern, H., & Doucette, J. (1994). Race and tardive dyskinesia among outpatients at a CMHC. *Hospital and Community Psychiatry, 45*, 38–42.

Grossman, I., Sullivan, P. F., Walley, N., Liu, Y., Dawson, J. R., Gumbs, C., et al. (2008). Genetic determinants of variable metabolism have little impact on the clinical use of leading antipsychotics in the CATIE study. *Genetic Medicine, 10*, 720–729.

Harding, C. M., Brooks, G. W., Ashikaga, T., Strauss, J. S., & Breier, A. (1987). The Vermont longitudinal study of persons with severe mental illness. I: Methodology, study sample, and overall status 32 years later. *American Journal of Psychiatry, 144,* 718–726.

Harrison, G., Hopper, K., Craig, T., Laska, E., Siegel, C., Wanderling, J., et al. (2001). Recovery from psychotic illness: A 15- and 25-year international follow-up study. *British Journal of Psychiatry, 178,* 506–517.

Herbeck, D. M., West, J. C., Ruditis, I., Duffy, F. F., Fitek, D. J., Bell, C. C., et al. (2004). Variations in use of second-generation antipsychotic medication by race among adult psychiatric patients. *Psychiatry Services, 55*(6), 677–684.

Jablensky, A., Sartorius, N., Ernberg, G., Anker, M., Korten, A., Cooper, J. E., et al. (1992). Schizophrenia: Manifestations, incidence and course in different cultures. A World Health Organization ten-country study. *Psychological Medicine Monograph Supplement, 20,* 1–97.

Jeste, D. V., Caligiuri, M. P., & Paulsen, J. S. (1995). Risk of tardive dyskinesia in older patients: A prospective longitudinal study of 266 patients. *Archives of General Psychiatry, 52,* 756–765.

Jones, B. E., & Gray, B. A. (1986). Problems in diagnosis schizophrenia and affective disorders among Blacks. *Hospital and Community Psychiatry, 37,* 61–65.

Kelly, D. L., Dixon, L. B., Kreyenbuhl, J. A., Medoff, D., Lehman, A. F., Love, R. C., et al. (2006). Clozapine utilization and outcomes by race in a public mental health system: 1994–2000. *Journal of Clinical Psychiatry, 67,* 1404–1411.

Kessler, R. C., Birnbaum, H., Demler, O., Falloon, I. R., Gagnon, E., Guyer, M., et al. (2005). The prevalence and correlates of nonaffective psychosis in the National Comorbidity Survey Replication (NCS-R). *Biological Psychiatry, 58,* 668–676.

Kessler, R. C., McGonogle, K. A., Zhao, S., Nelson, C. B., Hughes, M., Eshleman, S., et al. (1994). Lifetime and 12-month prevalence of DSM III-R psychiatric disorders in the United States. *Archives of General Psychiatry, 51,* 8–19.

Kuno, E., & Rothbard, A. B. (2005). The effect of income and race on quality of psychiatric care in community mental health centers. *Community Mental Health Journal, 41,* 613–622.

Lawson, W. B. (1986). The Black family and chronic mental illness. *American Journal of Social Psychiatry, 6,* 57–61.

Lawson, W. B. (2002). Mental health issues for African Americans. In B. Guillermo, J. E. Trimble, A. K. Burlow, & F. T. I. Leong (Ed.), *Handbook of racial and ethnic minority psychology* (pp. 561–570). Thousand Oaks, CA: Sage.

Lawson, W. B., Hepler, N., Holladay, J., & Cuffel, B. (1994). Race as a factor in inpatient and outpatient admissions and diagnosis. *Hospital and Community Psychiatry, 45,* 72–74.

Lawson, W. B., Yesavage, J. A., & Werner, R. D. (1984). Race, violence, and psychopathology. *Journal of Clinical Psychiatry, 45,* 294–297.

Le-Niculescu, H., Balaraman, Y., Patel, S., Tan, J., Sidhu, K., Jerome, R. E., et al. (2007). Towards understanding the schizophrenia code: An expanded convergent functional genomics approach. *American Journal of Medical Genetics, 144B,* 129–158.

Lieberman, J. A., Drake, R. E., Sederer, L. I., Belger, A., Keefe, R., Perkins, D., et al. (2008). Science and recovery in schizophrenia. *Psychiatric Services, 59,* 487–496.

Lieberman, J. A., Stroup, T. S., McEvoy, J. P., Swartz, M. S., Rosenheck, R. A., Perkins, D.

O., et al. (2005). Effectiveness of antipsychotic drugs in patients with chronic schizophrenia. *New England Journal of Medicine, 353*, 1209–1223.

Mark, T. L., Palmer, L. A., Russo, P. A., & Vasey, J. (2003). Examination of treatment pattern differences by race. *Mental Health Services Research, 5*, 241–250.

Moeller, F. G., Chen, Y. W., & Steinberg, J. L. (1995). Risk factors for clozapine discontinuation among 805 patients in the VA hospital system. *Annals of Clinical Psychiatry, 7*, 167–173.

Morgenstern, H., & Glazer, W. M. (1993). Identifying risk factors for tardive dyskinesia among long-term outpatients maintained with neuroleptic medications: Results of the Yale Tardive Dyskinesia Study. *Archives of General Psychiatry, 50*, 723–733.

Mueser, K. T., & McGurk, S. R. (2004). Schizophrenia. *Lancet, 363*, 2063–2072.

Opolka, J. L., Rascati, K. L., Brown, C. M., & Gibson, P. J. (2004). Ethnicity and prescription patterns for haloperidol, risperidone, and olanzapine. *Psychiatry Services, 55*, 151–156.

Paul, G. L., & Menditto, A. A. (1992). Effectiveness of inpatient treatment programs for mentally ill adults in public psychiatric facilities. *Applied and Preventive Psychology: Current Scientific Perspectives, 1*, 41–63.

Primm, A. B., Ogden, F. C., & Gomez, M. B. (2005). Race and ethnicity, mental health services and cultural competence in the criminal justice system: Are we ready to change? *Community Mental Health Journal, 41*, 557–569.

Robins, L. N., Locke, B., & Regier, D. A. (1991). An overview of psychiatric disorders in America. In L. N. Robins & D. A. Regier (Eds.), *Psychiatric disorders in American. The Epidemologic Catchment Area Study* (pp. 328–366). New York: Free Press.

Rosenfarb, I. S., Bellack, A. S., & Aziz, N. (2006a). Family interactions and the course of schizophrenia in African American and White patients. *Journal of Abnormal Psychology, 115*, 112–120.

Rosenfarb, I. S., Bellack, A. S., & Aziz, N. (2006b). A sociocultural stress, appraisal, and coping model of subjective burden and family attitudes toward patients with schizophrenia. *Journal of Abnormal Psychology, 115*, 157–165.

Seedat, S., Stein, M. B., & Forde, D. R. (2003). Prevalence of dissociative experiences in a community sample: Relationship to gender, ethnicity, and substance use. *Journal of Nervous and Mental Disease, 191*, 115–120.

Segal, S. P., Bola, J. R., & Watson, M. A. (1996). Race, quality of care, and antipsychotic prescribing practices in psychiatric emergency services. *Psychiatric Services, 47*, 282–286.

Strakowski, S. M., Keck, P. E., Jr., Arnold, L. M., Collins, J., Wilson, R. M., Fleck, D. E., et al. (2003). Ethnicity and diagnosis in patients with affective disorders. *Journal of Clinical Psychiatry, 64*, 747–754.

Strakowski, S. M., Lonczak, H. S., Sax, K., West, S. A., Crist, A., Mehta, R., et al. (1995). The effects of race on diagnosis and disposition from a psychiatric emergency service. *Journal of Clinical Psychiatry, 56*, 101–107.

Tollefson, G. D., Beasley, C. M., Jr., Tran, P. V., Street, J. S., Krueger, J. A., Tamura, R. N., et al. (1997). Olanzapine versus haloperidol in the treatment of schizophrenia and schizoaffective and schizophreniform disorders: Results of an international collaborative trial. *American Journal of Psychiatry, 154*, 457–465.

Tran, P. T., Lawson, W. B., Andersen, S., & Shavers, E. (1999). Treatment of the African

American patient with novel antipsychotic agents. In J. Herrera, W. B. Lawson, & J. Sramek (Eds.), *Cross cultural psychiatry* (pp. 131–138). Sussex, UK: Wiley.

U.S. Department of Health and Human Services. (2001). *Mental health: Culture, race, and ethnicity—A supplement to mental health: A report of the Surgeon General.* Rockville, MD: U.S. Department of Health and Human Services, Substance Abuse and Mental Health Services Administration.

Valenstein, M., Ganoczy, D., McCarthy, J. F., Myra K. H., Lee, T. A., & Blow, F. C. (2006). Antipsychotic adherence over time among patients receiving treatment for schizophrenia: A retrospective review. *Journal of Clinical Psychiatry, 67,* 1542–1550.

Weisman, A. G., Rosales, G. A., Kymalainen, J. A., & Armesto, J. C. (2006). Ethnicity, expressed emotion, and schizophrenia patients' perceptions of their family members' criticism. *Journal of Nervous and Mental Disease, 194,* 644–649.

Whaley, A. L. (2004). Ethnicity/race, paranoia, and hospitalization for mental health problems among men. *American Journal of Public Health, 94,* 78–81.

World Health Organization. (1979). *Schizophrenia: An international follow-up study.* Chichester, UK: Wiley.

Yang, M., Barner, J. C., Lawson, K. A., Rascati, K. L., Wilson, J. P., Crismon, M. L., et al. (2008). Antipsychotic medication utilization trends among Texas veterans: 1997–2002. *Annals of Pharmacotherapeutics, 42,* 1229–1238.

# 19

# Suicide

DONNA HOLLAND BARNES

This chapter provides an overview of suicide and reviews suicidal behavior, suicide attempts, and suicide completions within the African American population. There are more than 30,000 suicides a year in the United States and more than 1 million worldwide. The prevalence of suicide among African Americans has been of concern only recently. Suicide was thought to be a "White thing" for so long that it was difficult within the African American community to accept suicide as a serious concern by Black institutions, families, death certifiers, and the larger public. In fact, suicides were more likely to be misclassified for Blacks than for any other ethnic group (Crosby & Molock, 2006; Phillips & Ruth, 1993).

In 1938, Charles Prudhomme, a Black psychoanalyst, published an article in the *Psychoanalytic Review* entitled "The Problem of Suicide in the American Negro." He observed that suicide among African Americans increased as the Black population moved from rural communities to urban areas. He saw the close interpersonal ties among Blacks in rural areas as a protective factor that helped to explain the low rates of suicide among this population.

More recently, Alvin Poussaint, a Black psychiatrist at Harvard Medical School, has maintained that suicide has been an issue within Black society (Poussaint & Alexander, 2000). The difference is that suicide was never mentioned or admitted. It was classified as an accident by funeral directors and other death certifiers to protect families and often disguised as homicide or drug overdose. Today, Blacks have higher rates of homicides and drug-induced deaths than Whites (U.S. Department of Health and Human Services, Centers for Disease Control and Prevention, & National Center for Health Statistics, 2007). It is suggested that many of those homicides and drug overdoses are actually suicides (Poussaint & Alexander, 2000).

The rise in reported rates of suicide among Blacks in the 1980s and 1990s is attributed to a variety of factors, including internalization of failures, disrupted families and relationships, assimilation and acculturation issues into White lifestyles, feelings of discrimination and oppression, and loss of a belief system, mainly religious, or lack of religiosity (Lester, 1998; Poussaint & Alexander, 2000; Walker, Lester, & Joe 2006).

These explanations can be grouped within three broad theoretical constructs: sociological, psychological, and medical or psychiatric. The sociological construct interprets the suicidal act as emerging from the individual's relationship with others (i.e., society). Thus, difficulties arising from being a member of a minority and its treatment by the majority drive the suicidal ideation or acts (Cantor, 1999; Maris, Berman, & Silverman, 2000). The psychological framework uses negative internalization—internal drives found in low self-esteem and an internal negative locus of control—to explain suicidal thoughts and attempts. It is a conscious act of self-induced annihilation, best understood as a multidimensional malaise in a needful individual who perceives suicide as the best solution (Maris et al., 2000) to psychological or emotional pain brought on by unhappiness and hopelessness (Cantor, 1999). The medical or psychiatric model equates suicidal ideation or acts with mental illness (Cantor, 1999). Increasingly, this last model incorporates genetic or other biological factors into explanations for suicidal behavior.

Collectively, these constructs suggest that suicide is a multifaceted phenomenon and necessitates a multidimensional approach for prevention and for treatment of those who have attempted it (Jacobs, Brewer, & Klein-Benheim, 1999).

## DEFINITIONS

*Suicide* is a self-inflicted death with evidence that the person intended to die (American Psychiatric Association, 2003). A *suicide attempt* is a self-injurious behavior with a nonfatal outcome accompanied by evidence that the person intended to die. *Suicide ideations* are thoughts of serving as the agent of one's own death. Ideations may vary in seriousness depending on the specificity of suicide plans and degree of intent (American Psychiatric Association, 2003).

## INCIDENCE

The rate of suicide among African Americans has increased significantly during the 1980s and 1990s: For Black males between the ages of 15 and 24, it is the third leading cause of death after homicide and unintentional injuries, and for

Black females between the ages of 15 and 24, it is the fifth leading cause of death. It appears that Blacks attempt suicide at an earlier age than Whites (U.S. Department of Health and Human Services, Centers for Disease Control and Prevention, & National Center for Health Statistics, 2007).

The growth in the Black male suicide rate was first evident in 1993, when it jumped more than 8 points over the previous year (see Table 19.1).

Suicide rates are significantly lower for Black females compared with Black males (see Table 19.1). The large disparity prompts two questions: What prevents Black females from completing suicide? Do they even engage in suicidal behavior? Many theorists argue that Black females have a substantial amount of resiliency, which keeps them from spiraling to the level of hopelessness that drives people to suicide, and are more likely to defer their problems to God. Furthermore, often Black females have children to care for, serving as a protective factor against suicide. Friendship, kinship, social networks, and religion have been seen to be strong supports for African American females and, therefore, protective factors against hopelessness (Cook, 2002; Nisbet, 1996).

However, these low rates should not be misunderstood to indicate that Black females do not kill themselves or do not engage in suicidal behavior. They have high rates of attempts, comparable to those for White females, and their risk factors include partner abuse, family dysfunction, psychological and interpersonal issues, and childhood maltreatment (Kaslow et al., 1998, 2000; Twomey, Kaslow, & Croft, 2000).

**TABLE 19.1. Suicide Rates per 100,000 for Young (Ages 15–24) Black Males and Females**

| Year | Males | Females |
|------|-------|---------|
| 1990 | 14.53 | 2.37 |
| 1991 | 16.80 | 1.72 |
| 1992 | 18.40 | 2.18 |
| 1993 | 20.40 | 2.65 |
| 1994 | 20.89 | 2.65 |
| 1999 | 14.77 | 1.96 |
| 2000 | 14.59 | 2.26 |
| 2001 | 13.42 | 1.28 |
| 2002 | 11.56 | 1.69 |
| 2003 | 12.49 | 2.03 |
| 2004 | 12.36 | 2.23 |
| 2005 | 11.91 | 1.72 |
| 2006 | 10.94 | 1.79 |

*Note.* Data from Centers for Disease Control and Prevention.

## BIOLOGICAL/GENETIC FACTORS

Mental health scholars report that 90% or more of suicides are due to some form of mental disorder believed to have strong genetic components, such as bipolar and unipolar disorders or schizophrenia (Institute of Medicine, 2002). Neurobiological changes can occur when personality traits such as impulsivity and aggressive behavior interact with trauma, substance abuse, and chronic stress (Mann & Arango, 1999).

Studies suggest that impulsive and aggressive behaviors are related in part to lower levels of reduced central nervous system serotonergic function (Oquendo & Mann, 2000). Serotonin (5-hydroxytryptamine) is one of several neurotransmitters found in the brain influence brain functions such as appetite, sleep, and mood. Decreased levels of serotonin in the brain have been linked to depression. Increasing serotonin levels, often with medications such as selective serotonin reuptake inhibitors (SSRIs), can reverse this effect. Individuals who suffer from serotonin-related clinical depression that goes untreated have a 15% risk of suicide (Institute of Medicine, 2002).

To date, no one gene or genetic element has been identified as predisposing a person to suicide or suicidal behavior. Rather, it appears that an interaction between a critical mass of stress-producing life events and depression or another illness with a genetic component may trigger the event (Jamison, 1999). Vulnerability factors that influence the predisposition to complete or attempt suicide include a family history of low serotonergic functioning in the brain, aggressiveness, impulsivity, and chronic substance abuse (Mann, Waternaux, Haas, & Malone, 1999). More specifically, a clinical phenotype of suicidality shows genetic liability from two sources: (1) a genetic liability to mental illness and (2) a genetic liability to impulsive aggression. When both come together, the risk for suicide is high (Institute of Medicine, 2002).

## INDIVIDUAL FACTORS INFLUENCING RISK AND RESILIENCY

Several factors can increase a person's risk of suicide: emotional disorders, substance abuse, childhood and adult trauma, social isolation, economic hardships, relationship loss, previous suicide attempts, and psychological traits such as hopelessness.

### Mental Illness

As noted earlier, there is strong evidence linking mental illness to many but not all suicides (National Strategy of Suicide Prevention, 2001).

- An estimated 2–15% of persons who have been diagnosed with major depression die by suicide. Suicide risk is highest in depressed individuals who feel hopeless about the future, those who have just been discharged from the hospital, those who have a family history of suicide, and those who have attempted suicide in the past.

- An estimated 3–20% of persons who have been diagnosed with bipolar disorder die by suicide. Hopelessness, recent hospital discharge, family history, and prior suicide attempts all raise the risk of suicide in these individuals.

- An estimated 6–15% of persons diagnosed with schizophrenia die by suicide. In fact, suicide is the leading cause of premature death in this population. Between 75 and 95% of these individuals are male.

- Also at higher risk are individuals who suffer from depression and a comorbid mental illness, specifically substance abuse disorder, anxiety disorder, schizophrenia, and bipolar disorder.

- People with personality disorders are approximately three times as likely to die by suicide than those without. Between 25 and 50% of these individuals also have a substance abuse disorder or major depressive disorder.

## Adult and Childhood Trauma

Evidence shows that traumatic events such as sexual abuse, military combat, sexual assault, and domestic violence increase a person's risk for suicide (Goldman, Silverman, & Alpert, 1998; Tedeschi, 1999; Thompson et al., 1999). This risk may be due to the actual experience of the trauma or a related psychiatric condition that is expressed following the trauma (National Center for PTSD, 2007). Recent work with returning armed forces personnel suggests that an interaction among a variety of factors places veterans at risk, among them:

- Gender
- Alcohol abuse
- Family history of suicide
- Older age
- Poor social-environment support (homelessness and unmarried status)
- Familiarity with firearms and other weapons

The trauma of childhood abuse has been linked to suicidal behavior when depression is present. Several studies suggest that childhood sexual abuse may produce lasting alterations in the brain that can lead to increased risk of suicide (Perroud et al., 2007; Roy, Hu, Janal, & Goldman, 2007). Continual exposure to violence can have negative psychological effects, including depression, posttraumatic stress, anger, aggression, violent behavior, and suicidal behavior (Garbarino, Bradshaw, & Vorrasi, 2002; Gorman-Smith & Tolan, 1998).

Studies at the Grady Health System, Emory University, with African American women who had attempted suicide reported that childhood maltreatment had short- and long-term consequences on mental health. This included a strong cor-relation between childhood abuse and suicidality (Anderson, Trio, Price, Bender, & Kaslow, 2002; Thompson, Kaslow, Lane, & Kingree, 2000).

## Economic Hardship, Social Isolation, and Relationship Loss

Stressors, whether acute like sudden unemployment or the unexpected loss of a loved one, or chronic, like social alienation, discrimination, and oppression, can increase the risk of suicidality. When acute or chronic stressors accumulate and reach an individual's critical mass for handling them, the risk of suicide increases. For instance, when one loses a job unexpectedly, it can become more than just a lost job. It can generate economic hardship, relationship discord, and unstruc-tured time, which can lead to risky behavior and social isolation.

It is important to be aware that life events affect individuals differently. While some can become stronger and more faith based because of the hardships, others can become fearful and depressed, particularly if their typical coping mechanisms prove inadequate to handle stressful events.

## Previous Suicide Attempts

Of those who have attempted suicide, 10–15% will go on to complete suicide (Jamison, 1999). Any attempt must be taken seriously because predicting who will eventually succeed is impossible. Individuals who present with a history of attempts should be considered to be at risk for suicide. Some individuals are relieved to have survived while others regret having not been able to complete the act and become more depressed (Taylor, 2002).

## Hopelessness

When life loses its meaning and one cannot see beyond the present moment, people experience overwhelming hopelessness and see no reason for life. Studies indicate that hopelessness mediates the relation between suicidal ideation and depression, increasing the likelihood of a suicide attempt (Beck, Kovacs, & Weiss-man, 1975; Chioqueta & Stiles, 2007; Cole, 1988; Hendin, Maltsberger, & Szanto, 2007; Minkoff, Bergman, Beck, & Beck, 1973). This psychological pain is accom-panied by severe anxiety, shame or humiliation, psychological turmoil, decreased self-esteem, or agitation (American Psychiatric Association, 2003). Feelings of sadness, desperation, guilt, worthlessness, loneliness, and helplessness contrib-ute to feelings of hopelessness.

## Factors That Decrease Suicidality (Protective Factors)

The flipside of hopelessness is resiliency, a protective factor. Resiliency can come from within, when individuals develop positive attitudes with high expectations about their life. Resilient individuals generally have high tolerance levels, tenacity, and a sense of humor; are self-reliant and independent (Werner & Smith, 2001); and possess good coping skills. These coping skills are honed and strengthened by a strong social support system that can be found in the family, the community, and schools, or at work.

The more individuals are involved with their surroundings, attached to family, committed to work or school, and possess a strong belief system, the more likely it is that they will be resilient. Just as social isolation is a risk factor, social integration is a protective factor.

## FAMILY FACTORS INFLUENCING RISK AND RESILIENCY

Family factors that increase suicidal risk include aggressive and delinquent family members, suicide attempts or completion by another family member, a family environment marked by physical violence and with few resources, and emotionally unsupportive family members in the household (Centers for Disease Control and Prevention, 2007). The following case report from a state mental health center in Maryland serves as an example of this last point: A 17-year-old African American boy was referred to a psychiatrist by his teacher. The psychiatrist diagnosed him with schizophrenia and prescribed medication. When the young man came home with medication, his father poured the pills down the sink and told his son he didn't want him taking that "crap." The young boy ended his life 2 weeks later. As another example, based on police reports at the state of Maryland's coroner's office, a young Black 15-year-old boy was called for dinner. When he did not respond, his brother went to his room to get him, but instead found him hanging by a belt. The suicide victim left a note cursing the whole family.

Race is not the issue in either of these examples. Rather, in the first instance, a father rejected his son's medical needs, and in the second case there was a disconnection between the suicide victim and his family. I observe that too often African American families are afraid to take suggestions from the dominant culture regarding their children's well-being if it appears to be of a negative nature. Too often African Americans mistrust the system, and professional recommendations are seen as little more than glorified attempts to keep "the brother down," or, worse, to dupe them into engaging in a "Tuskegee" scheme.

Black males especially have a tendency to not seek mental health treatment. If they do seek treatment, they are unlikely to comply with or complete treatment (Poussaint & Alexander, 2000), increasing their risk for suicide. Family support is needed to encourage compliance. Toward this end, two factors are critical: (1) education for families regarding the diagnosis, treatment, and support, and, more importantly, (2) the cultivation of trust in a system whose history has engendered African American skepticism for decades.

While genetic factors can influence suicide attempts or completions, suicide thoughts and behavior can be influenced by other family members who have attempted or completed a suicide, particularly if no explanatory note was left behind. A relative's suicide can serve as a model, making imitation more likely (Institute of Medicine, 2002). Often the pain of losing a loved one to suicide engenders guilt, shame, and blame among surviving family members, especially if he or she did not leave a note explaining why. Among those who complete suicide, no more than 10% leave a note. Families left without notes are often in turmoil as they try to figure out why the suicide occurred and whether they may have contributed to the life-ending decision. Their despair can increase their own risk for suicidal ideation. As a case in point, in a support group for families who have lost loved ones to suicide, one parent shared that, although her 27-year-old son's suicide was devastating, she was spared guilt and its resulting turmoil because he left a note that was full of love and compassion for her.

Several studies suggest that positive expectations for children can encourage the development of their own strong sense of resiliency (Masten & Gewirtz, 2006; Werner, 1995). Some children appear to be born with resilient characteristics, while others need help to develop them (Masten & Gewirtz, 2006). According to Frey (1998), boys and girls have different needs at different times in their life cycles. Because of their physical immaturity, boys are more at risk for suicidal ideation earlier in life and girls are more at risk during their second decade because of their emerging sexuality and gender-culture expectations. Resiliency cultivated early in life serves as a protective factor.

## SOCIAL AND COMMUNITY FACTORS INFLUENCING RISK AND RESILIENCY

Numerous societal factors increase suicidal risk, among them poverty; norms that support sexual violence, especially male superiority and sexual entitlement; norms that maintain women's inferiority and sexual submissiveness; neighborhoods with high crime and drug misuse; and poor schools. Simply put, environments that harbor negative activities and support deviant behavior exercise a strong influence that can contribute to a decision to end one's life.

Such environments encourage fatalism, hopelessness, and helplessness, which can lead to risky, life-jeopardizing behavior, for example, waving a gun at a police officer, starting a fight with someone who has already threatened your life, or joining a violent gang that is known for homicidal behavior. Not surprisingly, rates of homicide and drug-related death are high within these neighborhoods. Poussaint and Alexander (2000) argue that many of these homicides are more accurately identified intentional suicides, that is, people have purposely placed themselves in harm's way.

Countering this exposure to harm is the reality that healthy elements within a community can provide a degree of protection. As noted earlier, a truly caring family is protective. A truly caring extended family is protective. A strong caring faith community is protective. Possessing characteristics like a sense of humor, intelligence, and attractiveness increases the likelihood that individuals will gain inclusion, respect, and recognition in even suboptimal school environments (Hammack, Richards, Luo, Edlynn, & Roy, 2004). This sense of well-being is protective.

## EVIDENCE-BASED TREATMENT INTERVENTIONS

### What Works

The objective of treatment intervention programs is to prevent the suicide from happening. However, where suicide is not predictable, the solutions are just as complex as the problem. Evidence-based treatments for suicide are inconclusive. There are standard practices, such as hospitalization or medication, but no scientific evidence that they prevent immediate or eventual suicide (Kalafat, 2003; Zemetkin, Alter, & Yemini, 2001).

### What Might Work

Treatment efforts generally start by reducing risk factors and promoting protective factors as much as possible. Ideally, the intervention should address factors at all levels of influence: individual, relationship, community, and society. Although many of the promising approaches to reducing suicide have not been tested at least three times successfully and certainly not tested on African Americans, efforts that reduce risk factors and promote protective factors should work with any population. The clinician needs to understand that what are considered risk factors and protective factors can vary depending on the culture. Assessment is key: Asking all the right questions, knowing when to stop, and letting the client know that you do not understand and you need further explanation.

Many times treating a suicidal client will mean short-term hospitalization. Generally, with hospitalization, the admitting physician needs to determine whether or not to take progressive or regressive therapeutic measures. With regressive therapeutic measures, the client is kept free of any responsibility: generally, no visits or phone calls home, no discussion of family conflicts, and no contact with his or her work environment. With progressive therapeutic measures, the client is given independence gradually as the suicidal ideations and depression wane. The client has complete independence throughout the hospitalization and normal contact with family, and his or her social problems are discussed. Generally, regressive measures are next to impossible for the impoverished client who is the head of household and has an ample amount of responsibility that cannot go without attention. In these cases, it is good practice to ask the client to collaborate with the therapist in an effort to minimize stress and to enhance the protective factors.

## *Counseling Approaches for Survivors of Attempts*

The overall process for managing a suicidal client includes assessment, treatment planning, and management of risk. According to Jobes (2006), a clinical approach strives to keep clients out of inpatient hospital settings and works toward developing clients' inner strength to take responsibility for their feelings. Jobes builds a client collaboration system that includes a treatment plan set up by the clinician that is time limited. A treatment plan with a suicidal client needs to be comprehensive because it is developed based on the fact that the client considers death to be an option. These thoughts are generally temporary, so the treatment plan can also be temporary because its focus is on the client thinking of suicide. Plus, the time limitation gives the client a feeling that he or she is working toward a final goal and not something that has to go on indefinitely. Once a time limit is established, the therapist develops the following:

1. A comprehensive assessment that measures the status of the client's suicidal thinking.

2. A contract between the client and the clinician whereby the client agrees to certain conditions such as not abusing alcohol or drugs if he or she is prone to do so or agreeing to restrict the means to suicide (e.g., by getting rid of a gun in the house).

3. A list of activities the client enjoys and that make him or her feel good, such as walking, bowling, knitting, drawing, or working in the yard. The client is encouraged to keep this list handy and to engage in these behaviors when feeling depressed. If the depression worsens, the client is encouraged to seek help.

In clinicians' assessments of African Americans, the incorporation of cultural considerations is essential for accurate diagnoses and effective care. According to the American Psychiatric Association, clinicians should always be cognizant of the following:

- Cultural identity of the individual
- Cultural explanations of the individual's illness
- Cultural factors related to psychosocial environment and levels of functioning
- Cultural elements of the relationship between the individual and the clinician

As Primm (2000) explains in her presentation and video *Black & Blue*, African American women will often refer to mental illness, ranging from depression to schizophrenia, as "bad nerves." It is a polite and socially acceptable code word and is less stigmatizing than the actual diagnosis.

## Therapy after an Attempt

One promising intervention developed by Guthrie and colleagues (2001) provides four sessions of psychotherapy for adults who have attempted suicide by poisoning. The unique aspect of this intervention is that it is home based and provided by a nurse therapist. Results achieved with this intervention were statistically significant when compared with treatment as usual. At the 6-month follow-up, only 9% of clients in the home-based model had harmed themselves compared with 28% who received treatment as usual.

Another promising approach involves the use of cognitive therapy. In a study at the University of Pennsylvania, 120 adult participants underwent a 10-session cognitive therapy intervention to prevent repeat suicide attempts. After 18 months only 13 patients who received cognitive therapy attempted again compared with 24 who received standard treatment (Brown et al., 2005).

## What Does Not Work

Techniques such as tough love that are based on withholding of empathy are ineffective for managing people in suicidal crisis. Most people in suicidal crisis do not want to die and are ambivalent right up to the last moment. Sneiden (1978) at the University of California at Berkeley interviewed survivors of a jump from the Golden Gate Bridge and found that the majority were glad to be alive and recalled thinking on their return from the bridge or during the jump that they wanted to live. In essence, suicidal individuals generally want only to kill the emotional pain that has become too difficult to manage. Self-destructive behavior among young adults is becoming a monumental problem. They don't want to kill themselves; rather, they want to murder the sadness. Being tough or providing tough love does not always work.

## PSYCHOPHARMACOLOGY AND SUICIDE

As mentioned, several researchers have linked low levels of the brain chemical serotonin to suicidal behavior. In unipolar depression, evidence suggests that medications (particularly SSRIs) can have a positive impact on reducing the chemical imbalance that partially explains the depression and improve the client's affect. Likewise, the use of medication has been helpful with individuals with bipolar disorders (Borne, 1994). In both instances, medication alone does not appear to be as effective as medication in combination with counseling.

## PREVENTION OF SUICIDE

Suicide is the most preventable cause of death if signs are properly recognized and caution prevails. If an individual is suffering from major depression, goes on a drinking binge, and has a gun available, think suicide. If an individual has borderline personality traits, relationship discord with the family, is on the verge of losing a job, and just got into a car accident, think suicide. If an individual just suffered the death of a close parent, is doing poorly in school, feels socially unacceptable, think suicide. It is never harmful to present individuals with your feelings of concern and ask them directly whether they are thinking of killing themselves. Asking the question will not put the idea in their head: Asking the question will make them feel that you are concerned and will give them relief in that they can now discuss their internal frustration or emotional pain. Ask the question in a manner that is sympathetic. Do not pass judgment. Do not ask the question as if to suggest it is a *stupid* or *crazy* idea. Ask the question with great understanding and compassion.

## What Works

A search of the literature did not identify a program that met the criteria for inclusion in this section.

## What Might Work

In general, school-based programs appear to be excellent prevention initiatives because they reach kids at early stages in their lives (Weissberg & Greenburg, 1997). The *Columbia University TeenScreen Program* is designed to identify youth who are at risk for suicide and potentially suffering from mental illness. Youth who are found to be suffering from a mental illness or in a suicidal crisis receive a complete evaluation generally after parental consent. Screening programs can take place anywhere as long as they are conducted by qualified practitioners, for example, churches, conventions, juvenile justice facilities, shelters, anywhere where people are seen on a daily basis or clustered.

The SOS Program: Signs of Suicide incorporates two prominent suicide prevention strategies into a single program: a curriculum that aims to raise awareness of suicidal signs and related issues and a brief screening for depression and other risk factors associated with suicidal behavior. It promotes the concept that suicide is directly related to mental illness, typically depression, and that it is not a normal reaction to stress or emotional states. The goal of this program is to teach students how to recognize the signs of suicide among their peers and respond to the signs as an emergency, just as one would do with cardiopulmonary resuscitation for a heart attack.

The Reconnecting Youth Class targets young people in grades 9–12 who show signs of poor school achievement, potential for school dropout, and other at-risk behaviors, including suicide risk behaviors. This program teaches skills to build resiliency with respect to risk factors and to moderate early signs of substance abuse and depression/aggression. The program includes social support and life skills training. It has been recognized by several governmental agencies as an effective, model program for reducing substance abuse and similar at-risk behaviors among youth.

The *Prevention of Suicide in Primary Care Elderly: Collaborative Trial* (PROSPECT; *www.nrepp.samhsa.gov/programfulldetails.asp?PROGRAM_ID=113*) aims to prevent suicide among older primary care patients by reducing suicidal ideation and depression. The intervention components are (1) recognition of depression and suicide ideation by primary care physicians; (2) application of a treatment algorithm for geriatric depression, which assists primary care physicians in making appropriate care choices during the acute, continuation, and maintenance phases of treatment; and (3) treatment management by health specialists (e.g., nurses, social workers, and psychologists), who collaborate with physicians to monitor patients and encourage patient adherence to recommended treatments. Patients are treated and monitored for 24 months.

Implementation of the program relies on educating primary care physicians to recognize symptoms and apply a clinical algorithm based on depression treatment guidelines for older patients from the American Psychiatric Association, the Agency for Healthcare Research and Quality, and the Texas Department of Mental Health. The recommended first-line treatment is citalopram (Celexa), an SSRI. If citalopram does not achieve the desired result, other medications may be added or substituted. Interpersonal psychotherapy may also be used in addition to or instead of pharmacological treatment.

Randomized primary care trials concluded that suicidal ideation resolved more quickly in patients who were randomly assigned to receive the intervention compared with those receiving standard usual care. "The impact of the intervention on depressive symptoms was greater among patients with major depression than for patients with mild depression unless suicidal ideation was also present" (Bruce et al., 2004).

## RECOMMENDED BEST PRACTICES

One approach for developing treatment and prevention interventions is to examine the profiles of individuals who committed suicide. In such a study, I examined coroner reports on 46 suicides by African American males younger than age 25 (Barnes, 2006). I found that the major issues in their life at the time of their suicide were disruptive families, relationship discord, and unemployment. These conditions, if lining up like lucky 7 on a slot machine, can cause desperation, hopelessness, rage, anxiety, feelings of abandonment, loneliness, guilt, humiliation, and on and on.

Although some suicides are the result of a mental disorder, others are not. For the former group, the National Institute of Mental Health (Rice et al., 1989) reported four major profiles:

1. Agitation, severe anxiety, associated with psychosis
2. Symptoms of anxiety and undiagnosed depression

3. Suicidal acting out in borderline disorder associated with anxiety and anticipated loss

4. Interpersonal loss in depression, associated with a history of drug or alcohol abuse and impulsive behavior

When delivered in a culturally appropriate manner and setting, the treatment interventions described earlier and the appropriate use of medication represent current best practice for African Americans.

The prevention of suicide, in my opinion, is less focused on intrapsychic factors and more on interpersonal factors and the environment. From an interpersonal perspective, what do we need to do? Not fire anyone, not divorce anyone, not cause anyone to get upset or anxious? How, in the world that we live in today, do we stop suicide? Many of these conditions can be caused by a lack of understanding, a lack of insurance, and a lack of assistance. Can we change the conditions of society overnight? The only thing we can do to decrease suicidal behavior is very simple: Recognize the risk factors and help to alleviate them.

## REFERENCES

American Psychiatric Association. (2003). *Practice guideline for the assessment and treatment of patients with suicidal behaviors.* Washington, DC: Author.

Anderson, P. L., Trio, J. A., Price, A. W., Bender, M. A., & Kaslow, N. J. (2002). Additive impact of childhood emotional, physical, and sexual abuse on suicide attempts among low-income African American women. *Suicide and Life-Threatening Behavior,* 32(2), 131–138.

Barnes, D. (2006). *Study on suicide among African American males under the age of 25.* Unpublished manuscript, Baltimore, MD.

Beck, A. T., Kovacs, M., & Weissman, A. (1975). Hopelessness and suicidal behavior: An overview. *Journal of the American Medical Association, 234,* 1146–1149.

Borne, R. (1994, October 10). Serotonin: The neurotransmitter for the 90's. *Drug Topics,* p. 108.

Brown, G., Ten Have, T., Henriques, G. R., Xie, S., Hollander, J., & Beck, A. (2005). Cognitive therapy for the prevention of suicide attempts: A randomized controlled trial. *Journal of the American Medical Association, 294*(5), 563–70.

Bruce, M., Ten Have, T., Reynolds, C., Katz, K., Schulberg, H., Mulsant, B., et al. (2004). Reducing suicidal ideation and depressive symptoms in depressed older primary care patients: A randomized controlled trial. *Journal of the American Medical Association, 291*(9), 1081–1091.

Cantor, P. (1999). Can suicide ever be eradicated: A professional journey. In D. G. Jacobs (Ed.), *The Harvard Medical School guide to suicide assessment and intervention* (pp. 239–248). San Francisco: Jossey-Bass.

Centers for Disease Control and Prevention. (2007). *Suicide: Risk and protective factors.* Atlanta, GA: Centers for Disease Control and Prevention, National Centers for Injury Prevention and Control, Division of Violence Prevention. Retrieved November 11, 2007, *www.cdc.gov/ViolencePrevention/suicide/riskprotectivefactors/html.*

Chioqueta, A., & Stiles, T. (2007). The relationship between psychological buffers, hopelessness and suicidal ideation: Identification of protective factors. *Crisis*, *28*(2), 67–73.

Cole, D. A. (1988). Hopelessness, social desirability, depression, and parasuicide in two college student samples. *Journal Consulting and Clinical Psychology*, *56*, 131–136.

Cook, J. M., Pearson, J. L., Thompson, R., Black, B. S., & Rabins, P. V. (2002). Suicidality in older African Americans: Findings from the EPOCH Study. *American Journal of Geriatric Psychiatry*, *10*(4), 437–446.

Crosby, A., & Molock, S. (2006). Suicidal behaviors in the African American community. *Journal of Black Psychology*, *32*(3), 253–261.

Frey, K. (1998). Introduction to resiliency. Retrieved December 28, 2009, from *www.westga.edu/~gadmh/ResourcesPublications/UnderstandingTrauma/Introduction%20to%20Resiliency.pdf.*

Garbarino, J., Bradshaw, C., & Vorrasi, J. (2002). Mitigating the effects of gun violence on children and youth. *The Future of Children*, *12*(2), 72–85.

Goldman, L., Silverman, M., & Alpert, E. (1998). Violence and aggression. In L. S. Goldman, T. Wise, & D. Brody (Eds.), *Psychiatry for primary care physicians* (pp. 273–284). Chicago: American Medical Association.

Gorman-Smith, D., & Tolan, P. (1998). The role of exposure of violence and developmental problems among inner-city youth. *Development and Psychopathology*, *10*, 101–116.

Guthrie, E., Kapur, N., Mackay-Jones, K., Chew-Graham, C., Moorey, J., Mendel, E., et al. (2001). Randomised controlled brief psychological intervention after deliberate self-poisoning. *British Medical Journal*, *323*, 1–5.

Hammack, P., Richards, M., Luo, Z., Edlynn, E., & Roy, K. (2004). Social support factors as moderators of community violence exposure among inner-city African American young adolescents. *Journal of Clinical Child and Adolescent Psychology*, *33*(3), 450–462.

Hendin, H., Maltsberger, J., & Szanto, K. (2007). The role of intense states in signaling a suicide crisis. *Journal of Nervous and Mental Disease*, *195*(5), 363–368.

Institute of Medicine. (2002). *Reducing suicide: A national imperative*. Washington, DC: National Academies Press.

Jacobs, D., Brewer, M., & Klein-Benheim, M. (1999). Suicide assessment: An overview and recommended protocol. In D. G. Jacobs (Ed.), *The Harvard Medical School guide to suicide assessment and intervention* (pp. 3–39). San Francisco: Jossey-Bass.

Jamison, K. (1999). *Night falls fast: Understanding suicide*. New York: Random House.

Jobes, D. A. (2006). *Managing suicide risk: A collaborative approach*. New York: Guilford Press.

Kalafat, J. (2003). Suicide, adolescence. In T. P. Gullotta & M. Bloom (Eds.), *Encyclopedia of primary prevention and health promotion* (pp. 1099–1105), New York: Kluwer Academic/Plenum.

Kaslow, N. J., Thompson, M. P., Meadows, L., Chance, S., Puett, R., Hollins, L., et al. (2000). Risk factors for suicide attempts among African American women. *Depression and Anxiety*, *12*, 13–20.

Kaslow, N. J., Thompson, M. R., Meadows, L. A., Jacobs, D., Chance, S., Gibb, B., et al. (1998). Factors that mediate and moderate the link between partner abuse and suicidal behavior in African American women. *Journal of Consulting and Clinical Psychology*, *66*(3), 533–540.

Lester, D. (1998). *Suicide in African Americans.* Commack, NY: Nova Science.

Mann, J., & Arango, V. (1999). The neurobiology of suicidal behavior. In D. G. Jacobs (Ed.), *Guide to suicide assessment and intervention* (pp. 98–114). San Francisco: Jossey-Bass.

Mann, J., Waternaux, C., Haas, G., & Malone, K. (1999). Toward a clinical model of suicidal behavior in psychiatric patients. *American Journal of Psychiatry, 156,* 181–189.

Maris, R. W., Berman, A. L., & Silverman, M. M. (2000). *Comprehensive textbook of suicidology.* New York: Guilford Press.

Masten, A., & Gewirtz, A. (2006). *Resilience in development: The importance of early childhood.* Montreal, Quebec: Centre of Excellence for Early Childhood Development. Retrieved December 12, 2007, from *www.excellence-earlychildhood.ca/documents/Masten-GewirtzANGxp.pdf.*

Minkoff, K., Bergman, E., Beck, A., & Beck, R. (1973). Hopelessness, depression, and attempted suicide. *American Journal of Psychiatry, 130,* 455–457.

National Center for PTSD. (2007). *How is PTSD measured?* Retrieved November 2, 2007, from *www.ncptsd.va.gov/ncmain/ncdocs/fact_shts/fs_lay_assess.html.*

National Strategy for Suicide Prevention. (2001). *Goals and objectives for action.* Rockville, MD: U.S. Department of Health and Human Services.

Nisbet, P. A. (1996). Protective factors for suicidal Black females. *Suicide and Life Threatening Behavior, 26*(4), 325–341.

Oquendo, M., & Mann, J. (2000). The biology of impulsivity and suicidality. *Psychiatric Clinics of North American, 23*(1), 11–25.

Perroud, N., Courtet, P., Vincze, I., Jaussent, I., Jollant, F., Bellivier, F., et al. (2007). Interaction between the brain and childhood trauma on adult's violent suicide attempt. *Genes Brain Behavior, 19,* 314–322.

Phillips, D., & Ruth, T. (1993). Adequacy of official suicide statistics for scientific research and public policy. *Suicide and Life-Threatening Behavior, 23*(4), 307–319.

Poussaint, A., & Alexander, A. (2000). *Lay my burden down: Unraveling suicide and the mental health crisis among African Americans.* Boston: Beacon Press.

Primm, A. (2000). *Black & blue: Depression in the African American community* [Videotape]. Baltimore: Bluerock Productions.

Prudhomme, C. (1938). The problem of suicide in the American Negro. *Psychoanalytic Review, 25,* 187–204.

Rice, J., Andreasen, N. C., Coryell, W., Endicott, J., Fawcett, J., Hirschfeld, R. M., et al. (1989). NIMH collaborative program on the psychology of depression: Clinical. *Genetic Epidemiology, 6*(1), 179–182.

Roy, A., Hu, X. U., Janal, M. N., & Goldman, D. (2007). Interaction between childhood trauma and serotonin transporter gene variation in suicide. *Neuropsychopharmacology, 32*(9), 2046–2052.

Sneiden, R. (1978). Where are they now? *Suicide and Life Threatening Behavior, 8*(4), 1–13.

Taylor, K. (2002). *Seduction of suicide: Understanding and recovering from addiction to suicide.* Nashville, TN: 1st Books Library.

Tedeschi, R. (1999). Violence transformed: Posttraumatic growth in survivors and their societies. *Aggression and Violent Behavior, 4*(3), 319–341.

Thompson, M., Kaslow, N., Kingree, J., Puett, R., Thompson, N., & Meadows, L. (1999). Partner abuse and posttraumatic stress disorders as risk factors for suicide attempts in a sample of low-income, inner-city women. *Journal of Traumatic Stress, 12*(1), 59–72.

Thompson, M., Kaslow, N., Lane, D., & Kingree, J. (2000). Childhood maltreatment, PTSD, and suicidal behavior among African American females. *Journal of Interpersonal Violence, 15*(1), 3–15.

Twomey, H., Kaslow, N., & Croft, S. (2000). Childhood maltreatment, object relations, and suicidal behavior in women. *Psychoanalytic Psychology, 17*(2), 313–335.

U.S. Department of Health and Human Services, Centers for Disease Control and Prevention, and National Center for Health Statistics. (2007). *Health, United States, 2007 with chartbook on trends in the health of Americans* (DHHS Publication No. 2007-1232). Hyattsville, MD: Author.

Walker, R., Lester, D., & Joe, S. (2006). Lay theories of suicide: An examination of culturally relevant suicide beliefs and attributions among African Americans and European Americans. *Journal of Black Psychology, 32*(3), 320–334.

Weissberg, R., & Greenburg, T. (1997). School and community competence enhancement and prevention programs. In E. Sigel & K. A. Renninger (Eds.), *Handbook of child psychology: Vol. 4. Child psychology in practice* (5th ed., pp. 877–954). New York: Wiley.

Werner, E. (1995). Resilience in development. *Current Directions in Psychological Science, 4*(3) 81–85.

Werner, E., & Smith, R. (2001). *Journey from childhood to midlife: Risk, resilience, and recovery.* Ithaca, NY: Cornell University Press.

Zemetkin, A. J., Alter, M. R., & Yemini, T. (2001). Suicide in teenagers: Assessment, management, and prevention. *Journal of the American Medical Association, 286,* 3120–3125.

# 20

# Child Maltreatment

Brenda Jones Harden
Jamell White

The maltreatment of children has left an indelible mark on human history, with adverse consequences for individuals, families, and even societies (Hampton & Gullotta, 2006; Myers et al., 2002). Child maltreatment has no boundaries, affecting children across all nations, all socioeconomic strata, and all racial/ethnic groups. Although the incidence of child maltreatment is no higher in the African American community than it is in other groups (Sedlak & Schultz, 2005), practitioners and scholars committed to promoting optimal outcomes for African American children must be concerned with understanding and eradicating it.

This chapter addresses the definitional issues, epidemiological trends, and risk and protective factors associated with child maltreatment in the African American community. Furthermore, it elucidates effectively prevention and treatment interventions, specifically those that have been tested with the African American population. Although addressing the developmental consequences to children is critical, this chapter focuses on the perpetrators of child maltreatment and strategies for reducing the abusive and neglectful behaviors that have such a major impact on affected children.

## DEFINING CHILD MALTREATMENT

The national definition of child maltreatment is "an act or failure to act by a parent, caregiver, or other person as defined under State law that results in physical abuse, neglect, medical neglect, sexual abuse, emotional abuse, or an act or failure to act which presents an imminent risk of serious harm to a child" (Administration for Children and Families [ACF], 2008, p. 104). Ambiguity continues to exist in the clinical and empirical literatures, however, regarding what constitutes child maltreatment in general as well as specific types of maltreatment.

For example, because the majority of American parents utilize corporal punishment in some form at some point in their children's lives (Benjet & Kazdin, 2003; Straus, 2000), there is considerable controversy regarding at what point corporal punishment becomes physically abusive behavior. Perhaps an even greater challenge lies with the definition of neglect, which varies among reporters, cultures, socioeconomic classes, and other groups (Rose, 1999). Given some evidence pointing to the co-occurrence of different forms of maltreatment (Lynch & Cicchetti, 1998), there is also the question of whether to address child maltreatment more broadly or to focus on specific subtypes. Finally, a major conundrum in the field is the specific criteria that should be used to determine whether or not child maltreatment has occurred. Currently, there is no national standard for decision making regarding the substantiation of child maltreatment.

Despite the definitional controversy surrounding child maltreatment, it is useful for practitioners to understand what constitutes different forms of child maltreatment. The general consensus is that there are four major forms of child maltreatment: physical abuse, neglect, sexual abuse, and emotional maltreatment (Administration for Children and Families, 2008). According to the National Incidence Study (NIS) of Child Abuse and Neglect (NIS-3; Sedlak & Broadhurst, 1996), physical abuse occurs when a child has experienced a nonaccidental injury as a result of having been hit with a hand or other object or of having been kicked, shaken, thrown, burned, stabbed, or choked by a parent or parent surrogate regardless of whether the intent was to injure the child. Physical abuse lies on a continuum from mild (e.g., bruise) to severe (e.g., broken bones, skull fractures, fatally). Typically excluded in this definition is physical discipline that does not cause bodily injury (e.g., spanking).

Neglect is defined as the omission of specific caretaking behaviors, which has a detrimental impact on child health, development, and functioning (Administration for Children and Families, 2008; Sedlak & Broadhurst, 1996). Some scholars have argued that a determination of neglect should be predicated on whether a child's needs are met, such as the need for shelter, food, medical care, and intellectual stimulation (Dubowitz, Black, Starr, & Zuravin, 1993; English, Edelson, & Herrick, 2005). Research on child maltreatment suggests that there are two subtypes of neglect: failure to supervise and failure to provide (Barth, 1991; Coohey, 2003). Failure to provide may be in the physical, medical, educational, or emotional realm (Cicchetti & Bartnett, 1991).

The definition of sexual abuse is somewhat more straightforward. Generally, it includes any sexual contact between a child and a parent or caregiver that provides sexual gratification or financial benefit to the adult (Berliner & Elliott, 2002). Activities such as fondling a child's genitals, penetration, incest, rape, sodomy, indecent exposure, and exploitation through prostitution, the Internet, or the production of pornographic materials constitute sexual abuse (Berliner & Elliott, 2002; Feerick, Knutson, Trickett, & Flanzer, 2006).

There is considerable ambiguity regarding the definition of emotional maltreatment. One assertion is that emotional maltreatment is related to all other forms of maltreatment, in that one cannot physically abuse or neglect children without emotionally harming them as well (Browne & Fereti, 1996; Cicchetti, Toth, & Hennessy, 1989; Garbarino, Guttman, & Seeley, 1986; Jaffee, Wolfe, & Wilson, 1990). In general, rejection and hostile treatment of the child is considered emotional abuse. The American Professional Society on the Abuse of Children (APSAC) delineates six categories of emotional maltreatment: (1) spurning; (2) terrorizing; (3) isolating; (4) exploiting or corrupting; (5) denying emotional responsiveness; and (6) mental health, medical, and educational neglect (Hart, Brassard, Binggeli, & Davidson, 2002). Finally, scholars and practitioners have suggested that indirect exposure to violence and other negative events in the home through witnessing these events also constitutes emotional maltreatment.

This definitional complexity extends to how child maltreatment is understood in the mental health community. Based on a medical-diagnostic definition, child maltreatment has been historically linked to the behavior of the abuser, not the experience of the child, among mental health providers (Aber & Zigler, 1981). As such, child maltreatment is considered a possible symptom or consequence of mental illness in parenting individuals, with the diagnosis of child maltreatment as a corollary of some other diagnostic category (e.g., dysthymia, hypersexual behavior, anxiety, antisocial disorder).

The most recent (fourth edition, text revision) *Diagnostic and Statistical Manual of the American Psychiatric Association* (DSM-IV-TR; American Psychiatric Association, 2000) does include specific V codes that pertain to child maltreatment, v61.21 for any perpetrator of child maltreatment; and v61.21 when there is a problem with the quality of parental nurturing. If the victim of child maltreatment is receiving clinical services, there are three relevant codes: 995.54 for physical abuse, 995.53 for sexual abuse, and 995.52 for neglect. Another diagnostic category related to the youngest victims of maltreatment is reactive attachment disorder of infancy or early childhood (313.89). Additionally, some victims of maltreatment receive a diagnosis of posttraumatic stress disorder (309.81; American Psychiatric Association, 2000).

## EPIDEMIOLOGY OF CHILD MALTREATMENT

Approximately 1 million children are victims of maltreatment annually in the United States. There are two major national strategies for determining the incidence of child maltreatment, which have yielded divergent incidence rates. The NIS (the most recent data are on the third study [Sedlak & Broadhurst, 1996], and the fourth study is currently underway) is a comprehensive research effort that interviews professionals and community members to determine the overall incidence of child maltreatment in the United States. The NIS-3 reported that 1,553,800 children were harmed by abusive and neglectful caregivers (Sedlak & Broadhurst, 1996). The other major source for child maltreatment statistics is the cumulative state-level data that form the National Child Abuse and Neglect Data System (NCANDS). Based on the most recent national data from NCANDS, 905,000 American children were found to be victims of child maltreatment in 2006 (Administration for Children and Families, 2008).

The discrepancy between NIS and NCANDS incidence rates is attributable to the fact that NCANDS only includes children who have been investigated by the state child protection agency, whereas NIS includes all children who have been maltreated. Furthermore, although the majority of cases that are referred to the child welfare system are investigated, child maltreatment is substantiated (i.e., has sufficient evidence to determine maltreatment) in only about one-third (Administration for Children and Families, 2008). Taken together, these findings suggest that many children at risk for maltreatment and their families are not served by the child welfare system.

Maltreatment rates vary by type, reported by NCANDS as follows: physical neglect, 64.1%; physical abuse, 16.0%; sexual abuse, 8.8%; psychological abuse, 6.6%; and medical neglect, 2.2% (Administration for Children and Families, 2008). The remaining 15.1% fall in an "other" category, which includes children who were not victimized by the major forms of maltreatment but may have been abandoned or born prenatally substance exposed. Some children are victims of multiple forms of maltreatment, which brings the overall cumulative percentage over 100% (Administration for Children and Families, 2008).

According to the most recent federal data (Administration for Children and Families, 2008), there are demographic factors that lead to differential rates of child maltreatment within the U.S. population. For example, children younger than age 3 had the highest rates of victimization, comprising 30% of the maltreated population. This becomes even more pronounced with children younger than age 1, who experience twice the rate of maltreatment than their older counterparts. Overall, children between 1 and 3 years of age have a child maltreatment incidence rate of 14.2 per 1,000, and those between birth and 1 year of age have a rate of 24.4 per 1,000. Regarding gender, slightly more than half the children victimized were female (51.5%). Almost 8% of the children had a reported disability.

The evidence regarding racial disparities in child maltreatment rates is much more complex (see Derezotes, Poertner, & Testa, 2005). Extant research indicates that, compared with their counterparts in other racial/ethnic groups, African American children are no more likely to be the victims of child maltreatment. The strongest data supporting this conclusion emanate from the NIS-3 (Sedlak & Broadhurst, 1996), which has documented that there is no difference, on a community level, in the incidence or prevalence of maltreatment between African Americans and other demographic groups (Sedlak & Broadhurst, 1996; Sedlak & Schultz, 2005).

Nevertheless, the response from the child welfare system toward African American families is substantially different from its response to other racial/ethnic populations. Specifically, African American children have higher rates of substantiation of abuse or neglect following a child protective service investigation than any other group. Federal data indicate that African American children are victimized by maltreatment at a rate of 19.8 per 1,000 compared with a national rate of 12.1 per thousand (Administration for Children and Families, 2008). Interestingly, the disparities between substantiation rates for African American and White children are greatest in areas where poverty is less severe (Wulczyn, Barth, Yuan, Jones Harden, & Landsverk, 2005). Furthermore, African American perpetrators may be differentially treated. For example, in a study of judicial system involvement in cases of child abuse, Keenan, Nocera, and Runyan (2008) found that minority perpetrators received more severe sentencing than White perpetrators of the same level of maltreatment.

As a result of these racial disparities, scholars have called for more careful monitoring of the child welfare trajectories of African American children and families and specialized attention to the services they receive while in that system. In fact, there is evidence for differential treatment of African American children throughout the course of their child welfare involvement. They are more likely to experience foster care placement, tend to have longer durations of foster care, are less likely to be reunified with their families, and receive fewer and lower-quality services while involved with the child welfare system (Derezotes et al., 2005; Jones Harden, 2008). Such disparities in the child welfare trajectories of African American children clearly have implications for their developmental outcomes, which may be worse than those of other demographic groups (Jones Harden & Nzinga-Johnson, 2006; Wulczyn et al., 2005).

## THEORETICAL APPROACHES

Many theories have been applied to scholarly and clinical work on child maltreatment, including attachment theory (Dozier, Stovall, Albus, & Bates, 2001; Lyons-Ruth, Easterbrooks, & Cibelli, 1997) and cognitive theory (Azar, Breton, & Miller, 1998; Azar, Robinson, Hekimian, & Twentyman, 1984). Building on an ecological framework (Bronfenbrenner, 1979), Belsky (1980, 1993) and Cicchetti (Cicchetti & Rizley, 1981; Cicchetti, Toth, & Maughan, 2000; Cicchetti & Valentino, 2006) have proffered two commonly cited theoretical approaches to explain the etiology and process of child maltreatment.

Belsky's ecological conceptualization of the etiology of maltreatment (1980, 1993) proposes four interactive levels: ontogenic, microsystem, exosystem, and macrosystem. The *ontogenic* level entails the individual characteristics of the parents, such as a history of being maltreated themselves and mental health difficulties. The *microsystem* is defined as the immediate environment of the child and includes features specific to the lives of maltreating families such as spousal conflict and violence and high familial stress levels. The *exosystem* encompasses larger contextual factors, such as poverty, community violence, and social isolation. Finally, the *macrosystem* reflects cultural ideologies, such as the larger society's attitude toward violence and corporal punishment and perspectives on the rights of children and proper childrearing.

An important feature of this formulation is that parenting quality is perceived to be on a continuum from normal to abnormal, with maltreatment at the extreme. Parental quality is determined by three primary forces: (1) individual child characteristics; (2) parents' developmental history and personal psychological resources; and (3) social-contextual sources of stress and support.

Extending these conceptualizations, Cicchetti and colleagues (Cicchetti & Rizley, 1981; Cicchetti et al., 2000; Cicchetti & Valentino, 2006) developed an ecological-transactional framework for understanding the causes, consequences, and processes of child maltreatment. Their multilevel model emphasizes the transactions between potentiating (risk) and compensatory (protective) factors at the level of the child and at different levels of the child's ecology, which increase or decrease the probability of maltreatment. Risk factors that render children more vulnerable to maltreatment include (1) biological influences such as illness or mental retardation; (2) historical influences such as the parents' experience of being maltreated; (3) psychological influences such as parental mental illness; (4) familial influences such as spousal violence; (5) sociological influences such as poverty; and (6) cultural influences such as the societal acceptance of physical punishment.

Protective factors can also be found in each of these domains and serve to buffer children against maltreatment. These include a child's easy temperament and high intellectual capacity, positive family relationships, and supportive social networks. This theory also proposes a temporal dimension to maltreatment, in which they acknowledge the existence of transient and enduring influences on the probability of maltreatment, such as the temporary lack of child care (i.e., transient vulnerability factor) or the parent's history of receiving high-quality parenting (i.e., enduring protective factor).

Specific to African American families, racially salient risk and protective factors may be found at the level of the individual, family, and community. On an individual level, how African American parents cope with the stressors of racism and their racial identity may promote or hinder their parenting capacities (McAdoo, 1982). The culturally based childrearing values (e.g., child centeredness) and practices (e.g., use of corporal punishment) of a family could increase or decrease the likelihood of child maltreatment (Giles-Sims & Lockhart, 2005). Finally, the African American community's sanction of specific childrearing practices and its experience of institutional racism are two factors rooted in the larger ecology that might affect the emergence of child maltreatment (Dodge, McLoyd, & Lansford, 2005).

Each of these ecologically oriented frameworks acknowledges that individual, interpersonal, and broader environmental factors conspire to increase the likelihood that child maltreatment will emerge in a particular family system. As such, these theories also help us to understand more fully the processes that are characteristic of maltreating families and the strategies that may be effective in eradicating maltreatment. The emphasis on the larger ecology allows for a consideration of the structural variables (e.g., poverty) that inequitably affect African American families and contribute to the manifestation of child maltreatment in the African American community.

## RISK AND PROTECTIVE FACTORS FOR CHILD MALTREATMENT: A BIOECOLOGICAL, TRANSACTIONAL VIEW

Consonant with the theories on maltreatment described in this chapter, there are multiple risk and protective factors for maltreatment that emerge at different levels of children's ecology (i.e., family, community, society) as well as within the children themselves (i.e., biological and psychological characteristics). As Belsky (1993) observes, the etiology of maltreatment is multifaceted and transactional. Child maltreatment is the result of the complex interplay among multiple child, parent, family, societal, and cultural factors. It is difficult to disentangle which factors are the causes or consequences of maltreatment. For example, just as the bidirectionality of parenting processes has been widely documented (i.e., child and parent factors contribute to outcomes; Campbell, Shaw, & Gilliom, 2000), bidirectional processes are determinants of child maltreatment as well.

### Biological Factors

Psychology's emphasis on the biological bases of behavior has, to some extent, shaped research on child maltreatment. However, the bulk of this research addresses the biological sequelae of maltreatment rather than biologically based, etiological factors (e.g., Ayoub & Rappolt-Schlichtmann, 2007; Kaufman, 2008). In this section, we examine the small literature on biological precursors to child maltreatment and studies from other fields that inform our understanding of this phenomenon. Additionally, we briefly consider the research on biological consequences of child maltreatment because of their potential influence on the intergenerational transmission of maltreatment and the salience of these studies for the development of future research on the biological antecedents of child maltreatment.

#### *Prenatal Development*

The vastly complex prenatal process commences the development of the human being (for a more comprehensive discussion of prenatal development, see Lecanuet, Fifer, Krasnegor, & Smotherman, 1995; Moore & Persaud, 1993). In an ideal situation, the uterine environment provides all that the developing fetus needs to thrive. For children at risk for maltreatment, their environments are often compromised from the moment of conception through the time of their births and beyond. Their developing systems may be exposed to a number of stressors, including malnutrition (Shanklin, 2000), maternal physical illnesses (Crum, Hogan, Chapple, Browne, & Greene, 2005), teratogens and toxins (Canfield, Gendle, & Cory-Slechta, 2004; Takser, Mergler, & Lafond, 2005), and maternal psychological vulnerability (King & Laplante, 2005). Each of these stressors impacts the developing organism in unique and potentially devastating ways.

The vulnerability of children experiencing prenatal stressors makes them more susceptible to maltreatment (DePanfilis & Zuravin, 1999; Jaudes & Mackey-Bilaver, 2008). Children with such prenatal risks are often born early and small, have more physical illnesses, exhibit developmental delays, and present with neurobehavioral difficulties. Each of these factors has been linked to maltreatment rates that are higher than those in the general population. Because these factors are manifested early in life, they contribute to the particular vulnerability of infants to experiences of maltreatment (see Jones Harden, 2007).

Prenatal substance exposure has particularly pernicious effects on affected children in terms of their psychological functioning as well as their susceptibility to maltreatment. A plethora of evidence points to the linkage between parental substance abuse and child maltreatment (see following sections). Current estimates indicate that substance use is implicated in upward of 80% of child welfare cases (Besinger, Garland, Litrownik, & Landsverk, 1999; Chaffin, Kelleher, & Hollenerg, 1996; Jaudes, Ekwo, & Voorhis, 1995). This potentially translates into high numbers of children who have been exposed prenatally to substances such as nicotine, alcohol, and illicit and legal drugs.

Multiple studies have documented the numerous negative developmental sequelae of prenatal substance exposure (Frank, Augustyn, Grant Knight, Pell, & Zuckerman, 2001; Jones Harden, 1998). Although there are distinct outcomes associated with particular substances (e.g., facial dysmorphology and cardiac problems from high levels of prenatal alcohol exposure; Coles & Platzman, 1993), general sequelae to prenatal substance exposure include prematurity, cognitive delays, and behavioral problems (Coles & Black, 2006; Jones Harden, 1998; McGuinness & Schneider, 2007). The impaired psychological and parenting capacity of drug-using individuals, in combination with the physical and psychological vulnerability of drug-affected children, elevates the likelihood that child maltreatment will occur (Seifer et al., 2004; Smith, Johnson, Pears, Fisher, & DeGarmo, 2007; Young, Boles, & Otero, 2007).

### Parental Physical Health

The behaviors of parents who are found to maltreat their children (e.g., drug use, sexual promiscuity) often lead to their poor physical health (Culbertson & Schellenbach, 1992). Although the research on the physical health of mothers who are involved in the child welfare system is limited, the evidence regarding mothers living in poverty is informative, particularly given the documented link between poverty and child maltreatment (Sedlak & Broadhurst, 1996; see social/community section). Mothers from impoverished backgrounds have higher rates of physical illness and are less likely to receive health-related services (Crum et al., 2005; Howell, Pettit, & Kingsley, 2005).

Although this linkage has not been extensively studied, there is evidence that parents who are physically ill are more likely to maltreat their children (Holden, Willis, & Corcoran, 1992). By and large, this finding emanates from literature on neglecting families. Additionally, impoverished mothers are more likely to have pregnancy-related health risks, yet are less likely to receive prenatal care (Crum et al., 2005; Howell et al., 2005). This set of circumstances leads to adverse physical, cognitive, and neurobehavioral outcomes in affected children (Crum et al., 2005; Kahn, Wilson, & Wise, 2005), which, in turn, precipitates elevated maltreatment rates.

## Physiology and Parental Psychological Functioning

Just as the mother's physical state impacts the developing fetus, her emotional functioning also influences the development of her unborn child. Maternal stress leads to reduced oxygen and nutrients carried in the bloodstream to the fetus and to increased stress hormones, which can raise fetal heart rate and activity level. Additionally, maternal stress is related to a variety of negative behaviors, such as smoking and drinking, which have their own physiological implications (see prior discussion on maternal substance use). Maternal psychological difficulty during pregnancy places children at risk for a variety of adverse health and developmental outcomes, such as prematurity, low birthweight, failure to thrive, physical illness, and compromised cognitive development (King & Laplante, 2005; Singer et al., 2002). Again, these child-level factors render children more susceptible to abuse and neglect.

Furthermore, parental mental illness is a strong parent-level predictor of abusive and neglectful behavior (Chaffin Kelleher, Harber, & Harper, 1994; see following section). Thus, parents' genetic predisposition to mental illness can be viewed as an important biological risk factor for child maltreatment (Kaufman, 2008; Kaufman & Henrich, 2000; Seifer & Dickstein, 2000). Genetic research has yielded evidence for genetic involvement in schizophrenia, depression, and substance use (Agrawal & Lynskey, 2008; Anisman, Merali, & Stead, 2008; Carter, Schulsinger, Parnas, Cannon, & Mednick, 2002; Ducci & Goldman, 2008), all of which are implicated in child maltreatment (Browne et al., 1999; Chaffin et al., 1994). Furthermore, there is some evidence for a genetic contribution to parental maltreating behavior (Kaufman, 2008).

Although the data are very limited, there has been conceptual and empirical interest in the biological underpinnings of the specific behaviors of maltreating parents (Ayoub & Rappolt-Schlichtmann, 2007; Daly & Wilson, 1999). The strongest body of research on the physiology of child maltreatment emanates from studies of physical abuse. Scholars suggest that parents who have a genetic predisposition to antisocial behavior (i.e., aggression) may have an increased propensity to abuse their children (Jaffee, Caspi, Moffitt, & Taylor, 2004; Milner & Dopke, 1997). Additionally, a few studies have documented that abusive parents have higher physiological reactivity to stressful stimuli McCanne & Milner, 1991). For example, their hyperarousal to stressful child-related stimuli (e.g., infant cries) has been found in studies using skin conductance and heart rate measures (Friedrich, Taylor, & Clark, 1985; Frodi & Lamb, 1980; Wolfe, Fairbanks, Kelly, & Bradlyn, 1983).

## Brain Development

Although there is a dearth of research that investigates brain functioning in maltreating parents, there has been substantial advancement in the knowledge about the impact of maltreatment on the developing brain. Broadly speaking, maltreatment seems to be associated with impaired brain growth and a general dampening of brain processing and efficiency (DeBellis, Hooper, & Sapia, 2005; Nelson et al., 2007). Additionally, brain research suggests that maltreatment experiences have an impact on brain structures and processes that give rise to a number of psychological difficulties (DeBellis, 2004, 2005; DeBellis et al., 2005; Nemeroff, 2004). For example, the impact of maltreatment has been observed in the frontal regions of the cortex, which control higher cognitive functioning; the corpus callosum, which contains the fibers between the two hemispheres of the brain that allow for faster mental processing; and the limbic system, which constitutes the brain's emotion center (DeBellis, 2004; DeBellis et al., 1999, 2005).

Many studies have implicated the hypothalamic–pituitary–adrenal axis and its associated hormonal processes in the impact of trauma on psychological functioning. These studies have found altered patterns of cortisol secretion, a process involved in stress reactivity, in maltreated children compared with controls (DeBellis et al., 1999; Gunnar, 1998). Furthermore, impairments in neurophysiological functioning have been documented, such as decreased serotonin and increased dopamine and testosterone (DeBellis et al., 1999, 2005; Lewis, 1992).

Although this evidence regarding alterations in brain structure and functioning applies to child maltreatment victims, the documented linkage between victimization and perpetration (Buchanan, 1998) suggests that the brain and neuropsychological functioning of maltreating parents may be impaired (Milner & Dopke, 1997). Similarly relevant is the research on the brain functioning of maltreating parents with specific mental illnesses. For example, studies on the biological bases of substance abuse, a disorder that is prevalent in the maltreating population, have documented dysfunction in the orbitofrontal cortex, an area of the brain involved in the control of behavior according to consequences (Koob & LeMoal, 2008; Schoenbaum & Shaham, 2008). Substance abuse disorder is also related to many other psychiatric disorders, which have their own physiological profiles (Baker & Belleman, 2007).

Also common among maltreating individuals are depressive disorders. Parents with disorders along this spectrum may exhibit overall dysfunction in the prefrontal regions of the brain, with specific regions of the brain affected, including the hippocampus, amygdala, basal ganglia, and anterior cingulate (Mayberg, 2003; Subbarao et al., 2008). Although a rare disorder, schizophrenia may be implicated in severe cases of maltreatment given its severity as a mental illness. Research on schizophrenia has yielded multiple findings regarding brain dysfunction, including reduced hippocampal gray matter and corpus callosum, as well as distinct morphology in the frontal and temporal lobes, hypothalamus, thalamus, and amygdala (Bray, 2008; Goldman et al., 2008).

## Individual Factors

### Child-Specific Factors

There are multiple individual-level factors that render children vulnerable to the experiences of maltreatment and associated negative outcomes. Regarding child-specific factors, young age (i.e., infancy) is a major risk factor for maltreatment, at least for physical abuse, neglect, and emotional abuse. Research has documented that children' low birthweight, prematurity, and poor health render them more susceptible to maltreatment (Browne & Herbert, 1997; Kotch et al., 1995; Sidebotham, Heron, & the ALSPAC Study Team, 2003). In addition, children are more likely to be maltreated if they have developmental problems, especially a diagnosed disability (Sidebotham et al., 2003; Sullivan & Knutson, 1998). Additionally, children with difficult temperaments (i.e., difficult to console, irritable) seem to be particularly victimized (Kotch et al., 1995).

There are mixed findings relative to the effect of gender on child maltreatment. Most studies conclude that boys and girls are equally victimized by child maltreatment (Arata, Langhinrichsen-Rohling, Bowers, & O'Brien, 2007). National data combining all forms of maltreatment suggest that girls may be victimized at a slightly higher rate than boys (Administration for Children and Families, 2008). The gender of the child also appears to influence the intensity and type of maltreatment. Nationally, girls are three times more likely to be victims of sexual abuse, whereas boys have increased rates of emotional neglect and serious injury (Administration for Children and Families, 2008). One study attempted to examine the higher risk of physical injury in male victims of child maltreatment and found that boys may be more susceptible to supervisory neglect and the adverse consequences thereof (Bernardo, 1996).

Just as specific individual factors render children at higher risk for maltreatment, they can protect children against the negative outcomes of this experience. For example, a child's gender might influence her resiliency to maltreatment. Some research has documented that girls who experience maltreatment tend to demonstrate better outcomes than affected boys (McGloin & Widom, 2001). Additionally, extant literature implies that children who demonstrate greater resiliency to maltreatment tend to share the characteristics of high self-esteem, above-average intelligence, self-reliance, and higher recognition of their efforts contributing to personal success (Cicchetti & Rogosch, 1997; Cicchetti, Rogosch, Lynch, & Holt, 1993; Herrenkohl, Herrenkohl, & Egold, 1994; Moran & Eckenrode, 1992).

### Parent–Specific Factors

National data confirm that the overwhelming majority (80%) of perpetrators of child maltreatment are parents of affected children. Many individual-level parent characteristics have been associated with child maltreatment. Whether the mother planned her pregnancy and how positively she perceives her newborn affect the likelihood of maltreatment (Sidebotham et al., 2003). Young maternal age (i.e., adolescent parenthood) has been associated with maltreatment in multiple studies (Browne, Catellier, Dufort, Kotch, & Winsor, 1999; Stier, Leventhal, Berg, Johnson, & Mezger, 1993). Furthermore, in the NCANDS study, 45.3% of maltreating mothers were younger than 30 years. Other demographic factors that have been linked to child maltreatment include single parenthood, low parental education, and being a nonbiological parent (Brown, Cohen, Johnson, & Salzinger, 1998; Christman, Wodarski, & Smokowski, 1996; Milner, 1998).

The effect of gender on child maltreatment perpetration is much clearer than what we know of its impact on victimization. Based on national data (NCANDS), it seems that overall the majority of child maltreatment perpetrators are women (57.9%). Fathers or male members of the household are more likely to commit physical abuse (Sedlak & Broadhurst, 1996). The propensity of males to maltreat is particularly salient in cases of severe abuse (Cavanagh, Dobash, & Dobash, 2007; Ricci, Giantris, Merriam, Hodge, & Doyle, 2003). Although somewhat conflictual, there is evidence that stepfathers are more likely to inflict harm on children in their care than are biological fathers (Cavanagh et al., 2007; Starling, Sirotnak, Heisler, & Barnes-Eley, 2007).

Maternal psychopathology has been strongly related to all forms of maltreatment (Browne et al., 1999). In a large national survey, several psychiatric disorders were associated with child maltreatment, including substance use disorder, major depressive disorder, antisocial and other personality disorders, and obsessive–compulsive disorder (Chaffin et al., 1996). Maternal depression has been linked to inadequate childrearing and maltreatment in multiple studies (Erickson & Egeland, 1987, 2002; Kotch, Browne, Dufort, Winsor, & Catellier, 1999; Lyons-Ruth, Alpern, & Repacholi, 1993; Windham et al., 2004). However, Chaffin and colleagues (1996) found that depression was only predictive of child physical abuse and was not related to neglect once substance abuse disorder was controlled.

Substance use has been implicated in the majority of cases of child maltreatment nationwide (Besinger et al., 1999; Kelleher, Chaffin, Hollenberg, & Fischer, 1994). Research has documented that children born to mothers who used drugs are more likely to be maltreated, particularly neglected (Hartley, 2002; Jaudes et al., 1995; Ondersman, 2002). In the Chaffin and colleagues study (1996), substance use disorder was the only disorder predictive of both child abuse and neglect. Substance use disorder has also been associated with maternal affiliation with antisocial male partners (Mezzich et al., 1997) and with other psychiatric disorders (e.g., depression, personality disorders) (Baker & Belleman, 2007; Chaffin et al., 1996; Rutter, 1992, 1997), all of which have been linked with child maltreatment.

Aspects of psychological functioning, which do not reach the level of mental illness, have also been implicated in the manifestation of child maltreatment. For example, parental coping style, locus of control, and ego strength are psychological variables that have been linked to child maltreatment (Brown et al., 1998; Erickson & Egeland, 2002; Wolfe, 1993). Maltreating parents may have less motivation (Coohey, 1998), lower self-esteem (Brown et al., 1998), impaired perspective taking and empathy (Crittenden, 1999), and fewer problem-solving and social skills (Coohey, 1998). Child maltreatment is also more likely when caregivers experience increased parental and life stress (Casady & Lee, 2002; DePanfilis, 1999; Pianta, Egeland, & Erickson, 1989).

## Family Factors

Specific features of the family constellation have been connected to child maltreatment. Children living in a family system that includes the mother's boyfriend, who is not the biological father, are at increased risk of being maltreated (Administration for Children and Families, 2005a). Large family size, particularly if other young children live in the home, also increases the likelihood of child maltreatment (Kotch et al., 1999; Ovwigho, Leavitt, & Born, 2003). If the mother was separated from her own mother as a young adolescent, she is more likely to maltreat her child as well (Kotch et al., 1999). Elevated rates of maltreatment have also been documented in foster families compared with the general population (DePanfilis & Girvin, 2004), perhaps because of the increased monitoring of these families, the developmental and behavioral challenges presented by the children, or the lack of a biological connection between parent and child.

The psychological difficulties observed with maltreating parents extend to their parenting behaviors. They demonstrate reduced knowledge of child development (Ammerman, Hersen, Van Hasselt, & Lubetsky, 1994) and inaccurate perceptions and expectations of their children (Azar, 1997; Azar et al., 1984; Bugental, Mantyla, & Lewis, 1989; Erickson & Egeland, 2002; Nayak & Miller, 1998). They may exhibit inconsistent childrearing practices (Susman, Trickett, Ianotti, Hollenbeck, & Zahn-Walker, 1985), critical, hostile, and aggressive styles of child management (Trickett & Kuczynski, 1986; Whipple & Webster-Stratton, 1991), as well as limited attention and problematic affect (Youngblade & Belsky, 1990). In general, maltreating parents tend to be unresponsive to children's needs and have more problematic parenting skills overall (Brayden, Altemeier, Tucker, Dietrich, & Vietze, 1992; Caselles & Milner, 2000; Erickson & Egeland, 2002).

Beyond parenting behaviors, family factors that have been implicated in cases of child maltreatment include a family context of hostility (Claussen & Crittenden, 1991; Wolfe, 1987) as well as heightened conflict and decreased cohesion (Azar et al., 1998; Mollerstrom, Patchner, & Milner, 1992). A lack of the ability to communicate, express feelings, and maintain emotional closeness has also been reported (Elliott, 1994; Gaudin, Kilpatrick, Polansky, & Chilton, 1996; Mannarino & Cohen, 1996). Inadequate social support and social isolation have been documented in multiple studies to increase the risk of child maltreatment (Coohey, 2000; DePanfilis & Zuravin, 1999; Kotch et al., 1997; Sidebotham, Heron, Golding, & ALSPAC Study Team, 2002). Additionally, the intergenerational transmission of abusive and neglectful behavior has been posited as an important etiological factor in child maltreatment (Christman et al., 1996; Dunn et al., 2002; Straus, 1994). Children who have experienced abuse are more likely to be perpetrators of abuse in adulthood (Caliso & Milner, 1992; Milner, Robertson, & Rogers, 1990).

The quality of the relationship between the adults in children's homes has a major impact on the likelihood of child maltreatment. Parental conflict and poor marital quality have been associated with child maltreatment (Baumrind, 1994; Brown et al., 1998; Noll, Horowitz, Bonanno, Trickett, & Putman, 2003). On the extreme of the marital relationship continuum, domestic violence is largely implicated in the emergence of child maltreatment, specifically, the co-occurrence of interadult violence, particularly woman battering, with child maltreatment has been documented (Edleson, 1999; Hartley, 2002). Domestic violence seems to have a particular effect on the occurrence of child physical abuse (Ricci et al., 2003; Windham et al., 2004). In contrast, positive paternal involvement, as well as the presence of another adult (e.g., grandmother), may protect a family against maltreatment (Brown et al., 1998; Dubowitz, Black, Harrington, Kerr, & Starr, 2000).

Studies have found that certain family characteristics, such as the level of emotional support, serve not only as risk factors but also as protective factors (Higgins, McCabe, & Ricciardelli, 2003; Wind & Silvern, 1994). In a study of adults who where maltreated as children, Higgins and colleagues (2003) found that family cohesiveness mediated the relationship between maltreatment and the individual's symptoms of trauma and self-depreciation. Similarly, parental affection and the quality of the parent–child relationship were moderators of the relation between child maltreatment and child psychological adjustment.

From a resilience perspective, the experiences and outcomes of physical abuse in the African American community merit special consideration. For example, because physical discipline is more common within the African American community, it is important to disentangle that which constitutes physical abuse and that which produces poor outcomes. Some scholars define any physical discipline as physical abuse (e.g., Straus, 2000). However, the use of physical discipline has been shown to have cultural significance and possible benefits to African

American adolescents in particular (Ispa & Halgunseth, 2004). Notably, the link between positive child outcomes and corporal punishment has been found when African American children are reared in an overall context of family warmth (Horn, Joseph, & Cheng, 2004).

Finally, there is converging evidence that maltreated children with stronger relationships with family members, other significant adults, and their personal social network exhibit greater resilience (Cicchetti & Rogosch, 1997; Heller, Larrieu, D'Imperio, & Boris, 1999; Widom, 1991). The strong social networks that are found in African American communities, regardless of class, may protect African American children from the adverse experiences and outcomes typically associated with maltreatment (McAdoo, 1982). For example, Hill (1998) has documented that extended family involvement and relative care of children continue to be more likely among African Americans than the majority population. Thus, despite their socioeconomic vulnerability, African American families may still have access to important family and social resources that prevent maltreatment and the subsequent foster care placement of maltreated children.

## Social/Community Factors

Although the microlevel family characteristics and interactions play the larger role in the experiences and outcomes of children at risk for maltreatment (Belsky, 1993; Higgins & McCabe, 1994), there are broader ecological factors that increase the likelihood of maltreatment. Poverty has been linked to all forms of child maltreatment (Drake & Pandey, 1996; Gillham et al., 1998; Kotch et al., 1997, 1999; Sedlak & Broadhurst, 1996; Sidebotham et al., 2002). Some studies suggest that particular aspects of being impoverished are precipitants for child maltreatment, such as employment status, housing situation, and material benefits (Gillham et al., 1998; Sidebotham et al., 2002). In a study examining families as they exited the Temporary Assistance for Needy Families program, a longer history of cash assistance and when they exited the program were major predictors of risk for child maltreatment (Ovwigho et al., 2003).

There is some evidence that income status is differentially related to distinct experiences of maltreatment. For example, many studies have documented the strong association between poverty and child neglect (Drake & Pandey, 1996; Sedlak & Broadhurst, 1996). In another study, male unemployment was found to be more related to physical abuse than to neglect and sexual abuse (Gillham et al., 1998). There seems to be less of a relation between income and sexual abuse (Berliner & Elliott, 2002). Finally, studies of the impact of poverty on child development have documented that poverty in the early years of life (i.e., infancy and early childhood) is more detrimental to child outcomes than poverty's impact at other points in childhood and adolescence (Duncan, Hubble, & Rusk, 1994; McLoyd, 1998).

The stigma of poverty often casts a negative light on the family practices within impoverished African American families. First, African American families are more likely to be poor than their White counterparts (U.S. Census Bureau, 2008). Furthermore, poor families are more likely to be reported to child protective services. Two reasons for this have been postulated: (1) Poor, minority families are under more scrutiny or (2) there is actually a higher rate of abuse and neglect occurring in families living in extreme poverty (Coulton, Korbin, Chow, & Su, 1995; Ernst, 2001; Garbarino & Kostelny, 1992; Hampton & Newberger, 1985). The racism and oppression that many African American families experience may exacerbate the stressors associated with poverty (Baumrind, 1995; Peters & Massey, 1983). On the other hand, some studies have found that abuse is actually less likely to occur within African American families when income is controlled (Cazenave & Straus, 1979, as cited in Baumrind, 1994).

Societal and cultural views about abuse and family practices also shape the public response to child maltreatment and discipline and perhaps the likelihood that parents will inflict harm on their children. A cultural phenomenon that is particularly germane to African American families is corporal punishment, which they are more likely to use (Benjet & Kazdin, 2003; Westbrook, Jones Harden, Vick, Meisch, & DeTaillade, 2009). As stated previously, there is evidence that the negative outcomes typically associated with this disciplinary practice in White families are not as salient in African American families (Deater-Deckard, Dodge, Bates, & Pettit, 1996; Deater-Deckard, Dodge, & Sorbring, 2005). The use of strict discipline and corporal/physical punishment in African American families has the potential of being misinterpreted as abuse if one is not aware of the cultural value this has been shown to have for the success of the community members. Such practices not only have been used to teach obedience, to teach respect for authority, and to modify behavior but have also been found to have a protective role in teaching children the skills needed (e.g., guardedness, appropriate aggressiveness) to survive in a hostile environment that is a reality for many African American youth (Ogbu, 1981).

The interaction of these factors can increase or decrease the likelihood of maltreatment of children. Extant literature underscores the complex interplay of factors that predispose a family to maltreatment, including individual, familial, and societal factors. The cumulative impact of these factors should also be underscored. As in the cumulative risk research (Sameroff & Fiese, 2000), child maltreatment research has documented that as the number of risk factors affecting families increases, the likelihood of child maltreatment increases markedly (Brown et al., 1998).

Whereas risk factors may be manifested within the individual, family, and the larger community, a child's resiliency to adversity is equally influenced by these same issues (Jaffee, Caspi, Moffitt, Polo-Tomas, & Taylor, 2007). Specifically, maltreated children who have been able to form supportive relationships with nonfamilial adults, including in foster care placements, have been found to demonstrate higher levels of resiliency (Cicchetti & Rogosch, 1997; Davidson-Arad, Englechin-Segal, & Wozner, 2003). Because child maltreatment may be an indicator of a family's ability to adapt to its environment and related stressors (Ernst, 2001), it is important that programs aimed at serving these families attempt to reduce the stressors that families experience and enhance their ability to adapt to the stressful situations that befall them.

## THE EVIDENCE BASE FOR THE PREVENTION OF CHILD MALTREATMENT

Given the large number of maltreated children who do not come to the attention of the child welfare system (Sedlak & Broadhurst, 1996), a service delivery system to prevent abuse and neglect is an imperative. Similarly, because the majority of maltreated children remain in the homes of their birth families (Barth, Landsverk, & Chamberlain, 2005), it is essential to develop effective in-home preventive services. However, the child welfare field expends a relatively small portion of its dollars on programs to prevent child abuse and neglect (Bess, 2002). Furthermore, child welfare systems typically offer extremely limited in-home services following maltreatment substantiation (Kohl & Barth, 2007). By design, intensive support services for birth families can accomplish both child welfare system goals: Prevent child maltreatment and maintain children within their birth families.

Attributable in large part to the emergence of the field of prevention science, there has been a proliferation of prevention programs serving high-risk children and their families in the last few decades (see Weissberg, Kumpfer, & Seligman, 2003). Similarly, the number of programs to reduce child maltreatment has rapidly increased since the passage of the comprehensive child welfare legislation in 1980 (PL 96-272). Despite an abundance of these prevention programs, few programs have been directed specifically at the child welfare population, and even fewer have been found to be effective in reducing the incidence of maltreatment (Barth et al., 2005; Wulczyn et al., 2005).

Recent meta-analyses of child maltreatment prevention programs have shown variation in the benefits of these programs (Lee, Aos, & Miller, 2008; MacLeod & Nelson, 2000; Sweet & Appelbaum, 2004). MacLeod and Nelson (2000) suggested that more effective programs were begun during the prenatal or infancy periods, were of longer duration and intensity, and had a primary prevention focus (i.e., families at risk for maltreatment, not yet identified as abusive or neglectful). Additionally, program effects were stronger when participants were of mixed socioeconomic status than when participants were primarily poor. In their meta-analysis of home visiting programs, Sweet and Appelbaum (2004) documented that, although overall home visiting programs did not affect the incidence of child abuse and neglect, programs with a specific goal of child maltreatment prevention were more likely to affect the potential for child maltreatment in participant families. Finally, the analysis conducted by the Washington State Institute for Public Policy (Lee et al., 2008) points to the increased benefit of specific programs, including home visiting, mental health, and early childhood programs.

Specific interventions, which have been found to be successful (MacLeod & Nelson, 2000), are often conducted as part of expensive clinical trials and have not been tested for effectiveness when delivered on the community level (Peterson, Tremblay, Ewigman, & Saldana, 2003). Another methodological challenge that has compromised maltreatment prevention research pertains to the use of abuse or neglect as a programmatic outcome. Because of increased surveillance of child maltreatment in prevention programs, there is a higher likelihood of its identification. The lack of effects in some evaluations of maltreatment prevention programs might be an artifact of this increased family monitoring (Brayden et al., 1993; Olds, Henderson, Kitzman, & Cole, 1995; Roberts, Kramer & Suissa, 1996). Finally, the research does not often include developmentally informed, comprehensive measurement of the functioning of the children participating in the studies.

## Programs That Work

Despite the previously delineated caveats, interventions exist that have been documented to be successful in preventing or reducing maltreatment (Centers for Disease Control and Prevention, 2003; Lee et al., 2008; MacLeod & Nelson, 2000). These interventions are often characterized by features of effective prevention programs in other fields, such as comprehensiveness, high levels of intensity, and a well-trained staff (Nation et al., 2003). These programs with proven efficacy can inform the child welfare field in its efforts to implement preventive interventions for all types of maltreatment at the community level.

The Nurse–Family Partnership (NFP) is a well-known and well-documented home visiting program with sites across the country. Originally implemented in a semirural community in upstate New York, the NFP employs nurses to provide a manualized home visiting intervention to high-risk primiparous mothers during the prenatal and infancy periods. Although the evaluation based on the entire sample showed no results related to maltreatment, in the group at greatest risk (i.e., low-income, unmarried adolescents), there was a trend suggesting that intervention mothers were less likely to abuse or neglect their children in the first 2 years of life (Olds, Henderson, Chamberlin, & Tatelbaum, 1986). No treatment–control differences were found regarding child abuse and neglect between 25 and 40 months of age, immediately after the end of intervention (Olds, Henderson, & Kitzman, 1994). Interestingly, at this time point, treatment mothers were documented to punish their children to a greater extent.

At a later follow-up of the whole sample (Olds et al., 1997), nurse-visited mothers had fewer substantiated child maltreatment reports 4 to 15 years after the birth of the child, particularly if they were unmarried and of low socioeconomic status. However, the program effects on the level of maltreatment were found to be attenuated by domestic violence, which has been shown to be a major risk factor for child maltreatment (Eckenrode et al., 2000). Furthermore, child maltreatment effects have not been reported for subsequent trials of this intervention in other sites (Olds, Hill, Robinson, Song, & Little, 2000).

The most visible and large-scale maltreatment prevention program is Healthy Families America (HFA). Based on the Hawaii Healthy Start model, HFA has hundreds of local affiliates across the country serving families and children from conception to 5 years. HFA principles inform the design of all local programs and include prenatal or immediate postnatal initiation of services, family assessment, voluntary nature of services, varying intensity of service depending on family need, long duration of services, and comprehensive services. Several principles relate to staffing of the program, including intensive training and supervision, cultural competence, and personal and employment-related competencies.

Several recent experimental and quasi-experimental evaluations of this model have been conducted. In some small-scale studies, which have been criticized for methodological shortcomings (Duggan et al., 1999; Gomby, 2007; Gomby, Culross, & Behrman, 1999), reductions in child maltreatment reports have been documented (Daro & Harding, 1999). However, three recent carefully administered, randomized control trials of the HFA model found no differences in levels of maltreatment in the intervention and control groups (San Diego, CA: Landsverk & Carrilio, 1995; Hawaii: Duggan, Fuddy, et al., 2004; Alaska: Duggan, McFarlane, et al., 2004; DuMont et al., 2008; Gessner, 2008).

In contrast, the rigorous evaluation of the Healthy Families program in New York did yield positive findings when participating children were 2 years of age (DuMont et al., 2008). Overall, control mothers reported that they committed four times as many acts of serious abuse than intervention mothers. In an analysis of program effects on subgroups, young, first-time mothers who began the intervention during the prenatal period were less likely to engage in minor physical aggression and harsh parenting with their children. Furthermore, "psychologically vulnerable" mothers who received the intervention were less likely to report engaging in serious abuse and neglect than their control group counterparts. It is important to note that, similar to other HFA evaluations, no differences were found between intervention and control families in regard to substantiated child protection reports.

Smaller programs have produced beneficial results in the child maltreatment arena. In an evaluation of a parent education program for urban adolescent, unmarried mothers, Britner and Reppucci (1997) found that, 3–5 years after the birth of their children, intervention mothers were less likely to have substantiated reports of child abuse and neglect than control mothers. Bugental and colleagues (2002) documented the impact of adding cognitive retraining to a 1-year, ongoing standard home visitation program for mothers identified during pregnancy or early in the postnatal period. A much lower proportion of mothers in the enhanced home visiting group were abusive than in the standard home visiting group and the control group.

Similarly, Peterson and colleagues (2003) implemented a 4-month cognitive-behavioral prevention model for mothers of children 18 months to 3 years that included group and home-based intervention. Intervention mothers demonstrated reductions in the use of harsh discipline, increased knowledge of the developmental needs of their children, less child-directed anger, understanding of their parental roles, higher levels of nurturance, and a higher sense of parenting efficacy. Child maltreatment was not directly measured in this study, but all these factors have been documented to be related to child maltreatment.

Zeanah and colleagues (2001) evaluated the impact of a preventive intervention designed to improve developmental and child welfare outcomes in maltreated children in foster care from birth to 48 months of age. Following an intensive assessment process, young children and their families were provided with treatment that was individualized to meet their specific needs. Based on an infant mental health approach, treatment potentially involved individual psychotherapy with parents, dyadic psychotherapy with parents and young children, and crisis intervention. It was found that birth mothers who received the intervention were less likely to maltreat their children than mothers who did not. However, fewer intervention children were reunified with their biological parents and more were freed for adoption, compared with those who did not receive the intervention.

Comprehensive child development programs have also been found to reduce maltreatment. A large longitudinal investigation of Title I Child–Parent Centers in Chicago, Illinois, documented a lower rate of child maltreatment, via court petitions and child protective service records, for early-intervention children than for children who received kindergarten intervention (Reynolds & Robertson, 2003). This finding held throughout childhood and adolescence and was more pronounced if the children had received 4–6 years of intervention. In another study, high-risk families participating in an interdisciplinary early-intervention program that included child development and mental health services were less likely to require child protection services and to have substantiated incidents of child abuse and neglect than a comparison group receiving standard care (Huxley & Warner, 1993). These families also reported more appropriate attitudes toward punishment and exhibited higher levels of emotional and verbal engagement with their children.

## Programs That Might Work

There are many programs that may not have directly affected maltreatment but may be promising in their approach. Such programs are typically defined as those that may have an impact on an intermediary outcome between intervention receipt and maltreatment (e.g., parenting stress) or those that have not been subject to evaluation of the highest rigor (e.g., randomized trial) but may be informed by the evidence (Chaffin & Friedrich, 2004). Although many descriptions of such programs exist in the literature, the following discussion focuses only on programs that address factors strongly related to the emergence of maltreatment and those that have used a quasi-experimental design to evaluate program effects.

An initiative alternately called Project 12-Ways or Project Safe Care represents one promising intervention for the prevention of child maltreatment (Lutzker & Bigelow, 2001; Lutzker, Bigelow, Doctor, Gershater, & Greene, 1998). Using an individualized, ecological-behavioral approach, this intervention is designed to build parental skills in a variety of areas, including child management and positive parent–child interaction. Typically, social workers or nurses would administer the intervention in the home, using videos, parent education, and skills practicing, with a focus on home safety, infant and child health care, and bonding and stimulation. Although a randomized, controlled trial of this preventive intervention has yet to be undertaken, several quasi-experimental and single-case design studies suggest that this program is effective in enhancing parental interaction with children, decreasing household hazards, and increasing parental knowledge of child health problems. Furthermore, families receiving this intervention were less likely to have a maltreatment recurrence and to have children removed than comparison families who received traditional child welfare services (Gershater-Molko, Lutzker, & Wesch, 2002).

Although follow-up data are not yet available, the Family Connections program in Baltimore, Maryland, has demonstrated effectiveness in its effort to prevent the neglect of school-age children. This community-based program uses an empowerment model to provide crisis services to families with a goal of building on their social support networks and enhancing parent–child relationships (Administration for Children and Families, 2003b). A rigorous evaluation of the program revealed a short-term impact on several family factors strongly related to child neglect, including decreases in substance use, depression, parenting, stress and child behavior problems and increases in appropriate parenting attitudes and perceptions of social support.

Despite the disappointing results that have been obtained in some evaluations of intensive family preservation and support programs (Littell & Schuerman, 2002), they nevertheless show promise in reducing child maltreatment (MacLeod & Nelson, 2000). These programs are explicitly designed to prevent the placement of children who have experienced or are at high risk for maltreatment. Family preservation programs that targeted a specific age group of children (e.g., infants) and delivered services consistent with the appropriate developmental period had an impact on maltreatment, placement, and participant well-being (Administration for Children and Families, 2001). In addition, more successful programs had higher levels of participant involvement, a strength-based approach, and a social support component (MacLeod & Nelson, 2000).

Crisis nurseries reflect another type of intervention that has been mounted to prevent the maltreatment of young children (Andrews, Bishop, & Sussman, 1999). This intervention provides emergency, temporary child care to families under stress to prevent formal placement. Child care may be provided during the day, or short-term residential child care can be provided. Parents using the facility require short-term hospitalization for mental health or substance use problems, are in school or are working and have not found or have lost a regular child care provider, or are stressed by the care of their children. Although no rigorous evaluation was conducted, a preliminary evaluation of a crisis nursery program in New York City, which compared one-time users of the facility with those who have used it multiple times, revealed that one-time families had only one unsubstantiated child protection report, and multiple-user families had five reports, only one of which was substantiated (Linares et al., 2006).

Infant mental health programs have been designed with the distinct purpose of addressing parenting difficulties often associated with child maltreatment and show promise for reducing child abuse neglect. These programs typically have a foundation in attachment theory and target families at risk for parent–child relationship disturbance (see Berlin, Ziv, Amaya-Jackson, & Greenberg, 2005). Unfortunately, very few have been subject to rigorous evaluation. A meta-analytic review of available evidence suggested that interventions that target parental sensitivity and that had less than a 16-week duration were more effective in promoting positive social-emotional outcomes in young children, even when the family was high risk (van IJzendoorn, 1995; van IJzendoorn, Bakermans-Kranenburg, & Juffer, 2005).

One attachment-based prevention program stands out because of its focus on high-risk families. One was a combination home- and clinic-based preventive child mental health program for mothers at psychological risk, in which psychotherapy, parent–child interaction, and developmental interventions were provided. In examining program effects, Heinicke and colleagues (Heinicke et al., 1999; Heinicke, Fineman, Ponce, & Guthrie, 2001) found that mothers receiving the intervention were less likely to be restrictive and punitive and more likely to promote their children's autonomy. Additionally, their children were less likely to be insecurely attached. Children also demonstrated a greater sense of a separate self and exhibited greater expectations that their needs would be effectively met.

Other prevention programs with home visiting as the primary service delivery mechanism show promise as well. In their examination of a program targeting high-risk mothers (i.e., those experiencing psychiatric illness, substance abuse, or domestic violence), Marcenko and Spence (1994; Marcenko, Spence, & Samost, 1996) documented a positive impact of paraprofessional home visiting. Intervention mothers reported less psychological distress and more social support over time; control mothers did not report these changes. However, their goal of reducing out-of-home placement for participant children was not achieved.

In a program for drug-abusing mothers from low-income backgrounds, trained nurses provided biweekly home visits for a 2-year period (Black et al., 1994). Mothers in the intervention group were less likely to report ongoing drug use, were more likely to complete pediatric appointments, and exhibited grater emotional and verbal responsiveness to their children. Gelfand, Teti, Seiner, and Jameson (1996) also used nurses to provide home visits to depressed mothers during their children's first year of life. Mothers in the treatment group exhibited fewer depressive symptoms and daily hassles than those in the control group. Additionally, control group mothers reported fewer social supports over time, and if depressed, became more punitive toward their children over time.

Parent education programs are arguably the most common intervention strategy for the prevention of child maltreatment and the enhancement of parenting behaviors. National estimates suggest that parents of nearly 400,000 children will participate in mandated or voluntary parent training on an annual basis (Administration for Children and Families, 2005b; Barth, Landsverk, & Chamberlain, 2005). Despite their wide usage, typically parent training interventions have not been subject to rigorous evaluation. Those programs documenting success often have methodological difficulties, such as the absence of a control group.

Despite these caveats, a 2006 meta-analysis of parent training programs suggests that most have moderate success (Lundahl, Nimer, & Parsons, 2006). The success of these programs increases if they have a behavioral component and include home visits (Lundahl et al., 2006). Education programs with high-risk parents have yielded benefits such as improvements in parental stress and parent–child interaction (Huebner, 2002) and more nurturing parenting attitudes (Cowen, 2001).

The evidence does suggest that parent education programs implemented in concert with more individualized therapeutic interventions may be more effective (Daro & Donnelly, 2002). For example, Peterson and colleagues' (2003) 4-month cognitive-behavioral prevention model for mothers of toddlers yielded reductions in the use of harsh discipline, increased knowledge of the developmental needs of their children, less child-directed anger, increased understanding of their parental roles, higher levels of nurturance, and a higher sense of parenting efficacy on the part of intervention mothers.

Additionally, parent education programs targeted at specific parenting problems have been used to avert child maltreatment. For example, educating new parents about how to cope with infant crying may be effective in reducing the incidence of abusive head trauma (Krugman, Lane, & Walsh, 2007). Parenting education interventions that utilize a cognitive-behavioral approach to reduce child behavior problems also are effective in reducing child maltreatment (Barth et al., 2005).

Specifically, The Incredible Years (TIY) model, aimed at reducing behavior problems in children from 2 to 8 years of age, has been tested in rigorous clinical trials with samples including large numbers of child welfare–involved children (Webster-Stratton & Hammond, 1997). This intervention consists of 12 weekly group sessions that educates parents on how to manage challenging children using a cognitive-behavioral approach. TIY has been found to be effective in promoting parenting competence in high-risk families, specifically in reducing negative parenting behaviors (e.g., harsh style) and increasing positive parenting behaviors (e.g., positive affect, praise).

## Programs That Do Not Work

Many programs have not yielded benefits for participating families. For example, Fraser, Armstrong, Morris, and Dadds (2000) conducted a randomized controlled trial of a child abuse and neglect home visiting intervention beginning early in the postnatal period. At follow-up (12–18 months postbirth), no differences were found in intervention and control families regarding parental stress, parenting competence, and quality of the home environment. Brayden and colleagues (1993) evaluated an intervention beginning in the prenatal period through age 2 and found no effects on maltreatment. The authors attributed the lack of effects to increased maltreatment detection in the intervention group of families. In an evaluation of paraprofessional home visitation to mothers at risk of child abuse during or soon after pregnancy, Barth (1991) did not find impacts on child abuse reports or on maternal self-report of functioning.

Furthermore, many generic child maltreatment prevention programs have not been successful. For example, extant literature suggests that global parenting education programs have limited effectiveness for families at risk for child maltreatment (Barth et al., 2005; Chalk & King, 1998). Additionally, parent groups that rely on didactic, informational, and discussion formats tend to be less effective (Daro, 1988; Durlak, 1997). Additionally, untargeted family preservation and support programs have not been found to reduce rates of maltreatment or placement (Chaffin & Schmidt, 2006; Littell & Schuerman, 2002).

Findings such as these have led to a call for the revamping of child maltreatment prevention programs, so that they deliver services that are informed by current evidence. For example, Chaffin (2004) suggests that these programs should target specific needs of families at risk for maltreatment, such as providing treatment for mental illness, substance abuse, and interpersonal violence. Other scholars have pointed to the importance of beginning these programs prenatally, focusing on implementation fidelity, selection of competent staff, and provision of sufficient dosage (Gomby, 2007; Olds et al., 2000).

## Prevention Programs and African American Families

Not all the effective and promising prevention programs just delineated have been found to be beneficial, or have even been tested, with African American populations. The two effective prevention programs that served primarily African American families were the Child–Parent Centers in Chicago and the Family Connections program in Baltimore. African American families are included in some of the Healthy Families evaluations but were not the targets of the interventions. When the Nurse–Family Partnership model was implemented in Memphis, Tennessee, with a predominantly African American sample, maltreatment effects were not documented per se (Olds et al., 2000). Reductions in health care encounters and hospitalizations for injuries and ingestions for intervention children were documented, which the authors suggested could reflect a decrease in child maltreatment incidents.

Two parenting programs targeted to African American families show promise in addressing maltreatment in this population. The Effective Black Parenting Program (EBPP; Alvy, 1994), grounded in theory about African American parenting, attempts to enhance parenting skills and strategies by incorporating African proverbs and other culture-specific narratives and artifacts. The program emphasizes helping African American parents enhance the quality of their relationships with their children and use parenting strategies and skills that research has shown to be most helpful in raising prosocial, competent, and healthy children. For parents of young children, the program does specifically address child maltreatment. EBPP has been field-tested with promising results documented regarding improving parental competencies (Alvy, 1994; Myers, Taylor, Alvy, Arrington, & Richardson, 1992).

The second intervention was designed as a supplement to the Nurturing Parenting Program (Bavolek, 2003), which has been widely used with child-maltreating parents with a goal of promoting positive parenting skills. The Enhancing Parenting Skills for African-American Families Program (Bass & Moody, 2003) incorporates such topics as diversity, Black history, transcending oppression, dual consciousness, spirituality, and accessing resources for Black children. The original version of the Nurturing Parenting Program has been field-tested and validated with diverse samples (Bavolek, 2003), but an evaluation of the curriculum adapted for African American parents has not been undertaken.

Possibly the only evidence-based prevention program to date that has specifically used a culture-based design to support African American families is not one that has maltreatment prevention as a goal. The Strong African-American Families Program is an intervention to prevent negative parenting processes and negative child outcomes among African American families in the rural South (Brody et al., 2004). Specifically, this program attempted to have an impact on parents' involvement with, socialization of, communication with, and expectations of their preadolescent children, which are all processes linked to child maltreatment (Belsky & Vondra, 1989; Milner & Crouch, 1993). A rigorous evaluation of this preventive intervention demonstrated its effectiveness in modifying parenting processes and ultimately promoting child protective factors (i.e., negative attitudes about alcohol/sex, acceptance of parental influence, future orientation).

The small number of effective interventions aimed at preventing maltreatment among African American families calls for an expansion of evidence-based programs targeted to this population. Such efforts should capitalize on the knowledge gained from the implementation of other programs and should avoid the methodological pitfalls that characterize evaluations of these programs. Specifically, prevention interventions should be tested with African American populations in randomized clinical trials. The design of these programs should be informed by evidence regarding the features of effective programs to prevent child maltreatment.

## EVIDENCE-BASED TREATMENT INTERVENTIONS

Treatment interventions have a goal of reducing the recurrence of maltreatment in abusive families. Whereas there is wide implementation as well as evaluation of child maltreatment preventive interventions, there is a dearth of treatment interventions for the parents of maltreated children. Most of the limited treatment interventions that have been tested focus on physically abusive parents and use a cognitive-behavioral approach. As such, the treatment involves addressing the perpetrators' cognitive distortions about the abusive behavior, increasing their empathy for their children, and developing their impulse control and child management skills to avoid abusing their children (Azar, 1997).

Evaluations of such treatment approaches have documented improved parental capacity to manage anger and aggression and reductions in the use of physical discipline (Kolko, 1996; Schinke et al., 1986). Additionally, Kolko (1996) reported that cognitive-behavioral therapy reduced parental distress and abuse risk and improved parental practices and overall family relationships. However, this treatment intervention did not have a significant impact on whether families experienced another child maltreatment report.

Two earlier studies reported reductions of child maltreatment. Wolfe, Edwards, Manion, and Koverola (1988) provided a behaviorally oriented parent–child interaction program to abusive parents of preschool children. Parents reported fewer child deviant behaviors and maternal adjustment difficulties. In addition, families' caseworkers reported reduced risk for child maltreatment among the intervention parents. In another study of a relatively small sample, maltreating parents who experienced a cognitive-behavioral group treatment model did not continue to maltreat their children at follow-up in comparison to a recidivism rate of 21% in a comparison group that received short-term insight-oriented treatment (Azar et al., 1984).

A recent rigorous evaluation of parent–child interaction therapy (PCIT) has been found to be effective in reducing the recurrence of maltreatment specifically. PCIT is an intensive treatment intervention that was designed to address behavior problems in young children (Eisenstadt, Eyberg, McNeil, Newcomb, & Funderburk, 1993), which has been adapted for use with families of young children who suffered physical abuse (Urquiza & McNeil, 1996). Families are coached *in vivo* by a trained therapist to respond to their children more appropriately during periods when the children exhibit challenging behavior and during more positive interactions. Evidence indicates that PCIT can improve parents' child management skills and reduce children's behavior problems (Chaffin & Valle, 2003). Moreover, PCIT has been found to reduce parents' re-abuse of their children (Chaffin et al., 2004).

A final model with promising results for the treatment of child physical abuse is multisystemic therapy (MST). This is a very intensive treatment program that typically targets families of adolescents and provides a wide array of services to address multiple systems in the life of the child (e.g., individual, family, school, community). Preliminary evidence suggests that MST improves parent–child interactions and child placement outcomes in maltreating families (Brunk, Henggeler, & Whelan, 1987; Chaffin & Schmidt, 2006).

Although the bulk of the research on sexual abuse treatment focuses on the effects on the victim and nonoffending parent, cognitive-behavioral treatment models have been attempted with sexual abuse perpetrators (Berliner & Elliott, 2002; Kolko, 2000). These interventions attempt to alter perpetrators' cognitive distortions about the sexual abuse, including their denial and minimization of their acts. Relapse prevention is typically a part of these treatment models, which include self-monitoring and behavioral reinforcement strategies. Unfortunately, the few rigorous evaluations of such programs have yielded disappointing results (Marquez, Wiederanders, Day, Nelson, & van Ommeren, 2005). The evidence from less rigorously designed studies is more positive, with findings of moderate decreases in sex offense recidivism (Hanson et al., 2002). It is important to note that these studies include a wide range of sex offenders against children, who are not always parent-to-child abusers, thus limiting our knowledge about sexual abuse treatment even further.

In sum, there is a dearth of evidence about effective treatment interventions for parents who have abused or neglected their children. Although the research base is slim, some progress has been made toward articulating appropriate treatment models for child abuse. In contrast, the very limited evidence on treatment of sexual abusers suggests that these interventions are not effective. Empirically based work on the treatment of neglect is virtually nonexistent, perhaps because of the complexity and subjectivity of its definition, the multiple parenting processes that constitute neglect, and neglect's correlation with global risks such as poverty. Furthermore, the benefit of these treatment modalities for African American families is not known. The need for more empirical testing of interventions that can inform the treatment of African American parents who abuse and neglect their children cannot be overstated.

## IMPLICATIONS OF RESEARCH FOR BEST PRACTICES

An understanding of the risk and protective factors related to child maltreatment is key for the development of effective interventions to serve affected families and children. Additionally, although the research on the benefits of prevention and treatment programs is limited in many ways, it is nevertheless informative about what approaches to child maltreatment show more promise. Here, we consider the implications of current evidence about child maltreatment processes and interventions for practice in psychology and other fields.

Regarding the prevention of child maltreatment, home visiting programs have been found to be effective when delivered with integrity and intensity by well-trained staff and when focused on the needs of targeted populations. Well-designed, long-term interventions begun during infancy seem to affect child maltreatment more than short-term programs with less conceptually sophisticated designs. However, it should be noted that these programs typically do not show maltreatment effects until later years, which may suggest more of an indirect program effect on maltreatment (Chaffin, 2004).

Comprehensive early childhood programs, which include center-based child development interventions and multigenerational services, also seem to be effective in reducing maltreatment. Such programs may have particular benefits for African American children and families (Administration for Children and Families, 2002). Thus, referrals of families to programs like Head Start, Early Head Start, and other early childhood interventions have the potential to enhance children's overall developmental functioning *and* reduce the risk for child maltreatment. The evidence on parent education programs is less compelling but does suggest that more experiential, interactive parent education programs that provide specific strategies to address specific child functioning factors can enhance parental behavior toward their children. Additionally, promising approaches for maltreated children and their families stem from mental health models, in which positive parental interaction with their children is promoted.

Overall, prevention programs with the following characteristics are most likely to benefit families at risk for maltreatment: (1) begun during pregnancy, infancy, or early childhood; (2) comprehensive in nature and address two generations; (3) intensive but not necessarily of long duration; (4) targeted to specific high-risk groups; (5) staffed by highly trained, professional staff; and (6) incorporate services to address specific risk factors. Furthermore, these programs should be culturally appropriate and build on the strengths of targeted community, specifically addressing the needs and cultural prescriptions of the African American population.

Although the evidence base is somewhat slim, some practice recommendations can be garnered from the evidence on treatment interventions for child abuse and neglect. Treatment interventions should be grounded in an appropriate theory that addresses a specific form of maltreatment. This is particularly apparent in the benefits documented with cognitive-behavioral treatments that address physical abuse. Because such approaches have not been successful with parents who sexually abuse or neglect their children, they may not have an impact regarding these types of child maltreatment. Practice approaches that go beyond treatment of the maltreating parent may be critical in these situations, such as intervening with the nonoffending parent in sexual abuse cases and case management in neglect cases.

Additionally, effective treatment interventions for child abuse and neglect often include a parent–child interaction component. The cognitive-behavioral treatments are often delivered in this context, in which parents' appropriate management of children's behavior is facilitated *while* they are interacting with their children. Although treatment of neglectful families has essentially been a neglected area of research, successful prevention programs have utilized a parent–child interaction approach that could be extended to treatment situations.

Furthermore, given that risk factors for child neglect (as explicated earlier in this chapter) are often in the parent/family mental health domain (e.g., substance abuse, depression, family violence), parent receipt of mental health treatment may be as important as intervention directly targeting child neglect.

## CONCLUSION

Child maltreatment is a major public health issue that affects families of all classes and races (Centers for Disease Control and Prevention, 2008). Although the rate of child maltreatment in the African American community is similar to that of White families, African American families have distinct experiences once they are involved in the service system that is charged with protecting children (i.e., child welfare) (Administration for Children and Families, 2003a). In order to prevent and treat child abuse and neglect, it is important that services are designed to address the myriad needs of maltreating families, from the individual vulnerabilities that parents exhibit to the ecological risk factors they face. These services should be equitable, culturally grounded, and documented to be effective for African American families.

The field of child maltreatment has evolved considerably from the days when the pediatrician Henry Kempe (1985) put child abuse on the public agenda with his description of "battered child syndrome." Scholars have amassed substantial evidence about the etiology, processes, and consequences of child maltreatment. What is lacking is a solid knowledge base about how to prevent child maltreatment and how to treat the families in which abuse and neglect has happened. Given its focus on delivering effective clinical services to vulnerable individuals, as well as using empirical evidence to inform practice, psychology has much to offer in the area of child maltreatment. Implementing effective services to intervene in the lives of families experiencing abuse and neglect represents an important use of psychology to promote the well-being of individual children whose development is hindered through parental victimization and to benefit the larger society upon which child maltreatment levies many psychological, social, and economic costs.

## REFERENCES

Aber, J. L., & Zigler, E. (1981). Developmental considerations in the definition of child maltreatment. *New Directions for Child Development, 11*, 1–29.

Administration for Children and Families. (2001). *Evaluation of family preservation and reunification programs: Interim report.* Washington, DC: U.S. Department of Health and Human Services.

Administration for Children and Families. (2002). *Making a difference in the lives of infants and toddlers and their families: The impacts of Early Head Start.* Washington, DC: U.S. Department of Health and Human Services.

Administration for Children and Families. (2003a). *Children of color in the child welfare system: Perspectives from the child welfare community.* Washington, DC: U.S. Department of Health and Human Services.

Administration for Children and Families. (2003b). *Emerging practices in the prevention of child abuse and neglect.* Washington, DC: U.S. Government Printing Office.

Administration for Children and Families. (2005a). *Male perpetrators of child maltreatment: Findings from NCANDS.* Washington, DC: U.S. Department of Health and Human Services.

Administration for Children and Families. (2005b). *National Survey of Child and Adolescent Well-Being: CPS sample component Wave 1 data analysis report.* Washington, DC: U.S. Department of Health and Human Services.

Administration for Children and Families. (2008). *Child maltreatment 2006 report.* Washington, DC: U.S. Department of Health and Human Services.

Agrawal, A., & Lynskey, M. T. (2008). Are there genetic influences on addiction: Evidence from family, adoption, and twin studies. *Addiction, 103*(7), 1069–1081.

Alvy, K. T. (1994). *Parent training today: A social necessity.* Studio City, CA: Center for the Improvement of Child.

American Psychiatric Association. (2000). *Diagnostic and statistical manual of mental disorders* (4th ed., text rev.). Washington, DC: Author.

Ammerman, R. T., Hersen, M., Van Hasselt, V. B., & Lubetsky, M. J. (1994). Maltreatment in psychiatrically hospitalized children and adolescents with developmental disabilities: Prevalence and correlates. *Journal of the American Academy of Child and Adolescent Psychiatry, 33*(4), 567–576.

Andrews, B., Bishop, A. R., & Sussman, M. S. (1999). Emergency child care and overnight respite for children from birth to 5 years of age: Development of a community-based crisis nursery. In J. A. Silver, B. J. Amster, & T. Haecker (Eds.), *Young children and foster care: A guide for professionals* (pp. 325–345). Baltimore: Brookes.

Anisman, H., Merali, Z., & Stead, J. D. H. (2008). Experiential and genetic contributions to depressive- and anxiety-like disorders: Clinical and experimental studies. *Neuroscience and Biobehavioral Reviews, 32*(6), 1185–1206.

Arata, C. M., Langhinrichsen-Rohling, D., Bowers, D., & O'Brien, N. (2007). Differential correlates of multi-type maltreatment among urban youth. *Child Abuse and Neglect, 31*(4), 393–415.

Ayoub, C. C., & Rappolt-Schlichtmann, G. (2007). Child maltreatment and the development of alternate pathways in biology and behavior. In D. Coch, G. Dawson, & K. W. Fischer (Eds.), *Human behavior, learning, and the developing brain: Atypical development* (pp. 305–330). New York: Guilford Press.

Azar, S. (1997). A cognitive behavioral approach to understanding and treating parents who physically abuse their children. In D. A. Wolfe, R. J. McMahon, & R. Peters (Eds.), *Child abuse: New directions in prevention and treatment across the lifespan* (pp. 79–101). Thousand Oaks, CA: Sage.

Azar, S., Breton, S., & Miller, L. (1998). Cognitive-behavioral group work and physical child abuse: Intervention and prevention. In K. Stoiber & T. Kratochwill (Eds.), *Handbook of group intervention for children and families* (pp. 376–400). Needham Heights, MA: Allyn & Bacon.

Azar, S., Robinson, D., Hekimian, E., & Twentyman, C. (1984). Unrealistic expectations and problem-solving ability in maltreating and comparison mothers. *Journal of Consulting and Clinical Psychology, 52*, 687–691.

Baker, A., & Belleman, R. (2007). *Clinical handbook of co-existing mental health and drug and alcohol problems.* New York: Routledge/Taylor & Francis.

Barth, R. (1991). An experimental evaluation of in-home child abuse prevention services. *Child Abuse and Neglect, 15*(4), 363–375.

Barth, R. P., Landsverk, J., & Chamberlain, P. (2005). Parent-training programs in child welfare services: Planning for a more evidence-based approach to serving biological parents. *Research on Social Work Practice, 15*, 353–371.

Bass, L., & Moody, D. (2003). *Nurturing parenting skills for African American families: A program guide.* Park City, UT: Family Development Resources.

Baumrind, D. (1994). The social context of child maltreatment. *Family Relations, 43*, 360–368.

Baumrind, D. (1995). *Child maltreatment and optimal caregiving in social contexts.* New York: Garland.

Bavolek, S. (2003). *Research and validation of the Nurturing Parenting Programs.* Park City, UT: Family Development Resources.

Belsky, J. (1980). Child maltreatment: An ecological integration. *American Psychologist, 35*, 320–335.

Belsky, J. (1993). Etiology of child maltreatment: A developmental–ecological analysis. *Psychological Bulletin, 114*, 413–434.

Belsky, J., & Vondra, J. (1989). Lessons from child abuse: The determinants of parenting. In D. Cicchetti & V. Carlson (Eds.), *Child maltreatment: Theory and research on the causes and consequences of child abuse and neglect* (pp. 153–202). New York: Cambridge University Press.

Benjet, C., & Kazdin, A. E. (2003). Spanking children: The controversies, findings and new directions. *Clinical Psychology Review, 23*(2), 197–224.

Berlin, L. J., Ziv, Y., Amaya-Jackson, L., & Greenberg, M. T. (Eds.). (2005). *Enhancing early attachments: Theory, research, intervention, and policy.* New York: Guilford Press.

Berliner, L., & Elliott, D. M. (2002). Sexual abuse of children. In J. E. B. Myers, L. Berliner, J. Briere, C. T. Hendrix, C. Jenny, & T. A. Reid (Eds.), *APSAC handbook on child maltreatment* (2nd ed., pp. 55–78). Thousand Oaks, CA: Sage.

Bernardo, L. (1996). Parent-reported injury-associated behaviors and life events among injured, ill, and well preschool children. *Journal of Pediatric Nursing, 11*, 100–110.

Besinger, B., Garland, A. F., Litrownik, A. J., & Landsverk, J. A. (1999). Caregiver substance abuse among maltreated children placed in out-of-home care. *Child Welfare, 78*, 221–239.

Bess, R. (2002). *The cost of protecting vulnerable children.* Washington, DC: Urban Institute.

Black, M., Nair, P., Kight, C., Wachtel, R., Roby, P., & Schuler, M. (1994). Parenting and early development among children of drug-abusing women: Effects of home intervention. *Pediatrics, 94*, 440–448.

Bray, N. (2008). Gene expression in the etiology of schizophrenia. *Schizophrenia Bulletin, 34*(3), 412–418.

Brayden, R., Altemeier, W., Dietrich, M., Tucker, D., Christensen, M., McLaughlin, F., et al. (1993). A prospective study of secondary prevention of child maltreatment. *Pediatrics, 122*(4), 511–516.

Brayden, R., Altemeier, W., Tucker, D., Dietrich, M., & Vietze, P. (1992). Antecedents of child neglect in the first two years of life. *Journal of Pediatrics, 120*, 426–429.

Britner, P., & Reppucci, N. (1997). Prevention of child maltreatment: Evaluation of a parent education program for teen mothers. *Journal of Child and Family Studies*, 6(2), 165–175.

Brody, G., Murry, V., Gerard, M., Gibbons, R., Molgaard, V., McNair, L., et al. (2004). The Strong African American Families Program: Translating research into prevention programming. *Child Development*, 75(3), 900–917.

Bronfenbrenner, U. (1979). *The ecology of human development: Experiments by nature and design.* Cambridge, MA: Harvard University Press.

Brown, J., Cohen, P., Johnson, J., & Salzinger, S. (1998). A longitudinal analysis of risk factors for child maltreatment: Findings of a 17-year prospective study of officially recorded and self-reported child abuse and neglect. *Child Abuse and Neglect*, 22, 1065–1078.

Browne, D., Catellier, D., Dufort, V., Kotch, J., & Winsor, J. (1999). Predicting child maltreatment in the first 4 years of life from characteristics assessed in the neonatal period. *Child Abuse and Neglect*, 23, 305–319.

Browne, K., & Fereti, I. (1996). Growing up in a violent family. In S. Nakou & S. Pantelakis (Eds.), *The child in the world of tomorrow: The next generation* (pp. 96–105). Elmsford, NY: Pergamon.

Browne, K., & Herbert, M. (1997). *Preventing family violence.* Chichester, UK: Wiley.

Brunk, M., Henggeler, S., & Whelan, J. (1987). Comparison of multisystemic therapy and parent training in the brief treatment of child abuse and neglect. *Journal of Consulting and Clinical Psychology*, 16, 243–258.

Buchanan, A. (1998). Intergenerational child maltreatment. In Y. Danielli (Ed.), *International handbook of multigenerational legacies of trauma* (pp. 535–552). New York: Plenum.

Bugental, D., Ellerson, P., Lin, E., Rainey, B., Kokotovic, A., & O'Hara, N. (2002). A cognitive approach to child abuse prevention. *Journal of Family Psychology*, 16(3), 243–258.

Bugental, D. B., Mantyla, S. M., & Lewis, J. (1989). Parental attributions as moderators of affective communication to children at risk for physical abuse. In D. Cicchetti & V. Carlson (Eds.), *Child maltreatment: Theory and research on the causes and consequences of child abuse and neglect* (pp. 254–279). New York: Cambridge University Press.

Caliso, J., & Milner, H. (1992). Childhood history of abuse and child abuse screening. *Child Abuse and Neglect*, 16, 647–659.

Campbell, S. B., Shaw, D. S., & Gilliom, M. (2000). Early externalizing behavior problems: Toddlers and preschoolers at risk for later maladjustment. *Development and Psychopathology*, 12(3), 467–488.

Canfield, R. L., Gendle, M. H., & Cory-Slechta, D. A. (2004). Impaired neuropsychological functioning in lead-exposed children. *Developmental Neuropsychology*, 26(1), 513–540.

Carter, J. W., Schulsinger, F., Parnas, J., Cannon, T., & Mednick, S. A. (2002). A multivariate prediction model of schizophrenia. *Schizophrenia Bulletin*, 28(4), 649–682.

Casady, A. M., & Lee, R. E. (2002). Environments of physically neglected children. *Psychological Reports*, 91(3), 711–721.

Caselles, C. E., & Milner, J. S. (2000). Evaluations of child transgressions, disciplinary choices, and expected child compliance in a no-cry and a crying infant condition in physically abusive and comparison mothers. *Child Abuse and Neglect, 24*(4), 477–491.

Cavanagh, K., Dobash, R. E., & Dobash, R. P. (2007). The murder of children by fathers in the context of child abuse. *Child Abuse and Neglect, 31*(7), 731–746.

Centers for Disease Control and Prevention. (2003). First reports evaluating the effectiveness of strategies for preventing violence: Early childhood home visitation: Findings from the Task Force on Community Preventative Services. *Morbidity and Mortality Weekly Report, 52,* 1–9.

Centers for Disease Control and Prevention. (2008). *Understanding child maltreatment: Factsheet.* Atlanta, GA: Author. Retrieved June 22, 2008, from *www.cdc.gov/violence prevetion/pdf/CM-FactSheet-a.pdf.*

Chaffin, M. (2004). Is it time to rethink Healthy Start/Healthy Families? *Child Abuse and Neglect, 28*(6), 589–595.

Chaffin, M., & Friedrich, B. (2004). Evidence-based treatments in child abuse and neglect. *Children and Youth Services Review, 26*(11), 1097–1113.

Chaffin, M., Kelleher, K., Harber, G., & Harper, J. (1994). Impact of substance abuse and child maltreatment training on service utilization in a rural setting. *Journal of Child and Family Studies, 3*(4), 379–387.

Chaffin, M., Kelleher, K., & Hollenerg, J. (1996). Onset of physical abuse and neglect: Psychiatric, substance abuse, and social risk factors from prospective community data. *Child Abuse and Neglect, 20*(3), 191–203.

Chaffin, M., & Schmidt, S. (2006). An evidence-based perspective on interventions to stop or prevent child abuse. In J. Lutzker (Ed.), *Preventing violence: Research and evidence-based intervention strategies* (pp. 49–68). Washington, DC: American Psychological Association.

Chaffin, M., Silovsky, J. F., Funderburk, B., Valle, L. S., Brestan, E. V., Balachova, T., et al. (2004). Parent–child interaction therapy with physically abusive parents: Efficacy for reducing future abuse reports. *Journal of Consulting and Clinical Psychology, 72*(3), 500–510.

Chaffin, M., & Valle, L. A. (2003). Dynamic prediction characteristics of the Child Abuse Potential Inventory. *Child Abuse and Neglect, 27,* 459–461.

Chalk, R., & King, P. A. (Eds.). (1998). *Violence in families: Assessing prevention and treatment programs.* Washington, DC: National Academy Press.

Christman, A., Wodarski, J. S., & Smokowski, P. R. (1996). Risk factors for physical child abuse: A practice theoretical paradigm. *Family Therapy, 23,* 233–248.

Cicchetti, D., & Bartnett, D. (1991). Toward the development of a scientific nosology of child maltreatment. In D. Cicchetti & W. Grove (Eds.), *Thinking clearly about psychology: Essays in honor of Paul E. Meehl* (pp. 346–377). Minneapolis: University of Minnesota Press.

Cicchetti, D., & Rizley, R. (1981). Developmental perspectives on the etiology, intergenerational transmission, and sequelae of child maltreatment. *New Directions for Child Development, 11,* 31–55.

Cicchetti, D., & Rogosch, F. A. (1997). The role of self-organization in the promotion of resilience in maltreated children. *Development and Psychopathology, 9,* 797–815.

Cicchetti, D., Rogosch, F. A., Lynch, M., & Holt, K. D. (1993). Resilience in maltreated children: Processes leading to adaptive outcome. *Development and Psychopathology, 5,* 629–647.

Cicchetti, D., Toth, S. L., & Hennessy, K. (1989). Research on the consequences of child maltreatment and its application to educational settings. *Topics in Early Childhood Special Education, 9*(2), 33–55.

Cicchetti, D., Toth, S. L., & Maughan, A. (2000). An ecological-transactional model of child maltreatment. In A. J. Sameroff, M. Lewis, & S. M. Miller (Eds.), *Handbook of developmental psychopathology* (2nd ed., pp. 689–722). New York: Kluwer.

Cicchetti, D., & Valentino, K. (2006). An ecological-transactional perspective on child maltreatment: Failure of the average expectable environment and its influence on child development. In D. Cicchetti & D. Cohen (Eds.), *Developmental psychopathology: Vol. 3. Risk, disorder and adaptation* (2nd ed., pp. 129–201). Hoboken, NJ: Wiley.

Claussen, A. H., & Crittenden, P. M. (1991). Physical and psychological maltreatment: Relations among the types of maltreatment. *Child Abuse and Neglect, 15*(1/2), 5–18.

Coles, C. D., & Black, M. M. (2006). Introduction to the special issue: Impact of prenatal substance exposure on children's health, development, school performance, and risk behavior. *Journal of Pediatric Psychology, 31*(1), 1–4.

Coles, C. D., & Platzman, K. A. (1993). Behavioral development in children prenatally exposed to drugs and alcohol. *International Journal of the Addictions, 28*(13), 1393–1433.

Coohey, C. (1998). Home alone and other inadequately supervised children. *Child Welfare Journal, 77*(3), 291–310.

Coohey, C. (2000). The role of friends, in-laws, and other kin in father-penetrated child physical abuse. *Child Welfare, 79*(4), 373–402.

Coohey, C. (2003). Defining and classifying supervisory neglect. *Child Maltreatment, 8,* 145–156.

Coulton, C. J., Korbin, J., Chow, J., & Su, M. (1995). Community level factors and child maltreatment rates. *Child Development, 66,* 1262–1276.

Cowen, P. (2001). Effectiveness of a parent education intervention for at-risk families. *Journal of the Society of Pediatric Nurses, 6*(2), 73–82.

Crittenden, P. M. (1999). Danger and development: The organization of self-protective strategies. *Monographs of the Society for Research in Child Development, 64,* 119–144.

Crum, L., Hogan, V., Chapple, T., Browne, D., & Greene, J. (2005). Disparities in maternal and child health in the United States. In J. Kotch (Ed.), *Maternal and child health* (pp. 299–346). Sudbury, MA: Jones & Bartlett.

Culbertson, J. L., & Schellenbach, C. L. (1992). Prevention of maltreatment in infants and young children. In D. J. Willis, E. W. Holden, & M. S. Rosenberg (Eds.), *Prevention in child maltreatment: Developmental and ecological perspectives* (pp. 47–77). Oxford, UK: Wiley.

Daly, M., & Wilson, M. (1999). *A Darwinian view of parental love: The truth about Cinderella.* New Haven, CT: Yale University Press.

Daro, D. (1988). *Confronting child abuse.* New York: Free Press.

Daro, D., & Donnelly, A. C. (2002). Child abuse prevention: Accomplishments and challenges. In J. E. B. Myers, L. Berliner, J. Briere, C. T. Hendrix, C. Jenny, & T. A. Reid (Eds.), *The APSAC handbook on child maltreatment* (2nd ed., pp. 431–448). Thousand Oaks, CA: Sage.

Daro, D., & Harding, K. (1999). Healthy Families America: Using research in going to scale. *Future of Children, 9*(1), 152–176.

Davidson-Arad, B., Englechin-Segal, D., & Wozner, Y. (2003). Short-term follow-up of children at risk: Comparison of the quality of life of children removed from home and children remaining at home. *Child Abuse and Neglect, 27*, 733–750.

Deater-Deckard, K., Dodge, K. A., Bates, J. E., & Pettit, G. S. (1996). Physical discipline among African American and European American mothers: Links to children's externalizing behaviors. *Developmental Psychology, 32*, 1065–1072.

Deater-Deckard, K., Dodge, K. A., & Sorbring, E. (2005). Cultural differences in the effects of physical punishment. In M. Rutter & M. Tienda (Eds.), *Ethnicity and causal mechanisms* (pp. 204–226). Cambridge, UK: Cambridge University Press.

DeBellis, M. (2004). Neurotoxic effects of childhood trauma: Magnetic resonance imaging studies of pediatric maltreatment-related posttraumatic stress disorder versus nontraumatized children with generalized anxiety disorder. In J. Gorman (Ed.), *Fear and anxiety: The benefits of translation research* (pp. 151–170). Washington, DC: American Psychiatric Publishing.

DeBellis, M. (2005). The psychobiology of neglect. *Child Maltreatment, 10*(2), 150–172.

DeBellis, M., Baum, A., Birmaher, B., Keshavan, M., Eccard, C., Boring, A., et al. (1999). Developmental traumatology: Part I. Biological stress systems. *Biological Psychiatry, 45*, 1259–1270.

DeBellis, M. D., Hooper, S. R., & Sapia, J. L. (2005). Early trauma exposure and the brain. In J. Vasterling & C. R. Brewin (Eds.), *Neuropsychology of PTSD: Biological, cognitive, and clinical perspectives* (pp. 153–177). New York: Guilford Press.

DePanfilis, D., & Girvin, H. (2004). Investigating child maltreatment in out-of-home care: Barriers to effective decision-making. *Children and Youth Services Review, 27*(4), 353–374.

DePanfilis, D., & Zuravin, S. J. (1999). Predicting child maltreatment recurrences during treatment. *Child Abuse and Neglect, 23*(8), 729–743.

DePanfilis, D. J. (1999). Intervening with families when children are neglected. In H. Dubowitz (Ed.), *Neglected children: Research, practice, and policy* (pp. 211–236). Thousand Oaks, CA: Sage.

Derezotes, D., Poertner, J., & Testa, M. F. (2005). *Race matters in child welfare: The overrepresentation of African American children in the system.* Washington, DC: Child Welfare League of America.

Dodge, K. A., McLoyd, V. C., & Lansford, J. E. (2005). The cultural context of physically disciplining children. In V. C. McLoyd, N. E. Hill, & K. A. Dodge (Eds.), *African American family life: Ecological and cultural diversity* (pp. 245–263). New York: Guilford Press.

Dozier, M., Stovall, K. C., Albus, K. E., & Bates, B. (2001). Attachment for infants in foster care: The role of caregiver state of mind. *Child Development, 72*(5), 1467–1477.

Drake, B., & Pandey, S. (1996). Understanding the relationship between neighborhood poverty and specific types of child maltreatment. *Child Abuse and Neglect, 20*(11), 1003–1018.

Dubowitz, H., Black, M., Harrington, D., Kerr, M., & Starr, H. (2000). Fathers and child neglect. *Archives of Pediatrics and Adolescent Medicine, 154*, 135–141.

Dubowitz, H., Black, M., Starr, R. H., & Zuravin, S. (1993). A conceptual definition of child neglect. *Criminal Justice and Behavior, 20*(1), 8–26.

Ducci, F., & Goldman, D. (2008). Genetic approaches to addiction: Genes and alcohol. *Addiction, 103*(9), 1414–1428.

Duggan, A., Fuddy, L., Burrell, L., Higman, S., McFarlane, E., Windham, A., et al. (2004). Randomized trial of a statewide home visiting program to prevent child abuse: Impact in reducing parental risk factors. *Child Abuse and Neglect, 28,* 623–643.

Duggan, A., McFarlane, E., Fuddy, L., Burrell, L., Higman, S. L., Windham, A., et al. (2004). Randomized trial of a statewide home visiting program to prevent child abuse: Impact in reducing child abuse and neglect. *Child Abuse and Neglect, 28,* 597–622.

Duggan, A., McFarlane, E., Windham, A., Rohde, C., Salkever, D., Fuddy, L., et al. (1999). Evaluation of Hawaii's Healthy Start Program. *Future of Children, 9,* 152–176.

DuMont, K., Mitchell-Herzfeld, S., Greene, R., Lee, E., Lowenfels, A., Rodriguez, M., et al. (2008). Healthy Families New York (HFNY) randomized trial: Effects on early child abuse and neglect. *Child Abuse and Neglect, 32*(3), 295–315.

Duncan, B. L., Hubble, M. A., & Rusk, G. (1994). To intervene or not to intervene?: That is not the question. *Journal of Systemic Therapies, 13*(4), 22–30.

Dunn, M., Kirisci, L., Kirillova, G., Mezzich, A., Tarter, R., & Vanyukov, M. (2002). Origins and consequences of child neglect and substance abuse in families. *Clinical Psychology Review, 22,* 1063–1090.

Durlak, J. A. (1997). *Successful prevention programs for children and adolescents.* New York: Plenum Press.

Edleson, J. (1999). The overlap between child maltreatment and woman battering. *Violence Against Women, 5,* 134–154.

Eisenstadt, T., Eyberg, S., McNeil, C., Newcomb, K., & Funderburk, B. (1993). Parent–child interaction therapy with behavior problem children: Relative effectiveness of two stages and overall treatment outcome. *Journal of Clinical Child Psychology, 22,* 42–51.

Elliott, D. M. (1994). Impaired object relations in professional women molested as children. *Psychotherapy, 21,* 79–86.

English, D. J., Edelson, J. L., & Herrick, M. E. (2005). Domestic violence in one's state's child protective caseload: A study of differential case dispositions and outcomes. *Children and Youth Services Review, 27*(11), 1183–1201.

Erickson, M. F., & Egeland, B. (1987). Developmental view of the psychological consequences of maltreatment. *School Psychology Review, 16*(2), 156–168.

Erickson, M. F., & Egeland, B. (2002). Child neglect. In J. E. B. Myers, L. Berliner, J. Briere, C. T. Hendrix, C. Jenny, & T. A. Reid (Eds.), *The APSAC handbook on child maltreatment* (2nd ed., pp. 3–20). Thousand Oaks, CA: Sage.

Ernst, J. (2001). Community-level factors and child maltreatment in a suburban county. *Social Work Research, 25*(3), 133–142.

Feerick, M. M., Knutson, J. F., Trickett, P. K., & Flanzer, S. M. (2006). *Child abuse and neglect: Definitions, classifications, & a framework for research.* Baltimore: Brookes.

Frank, D., Augustyn, M., Grant Knight, W., Pell, T., & Zuckerman, B. (2001). Growth, development, and behavior in early childhood following prenatal cocaine exposure. *Journal of the American Medical Association, 285*(12), 1613–1625.

Fraser, J., Armstrong, K., Morris, J., & Dadds, M. (2000). Home visiting intervention for vulnerable families with newborns: Follow-up results of a randomized controlled trial. *Child Abuse and Neglect, 24*(11), 1399–1429.

Friedrich, W., Taylor, J., & Clark, J. (1985). Personality and psychophysiological variables in abusive, neglectful, and low-income control mothers. *Journal of Nervous and Mental Disease, 170,* 577–587.

Frodi, A., & Lamb, M. (1980). Child abusers' responses to infant smiles and cries. *Child Development, 51,* 238–241.

Garbarino, J., Guttman, E., & Seeley, J. (1986). *The psychologically battered child: Strategies for identification, assessment and intervention.* San Francisco: Jossey-Bass.

Garbarino, J., & Kostelny, K. (1992). Child maltreatment as a community problem. *Child Abuse and Neglect, 16,* 455–464.

Gaudin, J., Kilpatrick, A., Polansky, N., & Chilton, P. (1996). Family functioning in neglectful families. *Child Abuse and Neglect, 20,* 363–377.

Gelfand, D., Teti, D., Seiner, S., & Jameson, P. (1996). Helping mothers fight depression: Evaluation of a home-based intervention program for depressed mothers and their children. *Journal of Clinical Child Psychology, 25,* 406–422.

Gershater-Molko, R., Lutzker, J., & Wesch, D. (2002). Using recidivism data to evaluate Project SafeCare: Teaching bonding, safety, and health care skills to parents. *Child Maltreatment, 7,* 277–285.

Gessner, B. (2008). The effect of Alaska's home visitation program for high-risk families on trends in abuse and neglect. *Child Abuse and Neglect, 32*(3), 317–333.

Giles-Sims, J., & Lockhart, C. (2005, March). Culturally shaped patterns of disciplining children. *Journal of Family Issues, 26*(2), 196–218.

Gillham, B., Tanner, G., Cheyne, B., Freeman, I., Rooney, M., & Lambie, A. (1998). Unemployment rates, single parent density, and indices of child poverty: Their relationship in different categories of child abuse and neglect. *Child Abuse and Neglect, 22*(2), 79–90.

Goldman, A., Pezawas, L., Mattay, V., Fischl, B., Verchinski, B., Zoltick, B., et al. (2008). Heritability of brain morphology related to schizophrenia: A large scale automated MRI segmentation study. *Biological Psychiatry, 63*(5), 475–483.

Gomby, D. (2007). The promise and limitations of home visiting: Implementing effective programs. *Child Abuse and Neglect, 31*(8), 793–799.

Gomby, D., Culross, P. L., & Behrman, R. (1999). Home visiting: Recent program evaluations-analysis and recommendations. *Future of Children, 9*(1), 4–26.

Gunnar, M. R. (1998). Quality of early care and buffering of neuroendocrine stress reactions: Potential effects on the development human brain. *Preventive Medicine, 27*(2), 208–211.

Hampton, R. L., & Gullotta, T. P. (2006). *Interpersonal violence in the African American community: Evidence-based prevention and treatment practices.* New York: Springer.

Hampton, R. L., & Newberger, E. H. (1985). Child abuse incidence and reporting in hospital: Significance of severity, class, and race. *American Journal of Public Health, 75,* 56–60.

Hanson, R., Gordon, A., Harris, A., Marquez, J., Murphy, W., Quinsey, V., et al. (2002). First report of the collaborative outcome data project on the effect of psychological treatment for sex offenders. *Sexual Abuse, 14,* 169–194.

Hart, S., Brassard, M., Binggeli, N., & Davidson, H. (2002). Psychological maltreatment. In J. E. B. Myers, L. Berliner, J. Briere, C. T. Hendrix, C. Jenny, & T. A. Reid (Eds.), *The APSAC handbook on child maltreatment* (pp. 79–104). Thousand Oaks, CA: Sage.

Hartley, C. C. (2002). The co-occurrence of child maltreatment and domestic violence:

Examining both neglect and child physical abuse. *Child Maltreatment, 7*(4), 349–358.

Heinicke, C., Fineman, N., Ponce, V., & Guthrie, D. (2001). Relation-based intervention with at-risk mothers: Outcomes in the second year of life. *Infant Mental Health Journal, 22*(4), 431–462.

Heinicke, C., Fineman, N., Ruty, G., Recchia, S., Guthrie, D., & Rodning, C. (1999). Relationship-based intervention with at-risk mothers: Outcome in the first year of life. *Infant Mental Health Journal, 20*(4), 349–374.

Heller, S. S., Larrieu, J. A., D'Imperio, R., & Boris, N. W. (1999). Research on resilience to child maltreatment: Empirical considerations. *Child Abuse and Neglect, 23*(4), 321–338.

Herrenkohl, E. C., Herrenkohl, R., & Egold, M. (1994). Resilient early school-age children from maltreating homes: Outcomes in late adolescence. *American Journal of Orthopsychiatry, 64,* 301–309.

Higgins, D. J., & McCabe, M. P. (1994). The relationship of child sexual abuse and family violence to adult adjustment: Toward an integrated risk-sequelae model. *Journal of Sex Research, 31,* 255–266.

Higgins, D. J., McCabe, M. P., & Ricciardelli, L. A. (2003). Child maltreatment, family characteristics, and adult adjustment: Mediating and moderating processes. *Journal of Aggression, Maltreatment and Trauma, 6*(2), 61–86.

Hill, R. (1998). Understanding Black family functioning: A holistic perspective. *Journal of Comparative Family Studies, 29*(10), 15–25.

Holden, E. W., Willis, D. J., & Corcoran, M. M. (1992). Preventing child maltreatment during the prenatal/perinatal period. In D. J. Willis, E. W. Holden, & M. S. Rosenberg (Eds.), *Prevention in child maltreatment: Developmental and ecological perspectives* (pp. 17–46). Oxford, UK: Wiley.

Horn, I. B., Joseph, J. G., & Cheng, T. L. (2004). Nonabusive physical punishment and child behavior among African-American children: A systematic review. *Journal of the National Medical Association, 96*(9), 1162–1168.

Howell, E., Pettit, K., & Kingsley, G. (2005). Trends in maternal and infant health in poor urban neighborhoods: Good news from the 1990s but challenges remain. *Public Health Report, 120,* 409–417.

Huebner, C. (2002). Evaluation of a clinic-based parent education program to reduce the risk of child and toddler maltreatment. *Public Health Nursing, 19*(5), 377–389.

Huxley, P., & Warner, R. (1993). Primary prevention of parenting dysfunction in high-risk cases. *American Journal of Orthopsychiatry, 63*(4), 582–588.

Ispa, J. M., & Halgunseth, L. C. (2004). Talking about corporal punishment: Nine low-income African American mothers' perspectives. *Early Childhood Research Quarterly, 19*(3), 463–484.

Jaffee, P. G., Wolfe, D. A., & Wilson, S. K. (1990). *Children of battered women.* Newbury Park, CA: Sage.

Jaffee, S., Caspi, A., Moffitt, T., & Taylor, A. (2004). Physical maltreatment victim to antisocial child: Evidence of an environmentally mediated process. *Journal of Abnormal Psychology, 113*(1), 44–55.

Jaffee, S. R., Caspi, A., Moffitt, T. W., Polo-Tomas, M., & Taylor, A. (2007). Individual, family, and neighborhood factors distinguish resilient from non-resilient maltreated children: A cumulative stressors model. *Child Abuse and Neglect, 31,* 231–253.

Jaudes, P., Ekwo, E., & Voorhis, J. (1995). Association of drug abuse and child abuse. *Child Abuse and Neglect, 19*(9), 1065–1075.

Jaudes, P. K., & Mackey-Bilaver, L. (2008). Do chronic conditions increase young children's risk of being maltreated? *Child Abuse and Neglect, 32*(7), 671–681.

Jones Harden, B. (1998). Building bridges for children: Addressing the consequences of exposure to drugs and to the child welfare system. In R. Hampton, V. Senatore, & T. P. Gullotta (Eds.), *Substance abuse, family violence, and child welfare: Bridging perspectives* (pp. 18–61). Thousand Oaks, CA: Sage.

Jones Harden, B. (2007). *Infants in the child welfare system: A developmental perspective on policy and practice.* Washington, DC: Zero to Three.

Jones Harden, B. (2008). Inequities in infancy: The overrepresentation of African American infants in the child welfare system. *Zero to Three, 28*(6), 5–12.

Jones Harden, B., & Nzinga-Johnson, S. (2006). Young, wounded and Black: The maltreatment of African American children in the early years. In R. Hampton & T. Gullotta (Eds.), *Interpersonal violence in the African American community* (pp. 17–46). New York: Springer.

Kahn, R., Wilson, K., & Wise, P. (2005). Intergenerational health disparities: Socioeconomic status, women's health conditions, and child behavior problems. *Public Health Report, 120,* 4399–4408.

Kaufman, J. (2008). Genetic and environmental modifiers of risk and resiliency in maltreated children. In J. J. Hudziak (Ed.), *Developmental psychopathology and wellness: Genetic and environmental influences* (pp. 141–160). Arlington, VA: American Psychiatric Publishing.

Kaufman, J., & Henrich, C. (2000). Exposure to violence and early childhood trauma. In C. H. Zeanah, Jr. (Ed.), *Handbook of infant mental health* (2nd ed., pp. 472–484). New York: Guilford Press.

Keenan, H., Nocera, M., & Runyan, D. (2008). Race matters in the prosecution of perpetrators of inflicted traumatic brain injury. *Pediatrics, 121*(16), 1174–1180.

Kelleher, K., Chaffin, M., Hollenberg, J., & Fischer, E. (1994). Alcohol and drug disorders among physically abusive and neglectful parents in a community-based sample. *American Journal of Public Health, 84,* 1586–1590.

Kempe, C. H. (1985). The battered-child syndrome. *Abuse and Neglect, 9*(2), 143–154.

King, S., & Laplante, D. P. (2005). The effects of prenatal maternal stress on children's cognitive development: Project Ice Storm. *International Journal on the Biology of Stress, 8*(1), 35–45.

Kohl, P., & Barth, R. (2007). Child maltreatment recurrence among children remaining in-home: Predictors of re-reports. In R. Haskins, F. Wulczyn, & M. B. Webb (Eds.), *Child protection: Using research to inform policy and practice* (pp. 207–225). Washington, DC: Brookings Institution Press.

Kolko, D. (1996). Individual cognitive-behavioral treatment and family therapy for physically abused children and their offending parents: A comparison of clinical outcomes. *Child Maltreatment, 1,* 322–342.

Kolko, D. (2000). Treatment research in child maltreatment: Clinical and research directions. *Journal of Aggression, Maltreatment, and Trauma, 4*(1), 139–164.

Koob, G., & LeMoal, M. (2008). Addiction and the brain anti-reward system. *Annual Review of Psychology, 59,* 29–53.

Kotch, J. B., Browne, D. C., Dufort, V., Winsor, J., & Catellier, D. (1999). Predicting child maltreatment in the first 4 years of life from characteristics assessed in the neonatal period. *Child Abuse and Neglect, 23*(4), 305–319.

Kotch, J. B., Browne, D. C., Ringwalt, C. L., Dufort, V., Ruina, E., Stewart, P. W., et al. (1997). Stress, social support, and substantiated maltreatment in the second and third years of life. *Child Abuse and Neglect, 21*(11), 1025–1037.

Krugman, S., Lane, W., & Walsh, C. (2007). Update on child abuse prevention. *Current Opinions in Pediatrics, 19*(6), 711–718.

Landsverk, J., & Carrilio, T. (1995). *San Diego Healthy Families America clinical trial.* San Diego, CA: Children's Hospital and Health Center.

Lecanuet, J., Fifer, W. P., Krasnegor, N. A., & Smotherman, W. P. (1995). *Fetal development: A psychobiological perspective.* Hillsdale, NJ: Erlbaum.

Lee, S., Aos, S., & Miller, M. (2008). *Evidence-based programs to prevent children from entering and remaining in the child welfare system: Benefits and costs for Washington* (Document No. 08-05-3902). Olympia: Washington State Institute for Public Policy.

Lewis, D. O. (1992). From abuse to violence: Psychophysiological consequences of maltreatment. *Journal of the American Academy of Child and Adolescent Psychiatry, 31,* 383–391.

Linares, T., Singer, L., Kirchner, H., Short, E., Min, M., Hussey, P., et al. (2006). Mental health outcomes of cocaine-exposed children at 6 years of age. *Journal of Pediatric Psychology, 31,* 85–97.

Littell, J. H., & Schuerman, J. R. (2002). What works best for whom?: A closer look at intensive family preservation services. *Children and Youth Services Review, 24*(9–10), 673–699.

Lundahl, B., Nimer, J., & Parsons, B. (2006). Preventing child abuse: A meta-analysis of parent training programs. *Research on Social Work Practice, 16*(3), 251–262.

Lutzker, J. R., & Bigelow, K. M. (2001). *Reducing child maltreatment: A guidebook for parent services.* New York: Guilford Press.

Lutzker, J. R., Bigelow, K. M., Doctor, R. M., Gershater, R. M., & Greene, B. F. (1998). An ecobehavioral model for the prevention and treatment of child abuse and neglect. In J. R. Lutzker (Ed.), *Handbook on child abuse research and treatment* (pp. 239–266). New York: Plenum Press.

Lynch, M., & Cicchetti, D. (1998). An ecological-transactional analysis of children and contexts: The longitudinal interplay among child maltreatment, community violence, and children's symptomotology. *Development and Psychopathology, 10*(2), 235–257.

Lyons-Ruth, K., Alpern, L., & Repacholi, B. (1993). Disorganized infant attachment classification and maternal psychosocial problems as predictors of hostile-aggressive behavior in the preschool classroom. *Child Development, 64*(2), 572–585.

Lyons-Ruth, K., Easterbrooks, M. A., & Cibelli, C. D. (1997). Infant attachment strategies, infant mental lag, and maternal depressive symptoms: Predictors of internalizing and externalizing problems at age 7. *Developmental Psychology, 33*(4), 681–692.

MacLeod, J., & Nelson, G. (2000). Programs for the promotion of family wellness and the prevention of child maltreatment: A meta-analytic review. *Child Abuse and Neglect, 24*(9), 1127–1149.

Mannarino, A. P., & Cohen, J. A. (1996). Family-related variables and psychological symptom formation in sexually abused girls. *Journal of Child Sexual Abuse, 5,* 105–120.

Marcenko, M., & Spence, M. (1994). Home visitation services for at-risk pregnant and postpartum women: A randomized trial. *American Journal of Orthopsychiatry, 64,* 468–476.

Marcenko, M., Spence, M., & Samost, L. (1996). Outcomes of a home visitation trial for pregnant and postpartum women at-risk for child placement. *Children and Youth Services Review, 18,* 243–259.

Marquez, J., Wiederanders, M., Day, D., Nelson, C., & van Ommeren, A. (2005). Effects of a relapse prevention program on sexual recidivism. Final results from California's sex Offender Treatment and Evaluation Project (SOTEP). *Sexual Abuse, 17*(1), 79–107.

Mayberg, H. (2003). Modulating dysfunctional limbic cortical circuits in depression: Towards development of brain-based algorithms for diagnosis and optimized treatment. *British Medical Bulletin, 65,* 193–207.

McAdoo, H. (1982). Stress absorbing systems in Black families. *Family Relations, 31*(4), 479–488.

McCanne, T., & Milner, J. (1991). Physiological reactivity of physically abusive and at-risk subjects to child-related stimuli. In J. Milner (Ed.), *Neuropsychology of aggression* (pp. 147–166). Boston: Kluwer Academic.

McGloin, J. M., & Widom, C. S. (2001). Resilence among abused and neglected children grown up. *Development and Psychopathology, 13,* 1021–1038.

McGuinness, T. M., & Schneider, K. (2007). Poverty, child maltreatment, and foster care. *Journal of the American Psychiatric Nurses Association, 13*(5), 296–303.

McLoyd, V. (1998). Socioeconomic disadvantage and child development. *American Psychologist, 53*(2), 185–204.

Mezzich, A. C., Tarter, R. E., Giancola, P. R., Lu, S., Kirisci, L., & Parks, S. (1997). Substance use and risky sexual behavior in female adolescents. *Drug and Alcohol Dependence, 44*(2–3), 157–166.

Milner, J., & Crouch, J. L. (1993). Physical child abuse. In R. L. Hampton (Ed.), *Family violence: Prevention and treatment* (pp. 25–55). Newbury Park, CA: Sage.

Milner, J., & Dopke, C. (1997). Child physical abuse: Review of offender characteristics. In D. Wolfe, R. McMahon, & R. Peters (Eds.), *Child abuse: New directions in prevention and treatment across the lifespan* (pp. 25–54). Thousand Oaks, CA: Sage.

Milner, J., Robertson, K., & Rogers, D. (1990). Childhood history of abuse and adult child abuse potential. *Journal of Family Violence, 5,* 15–34.

Milner, J. S. (1998). Individual and family characteristics associated with intrafamilial child physical and sexual abuse. In P. K. Trickett & C. J. Schellenbach (Eds.), *Violence against children in the family and community* (pp. 141–170). Washington, DC: American Psychological Association.

Mollerstrom, W. W., Patchner, M. M., & Milner, J. S. (1992). Family functioning and child abuse potential. *Journal of Clinical Psychology, 48*(4), 445–454.

Moore, K., & Persaud, T. (1993). *Before we are born* (4th ed.). Philadelphia: Saunders.

Moran, P. B., & Eckenrode, J. (1992). Protective personality characteristics among adolescent victims of maltreatment. *Child Abuse and Neglect, 16,* 743–754.

Myers, H., Taylor, S., Alvy, K., Arrington, A., & Richardson, M. (1992). Parental and family predictors of behavior problems in inner-city Black children. *American Journal of Community Psychology, 20*(5), 557–576.

Myers, J. E. B., Berliner, L., Briere, J., Hendrix, C. T., Jenny, C., & Reid, T. A. (Eds.). (2002). *The APSAC handbook on child maltreatment* (2nd ed.). Thousand Oaks, CA: Sage.

Nation, M., Crusto, C., Wandersman, A., Kumpfer, K., Seybolt, D., Morrissey-Kane, E., et al. (2003). What works in prevention: Principles of effective prevention programs. *American Psychologist, 58*(6/7), 449–456.

Nayak, M. B., & Milner, J. S. (1998). Neuropsychological functioning: Comparison of mothers at high-and low-risk for child abuse. *Child Abuse and Neglect, 22,* 687–703.

Nelson, C. A., Zeanah, C. H., Fox, N. A., Marshall, P. J., Smyke, A. T., & Guthrie, D. (2007). Cognitive recovery in socially deprived young children: The Bucharest Early Intervention Project. *Science, 318,* 1937–1940.

Nemeroff, C. B. (2004). Neurobiological consequences of childhood trauma. *Journal of Clinical Psychiatry, 65*(Suppl. 1), 18–28.

Noll, J. G., Horowitz, L. A., Bonanno, G. A., Trickett, P. K., & Putnam, F. W. (2003). Revictimization and self-harm in females who experienced childhood sexual abuse: Results from a prospective study. *Journal of Interpersonal Violence, 18*(12), 1452–1472.

Ogbu, J. (1981). Origins of human competence: A cultural-ecological perspective. *Child Development, 52,* 413–429.

Olds, D., Eckenrode, J., Henderson, C., Kitzman, H., Powers, J., Cole, R., et al. (1997). Long-term effects of home visitation on maternal life course and child abuse and neglect. *Journal of the American Medical Association, 278,* 637–643.

Olds, D., Henderson, C., Chamberlin, R., & Tatelbaum, R. (1986). Preventing child abuse and neglect: A randomized trial of nurse home visitation. *Pediatrics, 78,* 65–78.

Olds, D., Henderson, C., & Kitzman, H. (1994). Does prenatal and infancy nurse home visitation have enduring effects on qualities of parental caregiving and child health at 25 to 50 months of life? *Pediatrics, 93*(1), 89–98.

Olds, D., Henderson, C., Kitzman, H., & Cole, R. (1995). Effects of prenatal and infancy nurse home visitation on surveillance of child maltreatment. *Pediatrics, 95,* 365–372.

Olds, D., Hill, P., Robinson, J., Song, N., & Little, C. (2000). Update on home visiting for pregnant women and parents of young children. *Pediatrics, 30*(4), 105–148.

Ondersman, S. (2002). Predictors of neglect within low-SES families: The importance of substance abuse. *American Journal of Orthopsychiatry, 72,* 383–391.

Ovwigho, P. C., Leavitt, K. L., & Born, C. E. (2003). Risk factors for child abuse and neglect among former TANF families: Do later leavers experience greater risk? *Children and Youth Services Review, 25*(1–2), 139–163.

Peters, M., & Massey, G. (1983). Mundane extreme environmental stress in family stress theories: The case of Black families in White America. *Marriage and Family Review, 6,* 193–218.

Peterson, L., Tremblay, G., Ewigman, B., & Saldana, L. (2003). Multilevel selected primary prevention of child maltreatment. *Journal of Consulting and Clinical Psychology, 71*(3), 601–612.

Pianta, R., Egeland, B., & Erickson, M. (1989). The antecedents of child maltreatment: Results of the mother–child interaction research project. In D. Cicchetti & V. Carlson (Eds.), *Child maltreatment: Theory and research on the causes and consequences of child abuse and neglect* (pp. 203–252). New York: Cambridge University Press.

Reynolds, A., & Robertson, D. (2003). School-based early intervention and later child maltreatment in the Chicago Longitudinal Study. *Child Development, 74*(1), 3–26.

Ricci, L., Giantris, A., Merriam, P., Hodge, S., & Doyle, T. (2003). Abusive head trauma in

Maine infants: Medical, child protective, and law enforcement analysis. *Child Abuse and Neglect, 27*, 271–283.

Roberts, I., Kramer, M., & Suissa, S. (1996). Does home visiting prevent childhood injury?: A systematic review of randomised controlled trials. *British Medical Journal, 312*(7022), 29–33.

Rose, S. J. (1999). Reaching consensus on child neglect: African American mothers and child welfare workers. *Children and Youth Services Review, 21*(6), 463–479.

Rutter, M. (1992). Nature, nurture and psychopathology: A new look at an old topic. In B. Tizard & V. Varma (Eds.), *Vulnerability and resilience in human development* (pp. 21–38). Philadelphia: Jessica Kingsley.

Rutter, M. (1997). Anti-social behavior: Developmental psychopathology perspectives. In D. M. Stoff, J. Breiling, & J. D. Maser (Eds.), *Handbook of antisocial behavior* (pp. 115–124). New York: Wiley.

Sameroff, A. J., & Fiese, B. H. (2000). Models of development and developmental risk. In C. H. Zeanah, Jr. (Ed.), *Handbook of infant mental health* (pp. 3–19). New York: Guilford Press.

Schinke, S., Schilling, R., Kirkham, M., Gilchrist, L., Barth, R., & Blythe, B. (1986). Stress management skills for parents. *Journal of Child and Adolescent Psychotherapy, 3*, 293–298.

Schoenbaum, G., & Shaham, Y. (2008). The role of orbitofrontal cortex in drug addiction: A review of preclinical studies. *Biological Psychiatry, 63*(3), 256–262.

Sedlak, A. J., & Broadhurst, D. D. (1996). *Executive summary of the Third National Institute Study of Child Abuse and Neglect.* Washington, DC: U.S. Department of Health and Human Services.

Sedlak, A. J., & Schultz, D. (2005). Race differences in the risk of maltreatment in the general child population. In D. Derezotes, J. Poertner, & M. F. Testa (Eds.), *Race matters in child welfare: The overrepresentation of African American children in the system* (pp. 97–118). Washington, DC: Child Welfare League of America.

Seifer, R., & Dickstein, S. (2000). Parental mental illness and infant development. In C. H. Zeanah, Jr. (Ed.), *Handbook of infant mental health* (2nd ed., pp. 145–160). New York: Guilford Press.

Seifer, R., LaGasse, L., Lester, B., Bauer, C., Shankaran, S., Bada, H., et al (2004). Attachment status in children prenatally exposed to cocaine and other substances. *Child Development, 75*, 850–868.

Shanklin, D. (Ed.). (2000). *Maternal nutrition and child health* (2nd ed.). Springfield, IL: Charles C Thomas.

Sidebotham, P., Heron, J., & ALSPAC Study Team. (2003). Child maltreatment in the "children of the nineties": The role of the child. *Child Abuse and Neglect, 27*(3), 337–352.

Sidebotham, P., Heron, J., Golding, J., & ALSPAC Study Team. (2002). Child maltreatment in the "children of the nineties": Deprivation, class, and social networks in a UK sample. *Child Abuse and Neglect, 26*(12), 1243–1259.

Singer, L., Arendt, R., Minnes, S., Farkas, K., Salvator, A., Kirchner, H., et al. (2002). Cognitive and motor outcomes of cocaine-exposed infants. *Journal of the American Medical Association, 287*, 1952–1960.

Smith, D. K., Johnson, A. B., Pears, K. C., Fisher, P. A., & DeGarmo, D. S. (2007). Child maltreatment and foster care: Unpacking the effects of prenatal and postnatal parental substance use. *Child Maltreatment, 12*(2), 150–160.

Starling, S., Sirotnak, A., Heisler, K., & Barnes-Eley, M. (2007). Inflicted skeletal trauma and the relationship of perpetrators to their victims. *Child Abuse and Neglect, 31*(9), 993–999.

Stier, D. M., Leventhal, J. M., Berg, A. T., Johnson, L., & Mezger, J. (1993). Are children born to young mothers at increased risk of maltreatment? *Pediatrics, 91*(3), 642–648.

Straus, M. A. (1994). *Beating the devil out of them: Corporal punishment in American families.* Lexington, MA: Lexington Books.

Straus, M. A. (2000). Corporal punishment and primary prevention of physical abuse. *Child Abuse and Neglect, 24*(9), 1109–1114.

Subbarao, A., Rhee, S., Young, S., Ehreinger, M., Corley, R., & Hewitt, J. (2008). Common genetic and environmental influences on major depressive disorder and conduct disorder. *Journal of Abnormal Child Psychology, 36*(3), 433–444.

Sullivan, P. M., & Knutson, J. F. (1998). The association between child maltreatment and disabilities in a hospital-based epidemiological study. *Child Abuse and Neglect, 22*(4), 271–288.

Susman, E. J., Trickett, P. K., Ianotti, R. J., Hollenbeck, B. E., & Zahn-Walker, C. (1985). Child rearing patterns in depressed, abusive and normal mothers. *American Journal of Orthopsychiatry, 55*, 237–251.

Sweet, M. A., & Appelbaum, M. L. (2004). Is home visiting an effective strategy? A meta-analytic review of home visiting programs for families with young children. *Child Development, 75*(5), 1435–1456.

Takser, L., Mergler, D., & Lafond, J. (2005). Very low level environmental exposure to lead and prolactin levels during pregnancy. *Neurotoxicology and Teratology, 27*, 505–508.

Trickett, P. K., & Kuczynski, L. (1986). Children's misbehaviors and parental discipline strategies in abusive and nonabusive families. *Developmental Psychology, 22*(1), 115–123.

Urquiza, A., & McNeil, C. (1996). Parent–child interaction therapy: An intensive dyadic intervention for physically abusive families. *Child Maltreatment, 1*(2), 134–144.

U.S. Census Bureau. (2008). *Income, poverty, and health insurance coverage in the United States: 2007* (Report No. P60:235). Retrieved July 15, 2008, from *www.census.gov/prod/2008pubs/p60-235.pdf.*

van IJzendoorn, M. H. (1995). Adult attachment representations, parental responsiveness, and infant attachment: A meta-analysis on the predictive validity of the Adult Attachment Interview. *Psychological Bulletin, 117*, 387–403.

van IJzendoorn, M. H., Bakermans-Kranenburg, M. J., & Juffer, F. (2005). Why less is more: From the dodo bird verdict to evidence-based interventions in sensitivity and early attachments. In L. J. Berlin, Y. Ziv, L. Maya-Jackson, & M. T. Greenberg (Eds.), *Enhancing early attachments: Theory, research, intervention, and policy* (pp. 297–312). New York: Guilford Press.

Webster-Stratton, C., & Hammond, M. (1997). Treating children with early-onset conduct problems: A comparison of child and parent training interventions. *Journal of Consulting and Clinical Psychology, 65*(1), 93–109.

Weissberg, R., Kumpfer, K., & Seligman, M. (2003). Prevention that works for children and youth: An introduction. *American Psychologist, 58*(6–7), 425–432.

Westbrook, T., Jones Harden, B., Vick, J., Meisch, A., & DeTaillade, J. (2009). *Physical discipline use among African American families.* Manuscript submitted for publication.

Whipple, B. E., & Webster-Stratton, C. (1991). The role of parental stress in physically abusive families. *Child Abuse and Neglect, 15,* 279–291.

Widom, C. (1991). The role of placement experiences in mediating the criminal consequences of early childhood victimization. *American Journal of Orthopsychiatry, 61*(2), 195–209.

Wind, T. W., & Silvern, L. (1994). Parenting and family stress as mediators of the long-term effects of child abuse. *Child Abuse and Neglect, 18,* 439–453.

Windham, A. M., Rosenberg, L., Fuddy, L., McFarlane, E., Sia, C., & Duggan, A. K. (2004). Risk of mother-reported child abuse in the first 3 years of life. *Child Abuse and Neglect, 28*(6), 645–667.

Wolfe, D. (1987). *Child abuse: Implications for child development and psychopathology.* Newbury Park, CA: Sage.

Wolfe, D. (1993). Prevention of child neglect: Emerging issues. *Criminal Justice and Behavior, 20*(1), 90–111.

Wolfe, D., Edwards, B., Manion, I., & Koverola, C. (1988). Early intervention for parents at risk of child abuse and neglect. *Journal of Consulting and Clinical Psychology, 56,* 40–47.

Wolfe, D., Fairbanks, J. A., Kelly, J. A., & Bradlyn, A. S. (1983). Child abusive parents' physiological responses to stressful and non-stressful behavior in children. *Behavioral Assessment, 5,* 363–371.

Wulczyn, F., Barth, R., Yuan, Y., Jones Harden, B., & Landsverk, J. (2005). *Beyond common sense: Child welfare, child well-being and the evidence for policy reform.* New Brunswick, NJ: Aldine Transaction.

Young, N. K., Boles, S. M., & Otero, C. (2007). Parental substance use disorders and child maltreatment: Overlap, gaps, and opportunities. *Child Maltreatment, 12*(2), 137–149.

Youngblade, L. M., & Belsky, J. (1990). Social and emotional consequences of child maltreatment. In R. T. Ammerman & M. Hersen (Eds.), *Children at risk: An evaluation of factors contributing to child abuse and neglect* (pp. 109–146). New York: Plenum Press.

Zeanah, C., Larrieu, J., Heller, S., Valliere, J., Hinshaw-Fuselier, S., Aoki, Y., et al. (2001). Evaluation of a preventive intervention for maltreated children and toddlers in foster care. *Journal of the American Academy of Child and Adolescent Psychiatry, 40*(2), 214–221.

# 21

# Intimate Partner Violence

Jaslean J. La Taillade
Robert L. Hampton
Marcus Pope
April R. McDowell

Intimate partner violence (IPV) is considered a serious social and public health problem, with often devastating medical and psychological consequences for partners and family members, including physical injuries, clinical disorders, child abuse, and behavior problems (Holtzworth-Munroe, Meehan, Rehman, & Marshall, 2002; McCord, 1993). In general, IPV refers to "acts of violence that occur between current or former spouses, boyfriends, or girlfriends" (Hampton, Oliver, & Magarian, 2003, p. 535). There are two main forms of physical IPV: severe physical aggression and common couple violence (La Taillade, Epstein, & Werlinich, 2006). Severe physical aggression is seen less often in couples and has been defined as "male battering of a female partner for the purpose of dominating and controlling her, combined with relatively low-level female aggression, mostly for self-defense" (La Taillade et al., 2006, p. 394). In contrast, common couple violence is seen more frequently among couples, particularly distressed couples, and consists of mild to moderate forms of physical aggression (slapping, hitting, throwing objects) in which both the male and female partners are likely to be aggressors. IPV may also present in couples as psychological aggression, including threats of physical violence, withdrawal, and social or environmental restraints placed on one's partner.

National surveys indicate that African American[1] intimate relationships are at significantly greater risk for violence. The rate of IPV inflicted on Black women is 35% higher than for White women (Rennison, 2003), and rates of severe assault are 2.4 times that of their White counterparts (Hampton & Gelles, 1994). Statistics from the U.S. Department of Justice show that, between 1993 and 1998, 11.1 of every 1,000 Black women experienced nonlethal violence at the hands of an intimate partner. Furthermore, homicide by an intimate partner is the leading cause of death among African American women between the ages of 15 to 34 (Council on Scientific Affairs, 1992). In 2000, of the 1,247 women who were murdered by an intimate partner, 333, or 27%, were Black (Office of Justice Programs, Bureau of Justice Statistics, 2002). These figures have particular significance given that Black women account for only 13% of the U.S. female population (U.S. Census Bureau, 2003). Research findings have indicated that not only is IPV more frequent among Black Americans than White Americans, but it also tends to appear in a more reciprocal pattern between males and females. Specifically, rates of homicide between domestic partners are nearly even in terms of how often husbands and wives are the victims (Dawson & Langan, 1994, as cited in Hampton et al., 2003).

## RISK FACTORS ASSOCIATED WITH IPV

In developing effective intervention programs, it is important to consider those factors that may augment risk for IPV. Programs should include the goals of reducing risk factors as well as increasing protective factors against relationship violence (Coie et al., 1993). Information on the correlates of psychological and physical aggression is essential for both assessment and planning of interventions to reduce risk of future IPV among African Americans.

### Sociostructural Factors and Negative Life Events

Despite improvements in attitudes toward ethnic-minority groups among the dominant White culture, there is evidence that African Americans continue to be the object of intergroup racism, including ethnic discrimination in higher education, housing rentals and sales, and hiring practices (Clark, Anderson, Clark, & Williams, 1999). Research studies have shown that racism is a significant stressor for African Americans, and it is associated with psychological and physical health problems (Clark et al., 1999). In addition, African Americans are disproportionately exposed to specific negative life events, including joblessness and negative health outcomes (Clark et al., 1999; Tucker & Mitchell-Kernan, 1995). Research suggests that stress precipitates violence (Cano & Vivian, 2003; Straus,

---

[1]The terms *Black* and *African American* are used interchangeably within this chapter to describe persons of African descent residing in the United States.

1990). African American couples, by virtue of their ethnic-minority status, are more likely to experience stressors associated with IPV than their White counterparts, including experiences of joblessness, poverty, and racism, and as such are at increased risk for IPV.

The role of socioeconomic factors in explaining the incidence of IPV has been widely documented (Cazenave & Straus, 1990; Cunradi, Caetano, & Schafer, 2002; Fox, Benson, DeMaris, & Van Wyk, 2002; Hotaling & Sugarman, 1990; Lockhart, 1991). Among African Americans, poverty and joblessness are strongly associated with increased risk for IPV (Cunradi, Caetano, Clark, & Schafer, 2000) and predictive of conflictual spousal interactions, relationship distress, and future marital instability among African American couples in the early years of marriage (Hatchett, Veroff, & Douvan, 1995).

Although few studies have examined the impact of racism on African American couple relationships, there is evidence that these relationships are more likely to be exposed to such stressors, and that this may be associated with relationship difficulties. La Taillade (1999) found that reports of social and institutional experiences of discrimination among African American couples were negatively associated with use of constructive communication behaviors and positively associated with use of destructive forms of communication, such as verbal aggression and violence.

Research focused on White couples has shown support for a relationship between negative life events, marital interactions, and marital functioning. Occurrence of life events has been associated with greater interpersonal conflict and lower marital adjustment (Lavee, McCubbin, & Olson, 1987). Krokoff, Gottman, and Roy (1988) found that increases in negative affect during couple interactions were associated with husbands' report of job distress. According to Bolger, DeLongis, Kessler, and Wethington (1989), husbands who reported disagreements at work were more likely to report arguments with their wife at home during the evening (Cohan & Bradbury, 1997). Conger and colleagues (1990) found that economic strain was related to higher hostility among husbands, which was associated with decreased marital quality among wives. Overall, the combination of these findings suggest that economic marginalization and stressful circumstances encountered by African American couples are associated with difficulties in marital adjustment and abuse, potentially through increasing negative communication between spouses, creating new sources of marital conflict, or worsening existing conflicts (Cohan & Bradbury, 1997), which may increase the likelihood of violence.

## Psychological Correlates of Battering and IPV

In an attempt to understand the underlying dynamics of battering and design programs effective for both preventing and treating violence, researchers have sought to identify factors that place males at increased risk for IPV, in particular those factors that may be directly modifiable (Holtzworth-Munroe et al., 2002). Factors have included, but have not been limited to, witnessing violence as a child, difficulties with assertiveness and social skills deficits, hostile attitudes and attributions, psychopathology, use of alcohol and illegal substances, excessive jealousy, and dependence on one's partner. Research examining family of origin variables has revealed inconsistent findings, with history of child abuse victimization being an inconsistent predictor and witnessing parental violence a more consistent predictor across studies, varying only by the direction of violence witnessed (Dutton, 1988; Gottman et al., 1995). Some studies have found that violent men report significantly greater assertion problems than distressed nonviolent men (e.g., O'Leary & Curley, 1986) and are more likely to attribute hostile intentions to the partner's negative actions, allowing them to justify the aggression as a retaliation (Holtzworth-Munroe et al., 2002). In addition, when presented with hypothetical conflict situations, male abusers often provide less competent and more aggressive responses than nonviolent men and may be more likely to endorse hostile and adversarial attitudes toward their female partner (Holtzworth-Munroe, 2000). The presence of personality or Axis II disorders (e.g., antisocial personality disorder) and other psychological problems (e.g., anxiety, bipolar, and psychotic disorders) has been found to be more common in violent versus nonviolent men (e.g., Gottman et al., 1995; Magdol et al., 1997). Only a select few of these psychological variables have been studied within African American populations, however, as potential risk factors for violence.

Several researchers and theorists have suggested that men who are highly dependent on their partner are jealous and hypervigilant regarding threats, real or perceived, to the security of their relationship, resorting to violence when they fear the loss of their partner (Dutton & Golant, 1995). Compared with nonviolent men, those who use violence have been found to score higher on measures of jealousy (e.g., Holtzworth-Munroe, Stuart, & Hutchinson, 1997) and of fearful and preoccupied attachment to their partner (e.g., Holtzworth-Munroe et al., 1997; Murphy, Meyer, & O'Leary, 1994). Raj, Silverman, Wingood, and DiClemente (1999) found that African American males' sexual jealousy and perceptions of low empathy from his female partner were also significant predictors of IPV.

Alcohol-related problems among both male and female partners have been found to be important predictors of IPV across racial and ethnic groups (Campbell, Sharps, Gary, Campbell, & Lopez, 2002). Alcohol intoxication is a common factor in many incidents of domestic violence (Pan, Neidig, & O'Leary, 1994) and has been shown to increase husbands' negativity toward their spouse in a subsequent marital interaction, suggesting that alcohol may increase verbal aggression, which then increased the risk for physical aggression (Leonard & Roberts, 1998). Some researchers have found that, after controlling for demographic variables, alcohol-related problems among either partner remained the strongest risk factor for IPV among African American couples, but not White and Hispanic couples (e.g., Cunradi et al., 2000).

Although there has been much focus on factors that predict acts of IPV against women, there has been surprisingly little research on factors associated with African American women's vulnerability to victimization and on variables that may be associated with staying in violent relationships. However, we do know that one of the strongest predictors of IPV victimization among Black women is a history of interpersonal violence, including childhood sexual abuse and previous marital or dating violence (West, 2002). Another significant psychological factor is current or past illegal drug use, particularly crack cocaine, which significantly increases the risk of IPV victimization for Black women (Hampton, Oliver, & Magarian, 2003).

## Community and Social Support

Research has shown that integration into a network of friends and family as well as other social groups may buffer against relationship distress and violence (Straus, Gelles, & Steinmetz, 1980). More specifically, social support serves as a protective factor against IPV; social contacts are available to intervene and help the victim leave the abusive relationship. Conversely, social isolation may increase risk of victimization for female partners and is often used by perpetrators as a means of controlling access to their victims (Institute of Medicine, 1994). Hatchett, Veroff, and Douvan (1995) found that African American wives who maintained contact with extended family members were more likely to be in stable marriages. Overall, these findings indicate that the external environment can have a positive effect on couple relationships by providing emotional and instrumental support to the couple, increasing partners' satisfaction with the relationship, and promoting relationship stability.

## Couple Interaction Patterns and IPV

In an effort to fully understand the process by which conflicts escalate to violence, several researchers have used observational methodologies to examine how the interactions of violent couples are distinct from those of couples whose disagreements do not result in abuse. Several consistent findings have emerged across studies. During discussions of couple problems, violent men display more negative behaviors, including defensiveness and overtly hostile behavior, compared with nonviolent men (e.g., Margolin, Burman, & John, 1989). Even when compared with men in distressed but nonviolent couple relationships, men in domestically violent relationships display more hostile and provocative forms of anger (e.g., contempt and belligerence; Jacobson et al., 1994). Furthermore, both male and female partners in violent relationships are more likely to engage in negative reciprocity, that is, continuing the negative behavior once it has begun (Cordova, Jacobson, Gottman, Rushe, & Cox, 1993). However, consistent with clinical descriptions of violent arguments, once the violence starts, there is little the female partner can do to prevent escalation, and males are the perpetrators of violence (La Taillade & Jacobson, 1997).

Feminist theorists and researchers have posited that males' use of violence serves to establish or maintain power in the context of their relationships (e.g.,

Margolin & Burman, 1993; Straus, 1990). In support of this idea, some studies have found that men who abuse their partners report being more likely to use violence when they perceive themselves to be powerless and without control (Stets, 1988), and that both husbands and wives in violent relationships feel more coercively controlled by their partners than those in nonviolent relationships (Ehrensaft, Langhinrichsen-Rohling, Heyman, O'Leary, & Lawrence, 1999). Other researchers have attempted to operationalize dimensions of power in relationships—specifically socioeconomic resources (educational attainment, income, occupational status), decision-making power, and communication behaviors (e.g., withdrawal, belligerence, use of threats)—in order to ascertain how they may be differentially related to males' use of violence. Equal distributions of socioeconomic power have been associated with less relationship distress, increased ability to prevent conflict escalation, and lower risk of IPV (Goodyear-Smith & Laidlaw, 1999). Conversely, unequal distributions of socioeconomic power in which the husband has fewer resources than his wife, are associated with increased risk for IPV (Babcock, Waltz, Jacobson, & Gottman, 1993). In already distressed relationships, imbalances in socioeconomic status and decision-making power have been associated with higher incidences of violence (Babcock et al., 1993).

African American men have been acculturated to embrace patriarchal ideals but have been historically denied access to economic resources essential to reinforce this ideology (Ucko, 1994). The dehumanizing experience of enslavement and the subsequent structural limitations imposed through institutionalized racism have placed African American men disproportionately at risk for external and self-imposed perceptions of emasculation and powerlessness. Currently, a status discrepancy exists in which a greater number of Black women have obtained educational and occupational advancements relative to Black men, including bachelor's degrees and beyond (McKinnon, 2003). Thus, lacking such socioeconomic markers of masculinity have precipitated substantial numbers African American men to embrace unconventional expressions of masculinity, which often involve use of violence against others and their female partners as a means of gaining control and power in their relationship relative to the outside world (Hampton et al., 2003).

## EVIDENCE-BASED TREATMENT INTERVENTIONS

Despite our awareness that IPV is a significant public health problem particularly affecting the Black community, there is still little information regarding the effectiveness of interventions. Given the high physical and psychological tolls of IPV, design and implementation of effective interventions to target battering is essential. We next review the most utilized interventions for perpetrators and female victims, and discuss effectiveness of these interventions for African Americans.

## What Works

No treatment program thus far has completed three successful trials resulting in significant reduction or elimination of IPV among African Americans. However, several approaches may show future promise in being able to effectively treat IPV among African Americans. Next, we turn our attention to treatment programs that *may* work by examining programs with fewer than three successful trials.

## What May Work

### Arrest as an IPV Intervention

One of the most prominent studies of the use of arrest as an IPV treatment intervention is the Spouse Assault Replication Program (SARP). SARP is a project of the National Institute of Justice and it is the culmination of six individual studies conducted across the United States between 1981 and 1991 (Maxwell, Garner, & Fagan, 2001). The first SARP study (Minneapolis Domestic Violence Experiment) found that perpetrator arrest cut the rates of subsequent intimate partner battering in half over a 6-month period (Sherman & Berk, 1984, as cited in Maxwell et al., 2001). Following this report, five replication studies were then undertaken and the results pooled (Maxwell et al., 2001). It is important to note key demographic characteristics of the pooled sample, which included a total of 4,032 suspects. The race/ethnic background of the sample was as follows: African American, 51%; White, 38%; Hispanic, 11%; and Asian/other, 1%. At the onset of the original site studies, 72% of the sample was employed, 40% had prior arrests, and 45% reported use of intoxicants. In terms of their relationships with the victims, 57% were married, 2% were separated, 1% were divorced, and the remaining 40% were in current or had past intimate relationships (with no marital ties).

The results of the pooled study showed that arrest was consistently associated with reduced aggression toward victims. However, the relationship between suspect arrest and later offenses of IPV was not as strong as that between arrest and other factors, such as the male partner's age (older suspects committed fewer later offenses than younger suspects) or prior criminal record (suspects with prior arrests for any crime, on average, committed more later offenses than those without prior arrests). Furthermore, it was found that most suspects did *not* commit subsequent IPV offenses against their partner within the follow-up period regardless of whether or not they were in the arrest or nonarrest groups. Finally, there was *not* a significant relationship between arrest as an intervention and increased subsequent IPV offenses against the female partners; this has been noted as a concern regarding the use of arrest as an IPV intervention. Overall, it appears that arrest as an IPV intervention is not harmful to women survivors of IPV and actually may be helpful in many instances.

Results of the SARP study provide useful information for examining IPV within the African American community; 51% of the 4,032 suspects were Black males, and race was examined as one of the predictors of recidivism (Maxwell et al., 2001). The two sources of outcome data were victim interview reports and official police records. According to the victim reports, there was significantly less postintervention aggression when the suspect was non-White. However, this was not consistent with the analysis of official police records, which showed that White suspects had lower levels of subsequent IPV than non-White suspects (Maxwell et al., 2001). Although the authors note that those suspects assigned to the experimental arrest group tended to be White, potentially explaining why they may have had lower levels of subsequent IPV offenses than non-White participants, the fact that there is a discrepancy between victim reports and police records may reflect an underreporting by non-White, particularly African American, victims of later IPV offenses by their partners. Underreporting may have existed among Black victims because of cultural mistrust.

Hampton and colleagues (2003) report that African American women are more likely to endure abuse in their relationships than appeal to agencies and law enforcement for assistance. Furthermore, even when IPV becomes too intense for Black women to tolerate in silence, they are more likely to seek help from medical personnel and their social networks (Hampton et al., 2003). This may be reflective of African American women's "cultural mistrust" of the criminal justice system, which is often perceived as a racist institution based on the disproportionate numbers of African American males involved with it. As a result, many Black women may be unwilling to increase that number or may experience negative reactions from their family or community should they seek such assistance. In fact, reporting IPV to law enforcement officials in particular can place Black women into a cultural catch-22, where doing so represents racial disloyalty. Thus, even in communities where arrest is utilized properly and effectively as an IPV intervention, Black families may not reap the benefits.

### Community Advocacy as an IPV Intervention

Advocacy is one avenue by which communities throughout the United States are treating cases of IPV. According to the National Resource Center on Domestic Violence (1999),

> Advocacy efforts are generally classified as either individual-based (i.e., working specifically with or on behalf of individuals to ensure access to resources and opportunities) or systems-based (i.e., advocating to change and improve institutional responses) .. many advocacy efforts simultaneously involve assisting individuals [specifically women with abusive partners] and working to change systems. (p. 1)

Community intervention projects (CIPs) across the United States have the same common goal of intervening in male partner violence incidents against women. These projects involve collaborative and coordinated efforts between several systems and participants within local communities, including police officers, prosecutors, judges, probation officers, and volunteer advocates. In general, CIPs are structured such that law enforcement officers contact volunteer advocates once an incident of IPV has been reported to assist survivors in navigating the legal system and prosecuting their abusers. The overall results of CIP effectiveness studies show that incidents of IPV are significantly decreased (i.e., perpetrators are less prone to reoffend) when male perpetrators of IPV are both arrested and mandated to batterer interventions (Gamache, Edleson, & Schock, 1988; Steinman, 1990, and Syers & Edleson, 1992, as cited in the National Resource Center on Domestic Violence, 1999).

COMMUNITY ADVOCACY PROJECT

One example of a CIP that focuses on advocacy for survivors of IPV is the Community Advocacy Project (CAP) of Michigan (Sullivan, 1999, as cited in the National Resource Center on Domestic Violence, 1999). CAP provides one-on-one services for female survivors of IPV and helps them utilize the criminal justice and other local systems. CAP advocates work with survivors who have recently left domestic violence shelters for a 10-week period, 6 to 8 hours per week. The service areas addressed for women participating in CAP include, among many others, housing, employment, legal, child care, and social support. The results of an experimental study on the efficacy of CAP showed that over a 24-month postintervention time period "women who worked with advocates experienced less violence over time, reported higher quality of life and social support, and had less difficulty obtaining community resources over time" (Sullivan, 1999, p. 4, as cited in the National Resource Center on Domestic Violence, 1999). CAP proved to be effective for program participants compared with survivors in the control group (who received services as usual): 24% of survivors experienced no further IPV during the follow-up period.

## Culturally Focused Batterer Counseling

Although studies have demonstrated the effectiveness of arrest and community advocacy as IPV treatments, several scholars have noted the importance of using interventions that are *specific* to African Americans for the treatment of IPV (Gondolf & Williams, 2001; Oliver, 2000; Williams, 1992). Overall, research on the effectiveness of batterers' treatment programs indicates that existing intervention programs have limited success with ethnic minorities. A national survey of 142 batterer programs found that less than half made some special effort to address the needs of ethnic-minority populations, with only 24% of these incorporating three or more culturally appropriate interventions (Williams & Becker, 1994). Many batterer treatment programs, as they are currently being offered, erroneously assume that their interventions will be equally effective across all offenders regardless of race, ethnicity, or socioeconomic background (Babcock & La Taillade, 2000).

Culturally focused batterer counseling has been described by Gondolf and Williams (2001) as "specialized counseling for racially homogeneous groups that explicitly identifies and addresses cultural issues that may reinforce violence or present barriers to stopping violence. . . [Culturally focused batterer counseling] also promotes the positive aspects of culture that can strengthen a man's effort to be nonviolent" (p. 284). This approach is different from ethnically sensitive approaches because cultural issues and themes are explicit and integrated into the program's format. Indeed, there are three main components of culturally focused batterer counseling for African American men that set it apart from ethnically sensitive approaches. First, all participants are men who self-identify as African American. Second, the counselor is African American and is trained to address the culturally based themes that arise during the program. Last, cultural themes specific to African American men are discussed during sessions. Curriculum themes may include men's perceptions of law enforcement, perceptions of African American masculinity, and experiences with violence, prejudice, and discrimination (Gondolf & Williams, 2001).

The outcome research of culturally focused approaches is very limited and preliminary, with no definitive results yet available. The little research that does exist shows that counseling groups exclusive to African Americans and counselor–client racially matched treatment approaches have produced lower dropout rates for minority participants than traditional approaches in some cases, but no significantly greater improvements in outcomes such as lower posttreatment battering offenses (see Gondolf & Williams, 2001). These findings may reflect the fact that there is great diversity in cultural attitudes and degrees of cultural identification within the African American community that may not be addressed in existing culturally focused treatment programs for African American men. Furthermore, the levels of cultural sensitivity of individual counselors and program curriculums may vary from one program to the next, even in culturally focused programs designed specifically for African American men.

### Conjoint Treatment as Secondary Prevention: Targeting Psychological and Mild Physical Aggression

Secondary prevention strategies extend beyond those areas covered in marital distress prevention programs to address couples' early use of psychological as well as physically aggressive behaviors to prevent escalation to severe violence, battering, and injury to one or both partners. Research has shown that among couples seeking marital therapy more than 50% of the husbands have engaged in some form of physical aggression against their partner in the past year (Holtzworth-Munroe et al., 2002; O'Leary, Vivian, & Malone, 1992). However, couples coming to therapy rarely report physical violence as a presenting issue (Holtzworth-Munroe et al., 2002). As such, secondary prevention programs target couples in which one or both partners have used psychological or physical abuse but (1) do not engage in battering or severe violence, (2) desire to improve their relationship and remain together, and (3) are not fearful of participating in conjoint treatment.

PHYSICAL AGGRESSION COUPLES TREATMENT

Although several secondary IPV prevention programs have been developed for military couples (e.g., the Domestic Conflict Containment Program; Neidig & Friedman, 1984) and the population at large (see Low, Monarch, & Hartman, 2002, and Stith, Rosen, & McCollum, 2003, for reviews), only the Physical Aggression Couples Treatment (PACT) program (Heyman & Neidig, 1997; Heyman & Schlee, 2003; O'Leary, Heyman, & Neidig, 1999) has been subject to both short- and long-term empirical evaluation. The PACT program is directed at couples currently experiencing violence in their relationship and focuses on the prevention of negative escalation and conflict and on improvement of communication skills to prevent future violence. The PACT program is a conjoint approach using a group format targeted at couples who demonstrate psychological and physical aggression but not severe violence characteristic of battering. The goals of the program include educating couples about the cycle of violence; increasing personal responsibility for the use of violence; reducing and ultimately eliminating IPV through anger management and conflict resolution skill training; increasing relationship satisfaction and positive couple interactions through communication and problem-solving skill training; and educating couples about alternatives to IPV.

PACT was compared with gender-specific treatment in a longitudinal investigation of its efficacy in reducing and eliminating IPV. Husbands and wives who completed the PACT program had significantly higher marital adjustment scores posttreatment versus pretreatment. In addition, husbands scored lower on measures of both psychological and physical aggression at posttreatment. Furthermore, husbands reported significant increases in taking responsibility for their violence as well as significant decreases in blaming their wives for their own use of violence. Similarly, wives reported significant decreases in self-blame and taking responsibility for their husbands' use of aggression. One-year follow-up results indicated that husbands' use of physical aggression was significantly reduced, according to both husbands' and wives' reports. Husbands also demonstrated significant decreases in their use of psychological aggression. In addition, both husbands' and wives' reported significant increases in marital satisfaction at 1-year follow-up.

Contrary to the authors' hypotheses, however, both PACT and gender-specific treatment conditions were found to be equally effective on outcome measures. Although there were significant reductions in intensity and frequency of aggression, use of violence was not eliminated as a result of treatment; in fact, the cessation rate was 26% at 1-year follow-up for the PACT program. Furthermore, neither the short- nor long-term efficacy of PACT has been demonstrated with African Americans or other ethnic-minority populations.

## African American Popular Culture Interventions

Oliver (2000) argues that African American popular culture can be used as a psychoeducational prevention strategy to address the problem of IPV within the Black community, because it can enhance the degree to which African Americans can identity with, personalize, and endorse the messages being delivered. Oliver defines popular culture as "a major portion of a society's total way of life ... [including] articles and events, heroes, rituals, and popular arts" (p. 537). The fundamental components of Black popular culture that help to distinguish it from broader American culture include the emphasis on racial justice and equality, music, religion, and the Black Church (Oliver, 2000). Specific intervention strategies recommended by Oliver include the use of gospel musicals and radio campaigns.

Gospel music, or Black religious music, forms the basis of a gospel musical, which can be defined as "a theatrical production in which the plot is centered around the main characters' efforts to cope with a particular situation or adverse circumstances, including alcoholism, drug abuse, teenage pregnancy, female-headed families, domestic violence, poverty, and criminal behavior" (Oliver, 2000, p. 541). Although there are examples of specific gospel musicals that have included IPV as a major theme, we have found no IPV prevention programs that have used gospel musicals as their primary delivery platform. However, Oliver (2000) outlines five major advantages to using gospel musicals to address IPV in the Black community: (1) They can readily serve as primary prevention strategies by delivering IPV education to African Americans, (2) they can serve as secondary interventions by educating at-risk or current IPV victims and perpetrators on available services, (3) musical characters can model behavior by demonstrating appropriate conflict-management strategies or ways of handling IPV in social situations relevant to African Americans, (4) the popularity of gospel musicals can generate dialogue about IPV within the Black community, and (5) gospel musicals could be embedded into the curriculum of existing IPV interventions for victim and perpetrator groups.

Oliver (2000) also discusses the potential impact of Black radio on treating IPV among African Americans. One suggestion is for Black popular culture icons and celebrities to develop media campaigns and public service announcements aimed toward reducing and preventing IPV in the African American community. Another suggestion is for Black disc jockeys to get involved in such campaigns as well, because they often are viewed as having a significant influential and leadership role in both local communities and in the wider Black American community.

Oliver (2000) points to one example of a current radio campaign targeted to IPV in Black community. The *It's Your Business* campaign by the Family Violence Prevention Fund is a 12-week radio-based educational series that uses 90-second acting segments with fictional characters to depict the issue of IPV and educate listeners. The primary goals of the campaign include increasing awareness, educating listeners, generating dialogue, and encouraging more responsiveness to IPV among African Americans (Family Violence Prevention Fund, 2008; Oliver, 2000). The following is an example of a message that the campaign sends to its audience members: "The It's Your Business campaign is for brothers like you— African American men who value Black women and who believe in non-violent, respectful relationships" (Family Violence Prevention Fund, 2008). The campaign has been disseminated to approximately 250 Black radio stations across the country, and although plans for community evaluations were underway to determine its impact, it is unclear at this time whether these studies have been completed.

## What Does Not Work

Gender-specific treatment (GST) is a form of IPV treatment in which typically only the male battering partner attends treatment. Because the target population for GST is perpetrators who have engaged in moderate to severe forms of physical and psychological aggression, involving both male and female partners would be contraindicated and increase the risk of violence toward the victim. GST is usually administered in a group format for a period of 6 to 52 weeks depending on the particular program (Holtzworth-Munroe et al., 2002). The length and format of GST programs are standardized by states in some cases. The benefit of a group format is that it is cost-effective and provides opportunities for male batterers to support one another, model positive behavior, and form connections so that participants do not feel isolated. Furthermore, "referring the man to GST gives both partners the clear message that the man is responsible for his violence and for learning to become nonviolent" (Holtzworth-Munroe et al., 2002, p. 454).

GST programs are typically based on cognitive-behavioral and feminist theories. Programs based on a cognitive-behavioral approach focus on psychoeducation regarding partner violence and skills training, including anger management and relaxation techniques, and on challenging problematic cognitions that contribute to violent behavior. Those that also incorporate feminist theory into their curriculum focus on ending violent behavior toward women by examining power and control as they relate to male patriarchy, exploring the function of abusive behavior, and encouraging men to take personal responsibility for their violent behavior. With this approach, programs address both the societal and interpersonal implications of IPV (Babcock & La Taillade, 2000; Holtzworth-Munroe et al., 2002).

The outcome literature on GST has not provided clear support for the effectiveness of this form of treatment. Although there is evidence that GST is more effective in reducing IPV than no treatment at all for male batterers, some studies have found that the rates of reoffending did not significantly decrease for male participants compared with other forms of treatment (see Babcock & La Taillade, 2000; Holtzworth-Munroe et al., 2002). In fact, a high percentage of men who participate in such programs reoffend after treatment (Babcock & La Taillade, 2000). Furthermore, such programs have limited success with ethnic minorities, as reflected in lower participation and completion rates and increased recidivism (Babcock & Steiner, 1999; Saunders & Parker, 1989; Tolman & Bennett, 1990). However, in the absence of appropriate alternatives to treatment, GST is often recommended and court ordered for male perpetrators of IPV. As a result, efforts have been directed toward using criminal justice responses as interventions for IPV.

## PREVENTION OF IPV

In addition to a relative absence of cultural sensitivity in the design and administration of programs, there are other reasons why treatment programs, as they are currently being offered, may be ineffective in reducing IPV. First, current treatment and intervention programs target the most severe of batterers in terms of psychopathology, criminal history, severity of violence, and ability to instill fear in their partner. This population is likely to be less amenable to establishing and maintaining gains made in such programs. Furthermore, lifetime survey estimates suggest that 30% of couples experience physical aggression at least once in their marriage (Straus & Gelles, 1990). However, a much smaller segment of the female population, up to 2 million women, is severely assaulted by their male partners (Straus & Gelles, 1990). Couples whose relationships are not characterized by battering but may be at risk for future violence would not be appropriate for existing treatment programs.

Second, the occurrence and course of IPV varies across the life span. An inverse relationship between age and use of IPV has been demonstrated with longitudinal data (O'Leary, 1999), with rates of spousal abuse peaking in the late teenage years and early 20s and decreasing with age and the most significant decrease occurring from the 20s to the 30s (O'Leary, 1999). In the United States, adolescents begin to develop romantic relationships between the ages of 12 and 15 years, during their transition to junior high school, which coincides with reports of adolescent dating violence (Avery-Leaf, Cascardi, O'Leary, & Cano, 1997; O'Leary, 1999). Age-related changes in physical aggression appear to coincide with the developmental course of intimate relationships, from dating to marriage. Furthermore, research suggests that African American youth may be particularly vulnerable to dating violence victimization (Watson, Cascardi, Avery-Leaf, & O'Leary, 2001). Given that national survey data estimate that severe batterers constitute a relatively small proportion of the population of abusers, and that use of violence in intimate relationships may occur early in the life span, development of prevention programs that are both culturally sensitive and designed to reduce risk of IPV in the population at large, as well as those at greater risk for abuse, is warranted. We review now the effectiveness of several prevention approaches.

## What Works

Just as for adult intimate relationships, the use of psychological aggression, jealous and controlling behaviors, as well as difficulties with conflict resolution have been found to be associated with adolescent dating violence (Bookwala, Frieze, Smith, & Ryan, 1992; Cano, Avery-Leaf, Cascardi, & O'Leary, 1998). Attitudes and beliefs that youth have about the acceptability of aggression is one of the most consistent risk factors associated with use of physical aggression in dating relationships, particularly for young men (Avery-Leaf & Cascardi, 2002; Bookwala et al., 1992; Cano et al., 1998). It may be that adolescents' tendency to exaggerate gender-specific roles and endorse mythical ideas about romantic relationships makes them especially vulnerable to violence in their relationships (Prothrow-Stith, 1993). For African American adolescents in particular, adoption of hypermasculine behaviors (e.g., endorsing derogatory attitudes toward women, adopting threatening facial expressions and physical gestures) in an effort to appear tough and in control may make it difficult for a male to utilize nonviolent responses in a dispute with a girlfriend (Majors & Billson, 1992).

Given that patterns of IPV may begin as early as the transition to adolescence and dating, several researchers have targeted this population with programs designed to educate young persons about the prevalence, causes, and consequences of dating violence; modify attitudes related to the use of violence; teach skills for effective communication and conflict management that do not involve the use of violence; and increase available resources and adolescent help-seeking behaviors in efforts to curtail dating violence.

### *Building Relationships in Greater Harmony Program*

The Building Relationships in Greater Harmony (BRIGHT) program uses a psychoeducational, skills-based approach focusing on attitudinal changes and skills enhancement. This intervention developed for adolescents, regards dating violence as a multifactorial phenomenon, is sensitive to gender inequities (Cascardi & Avery-Leaf, 1998), and yet acknowledges that both males and females may be victims or perpetrators within a dating relationship. The BRIGHT program has undergone several evaluations in both suburban high schools and urban middle schools settings. Two pilot studies conducted in an ethnically diverse high school and a primarily White high school indicated that students who participated in the intervention perceived dating violence as significantly less justified, whereas control students did not show attitudinal change. Furthermore, a larger study involving six ethnically diverse New York City high schools suggested that students participating in the program showed significant gains in knowledge and were significantly less accepting of attitudes that support dating violence. Additionally, program participants were more likely to report greater help-seeking intentions if they find themselves harmful relationships in the future.

An evaluation of the BRIGHT program by Cascardi, Avery-Leaf, and O'Leary (1999) was completed with five primarily African American inner-city middle schools (Cascardi et al., 1999). The students, more than 15,500 seventh and eighth graders, were assigned to one of three conditions: double-program-dose group, single-program-dose group, or control group. This study provided further evidence for the intervention's efficacy in that the single-dose group showed substantial gains in knowledge and help-seeking intentions as well as decreases in intent to use aggression; however, the double-dose group showed even greater improvements in behavioral intentions. Moreover, the double-dose group showed attitudinal changes not seen in the single-dose condition. Interestingly, both knowledge and help-seeking intention effects disappeared after the double dose. Possible explanations offered by the researchers were that students (1) may have perceived their immediate environment as not helpful, thus resulting in lower help-seeking intentions, or (2) may have perceived themselves as being less likely to be involved in a dating relationship characterized by aggression and, therefore, less likely to perceive the need for help. The results also suggest that a single dose of the program has the potential to decrease the frequency with which control tactics and verbal aggression are used against a partner. Finally, another finding suggests that receiving a single dose resulted in significantly less peer aggression and sexual harassment for male program participants than males assigned to the control condition.

### Safe Dates Program

Safe Dates is a school-based program designed to prevent the initiation of psychological, physical, and sexual abuse in adolescent dating relationships. The program is intended for male and female middle and high school students ranging in age from 12 to 18. Program goals include changing adolescent dating violence norms and overcoming gender stereotyping; improving conflict resolution skills; increasing awareness of community resources for dating violence; promoting help-seeking behaviors by both victims and perpetrators of dating violence; and promoting peer help-giving skills for those in abusive relationships. Safe Dates interventions consist of both school activities, which promote the primary prevention of violence, and community activities, which promote secondary prevention. School activities include (1) a theatre production performed by peers; (2) a curriculum of ten 45-minute sessions; and (3) a poster contest based on curriculum content. Community activities include special services for adolescents in abusive relationships (i.e., crisis hotline, support groups, materials for parents) and community service provider training. In addition to adolescent-focused interventions, both parents and teachers are encouraged to connect with available community resources and are provided with resources and information about dating violence among adolescents. As such, the program is comprehensive in including all social relationships and communities with which adolescents are involved in order to prevent dating violence more effectively.

The Safe Dates program is the most thoroughly researched prevention program to date, with follow-up data obtained 1 month and 1, 2, 3, and 4 years after the program's completion (Foshee et al., 1998, 2000, 2004). The program was evaluated in 14 primarily rural areas in North Carolina, with a sample consisting of 1,886 male and female adolescents in the eight or ninth grade, 77.1% of whom were White and 19.1% African American.

Evaluations of the program at 1 month and 1, 2, and 3 years postintervention found that, in comparison to controls, adolescents who participated in the Safe Dates program reported less psychological, physical, and sexual dating violence perpetration and less physical dating violence victimization at all four follow-up periods. Adolescents in the treatment group, compared with controls, were less supportive of prescribed dating violence norms, were more supportive of proscribed dating violence norms, perceived fewer positive consequences from using dating violence, used more constructive communication skills and responses to anger, were less likely to engage in gender stereotyping, and were more aware of victim and perpetrator services.

In addition, Safe Dates had both primary and secondary prevention effects on all outcome measures and was found to be equally effective for both genders and across all ethnic groups sampled. Program effects were mediated primarily by changes in dating violence norms, gender stereotyping, use of constructive communication skills, and awareness of community services for dating violence. Additional analyses found that program effects on victimization and perpetration were maintained 4 years after completion of the program, with treatment groups scoring 56–92% lower than controls on almost all outcome measures.

Three years after Safe Dates was implemented, a booster was implemented with a random half of the original treatment group (Foshee et al., 2004). The booster was an 11-page newsletter mailed to each adolescent, followed 4 weeks later by a telephone call from a health educator. The newsletter included information from the Safe Dates curriculum, such as indicators, or "red flags," that a relationship is abusive, effective communication strategies, and tips for safe dating. Contact by the health educator consisted of answering the adolescent's questions related to the newsletter, providing additional information when needed, and determining whether the adolescent read each informational component and completed the work sheets.

The booster did not improve the effectiveness of Safe Dates in preventing physical, serious physical, or sexual dating violence perpetration, and prior involvement in psychological abuse perpetration moderated the effect of the booster on psychological abuse perpetration. In fact, those adolescents high in prior psychological abuse perpetration who received the Safe Dates booster reported significantly more psychological abuse perpetration at follow-up than those who did not. With regard to victimization, analyses revealed no effects of the booster on psychological abuse victimization, and the effects of the booster on physical, serious physical, and sexual victimization were moderated by prior victimization; that is, when prior involvement in dating violence was high, adolescents exposed to the booster reported more serious physical and sexual victimization at follow-up than those who completed only Safe Dates. Overall, these findings indicate that the Safe Dates programs may be effective in preventing violence generally, but may be contraindicated for those adolescents demonstrating more severe dating violence behaviors.

## What May Work

### Southside Teens About Respect

Although additional clinical trials are warranted, the Southside Teens About Respect (STAR) program is another dating violence prevention program that shows promise in preventing IPV among African Americans. In a 2-year longitudinal study with a cohort of urban African American students, Schewe (2000) evaluated STAR, which is a 10-session curriculum dating violence prevention intervention targeting adolescents. The curriculum is a module that is part of a larger comprehensive community-based intervention involving a social marketing campaign, a hotline, parent and teacher training, and peer advocate training. The study consisted of 333 students in the original sample, of whom 118 had complete data at all four time points. A comparison of students who received 2 years of the curriculum, students who received 1 year, and students who did not participate demonstrated significant effects regarding conflict behavior, self-ratings of relationship skills, and help-seeking behavior. Although trends were headed in the right direction, in terms of attitudes supporting violence and justifying violence in relationships, they were not statistically significant. Additionally, data analyses for each year indicated that students were more likely to report an increase in their determination to engage in help-seeking behavior following abuse after only just 1 year of the curriculum. Collectively, these findings indicate that students who received the 2-year intervention benefited considerably more than those who did not receive the intervention and those who received the 1-year intervention.

### Prevention of Marital Distress

Research has consistently demonstrated a strong association between relationship discord and violence. Pan, Neidig, and O'Leary (1994) found that relationship discord was the most accurate predictor of physical aggression against a partner. Rogge and Bradbury (1999) found that reports of violence and psychological aggression were the strongest predictors of divorce in the first 4 years of marriage, and communication quality was the best predictor of marital satisfaction (Low et al., 2002). Longitudinal studies have demonstrated that destructive communication behaviors, such as negative reciprocity and withdrawal, are the leading risk factors for relationship distress (e.g., Markman & Hahlweg, 1993) and are characteristic of violent couples (e.g., Cordova et al., 1993; Jacobson et al., 1994).

Although nearly half of all couples are expected to divorce (Bray & Hetherington, 1993), rates of separation and divorce for African American couples have increased nearly fivefold in the last 30 years and are double the rate of the general population (Tucker & Mitchell-Kernan, 1995). The higher divorce rate has been attributed to several stressors that disproportionately affect African Americans, including economic instability, joblessness, exposure to poverty and violence, and continued experiences of discrimination, as well as the continued negative impact of the legacy of slavery. Given this association between discord and relational predictors of aggression, it is imperative to incorporate strategies to prevent marital discord and conflict in the design of IPV prevention programs for African Americans. Thus, the skills targeted in existing programs designed to prevent distress and divorce (e.g., communication and problem-solving skills training) may have implications for the prevention of IPV (Low et al., 2002). Despite the plethora of couple distress prevention programs available (see Berger & Hannah, 1999, for a review), only one such program has provided empirical evidence demonstrating its short- and long-term effectiveness.

## PREVENTION AND RELATIONSHIP ENHANCEMENT PROGRAM

The Prevention and Relationship Enhancement Program (PREP) (Markman, Stanley, & Blumberg, 2001) was developed in an effort to prevent the onset of marital distress and enhance adaptive functioning in couples. PREP is a 12-hour program designed for couples who are planning marriage, with the principal aim of helping them gain skills that protect the marriage from future distress (Low et al., 2002). PREP teaches couples communication skills designed to facilitate constructive conflict resolution and discussions, problem-solving skills, and self-regulation of affect (Markman, Floyd, Stanley, & Storaasli, 1988). Along with instruction in behavioral techniques, PREP targets key protective factors, such as maintaining friendship and commitment between partners, promoting sensual and spiritual connection, and the continuation of fun and pleasurable activities (Markman, Stanley, & Blumberg, 1994). In short, reducing negative interaction and maintaining positive elements of the relationship are the primary aims of prevention in this model (Stanley et al., 2001).

PREP is the most thoroughly researched of all relationship distress preventive programs to date; studies examining its effectiveness date back to past 20 years (Stanley, Markman, St. Peters, & Leber, 1995). Couples using the skills taught in the PREP workshops have reported greater satisfaction with conflict discussions, greater relationship satisfaction, and lower levels of conflict escalation compared with control couples receiving no premarital intervention (Low et al., 2002). Follow-up research has demonstrated that PREP is effective in lowering problem intensity, in decreasing the likelihood that couples will engage in negative communication behaviors, in decreasing likelihood of separation or divorce, and in lowering negative escalation as much as 4 years after participation in the program (Markman, Renick, Floyd, Stanley, & Clements, 1993). Additionally, a study evaluating a weekend version of PREP confirmed that the mechanism through which the program proposes to reduce distress—improvements in communication and problem-solving skills—was significant in producing longitudinal decreases in distress and effective for males in particular (Schilling, Baucom, Burnett, Allen, & Ragland, 2003).

With regard to preventing IPV, couples receiving PREP training were less likely to engage in physical aggression up to 4 years after program completion (Markman et al., 1993). Furthermore, over a 5-year period, couples who had participated in PREP premaritally had one-fourth the number of aggressive incidents compared with control couples (Markman et al., 1993).

However, there is concern that PREP may not be as effective for more distressed populations; some investigators believe that the samples used in the Markman and Hahlweg (1993) study were not at risk (Kelly & Fincham, 1999). Furthermore, to date, no research is available on the effectiveness of PREP with African American and other ethnic-minority populations. Only recently has the program been tested with ethnic-minority and low-income populations. For example, in an evaluation of the effectiveness of PREP with military personnel, investigators found successful outcomes for lower income persons and couples in which at least one member was an ethnic minority (Stanley, Markman, & Sair, 2003). In addition, through the Temporary Assistance to Needy Families program and the Oklahoma Marriage Initiative, PREP was adopted statewide to determine its effectiveness in reducing divorce among at-risk low-income couples. Finally, ProSAAM (Program for Strong African American Marriages), an intervention designed to strengthen the marriages of African American couples using a format based on the PREP curriculum, has set out to evaluate the effectiveness of their program (University of Georgia, 2008). ProSAAM expands on PREP by incorporating religious behaviors, such as praying, as both an alternative to psychological and physical aggression and a means of increasing closeness between partners.

## What Does Not Work

In our review, we found no IPV preventive approaches that have been found successful to some extent among African Americans. Thus, for prevention, we place no programs or approaches in this category.

## ADDRESSING IPV AMONG AFRICAN AMERICANS: BEST-PRACTICE RECOMMENDATIONS

Of the programs reviewed in this chapter, it appears that GST programs are not consistently effective in reducing recidivism among African Americans. Additionally, programs targeting relationship distress and mild psychological and physical aggression have not been evaluated with African American couples; as such, it is unknown whether such programs, as currently designed, will be effective in preventing IPV in this population. It is recommended that further clinical trials on conjoint approaches such as the PACT program be implemented with African American couples to ascertain their potential effectiveness in addressing IPV.

In contrast, the greatest results may be seen in community advocacy efforts and in dating violence prevention programs (Safe Dates, the BRIGHT program, as cited in Cascardi & Avery-Leaf, 1998) initiated in adolescence that are focused on shaping knowledge, and modifying attitudes and behaviors associated with violence and are multisystemic in their inclusion of scholastic, parental/family, and community arenas in addressing IPV in dating relationships. The continuance of these programs is recommended. Further research is needed, however, to determine their impact on rates of exposure and use of violence among African American victims and adolescents in the long term. More studies are needed to determine not only whether prevention and intervention programs are longitudinally effective in reducing violence and related outcome behaviors but also *how* such programs work to effectively reduce and eliminate violence among Black couples and families; in other words, what are the "essential ingredients" that produce desired treatment effects?

We next offer our recommendations for improving the effectiveness of current and future IPV treatment and prevention programs.

## Integrating Treatment and Prevention Programs in Communities of Color

Grounding treatment and prevention programs in communities of color is essential in the overall effort to eliminate IPV. Natural networks of kinship, family, neighborhood, and community often remain available after crises subside and interventions cease; as such, these sources of support are essential to maintaining gains that may result from more formal interventions (Budde & Schene, 2004; Rzepnicki, 1991). Community-based approaches have the ability to impact multiple aspects of the social environment in which African American couples and families reside, including community attitudes, norms, and policies regarding violence. Such approaches foster the involvement of individuals and organizations (e.g., adolescents, parents, couples, religious leaders, educators, law enforcement, health care professionals, policymakers), who can all work together toward the shared goal of eliminating violence. Finally, a community-based approach allows the community to invest and take ownership of the interventions, thus ensuring that its residents likewise take ownership and assume responsibility for the continuance of and participation in IPV programs (McElhaney & Effley, 1999).

## Altering Program Content to Reflect Experiences of African American Couples and Families

Existing treatment and prevention programs fail to consider environmental conditions that potentially exacerbate couple distress and conflict among African

Americans, specifically joblessness, poverty, community violence, and racism, thus rendering current efforts inapplicable to "all but the most assimilated people of color" (Cross, Bazron, Dennis, & Issacs, 1989, p. 23). Although such situational factors may not directly address causal mechanisms in the development and continuance of distress and violence, the fact that many African American couples are disproportionately exposed to such stressors suggests the need for programs to develop culture-specific interventions that aid Black men and women in successfully adapting to such stressors.

In addition, programs must be vigilant in addressing the dynamics of sex, gender, power, and violence in African American relationships. Research has shown that status discrepancies between partners, in which Black males have fewer economic resources than their female partners, is associated with males' use of violence as a means of asserting power and control in the face of perceived powerlessness, in both their intimate relationships and society at large. Such issues must be incorporated in programs to both elucidate the cycle of violence among Black couples and assist males and females in developing constructive approaches to conflicts reflective of themes of relative power in relationships.

## Increasing Cultural Competence of Intervention and Treatment Providers

The lower effectiveness of IPV intervention programs among Black participants may be due to their non-culturally relevant foundation or the facilitators' lack of African American cultural knowledge. Black males in batterer programs may not readily identify with the themes found in mainstream programs or may even mistrust the motives of such programs, which often feel stigmatizing to participants (Williams, 1992).

Williams outlines three stages of cultural competence of program facilitators (from least to most advanced): cultural resistance, color blindness, and cultural sensitivity. In the cultural resistance stage, practitioners deny and minimize the need to incorporate cultural competence into practice, limit their own opportunities to learn from minority clients, and use mainstream approaches, which may support assimilation of minority clients into majority culture. Practitioners in the color blindness stage are more advanced because they recognize the need for ethnically sensitive practice but lack the appropriate cultural knowledge and skills to achieve success with minority clients. Program facilitators in the most advanced stage, cultural sensitivity, "demonstrate humanistic values and cultural sensitivity ... continually examine their behavior to determine how their attitudes and feelings influence their relationships with clients ... [remain] aware that, for some African American men who batter, violent behavior may be the result of having been the target of hostile social interactions ... [and] include minority clients in the treatment process (Williams, 1992, p. 591). African Americans stand to gain the most benefit from IPV programs that are guided by these principles. It is important that cultural congruence between program participants and facilitators be considered during treatment. Although Black facilitators may in some ways have advantages in working with Black participants, practitioners of any background can work with this population as long as cultural sensitivity is understood and practiced.

## Incorporating Protective Factors Used by African American Couples and Families

The majority of prevention programs reviewed have incorporated protective factors common across couples, regardless of racial or ethnic background, that may buffer against distress and IPV. However, none of the programs have included the protective factors unique to the ethnic and cultural experiences that are associated with positive functioning in African American couple relationships. For example, research examining the relationship between aspects of ethnic identity and relationship quality has found that positive feelings toward one's ethnic group and heritage were associated with relationship satisfaction and support; conversely, internalized racism was associated with relationship distress (e.g., Bell, Bouie, & Baldwin, 1998; Kelly & Floyd, 2001; Taylor & Zhang, 1990). Positive feelings toward one's ethnic group may counteract negative racial stereotypes associated with perceptions of powerlessness that precipitate use of violence, and may protect African Americans against the deleterious effects of discrimination and other stressful events.

In addition to psychological factors associated with ethnic-minority status, African Americans' use of informal sources of social support, such as churches and community networks, are additional protectors associated with decreased risk of violence and should be incorporated in existing prevention programs. Further research is needed, however, to clarify additional protective factors that may be utilized by this population.

Although the domestic violence field has made much progress in recognizing the seriousness of domestic violence in African Americans, we have long way to go in eliminating abuse among African American couples. We have limited knowledge of the relationship between ethnic-minority status and the social, cultural, situational, and interpersonal factors that interact to augment risk of violence. In addition, the process of developing effective treatment and prevention programs has thus far moved in separate and parallel directions, with researchers moving along one path and African American communities taking alternate routes to mobilize local resources. Recent governmental policy initiatives, however, have encouraged grassroots community organizations, religious leaders, clinicians, and researchers who share a common goal of preventing distress and violence to work together toward promoting the health and well-being of ethnic minority couples and families. It is our hope that researchers and clinicians will continue to work collaboratively with communities of color to develop programs that are culturally sensitive, community-based, and effective in eliminating IPV in African American families.

# REFERENCES

Avery-Leaf, S., & Cascardi, M. (2002). Dating violence education: Prevention and early intervention strategies. In P. A. Schewe (Ed.), *Preventing violence in relationships: Interventions across the lifespan* (pp. 79–105). Washington, DC: American Psychological Association.

Avery-Leaf, S., Cascardi, M., O'Leary, K. D., & Cano, A. (1997). Efficacy of a dating violence prevention program on attitudes justifying aggression. *Journal of Adolescent Health, 21,* 11–17.

Babcock, J. C., & La Taillade, J. J. (2000). Evaluating interventions for men who batter. In J. Vincent & E. N. Jouriles (Eds.), *Domestic violence: Guidelines for research-informed practice* (pp. 37–77). London: Jessica Kingsley.

Babcock, J. C., & Steiner, R. (1999). The relationship between treatment, incarceration, and recidivism of battering: A program evaluation of Seattle's coordinated community response to domestic violence. *Journal of Family Psychology, 13,* 46–59.

Babcock, J. C., Waltz, J., Jacobson, N. S., & Gottman, J. M. (1993). Power and violence: The relation between communication patterns, power discrepancies, and domestic violence. *Journal of Consulting and Clinical Psychology, 61*(1), 40–50.

Bell, Y. R., Bouie, C. L., & Baldwin, J. A. (1998). Afrocentric cultural consciousness and African American male-female relationships. In J. Hamlet (Ed.), *Afrocentric visions: Studies in culture and communication* (pp. 47–71). Thousand Oaks, CA: Sage.

Berger, R., & Hannah, M. T. (1999). *Preventive approaches in couples therapy.* Philadelphia: Brunner/Mazel.

Bolger, N., DeLongis, A., Kessler, R. C., & Wethington, E. (1989). The contagion of stress across multiple roles. *Journal of Marriage and the Family, 51,* 175–183.

Bookwala, J., Frieze, I. H., Smith, C., & Ryan, K. (1992). Predictors of dating violence: A multivariate analysis. *Violence and Victims, 7,* 297–311.

Bray, J. H., & Hetherington, E. M. (1993). Families in transition: Introduction and overview. *Journal of Family Psychology, 7,* 3–8.

Budde, S., & Schene, P. (2004). Informal social support interventions and their role in violence prevention: An agenda for future evaluation. *Journal of Interpersonal Violence, 19,* 341–355.

Campbell, D. W., Sharps, P. W., Gary, F., Campbell, J. C., & Lopez, L. M. (2002). Intimate partner violence in African American women. *Online Journal of Issues in Nursing, 7*(1), 5. Retrieved September 1, 2004, from *www.nursingworld.org/MainMenuCategories/ANAMarketplace/ANAPeriodicals/OJIN/TableofContents/Volume72002/No1Jan2002/AfricanAmericanWomenPartnerViolence.aspx.*

Cano, A., Avery-Leaf, S., Cascardi, M., & O'Leary, K. D. (1998). Dating violence in two high school samples: Discriminating variables. *Journal of Primary Prevention, 18,* 431–446.

Cano, A., & Vivian, D. (2003). Are life stressors associated with marital violence? *Journal of Family Psychology, 17,* 302–314.

Cascardi, M., & Avery-Leaf, S. (1998). *Building relationships in greater harmony together (BRIGHT) program.* Glen Ridge, NJ: DVPP.

Cascardi, M., Avery-Leaf, S., & O'Leary, K. (1999). Factor structure and convergent validity of the Conflict Tactics Scale in high school students. *Psychological Assessment, 11,* 546–555.

Cazenave, N. A., & Straus, M. A. (1990). Race, class, network embeddedness, and family violence: A search for potent support systems. In M. A. Straus & R. J. Gelles (Eds.), *Physical violence in American families: Risk factors and adaptations to violence in 8,145 families* (pp. 321–339). New Brunswick, NJ: Transaction.

Clark, R., Anderson, N. B., Clark, V. R., & Williams, D. R. (1999). Racism as a stressor for African Americans: A biopsychosocial model. *American Psychologist, 54,* 805–816.

Cohan, C. L., & Bradbury, T. N. (1997). Negative life events, marital interaction, and the longitudinal course of newlywed marriage. *Journal of Personality and Social Psychology, 73,* 114–128.

Coie, J., Watt, N., West, S. G., Hawkins, J. D., Asarnow, J. R., Markman, H. J., et al. (1993). The science of prevention: A conceptual framework and some directions for a national research program. *American Psychologist, 48,* 1013–1022.

Conger, R., Elder, G., Lorenz, F., Conger, K., Simons, R., Whitbeck, L., et al. (1990). Linking economic hardship to marital quality and instability. *Journal of Marriage and the Family, 52,* 643–656.

Council on Scientific Affairs. (1992). Violence against women: Relevance for medical practitioners. *American Medical Association, 267,* 3184–3189.

Cordova, J. V., Jacobson, N. S., Gottman, J. M., Rushe, R., & Cox, G. (1993). Negative reciprocity and communication in couples with a violent husband. *Journal of Abnormal Psychology, 102,* 559–564.

Cross, T., Bazron, B., Dennis, K., & Issacs, M. (1989). *Towards a culturally competent system of care.* Washington, DC: CASSP Technical Assistance Center.

Cunradi, C. B., Caetano, R., Clark, C., & Schafer, J. (2000). Neighborhood poverty as a predictor of intimate partner violence among Caucasian, African American, and Hispanic couples in the United States: A multilevel analysis. *Annals of Epidemiology, 10,* 297–308.

Cunradi, C. B., Caetano, R., & Schafer, J. (2002). Socioeconomic predictors of intimate partner violence among White, Black, and Hispanic couples in the United States. *Journal of Family Violence, 17*(4), 377–389.

Dutton, D. G. (1988). *The domestic assault of women: Psychological and criminal justice perspectives.* Boston: Allyn & Bacon.

Dutton, D. G., & Golant, S. K. (1995). *The batterer: A psychological profile.* New York: Basic Books.

Ehrensaft, M. K., Langhinrichsen-Rohling, J., Heyman, R. E., O'Leary, K. D., & Lawrence, E. (1999). Feelings controlled in marriage: A phenomenon specific to physically aggressive couples? *Journal of Family Psychology, 13,* 20–32.

Family Violence Prevention Fund. (2008). *It's your business.* San Francisco: Author. Retrieved June 5, 2008, from *www.endabuse.org/section/programs/public_communications/_multimedia#business.*

Foshee, V. A., Bauman, K. E., Arriaga, X. B., Helms, R. W., Koch, G. G., & Linder, G. F. (1998). An evaluation of Safe Dates, an adolescent dating violence prevention program. *American Journal of Public Health, 88,* 45–50.

Foshee, V. A., Bauman, K. E., Ennett, S. T., Linder, G. F., Benefield, T., & Suchindran, C. (2004). Assessing the long-term effects of the Safe Dates program and a booster in preventing and reducing adolescent dating violence victimization and perpetration. *American Journal of Public Health, 94,* 619–624.

Foshee, V. A., Bauman, K. E., Greene, W. F., Koch, G. G., Linder, G. F., & MacDougall, J. E.

(2000). The Safe Dates program: 1-year follow-up results. *American Journal of Public Health, 90,* 1619–1622.

Fox, G. L., Benson, M. L., DeMaris, A. A., & Van Wyk, J. (2002). Economic distress and intimate violence: Testing family stress and resources theories. *Journal of Marriage and the Family, 64*(3), 793–807.

Gondolf, E. W., & Williams, O. J. (2001). Culturally focused batterer counseling for African American men. *Trauma, Violence, and Abuse, 2,* 283–295.

Goodyear-Smith, F., & Laidlaw, T. M. (1999). Aggressive acts and assaults in intimate relationships: Towards an understanding of the literature. *Behavioral Sciences and the Law, 17,* 285–304.

Gottman, J. M., Jacobson, N. S., Rushe, R. H., Shortt, J. W., Babcock, J. C., La Taillade, J. J., et al. (1995). The relationship between heart rate activity, emotionally aggressive behavior and general violence in batterers. *Journal of Family Psychology, 9,* 227–248.

Hampton, R. L., & Gelles, R. J. (1994). Violence towards Black women in a nationally representative sample of Black American families. *Journal of Comparative Family Studies, 25,* 105–119.

Hampton, R. L., Oliver, W., & Magarian, L. (2003). Domestic violence in the African American community: An analysis of social and structural factors. *Violence Against Women, 9*(5), 533–557.

Hatchett, S., Veroff, J., & Douvan, E. (1995). Marital instability among Black and White newlyweds. In M. B. Tucker & C. Mitchell-Kernan (Eds.), *The decline in marriage among African Americans* (pp. 177–218). New York: Russell Sage Foundation.

Heyman, R. E., & Neidig, P. H. (1997). Physical aggression in couples treatment. In W. K. Halford & H. J. Markman (Eds.), *Clinical handbook of marriage and couples intervention* (pp. 589–617). New York: Wiley.

Heyman, R. E., & Schlee, K. (2003). Stopping wife abuse via physical aggression couples treatment. *Journal of Aggression, Maltreatment, and Trauma, 7,* 135–157.

Holtzworth-Munroe, A. (2000). Social information processing skills deficits in maritally violent men: Summary of a research program. In J. P. Vincent & E. N. Jouriles (Eds.), *Domestic violence: Guidelines for research-informed practice* (pp. 13–36). London: Jessica Kingsley.

Holtzworth-Munroe, A., Meehan, J. C., Rehman, U., & Marshall, A. D. (2002). Intimate partner violence. In A. S. Gurman & N. S. Jacobson (Eds.), *Clinical handbook of couple therapy* (3rd ed., pp. 441–465). New York: Guilford Press.

Holtzworth-Munroe, A., Stuart, G. L., & Hutchinson, G. (1997). Violent versus nonviolent husbands: Differences in attachment patterns, dependency, and jealousy. *Journal of Family Psychology, 11,* 314–331.

Hotaling, G. T., & Sugarman, D. B. (1990). A risk marker analysis of assaulted wives. *Journal of Family Violence, 5,* 1–13.

Institute of Medicine. (1994). *Reducing risks for mental disorders: Frontiers for preventive intervention research.* Washington, DC: National Academy Press.

Jacobson, N. S., Gottman, J. M., Waltz, J., Rushe, R., Babcock, J., & Holtzworth-Munroe, A. (1994). Affect, verbal content, and psychophysiology in the arguments of couples with a violent husband. *Journal of Consulting and Clinical Psychology, 62,* 982–988.

Kelly, A. B., & Fincham, F. D. (1999). Preventing marital distress: What does research offer? In R. Berger & M. T. Hannah (Eds.), *Preventive approaches in couples therapy* (pp. 361–390). Philadelphia: Brunner/Mazel.

Kelly, S., & Floyd, F. (2001). The effects of negative racial stereotypes and Afrocentricity on Black couples. *Journal of Family Psychology, 15,* 110–123.

Krokoff, L., Gottman, J., & Roy, A. (1988). Blue-collar and White-collar marital interaction and communication orientation. *Journal of Social and Personal Relationships, 5,* 201–221.

La Taillade, J. J. (1999). *Predictors of satisfaction and resiliency in African American/White interracial relationships.* Unpublished doctoral dissertation, University of Washington.

La Taillade, J. J., Epstein, N. B., & Werlinich, C. A. (2006). Conjoint treatment of intimate partner violence: A cognitive behavioral approach. *Journal of Cognitive Psychotherapy, 20,* 393–410.

La Taillade, J. J., & Jacobson, N. S. (1997). Domestic violence: Antisocial behavior in the family. In D. M. Stoff, J. Breiling, & J. D. Maser (Eds.), *Handbook of antisocial behavior* (pp. 534–550). New York: Wiley.

Lavee, Y., McCubbin, H., & Olson, D. (1987). The effect of stressful life events and transitions on family functioning and well-being. *Journal of Marriage and the Family, 49,* 857–873.

Leonard, K. E., & Roberts, L. J. (1998). The effects of alcohol on the marital interactions of aggressive and nonaggressive husbands and their wives. *Journal of Abnormal Psychology, 107,* 602–615.

Lockhart, L. L. (1991). Spousal violence: A cross-racial perspective. In R. L. Hampton (Ed.), *Black family violence: Current research and theory* (pp. 85–101). Lexington, MA: Lexington Books.

Low, S. M., Monarch, N. D., Hartman, S., & Markman, H. J. (2002). Recent therapeutic advances in the prevention of domestic violence. In P. A. Schewe (Ed.), *Preventing violence in relationships: Interventions across the lifespan* (pp. 197–221). Washington, DC: American Psychological Association.

Magdol, L., Moffitt, T. E., Caspi, A., Newman, D. L., Fagan, J., & Silva, P. A. (1997). Gender differences in rates of partner violence in a birth cohort of 21-year-olds: Bridging the gap between clinical and epidemiological approaches. *Journal of Consulting and Clinical Psychology, 65,* 68–78.

Majors, R., & Billson, J. M. (1992). *Cool pose: The dilemmas of Black manhood in America.* Lexington, MA: Lexington Books.

Margolin, G., & Burman, B. (1993). Wife abuse versus marital violence: Different terminologies, explanations, and solutions. *Clinical Psychology Review, 13,* 77–84.

Margolin, G., Burman, B., & John, R. S. (1989). Home observations of married couples reenacting naturalistic conflicts. *Behavioral Assessment, 11,* 101–118.

Markman, H., Floyd, F., Stanley, S., & Storaasli, R. (1988). Prevention of marital distress: A longitudinal. *Journal of Consulting and Clinical Psychology, 56,* 210–217.

Markman, H. J., & Hahlweg, K. (1993). The prediction and prevention of marital distress: An international perspective. *Clinical Psychology Review, 13,* 29–43.

Markman, H. J., Renick, M. J., Floyd, F. J., Stanley, S. M., & Clements, M. (1993). Preventing marital distress through communication and conflict management training: A 4- and 5-year follow-up. *Journal of Consulting and Clinical Psychology, 61,* 70–77.

Markman, H. J., Stanley, S. M., & Blumberg, S. (1994). *Fighting for your marriage: Positive steps for a loving and lasting relationship.* San Francisco: Jossey-Bass.

Markman, H. J., Stanley, S. M., & Blumberg, S. (2001). *Fighting for your marriage: Positive steps for preventing divorce and preserving a lasting love*. San Francisco: Jossey-Bass.

Maxwell, C. D., Garner, J. H., & Fagan, J. A. (2001). *The effects of arrest on intimate partner violence: New evidence from the Spouse Assault Replication Program. Research in brief*. Washington, DC: U.S. Department of Justice.

McCord, J. (1993). Conduct disorder and antisocial behavior: Some thoughts about processes. *Developmental and Psychopathology, 5*, 321–329.

McElhaney, S. J., & Effley, K. M. (1999). Community-based approaches to violence prevention. In T. P. Gullotta & S. J. McElhaney (Eds.), *Violence in homes and communities: Prevention, intervention, and treatment* (pp. 269–299). Thousand Oaks, CA: Sage.

McKinnon, J. (2003). *The Black population in the United States: March 2002*. Retrieved August 3, 2004, from *www.census.gov/prod/2003pubs/p20-541.pdf*.

Murphy, C. M., Meyer, S., & O'Leary, K. D. (1994). Dependency characteristics of partner assaultive men. *Journal of Abnormal Psychology, 103*, 729–735.

National Resource Center on Domestic Violence. (1999). *Evaluations of advocacy efforts to end intimate male violence against women*. Harrisburg, PA: Author.

Neidig, P. H., & Friedman, D. H. (1984). *Spouse abuse: A treatment program for couples*. Champaign, IL: Research Press.

Office of Justice Programs, Bureau of Justice Statistics. (2002). *Bureau of Justice statistics homicide trends in the U.S.: Intimate homicide*. Retrieved September 1, 2004, from *www.bjs.ojp.usdoj.gov/content/homicide/intimates.cfm*.

O'Leary, K. D. (1999). Developmental and affective issues in assessing and treating partner aggression. *Clinical Psychology: Science and Practice, 6*, 400–414.

O'Leary, K. D., & Curley, A. D. (1986). Assertion and spouse abuse: Correlates of spouse abuse. *Journal of Marital and Family Therapy, 12*, 284–289.

O'Leary, K. D., Heyman, R. E., & Neidig, P. H. (1999). Treatment of wife abuse: A comparison of gender-specific and couples approaches. *Behavior Therapy, 30*, 475–505.

O'Leary, K. D., Vivian, D., & Malone, J. (1992). Assessment of physical aggression against women in marriage: The need for multimodal assessment. *Behavior Assessment, 14*, 5–14.

Oliver, W. (2000). Preventing domestic violence in the African American community: The rationale for popular culture interventions. *Violence Against Women, 6*, 533–549.

Pan, H., Neidig, P., & O'Leary, K. D. (1994). Predicting mild and severe husband-to-wife aggression. *Journal of Consulting and Clinical Psychology, 62*, 975–981.

Prothrow-Stith, D. (1993). *Deadly consequences*. New York: HarperPerennial.

Raj, A., Silverman, J. G., Wingood, G. M., & DiClemente, R. J. (1999). Prevalence and correlates of relationship abuse among a community-based sample of low-income African American women. *Violence Against Women, 5*, 272–291.

Rennison, C. M. (2003). *Intimate partner violence, 1993–2001*. Retrieved July 27, 2004, from *www.bjs.ojp.usdoj.gov/content/pub/pdf/ipv01.pdf*.

Rogge, R. D., & Bradbury, T. N. (1999). Till violence does us part: The differing roles of communication and aggression in predicting adverse marital outcomes. *Journal of Consulting and Clinical Psychology, 67*, 340–351.

Rzepnicki, T. L. (1991). Enhancing the durability of intervention gains: A challenge for the 1990s. *Social Service Review, 65*, 92–111.

Saunders, D. G., & Parker, J. C. (1989, September). Legal sanctions and treatment follow-through among men who batter: A multivariate analysis. *Social Work Research and Abstracts*, pp. 21–29.

Schewe, P. A. (2000, May). *Southside Teens about Respect (STAR): An intervention to promote healthy relationships and prevent teen dating violence.* Paper presented at the National Sexual Violence Prevention Conference, Dallas, TX.

Schilling, E. A., Baucom, D. H., Burnett, C. K., Allen, E. S., & Ragland, L. (2003). Altering the course of marriage: The effect of PREP communication skills acquisition on couples' risk of becoming maritally distressed. *Journal of Family Psychology, 17,* 41–53.

Stanley, S. M., Markman, H. J., Prado, L. M., Olmos-Gallo, A., Tonelli, L., St. Peters, M., et al. (2001). Community-based premarital prevention: Clergy and lay leaders on the front lines. *Family Relations, 50,* 67–76.

Stanley, S. M., Markman, H. J., & Sair, C. C. (2003, November). *Program evaluation of divorce prevention education in the U. S. Army: Insights on response and program satisfaction for minority and low-income couples.* Paper presented at the annual meeting of the Association for the Advancement of Behavior Therapy, Boston.

Stanley, S. M., Markman, H. J., St. Peters, M., & Leber, B. D. (1995). Strengthening marriages and preventing divorce: New directions in prevention research. *Journal of Applied Family and Child Studies, 44,* 392–401.

Stets, J. E. (1988). *Domestic violence and control.* New York: Springer-Verlag.

Stith, S. M., Rosen, K. H., & McCollum, E. E. (2003). Effectiveness of couples treatment for spouse abuse. *Journal of Marital and Family Therapy, 29,* 407–426.

Straus, M. A. (1990). Social stress and marital violence in a national sample of American families. In M. A. Straus & R. J. Gelles (Eds.), *Physical violence in American families: Risk factors and adaptations to violence in 8,145 families* (pp. 181–201). New Brunswick, NJ: Transaction.

Straus, M. A., & Gelles, R. J. (Eds.). (1990). *Physical violence in American families: Risk factors and adaptations to violence in 8,145 families.* New Brunswick, NJ: Transaction.

Straus, M. A., Gelles, R. J., & Steinmetz, S. K. (1980). *Behind closed doors: Violence in the American family.* Newbury Park, CA: Sage.

Taylor, J., & Zhang, X. (1990). Cultural identity in maritally distressed and nondistressed Black couples. *Western Journal of Black Studies, 14,* 205–213.

Tolman, R. T., & Bennett, L. (1990). A review of quantitative research on men who batter. *Journal of Interpersonal Violence, 5,* 87–118.

Tucker, M. B., & Mitchell-Kernan, C. (1995). *The decline in marriage among African Americans.* New York: Russell Sage Foundation.

Ucko, L. G. (1994). Culture and violence: The interaction of Africa and America. *Sex Roles, 31*(3–4), 185–204.

University of Georgia. (2008). *ProSAAM: About the project.* Retrieved July 15, 2008 from *www.uga.edu/prosaam/about/index.htm.*

U.S. Census Bureau. (2003). *U.S. Census Bureau, current population survey: The Black population in the United States, March 2002.* Retrieved August 31, 2004, from *www.census.gov/population/www/socdemo/race/ppl-164.html.*

Watson, J. M., Cascardi, M., Avery-Leaf, S., & O'Leary, K. D. (2001). High school students' responses to dating aggression. *Violence and Victims, 16,* 339–348.

West, C. M. (2002). Battered, Black, and blue: An overview of violence in the lives of Black women. *Women and Therapy, 25,* 5–27.

Williams, O. J. (1992). Ethnically sensitive practice to enhance treatment participation of African American men who batter. *Families in Society, 73*, 588–595.

Williams, O. J., & Becker, R. L. (1994). Domestic partner abuse programs and cultural competence: The results of a national survey. *Violence and Victims, 9*, 287–296.

# 22

## Pathways to Prison

DEBORAH J. BURRIS-KITCHEN

**F**rom the beginning, the colonization of the New World has been about the killing, beating, raping, and exploiting of any people with whom Europeans came into contact. Whether it was the Spanish in South America or the English and others in North America, the New World was built on the backs of enslaved Native Americans and, with their near extermination, then enslaved people of color.

This chapter discusses these early injustices and examines the present use of laws to justify the continued human rights violations, enslavement, and disenfranchisement and incarceration of people of color in the United States today. This chapter draws upon Marxist and neo-Marxist theory, and from those perspectives recommendations for change that impact health are made.

## HISTORICAL OVERVIEW

Most Americans understand African history from a Eurocentric view in which Africans are backward, dark, and animalistic. This perspective justified their victimization, contending that African people were a subspecies of the human race who were no better than the average farm animal. Ignoring evidence to the contrary that documented great African nations, European Americans used the labor of these people to construct a successful agrarian economy in the southern colonies (of what was later to become the United States), which was responsible for the early economic success of the colonies and later the fledgling nation.

536

It does not appear that American colonists consciously began with a plan to enslave the African people. It was much more cost-effective to use the indigenous natives. Rather, the introduction and spread of smallpox and other diseases to which Native American tribes were totally vulnerable so devastated the original inhabitants of the New World that colonists turned, out of economic necessity, to Africa to identify a labor force able to withstand the heat, humidity, and harsh conditions associated with raising first sugar cane and later tobacco and cotton.

Trading voyages from the New World to the African coast in the 1500s provided more than a chance to exchange economic goods. It afforded the opportunity to rationalize the capture, enslavement, and exportation of African people. From a Eurocentric perspective, Black stood for everything that was the exact opposite of White. European colonists viewed their dress, language, and morals as superior to those of the African people, who were savages in the same fashion as the Native American Indians (Takaki, 1994). English Christian leaders connected the slavery of the African people to the biblical curse of Ham and linked slavery to skin color (Parrillo, 1997). Christianity, the religion of European colonists, not only legitimized their "crusade" of spreading salvation but had resolved, centuries earlier, any possible moral dilemma over enslavement in favor of the Europeans. The stage was thus set for the brutal treatment of the African people that followed.

The legal exportation of slaves from Africa lasted from 1619 until 1808. Conditions were brutal, degrading, demoralizing, oppressive, and deadly. Slaves were shackled, packed into ships, and brought to North America. Many chose to end their lives by leaping into the sea rather than be enslaved. Newly delivered babies were ripped from their slave mothers' arms and cast overboard. Many slaves died of disease and starvation on these hell ships, with upward of 14% perishing before landing. Scholars of the slave trade have estimated that anywhere from 14 to 23% of slaves died in transport. However, these historians omitted the number of deaths that occurred during slave revolts, in port areas, and the lives lost to disease. They also did not have an accurate count of those who died in confinement while waiting to be sold (McMillin, 2004). Thus, the actual number of Africans who died in transit is likely much higher. The price captured Africans paid for escaping, or being aggressive toward their oppressor, was costly. They were beaten, lynched, or shot.

## Instituting Legal Disparity

As early as the 1600s, laws distinguished people of color from Whites to their detriment. For example, in the 1630s, laws were established prohibiting miscegenation and removing the previous property rights of Black slaves. "In 1699 Virginia became the first colony to declare that it was not a crime to kill an unruly slave in the ordinary course of punishment" (Davis & Mintz, 1998, p. 57). These and other acts contributed to a belief in the slave as property among White males in America, even those who entered this country as indentured servants themselves.

By 1704 the commitment to slavery was strong among southern landowners, with more than 10,000 Blacks enslaved in Virginia alone (Davis & Mintz, 1998).

Following the American Revolution, many White Americans were forced to rethink the consequences and humanity of slavery. Many states enacted emancipation laws, beginning with Vermont in 1777, followed by Pennsylvania in 1780 and Massachusetts, Connecticut, and Rhode Island soon thereafter. Although Thomas Jefferson proposed to exclude slavery from developing in the western territories after the 1800s, his wishes were not fulfilled (Davis & Mintz, 1998). Rather, the Missouri Compromise and other acts merely postponed the inevitable conflict between the promise in the Declaration of Independence and the reality of a nation that legally permitted slavery.

With the ratification of the Thirteenth Amendment to the U.S. Constitution, slavery was officially abolished. The Constitution stated that "neither slavery nor involuntary servitude, except as punishment for a crime whereof the party shall be duly convicted, shall exist within the United States, or any place subject to their jurisdiction" (Willoughby, 1910, p. 848). For the creative miscreant embracing neither the meaning nor the spirit of this act, this language permitted many Blacks to be found guilty of crimes by White legal authorities and returned to plantations as laborers to work off their fine for their criminal conviction. Not surprisingly, these Blacks were not afforded either due process or a jury of their peers. This behavior went unchallenged and unchanged until the 1964 Jury Selection Act was passed.

As this example suggests, the resolution of the conflict between a nation that simultaneously embraced individual freedom and permitted slavery was no assurance that people of color would be admitted into the clubhouse. Indeed, following the Civil War, proposals were put forth to establish a separate African reservation modeled after the nation's success with Native American reservations. Another proposal was the exportation of Africans to Africa, specifically Liberia, which was established for this very purpose. Neither proposal succeeded, and with both southerner and northerner fearful of miscegenation it was inevitable that

> groups who were anti-slavery and those who were pro-slavery both viewed the newly freed African-Americans as inferior to Whites. Reformers believed that the degradation, social and economic conditions of Blacks were a result of their own paucity. Slaves equaled Blackness; convicts also equaled slaves. Therefore the connection between slavery and Blackness became easily translated to an idea of Black criminality. The free African American population became more than just troublesome, they became dangerous; and dangerous people need to be imprisoned which became Whites' ultimate solution of what to do with free Blacks. (McIntyre, 1993, pp. 161–162)

By the turn of the 21st century, criminality was attached not just to an individual but to an entire race of people. The increased incarceration rates of Black males from 1972 to the present (> 1.3 million men in prison by the end of the 20th century) has led some researchers to claim that prison time has become a normal part of life for young Black males (Freeman, 1996; Irwin & Austin, 1997).

The ending of slavery was not the end of oppression, discrimination, and violence committed against Blacks in this country. A bit more than half century after *Brown v. the Board of Education of Topeka* (1954), many children of the South continue to be provided with an inferior education. Adults are still denied jobs and the opportunity to own property and businesses. Because of the history of legal segregation in the South, many Blacks fled to the North in hopes of economic prosperity and equal treatment, only to find that northern Whites were fearful of Blacks taking their jobs, thus decreasing the power of their newly founded labor unions. In the North, Blacks were, and still are, denied jobs, the opportunity to join unions, and the acquisition of loans and property. Racial segregation, criminalization, unemployment, and poverty quickly became a serious problem for Blacks in the North as well as in the South (Takaki, 1994).

## BIOLOGICAL/GENETIC FACTORS AND CRIMINAL BEHAVIOR

Explanations to account for the differences between the races are as old as the recognition that people differ in appearance. These pseudoscientific fantasy excursions have provided justifications for the momentarily powerful to exert their will over others. As the explanatory power of phrenology, facial characteristics, and body type fell into disfavor, the new science of DNA analysis reveals:

> There are more DNA variants among people of Africa than there are among peoples with recent ancestry from other continents, so two unrelated Black Africans or African Americans are less likely to possess genetic similarity than two people of other races. Yet, outside of Africa Blacks are frequently treated as a homogeneous group in a broad variety of social and scientific contexts. ... Blacks have the most internal genetic variation of any racialized population group yet are most likely to be treated as if they were genetically homogeneous. (Ossorio & Duster, 2005, p. 122)

The idea of criminal behavior being attached to skin color is not a new concept. Since the early works of Cesare Lombroso's (1876/2006) *Criminal Man*, physicians and other scientists have tried to tie together genetics and crime. Lombroso, an Italian physician coming out of the tradition of Darwin's theory of evolution, believed that the criminal man had a stigma related to being an atavistic criminal, a throwback to Neanderthal man. These born criminals could be identified by their excessive arm length; kinky, rough-textured hair; a flat, receding ape-like chin; swollen and protruding lips; large deep-set eyes; and excessive dimensions of cheekbones and jaw. Lombroso concluded that "many of the characteristics found in savages, and among the coloured races, are also to be found in habitual delinquents" (Lombroso, cited in Beirne & Messerschmidt, 2000, p. 77).

Klaatsch (1911), as cited in Bonger (1943/1969), took a position similar to Lombroso. He claimed that Europe was inhabited by two distinct racial categories: "the Aurignac and the Neanderthal" (Bonger, 1943/1969, p. 20). Klaatsch claimed that the descendants of the Neanderthal man were still living and the nature of the Neanderthal man was rough, whereas the nature of the Aurignac was noble. The Neanderthal was attached to populations of people who were descendents of Africa while the Aurignac's were descendants of Europe (Bonger, 1943/1969, p. 20).

These early biological explanations of criminal behavior were built on fatally flawed data gathered from convicted and incarcerated individuals. For example, Lombroso's autopsies were performed only on people who died while in prison. Lombroso assumed that those who were incarcerated were the most prone to criminality. However, scholars like Du Bois recognized early the error in this assumption. Justice has been blind to neither color nor economic status. Those who are the wealthiest experience the most leniency in the judicial system (e.g., diversion, parole) and, therefore, are the least likely to be incarcerated (Du Bois, 1903).

Today's scholars recognize that physical characteristics do not predict criminal behavior. Instead, it is influenced by socioeconomic position, educational attainment, mental capacity, social bonding, and other social and environmental conditions.

How is it, then, that race is used as an explanation for criminal behavior within mainstream American society? For African Americans who feel apart from that "mainstream," race is simply a way of profiling and justifying the overrepresentation of people of color in America's prisons. For people of color, race continues to matter when it comes to definitions of crime, profiling, and the criminal (Mann, 1993; Russell, 1998; Tonry, 1995; Walker, Sphon, & Delone, 2004).

Race matters when trying to understand racial distributions of crime and incarceration. Physical characteristics are still being used to identify racial categories and are continually used to criminalize those who fit the original description of Lombroso's "criminal man." "Race is a complex but empirically demonstrable stratifying practice that creates identity and hierarchy through social interaction" (Ossorio & Duster, 2005, p. 124). The reality is that societies that have significant racial stratification patterns also have visible social consequences that have led to the acceptance of many blatantly racist biological explanations for the alleged differences in criminal behavior by race. Unfortunately, "the practice of creating social hierarchy based on perceived race has deep and pervasive historical roots; racial stratification has been a significant aspect of the U.S. social and political landscape since this country's inception" (Ossorio & Duster, 2005, p. 125).

While the head bumps of phrenologists are relegated to the shelves of obscurity, the new darling of science DNA analysis bears careful watching lest it be misused to perpetuate the errors of the past. Fortunately, the theories of the late

19th century that attempted to explain crime by identifying similar physical characteristics of those who were in prison have been exposed for their blatant statements of European superiority and their unethical and unscientific methodological approaches (Du Bois, 1903; Siegel, 2008). To change the way people think about who and what is criminal will require persistent vigilance in the monitoring of the political and social constructs of American society.

Currently, the mapping of human DNA is used to link particular genotypes with risk for diseases like alcoholism. For African Americans, it is not a great leap of the imagination to assume that soon claims will be made linking genotypes with the risk for violent criminal behavior, like homicide, rape, aggravated assault, and robbery. Indeed, according to Ossorio and Duster (2005), correlating genotypes and violent criminal behavior took less than 30 months. DNA dragnets were used to round up a serial killer in San Diego, California, in addition to a serial rapist and a murder suspect in Ann Arbor, Michigan. DNA samples, like searches for illegal drugs, will include a disproportionate amount of samples from African Americans because they are arrested more frequently than Whites for similar offenses. This will lead many in the general public and those working within criminal justice agencies to conclude that if there are more DNA samples collected from African Americans, and more hits made from those samples, then Blacks must be more criminal.

Race will continue to have an impact on the physical and mental health of African Americans as well as their socioeconomic and political status, thus leaving many African Americans vulnerable to the racially stratified criminal justice system. Crime is especially seductive to study in the early 21st century thanks to the many current television dramas, such as *CSI*, *Cold Case*, and *Bones*, that have popularized investigative forensics. However, when the assumption that race is the primary predictor of criminal behavior becomes the norm, the social consensus is to get tough on African Americans through increased incarceration trends, resulting in a negative impact on the next generation of African Americans. "Like the phrenology of the 19th century, findings of genetic markers that correlate with criminalized behavior will likely be only that—correlations and not explanations of causes of violence or crime" (Ossorio & Duster, 2005, p. 121).

## INDIVIDUAL RISK FACTORS AND CRIMINAL BEHAVIOR

Alone, genetic and biological risk factors for involvement in criminal behavior have been critiqued as racist and inadequate for explaining crime. Rather, a multitude of circumstances interact to place a person at varying degrees of risk for engaging in criminal behavior. Biological and personality characteristics interact with parental control and guidance, peer pressure and influence, school achievement, and the neighborhood to influence a person's behavior (Siegel, 2008).

For example, consider the role malnutrition can play in antisocial behavior. Young children who maintain a healthy diet are more likely to experience normal brain development and functioning. A poor diet can lead to chemical imbalances, which can contribute to learning disabilities and antisocial behavior (Siegel, 2008). Poverty is the primary predictor of malnutrition and blood sugar disorders and is a problem that plagues the Black community. Whereas in 2005 the poverty rate for Whites was 8.6%, the rate for Black families and individuals was 23.8%. Even more shocking are poverty statistics for single-parent, female-led households: 19.9% for Whites versus 34.6% for Blacks (DeNavas-Walt, Proctor, & Smith, 2008).

Nutritional imbalances can lead to early problem behavior, especially when blood sugar levels fall below that necessary for the brain to function normally. Diane Fishbein (2000) correlated low blood sugar levels to high rates of violence. Other researchers have found a relationship between blood sugar level and antisocial behavior, including violence (Virkkunen, 1986; Yaryura-Tobias & Neziroglu, 1975).

ADHD has been linked not only to bullying, stubbornness, and aggression but also to school failure. Low intelligence and poor school performance are risk indicators for involvement in the criminal justice system. For African Americans, 79.2% of those older than age 25 have completed high school compared with 88.7% of their White counterparts (Muhammad, Davis, Lui, & Leondar-Wright, 2004). Intelligence is assessed through IQ tests, which only measure the amount of knowledge that has been taught, not what can be learned. We continue to segregate schools across social class and racial lines, thus isolating the poor and minorities into schools that are understaffed and underfunded. The conditions of these schools are horrible. Students are treated as criminals from the beginning and are monitored by surveillance cameras and metal detectors. In the classroom, teachers arrive late, and resources in the classrooms and libraries are inadequate (Carr, Gray, & Holley, 2007; Kozol, 1991).

Foucault (1995), in *Discipline and Punish: The Birth of the Prison*, draws similarities between prisons and schools, suggesting that racially segregated schools serving the poor function to prepare their students for prison life. Seeing how one in three African American males born in 2000 will be under some form of correctional control within the next 10 years, the assumption of state and federal legislators as well as elementary and secondary education staff is that we must not invest our time and money into lower income schools and students because they are on their way to prison anyway. The message to the students in these segregated and impoverished schools is that they are not in school to learn but rather are being warehoused until they enter the prison system (Burris-Kitchen, 2002).

Poor children are also impacted more often by the numerous environmental contaminants that can impact the ability of youth to think and behave rationally. These dangerous chemicals include nitrogen dioxide, chlorine, inorganic gases, copper, cadimium, and mercury. There is evidence that exposure to these chemicals can lead to violent and antisocial behavior. For example, lead poisoning has been linked to male delinquency (Dumont, 2000). Deborah Denno (1993) studied the cases of more than 900 African American juvenile delinquents and reported that lead poisoning was the most common factor among these youth. Harmful exposure to environmental contaminants is prevalent among the poor, especially minority youth, who often live in older houses with lead paint and in heavily congested traffic areas, thus being exposed to unsafe levels of carbon monoxide (see Table 22.1.)

## FAMILY FACTORS AND CRIME

Several family factors are predictors of incarceration, among them a lack of supervision by parents, lack of positive role models in the family and community, physical or sexual abuse by a family member, inconsistent or lack of discipline, family size, and family conflict (McCarthy, Laing, & Walker, 2004). However, the most important indicator of a future in crime and the future incarceration is having a parent who is incarcerated. There are more than 2 million children with one or more parents in prison (Wright & Seymour, 2000), an increase from 500,000 in 1991. The greater use of incarceration as a form of punishment politically, socially, and economically impacts the future of not only the children of inmates but also the community as a whole and Blacks more than Whites (Mumola, 2000; see Table 22.2). Almost 800,000 African American children will be without at least one parent for an average of 6½ years if the parent is serving time in a state prison or for more than 8 years if the parent is in a federal facility. Greater than 60% of

**TABLE 22.1. Percentage of Children Living in Counties in Which Air Quality Standards Were Exceeded, by Race/Ethnicity, 2004**

|  | All races/ ethnicities | White non-Hispanic | Black non-Hispanic | American Indian/Alaska Native non-Hispanic | Asian or Pacific Islander non-Hispanic | Hispanic |
|---|---|---|---|---|---|---|
| Ozone 8-hour standard | 41% | 33% | 45% | 17% | 50% | 61% |
| PM-10 | 6.7% | 5.2% | 6.9% | 8.2% | 4.9% | 11% |
| PM-2.5 | 16% | 11% | 22% | 5.6% | 19% | 26% |
| Carbon monoxide | 0.071% | 0.026% | 0.0072% | 0.070% | 0.025% | 0.27% |
| Lead | 0.0% | 0.0% | 0.0% | 0.0% | 0.0% | 0.0% |
| Sulfur dioxide | 0.0% | 0.0% | 0.0% | 0.0% | 0.0% | 0.0% |
| Nitrogen dioxide | 0.0% | 0.0% | 0.0% | 0.0% | 0.0% | 0.0% |
| Any standard | 46% | 37% | 52% | 22% | 53% | 66% |

*Note.* Data from U.S. Environmental Protection Agency, Office of Air and Radiation, Aerometric Information Retrieval System (2004).

**TABLE 22.2. Number of Minor Children in the U.S. Population with a Parent in Prison**

| | | |
|---|---|---|
| Black | 1,017,429 | 6.7% |
| White | 136,668 | 0.9% |
| Hispanic | 364,448 | 2.4% |
| Total | 1,518,545 | 2.3% |

*Note.* Children were assumed to have the same race/ethnicity as the incarcerated parent. Data from DeNavas et al. (2005).

these children's parents are imprisoned in facilities more than 100 miles from home (DeNavas-Walt, Proctor, & Lee, 2005).

Incarcerated parents are overwhelmingly male (93%) and in prison for non-violent offenses. About 14% have some mental deficiency, and greater than 70% did not have a high school diploma at the time of arrest. More than half of mothers in prison were unemployed at the time of arrest and 27% of fathers reported being unemployed. However, of those who were employed at the time of their arrest, only 46% reported incomes of at least $1,000 per month (DeNavas-Walt et al., 2005).

Not only is the incarceration of Black males and females devastating politically, economically, and socially to the children and community, but it is destructive to the health of the Black family as well (Arias, 2007). The increase in the incarceration rates of both Black males and females is associated with a rise in the number of their children who will end up in the juvenile justice system and eventually, like their parents, in an adult penal facility. For those who escape the inevitable chains of prison, their lives will be plagued with poverty and poor health.

> Increasing rates of drug arrest have led to prison overcrowding and more inmates with chronic and infectious diseases such as HIV, tuberculosis, hepatitis, which have overwhelmed the prison health system. Many inmates also go untreated for mental illnesses such as schizophrenia, anxiety disorder, post-traumatic stress disorder and depression. (Arias, 2007, p. 6)

It is important to understand that the majority of these parents will eventually be released from prison, and their poor health, lack of health care, lack of employable skills, and blatant employment discrimination against them (male or female) because of their criminal record will have a lasting, devastating effect on the other members of the community into which they are released. This impact will be felt most by the children of these ex-felons. The pain of social and physical death of these ex-inmates will be inflicted upon the innocent children of the community as a result of continued poverty, which is exacerbated by health care costs (Arias, 2007).

Poverty and powerlessness escalate physical and emotional abuse of children by parents. Whether it is a two-income or a one-income family, frustration resulting from the inability to provide adequately for one's children may lead to abuse. More than 70% of Black children are born to single mothers, who are more likely to be poor than mothers who are married. "The truth is that we are now a two-family nation, separate and unequal—one thriving and intact, and the other struggling, broken, and far too often African-American" (Hymowitz, 2005, p. 1). Poverty and fatherlessness correlate with high levels of child abuse and juvenile delinquency, joblessness, school failure, delinquency, and familial abuse (Hymowitz, 2005). The Children's Defense Fund (CDF) announced in 2004 that "it is morally and economically indefensible that a Black preschool child is three times as likely to depend solely on a mother's earnings." The CDF claimed that this is a case for natural disaster relief (Hymowitz, 2005). Recently, the trend has been to force mothers to raise their children without any government support. New welfare reforms and cutbacks have forced many women out of the house and into one (or multiple) minimum-wage jobs, leaving their children unsupervised. Many single mothers used to have access to Aid to Families with Dependent Children, but with the passage of welfare reform legislation by the Clinton administration in 1996, many recipients who were able to raise their children at home were now forced to join the working poor (Beirne & Messerschmidt, 2000).

Although poverty has been linked with child abuse and neglect, these findings may be due to disparities in reporting. Some people's lives are more private than others. Poor people cannot hide from the police or child protective services as easily as the wealthy. Nonetheless, neglect and abuse have a greater impact on the prediction of future criminal behavior among children from lower socioeconomic status families compared with those from higher income communities. It is possible that children from the middle and upper classes may have more positive role models than those living in economically and socially poor communities. Their abuse and neglect do not predict a future of street crime in the same way that the abuse and neglect impact children from poorer communities, because there are adults in the community who can offset the negative of abuse. In predominantly single-parent, low-income neighborhoods, positive role models may be limited in presence and influence (Currie & Tekin, 2004).

According to Currie and Tekin (2004), a future of crime was more predictable for neglected males and did not impact females with the same outcomes, such as an arrest for assault and a conviction. The more serious the abuse experienced by the child, the more likely that the abused male would become engaged in criminal activity, especially if the child came from a low-income community. They also noted higher reports of abuse from lower income communities. According to Shaffer and Ruback (2002), the higher the rates of violent victimization, the higher the probability of violent offending: "Violent victimization is indeed a warning signal for future violent offending among juveniles. Protecting juveniles against violent victimization may, therefore, reduce overall levels of juvenile violence" (p. 1).

Studies of incarcerated women have reported that high rates of victimization can lead to a significant risk of these women becoming perpetrators themselves. Many women in prison had experienced physical and sexual abuses throughout most of their lives, and within this population those who had been sexually abused had the highest rates of sexual revictimization: Once victims within the criminal justice system, these women are now defendants. Because of social class and racial discrimination, poor women, primarily those of color, are overrepresented as defendants in the criminal justice system. Drug enforcement in poor communities often leads to prison time and long sentences for women who are poor, undereducated, underemployed, and unemployed, most of whom are Black. "We need to document the extent of race, gender and class entrapment by abusers, laws, social policies and enforcement practices. The movement to end violence against women needs the leadership and expertise of women who experience criminalization, entrapment and enforcement abuse" (Gilfus, 2002, p. 7). Women under the supervision of state and federal departments of corrections are the most impoverished and violated population yet. They have no rights, no resources, and no advocates (Gilfus, 2002).

According to the Bureau of Justice Statistics (BJS), there are more than 65,600 mothers at midyear 2007 in the custody of the criminal justice system; at year-end, 987,427 mothers (DeNavas-Walt et al., 2008). Since 1986 the rate at which women are incarcerated has increased 400% and for women of color, in particular, 800%. Women of color make up almost 40% of the female prison population. This increase has impacted the lives of over 1.5 million children; "65% of women in state prisons were parents of minor children" (BJS, The Sentencing Project, 2008). Greater than 25% of these women have a history of mental illness, and more than 50% have been victims of sexual or physical abuse. Many of the children of these incarcerated mothers are between 7 and 12 years of age when their mother is arrested.

> As a result of their parents' incarceration, these children experience tremendous amounts of trauma, anxiety, guilt, shame, and fear. As children enter adolescence, their suffering frequently manifests itself in poor academic achievement, juvenile delinquency, gang involvement, violence and, eventually, adult criminal behavior—the final link in an intergenerational cycle of criminal justice involvement. (Women's Prison Association, 1995, p. 3)

Child maltreatment increases the likelihood that these children will enter a life of crime; the risk is greater for males than females and increases with greater severity of abuse. Lack of parental supervision and having an imprisoned parent increases a child's risk of becoming a career criminal and being incarcerated as an adult. Race and social class are predictors of a lack of parental supervision as well as the likelihood of a parent being under the watch of the criminal justice system (Currie & Tekin, 2004).

## SOCIAL AND COMMUNITY FACTORS AND CRIME

Several social and community factors can influence criminal behavior; among them poverty, racial composition of the community, quality of housing, community crime rates, level of community and family violence, transitions and mobility, laws and norms, and community disorganization. Poverty and race are the most significant predictors of substandard housing, crime, violence, mobility, legal sanctioning, and identification of a community as socially disorganized. As so eloquently expressed by Dr. Martin Luther King, Jr., in his sermon at the National Cathedral in Washington, DC, on March 31, 1968, "There is nothing new about poverty. What is new is that we now have the techniques and the resources to get rid of poverty. The real question is whether we will."

The Black community continues to pay a high price for America's history of racism and oppression. Although the rates of homicide, poverty, school dropout, homelessness, infant mortality, and crime still plague the Black community, at no time had their suffering been brought to the forefront of national consciousness as it was from the 1950s to the 1970s. This could not have been a scarier time for White men in power. America had seen the most violent riots break out in their urban centers, violence the likes of which had been unmatched in this country since the Civil War.

> Panthers—Black Marxists and fully armed—stormed the California state capitol. In Newark, Watts, and Chicago, Black people shot back at cops and National Guardsmen; in Detroit, transplanted urban hillbillies joined African American snipers. In New Mexico, armed Chicanos fired on a county court house, trying to kill the sheriff. Chants of Black Power, Brown Power, and Red Power rose from all quarters. Gay men, routinely pilloried as sissies, were knocking out cops during the pitched battles following a police raid on the Stonewall bar in New York City. Meanwhile, women burnt bras and more importantly, filed suits, protested against discrimination, and won the right to reproductive choice. (Parenti, 1999, p. 3)

These violent protests led to changes in both the North and South. Finally, segregation was seen as harmful, and civil rights legislation was passed to help enforce compliance to the fourth, sixth, eighth, fourteenth, and nineteenth Amendments to the U.S. Constitution. The introduction of the twenty-fourth Amendment in 1964, which ended the enforcement of a poll tax that had to be paid in order to be eligible to vote in any election, civil rights legislation of 1964, and the Voting Rights Act of 1965 were victories for women, Blacks, Latinos, Native Americans, Asians, and gays, but it was also a time of confusion for both Whites and Blacks (Lusane, 1991).

White political leaders felt threatened by the newly awarded political and economic power guaranteed to Blacks under the new amendments to the U.S. Constitution. The ending of long-time legal segregation and discrimination meant that White politicians, business leaders, and admission officers at universities would have to open their doors and minds to allow Blacks and women equal opportunities to compete in business, politics, and education. Many White males saw this as a threat to their firmly established White male networking, which allowed for them to progress economically and politically, with little competition from women and people of color; this threat led to a reevaluation of the situation at hand. Where do we go from here? The solution to maintaining economic and political control by the White dominate class would be a war on drugs. The war on drugs had worked effectively in the past, and so it would work again.

Waging a war against drugs, and targeting minorities and poor people as the enemies in this war, is nothing new. The criminalization of people of color is the direct result of the European colonial belief that these drugs affect people of color differently than Whites. This takes the White man's fear of darkness to a whole new level of legitimization made manifest in enslavement and violence against the Black man and woman. This time it appears that incarceration and isolation are necessary evils to protect the rest of society from falling victim to Black male innate rage, which is often believed to be exacerbated by drug use (McIntyre, 1993).

Race has always been at the forefront of discussions involving the enforcement and enactment of drug-related laws. In 1910, President Roosevelt appointed Hamilton Wright to investigate the effects of opium in order to convince the United States and other nations to stop the opium trade with Asia. This report is noteworthy because it had exaggerated not only figures regarding opium use but also its impact on Blacks. Wright's report described, in detail, the supposed superhuman powers and extreme behavior experienced by Blacks after ingesting cocaine. Wright reinforced the myth of the oversexed Black male by reporting that Black men were more likely to rape while under the influence of cocaine. News articles like that written in the *New York Times* stated that sheriffs had switched from .32 caliber guns to .38 pistols to protect themselves from the superhuman Blacks on cocaine (Lusane, 1991; Parenti, 1999).

The war on drugs has always targeted poor and minority communities and especially the Black and Latino populations. Consider, for example, that during the Great Depression federal authorities decided to label a plant smoked by Mexican Americans for recreational purposes (marijuana) as a narcotic and encouraged an illegal state effort to repatriate an estimated 500,000 Mexican Americans, many of whom were not illegal immigrants but citizens of the United States (Novas, 1994)!

The war on drugs reached new heights when Nixon assumed presidency. Ironically, only a few years after the signing and implementation of civil rights legislation, a document promising rights and freedoms denied African Americans for more than 400 years in this country, the greatest violation against our constitutional democracy took place, that is, at least the greatest violation of democracy against Blacks since slavery.

Nixon's war on drugs was an attempt to destroy and incarcerate the Black race. He linked crime and drugs to the corrosive nature of rebellion in urban centers. For Nixon, "Crime meant urban, urban meant Black, and the war on crime meant a bulwark built against the increasingly political and vocal racial other by the predominantly White race" (Parenti, 1999, p. 7). Nixon established the Office of Drug Abuse and Law Enforcement, organized to wage a street-level attack on dealers in low-income Black neighborhoods where riots had recently occurred following the assassination of Martin Luther King, Jr. Nixon played on the fear of White Americans that Blacks were taking over, and that recently introduced social programs were handouts to lazy Blacks who just didn't want to work. At the same time, he encouraged the Federal Bureau of Investigation's war against the Black Panthers and urged the Internal Revenue Service to audit the Urban Black League (Parenti, 1999).

Reagan continued the war on the poor and Blacks with the same intensity as Nixon, but his effort took an economic turn. This economic crunch brought on by Reaganomics led to more drug use, higher unemployment, and a greater need for an informal economy. William Julius Wilson (1997) noted that urban poverty is an age-old problem, but massive joblessness is not. Joblessness leads to Blacks falling victim to social control efforts by the predominantly White criminal justice system; in short, joblessness leads to criminalization (Parenti, 1999; Wilson, 1997). By 1987, more than 2 million Americans were homeless. Reagan created a whole new population of poor and desperate Americans. His corporate welfare, coupled with the cutting of social welfare programs, devastated rural and urban populations alike (Eitzen & Baca Zinn, 2003).

Of course, with economic destruction, there is a need to increase law enforcement efforts to control the populations left desperate, hungry, and homeless. The 1984 crime bill was just what was needed for local and state police to wage an all-out war against street vendors. This bill established minimum sentencing, allowed federal judges to deny bail, eliminated federal parole, and tightened the sentencing policy for federal felonies committed with a firearm. This crime bill allowed for the forfeiture of assets, making it very profitable for local police departments to bust drug dealers. "Nationwide the gross receipts of all seizures shot from about $100 million in 1981 to over $1 billion by fiscal year 1987" (Parenti, 1999, p. 51).

The 1986 Anti-Drug Abuse Act was probably the most damaging to Black offenders. This bill called for a mandatory minimum sentence of 5 years for the illegal possession of 100 grams of heroin, 500 grams of cocaine, and a mere 5 grams of crack. In 1980 Blacks made up about 12% of the U.S. population and 23% of the prison population. With the passage of the 1986 Anti-Drug Abuse Act, by the late 1980s Blacks made up 40% of the prison population. Of those, 60% were charged with possession of narcotics. The war was fought against not just dealers but users as well. By the end of the 1980s, the government budget for narcotics control was more than $8 billion, and more than 1 million people were in prisons and jails (Lusane, 1991; Parenti, 1999). "Of the 265,000 state prison inmates serving time for drug offenses in 2002, 126,000 (47%) were Black, 61,700 (23.27%) were Hispanic, and 64,500 (24.33%) were White" (McVay, 2007). Disturbingly, Black males represent only 13% of drug users and 38% of drug arrests, yet they make up 59% of the convictions for drug-related offenses (Drug Policy Alliance Network, 2006).

The abuses of civil rights continued through the 1990s under the watch of the Clinton administration. The 1994 crime control bill put 100,000 more police officers on city streets and helped mayors across the country wage an all-out "ass-kicking" war against the poor and drug users. Police from New York to Los Angeles broke down doors to apartments, raided apartments without warrants, and fatally beat and shot innocent people who got in the way. Blacks and Latinos paid, and are still paying, the highest price for this war (Clear & Cole, 2006; Lusane, 1991; Parenti, 1999).

Neo-Marxist criminologists focus primarily on the economic power struggles between the bourgeoisie and the proletariat and view the class struggle as the root cause of socially constructed definitions of crime, including drug violations. These definitions of street crimes and property crimes as the most dangerous and only forms of crime benefit those in positions of power and stem primarily from the class struggle between those who own the means of production (those in power) and those who are workers (the exploited labor class). Neo-Marxists view "real" crime as violations against human rights. Such violations include racism, sexism, imperialism, and capitalism. Human rights violations (according to neo-Marxists) are the most harmful forms of crime to all members of society (Siegel, 2008).

Neo-Marxists further suggest that punishment is a mechanism used by the dominate group to control those populations who are unemployed or unemployable or who are considered the lumpenproletariat (the flotsam of society). These theories view racial disparities in punishment as a result of social class position. Those who are poor are more likely to be arrested, be detained at pretrial, receive a public defender as opposed to a private attorney, be found guilty by a jury, and receive harsher penalties when convicted of a crime (Humphries, 1981; Jacobs; 1978; Rusche & Kircheimer, 1939/1968; Spitzer, 1981; Wallace & Humphries, 1981). "In societies and communities characterized by rigid economic stratification and heavy urban concentration of poor, elites are likely to use the administration of criminal justice to enforce laws which preserve economic order" (Bridges & Crutchfield, 1988, p. 701).

Increases in the economic gap between the owning class and the working class lead to increased efforts to control the poor. These increases in enforcement efforts lead to increases in the imprisonment of the working class, which expands the gap between the workers and the owners.

> If an indicator of inequality that is most sensitive to the gap between the poor and middle-income recipients predicts imprisonment better than alternative measures, the threat posed by an expanding economic underclass becomes a

more credible explanation for increased incarceration rates. (Jacobs & Helms, 1996, p. 328)

In America there is an overrepresentation of people of color living below the poverty line and, therefore, they are overrepresented in the prison population.

"The Black community is suffering record rates of homicide, infant mortality, school dropout, AIDS infection, hunger and homelessness" (Lusane, 1991, p. 11). Poverty is a heart-wrenching reality many Blacks must face everyday, especially considering all the social problems that go along with being poor. Almost 37 million people live below the official poverty line in the United States (Greenberg, Dutta-Gupta, & Minoff, 2007). However, if we drew a more realistic poverty line, keeping regional differences and cost of medical care and housing in mind, the number of people living below poverty would be about 52 million, or almost 18% of the U.S. population (Burtless, Corbett, & Primus, 1997).

Many of the social problems faced in inner-city Black communities are the result of the 1980s and 1990s exodus from these communities for the suburbs. As the middle class leaves, so do taxes and government-supported services. Urban disinvestment started with middle-class White abandonment of the city to suburbia following World War II. This "White flight" has increased racial and economic segregation. Crime and poverty grow in communities abandoned by people and businesses and without job opportunities. Race and crime become two words that mean the same thing for many Whites, including police officers. The shift from industrialized jobs to service work lowered the average wages and took away many benefits that came with unionized workers employed in industrialized jobs (Eitzen & Baca Zinn, 2003).

This job exodus hit the Black community the hardest. Blacks in inner cities had unemployment rates at least 50% higher than the national average (Eitzen & Baca Zinn, 2003). The kind of jobs left for low-skilled inner-city community residents are low-paying service work jobs that do not pay enough to pull them out of poverty. Although most Blacks are not poor or clustered in highly segregated communities, there are high concentrations of minorities in urban centers to the point where the media could use this concentration of people of color to socially construct an image of Blacks as solely urban and poor (Eitzen & Baca Zinn, 2003; Lusane, 1991).

## EVIDENCE-BASED TREATMENT INTERVENTIONS

The high concentrations of African Americans living in urban centers have left the Black population vulnerable to being labeled "drug addicts" and especially "crack heads." The flood of drugs that hit the Black and mostly impoverished communities during the late 1970s and 1980s has been called an attempt at Black genocide at the hands of a White racist society (Lusane, 1991; Parenti, 1999). At the end of the civil rights movement, Black unemployment was still twice as high as that of Whites. More than one-half of children born to single Black women were living in deep poverty. Basic needs were not, and still are not, being met in the Black community. As the Black power movement gained momentum, there was a sudden increase in the amount of illegal drugs that entered Black communities. One explanation is that poverty leads to a need to make money, which potentially leads to a need to sell drugs.

> Black people's need for money and consequent desire for psychological escape, exacerbated by the alienating and inequitable environment for poor communities, go a long way in explaining the drug crisis. That this situation would be exploited by those within and without these communities is not only a logical response under the capitalistic system, but a rational one. The structures and institutional mechanisms of capitalism, the systemic levers of racism accompanying it, are themselves explanation enough. (Lusane, 1991, pp. 13–14)

Economically on the margins and politically voiceless, Blacks and Latinos were the most likely to become victims of the war on drugs. Police are seven times more likely to arrest a Black male than a White male, and more than 30% of Black males between the ages of 18 and 24 are under the supervision of the criminal justice system (Muhammad et al., 2004).

The relationship between racism and the war on drugs is highlighted here as a necessary precursor to the prison crisis. The United States must figure out how to truly eliminate a racism that is so imbedded in our culture it allows not only Whites but Blacks as well to blame the Black community for the majority of drugs and crime. This is not reality but rather a myth.

As most of us know, it would be a difficult task to completely eliminate something as accepted as racial stereotyping in our society, but maybe we can address this reality that what we know leads to the overrepresentation of Blacks and Latinos in the criminal justice system.

First, we know that there is more police activity in communities with large populations of poor people of color. This behavior leads to more arrests by police simply because if they are looking for crime, they will find it. Alfred Blumstein (1993) has concluded that at least 24% of the racial disparities found within the criminal justice system are explained by racial bias and criminal histories. The other 67% of the disparities can be explained by the seriousness of the offense. Many criminologists have concluded that crime rates, policing practices, racial profiling, and sentencing legislation and practices lead to racial disparities in incarceration (Spohn & Holleran, 2000).

Once the decision is made to arrest someone and move them through the system, those in positions of power over the poor and criminalized have limited options as to how to help or penalize the person accused of a crime, especially a drug arrest.

For example, in pretrial release sentencing, it is important that the accused and convicted have a place to live with a steady job and a phone line. Most probation or early-release programs require electronic monitoring, which requires a home and a home telephone. For the very poor, this is not an option. Thus, they are sentenced to prison and are incarcerated longer.

Addiction treatment programs may be offered to those convicted of drug offenses; however, these programs are typically paid for by the accused. Before trial it may be advantageous to hire a psychologist and expert witnesses to prepare for a legal defense. These professionals are often not available to those who do not have money to pay for the services. Without money, the accused must be assigned a public defender, a disadvantage for poor people regardless of race: "Public defenders with high case loads may not be able to develop individualized alternative programs or sentencing options" (Schrantz & McElroy, 2000, p. 8).

Access to pretrial release is also important in the outcome of a trial. Whereas people with money can pay their bail or be released on their own recognizance, poor people will spend their days leading up to trial behind bars. When an inmate appears in court in a jail uniform, jurors may be more likely to assume the defendant's guilt (Schrantz & McElroy, 2000, p. 8).

It is the opinion of many that the leading cause of racial disparities in length of prison sentencing between Blacks and Whites has to do with legislation that has been passed over the last 30 years, primarily that regarding crack cocaine. This legislation has required minimum/maximum durations in prison for trafficking and possession charges, with most federal legislation mandating prison time for any felony conviction of possession with intent to sell crack. It has been obvious that law enforcement efforts have been targeting the Black community when it comes to arrest for possession of crack (Lusane, 1991; Parenti, 1999). The political fury over crack dealers has led to their increased housing in U.S., and especially federal, prisons. The latter were used to house primarily White-collar criminals and maximum security federal prisons, the most dangerous in our society. Now the majority of federal prison inmates are nonviolent drug offenders (Clear & Cole, 2006).

"As long as racism exists within society at large, it will be found within the criminal justice system. Racism fuels the overt bias which can show in language, attitude, conduct, assumptions, strategies and policies of criminal justice agencies" (Schrantz & McElroy, 2000, p. 10). It is important to guard against racism within the criminal justice system. Therefore, we must implement training programs and orientation programs for various cultures within every agency that has contact with the poor, people of color, and, importantly, those who are accused of criminal behavior. There must be a mechanism in place within each criminal justice institution that detects and corrects racial bias among criminal justice personnel (Schrantz & McElroy, 2000).

Keeping in mind that the ultimate goal is to eliminate racism altogether, there are other initiatives that may be effective in reducing the number of people in prison, especially those of color. First, criminal justice agencies must cooperate with leaders of minority communities to develop measures that will correct the racial injustices that exist in these communities. For example, police and community partnerships must intentionally be formed to develop positive relationships between poor communities of color and the predominantly White police officers who patrol those communities. Second, police and community leaders need to identify neighborhoods with high rates of arrest and work with community representatives to implement crime-reducing strategies. Third, it is important to study the impact of the "get-tough" policies on low-income neighborhoods of color. National and local leaders can investigate how these policies could be changed to reduce the impact of mandatory sentencing, for example. Finally, college professors need to incorporate into the curriculum of juris doctorate programs and policing programs courses that will sensitize students entering these professions to the issues and injustices that are a result of a racist society.

America is a drug-using culture, and it has a serious problem with the abuse of legal and illegal drugs (Clinard & Meier, 2008). According to Johnston, O'Malley, Bachman, and Schulenberg (2006), more than 50% of high school seniors have tried an illicit drug, 34% have smoked marijuana, 2% have tried LSD, 5% have used cocaine, and 0.8% have used heroin within the last year. Although we must encourage efforts to lower abuse and addiction in our country, Black genocide is not an option. Addiction should be seen as a national health issue, not the focus of our criminal justice system. Countries such as Canada and the Netherlands have been treating it as a medical issue for years, and their rates of addiction, use, and drug-related violence has declined. Additionally, both countries have seen a decrease in the number of people who have contracted AIDS as a result of free needle-exchange programs (Diamond, 1995; National Organization for the Reform of Marijuana Laws, 2003).

Treatment programs are the primary focus of countries that deal with drug use and addiction as a medical issue. Although many states in this country do offer treatment programs, the majority are paid for by the addict, penalizing those who cannot afford to receive this kind of help. Many who cannot afford treatment spend their time instead behind bars. For some inmates, treatment is available, but for many it is not (Clear & Cole, 2006; Clinard & Meier, 2008).

Available treatment programs include methadone maintenance for heroin addicts, which substitutes methadone for heroin and may or may not include counseling services, needle-exchange programs, and detoxification with counseling and/or halfway houses. The success of these programs varies, with recovery being an elusive and lifelong struggle for many (Clinard & Meier, 2008).

Treatment must be tailored to the individual seeking help for an addiction, and it must be available for the addict when the addict needs it. Most addicts are forced into treatment before they are ready to give up the addiction. The addict must be committed to treatment when it is being offered. The treatment must meet the multiple needs of the addict. Addiction can be fed by a combination of problems and stressors faced by the addict, for example, a family crisis, loss of a loved one, economic pressures, loss of a job, or work-related pressure. The treatment plans created for the individual addict must constantly be reviewed and revised based on his or her needs (National Institute on Drug Abuse, 2005).

Drug treatment is cost-effective when it comes to detouring and incarcerating drug offenders. According to the National Institute on Drug Abuse (2005), for every $1 spent on treatment programs, $4 to $7 are saved on drug-related crime. It should be noted that these savings do not take into consideration the costs related to lost productivity, health care for aging and health-failing addicts, and social services for the children of addicts.

Two other solutions to prison overpopulation, especially of African American inmates, are to improve school systems and reduce poverty. The poverty–crime connection was established earlier in this chapter; the education–crime correlation is just as significant. School suspensions have been used all too frequently over the past 25 years to decrease student violence, even though the data indicate that they are not effective. In fact, school suspensions typically lead to dropout, which, in turn, leads to increased interaction with the juvenile justice system, which eventually feeds the prison pipeline. Alternative school programming is one solution to counter high dropout rates and school failure. The objective of alternative schools is to increase the likelihood of youth graduation from high school, which, it is hoped, will be a protective factor against future involvement in the criminal justice system. Good programs offer after-school activities, leadership training, community service, and work skills and mentoring programs. Despite some successes, these programs must be implemented in conjunction with improvements in the sociopolitical environment (Weissman et al., 2005).

Urban poverty and school funding go hand in hand. Most of the poorest neighborhoods across the country have the least amount of funding and opportunities for their children. The lack of books and adequate supplies, transience of, teachers in the classroom, high student–teacher ratios, lack of funding for laboratories or advanced placement classes, and crumbling infrastructures render students ill equipped to learn. The conditions of these schools send the message to low-income families that education is not important. This, combined with the "police state" mentality found in many lower income schools, forms the perfect incubator for preparing these children for prison (Foucault, 1995; Kozol, 1991; Reiman, 2007).

We must develop a sense of safety in our schools and communities, reduce the impact of poverty, reduce racial stereotypes and the stigma of race, improve the quality of education, reduce addiction to illegal drugs, and keep children in school and keep them learning while they are there. We must "avoid the marginalization of the very students for whom education is the only ticket out of a lifetime of poverty and social problems" (Weissman et al., 2005, p. 13).

## MENTAL ILLNESS AND THE PATHWAY TO PRISON

The deinstitutionalization of mentally ill patients has led to their growing number among the prison population. Many prisons do not have the resources or skilled staff to help the mentally ill who are incarcerated in state and federal facilities.

More than one in six prisoners suffer from a mental illness. Often young people arrested for substance abuse are self-medicating for untreated mental health issues (Berkowitz, 2003). Many of the poor who are living without health benefits cannot afford the medical treatment they need, so they seek their drugs through the illegal market. In 2005 almost 47 million people were without health insurance: 14.1% of African Americans, 22.1% of Hispanics, and 11.4% of Asian children, and 7.3% of Whites (Johnson, 2008).

Illnesses that can promote self-medication through the use of illegal drugs include schizophrenia, bipolar disorder, and depression. Once arrested and incarcerated for possession of an illegal substance, most inmates do not receive adequate mental health or drug treatment services. The primary concern of the prison is punishment, not treatment:

> Over the past twenty years, the politics of lock-em-up-as-fast-as-possible became the anti-crime mantra of most politicians. Hundreds of thousands of victims of the "war on drugs" were imprisoned. As the rate of incarceration soared so did the prison population of mentally ill inmates. (Berkowitz, 2003, p. 2)

Prison can be a very brutal, dehumanizing place, especially for inmates with mental illnesses.

The cutting of state and federal dollars for mental health makes it even more difficult for inmates to receive the medical and psychological treatments they need. The dismantling of the U.S. mental health system has made it nearly impossible for the poor, and especially the incarcerated, to get help.

> We have to halt the heartless dismantling of the social safety net, including public mental health services. We have to end racism that's rampant in the criminal justice system. The Human Rights Watch report reminds us that prisoners are human beings, and we have a social responsibility to do something about their pain and suffering. (Berkowitz, 2003, p. 3)

## THE PREVENTION OF THE PATHWAY TO PRISON

W. E. B. Du Bois, as early as 1899, believed that the explanations for the overrepresentation of African Americans in the criminal justice system were obvious. He told his readers that African Americans were arrested for lesser offenses than Whites, spent more time behind bars once convicted, and were never given a trial to prove their guilt or innocence. He wrote, "The rich are always favored somewhat at the expense of the poor, the upper class at the expense of the unfortunate classes, and Whites at the expense of Negros" (p. 249). The unfairness of the criminal justice system based on race was so overt that even most Whites reported they felt that Blacks were treated unfairly by the criminal justice system. Unfortunately, these injustices are still present today, and race, especially when exacerbated by poverty, is still the primary predictor of a ticket to prison.

The political construction of the fear of the Black male in the United States is economic in origin. Jacobs and Helms (1996) suggest that as economic gaps widen between racial groups, danger is imminent. The risk of the minority predator rises as a result of rebellion against the exploitation and economic conditions of the group. Once the underclass starts challenging the position of the upper class, political and legal controls tighten, and ultimately so do the imprisonment rates of the lower class.

> The astronomical overrepresentation of Blacks in houses of penal confinement and the increasingly tight meshing of the hyperghetto with the carceral system suggest that, owing to America's adoption of mass incarceration as a queer social policy designed to discipline the poor and contain the dishonoured, lower-class African-Americans now dwell, not in a society with prisons as their White compatriots do, but in the *first genuine prison society* in history. (Wacquant, 2003, p. 201)

The social consequences of race and income on the overrepresentation of Blacks in prison are clear. Reducing the amount of economic disparity between Blacks and Whites and ending racism would be one obvious solution to address the issue of crime committed by racial minorities. It would also limit the racial disparities in sentencing and the amount of time served by Black males and females convicted of crimes. There also needs to be new policies to protect Blacks from racial profiling and discrimination once they enter the court system. In addition to eliminating racism and narrowing the economic gap between the rich and the poor in this country, real efforts to provide equal education to every American student, regardless of social class and skin color, must be made. Quality schools and commitment to educating our youth can lower dropout rates and ultimately decrease crime.

In addition to better schools and the elimination of racism and poverty, mental health issues must be addressed. There must be quality mental and physical health care available to all, regardless of race and social class. Finally, we need to revisit the impact of the injustice of drug laws that were put in place during the second half of the 20th century. Many of these laws are racist by design and fast-track young people of color to dead-end lives.

## RECOMMENDED BEST PRACTICES

Changes are necessary at the interpersonal, institutional, and structural levels. Interestingly, recommendations at the interpersonal level were promoted in a congressional report by Davis (2007–2008). This report advised several actions: drug treatment programs as alternatives to incarceration, substance abuse programs funded by grants and not by the offender, family-based treatment programs inside and outside the prison walls, improved educational and occupational skills for inmates during their incarceration, and career counseling for inmates upon release. It is evident that progressive approaches to the problem are known to others outside of the Black community. The question remains whether there is the will to enact them.

Schrantz and McElroy (2000) provide solid structural and institutional recommendations to reduce racial disparities. They include:

1. *For law enforcement*
   a. Develop community-policing approaches.
   b. Develop alternatives to arrest and incarceration.
   c. Develop educational programs on racial disparity for police departments and communities.

2. *For prosecutors*
   a. Examine the role of race in all cases.
   b. Collaborate with representatives from minority communities to identify the impact of a racially disparate criminal justice system.
   c. Examine the impact of drug policies (minimum and maximum sentencing) on minority communities.
   d. Engage in advocacy regarding racial disparities.
      • Take a position against historically racially biased legislation that leads to disparate treatment.
      • Develop pretrial release programs.
      • Incorporate race-related curricula into continuing education programs.
      • Encourage active recruitment of minorities into the legal profession.

3. *For the defense*
   a. Provide education on racial disparities in the criminal justice system and its impact on the Black family and community.
   b. Advocate for a more just and fair criminal justice system.
   c. Encourage more minorities to enter law school and become defense attorneys.

4. *For the judiciary*
   a. Provide sentencing options.
   b. Require pretrial reports from probation.
   c. Examine the role of racially based decision making at prior stages in the criminal justice process.
   d. Remain familiar with scholarly research on race relations.

5. *Incarceration*
   a. Be dedicated to addressing racial disparities in the prison system.
   b. Provide training for staff on racial sensitivity.
   c. Investigate racial disparities in parole release.
   d. Develop relationships with community-based organizations that pro-

vide alternatives to incarceration and with organizations that provide service for inmates reintegrating into the community.

   e. Develop race-based risk management skills for those in positions of leadership.

Most policing efforts focus on poor minority neighborhoods. Not surprisingly, there is a higher rate of arrest simply because the police are there and not elsewhere! Once a person of color is arrested, bail and pretrial release screenings are based on previous records, skin color, income, and quality of legal representation at the bail hearing. Many poor minorities are not released pretrial and spend their time in jail waiting for their court hearing. When a person appears for trial directly from a jail cell, it is assumed more often than not that he or she is guilty even before the case is heard before the court. These biases and injustices must be addressed if we are to reduce the overrepresentation of the poor and people of color in jails and prison.

Most drug laws are socially and racially biased. Consider the Anti-Drug Abuse Act of 1986, which required a mandatory minimum of 5-year sentences for possession of 5 grams of crack, 100 grams of heroin, and 500 grams of cocaine. The addition of the 1994 crime control bill, which put 100,000 more police officers on city streets, translated to a war on the Black community. Crack was seen as an inner-city Black drug of choice, and the police frequently searched for crack dealers and users in predominantly Black communities. After this policy was put into place, the criminal justice system saw a huge surge in the Black prison population, and for the first time in American history there were more nonviolent drug offenders in prison than violent offenders (Parenti, 1999).

Racial and social class bias in trial defense and sentencing must be corrected. The assignment of public counsel must take place before the arraignment of the case. There must be an available range of community-based program alternatives for those convicted. Sentencing a person in possession of 5 grams of crack cocaine to a mandatory 5-year prison sentence is not a solution to the U.S. drug problem, being akin to dropping a block-busting bomb to swat a single fly; it is an excessively large, costly overkill reaction. Instead, we need occupational training, educational opportunities, and drug treatment in place of prison terms. These approaches are not only less expensive but offer the real possibility that convicted individuals will rejoin society as taxpayers, not tax drainers. Finally, there needs to be a minority counsel serving as an overseer of the court jurisdiction to ensure that minority defendants have access to the same representation as their White counterparts (Schrantz & McElroy, 2000).

It is imperative that these criminal justice changes occur. Crime and poverty will continue to exist without an all-out effort to improve both the quality of education within our schools and the provision of living-wage jobs. If these actions are ignored, the gap between the rich and poor will widen even more. Law enforcement efforts to control the poor will increase. The prison population will continue to grow, and crime will continue to increase.

## REFERENCES

Arias, D. C. (2007, March 1). High rate of incarcerated Black men devastating to family health. *The Nation's Health*, p. 7. Retrieved January 1, 2010, from *www.donyacurrie. com/writing_samples/Donya_Currie_incarceration.doc*.

Beirne, P., & Messerschmidt, J. (2000). *Criminology* (2nd ed.). Boulder, CO: Westview Press.

Berkowitz, B. (2003, November 19). *Mad in the USA*. Retrieved January 1, 2010, from *www. prisonerlife.com/articles/articleID=51.cfm*.

Blumstein, A. (1993). Racial disproportionality of the U.S. prison population. *University of Colorado Law Review, 64*(3), 743–760.

Bonger, W. A. (1969). *Race and crime*. Montclair, NJ: Columbia University Press. (Original work published 1943)

Bridges, G., & Crutchfield, R. (1988). Law, social standing and racial disparities in imprisonment. *Social Forces, 66*(3), 699–724.

*Brown v. Board of Education of Topeka*, 347 U.S. 483 (1954).

Bureau of Justice Sentencing Project. (2007). Washington, DC: Bureau of Justice Statistics.

Burris-Kitchen, D. J. (2002). *Short rage: An autobiographical look at heightism in America*. Santa Barbara, CA: Fithian Press.

Burtless, G., Corbett, T., & Primus, W. (1997). *Improving the measurement of American poverty*. Washington, DC: Brookings Institution Press.

Carr, M. J., Gray, N. L., & Holley, M. J. (2007). Shortchanging disadvantaged students: An analysis of intra-district spending patterns in Ohio. *Journal of Educational Research and Policy Studies, 7*(1), 36–53.

Clear, T., & Cole, G. (2006). *American corrections* (7th ed.). Belmont, CA: Wadsworth.

Clinard, M. B., & Meier, R. (2008). *Sociology of deviant behavior* (13th ed.). Belmont, CA: Thomson/Wadsworth.

Currie, J., & Tekin, E. (2004). *Does juvenile delinquency cause crime?* Cambridge, MA: National Bureau of Economic Research.

Davis, D. (2007–2008). *Second Chance Act of 2007*. Retrieved April 9, 2008, from *www. govtrack.us/congress/bill.xpd?bill=h110-1593*.

Davis, D. B., & Mintz, S. (1998). *The boisterous sea of liberty*. New York: Oxford University Press.

DeNavas-Walt, C., Proctor, B. D., & Lee, C. H. (2005). *Income, poverty, and health insurance coverage in the United States: 2004*. Retrieved October 30, 2008, from *www.census.gov/prod/2005pubs/p60_229.pdf*.

Denno, D. (1993). Considering lead poisoning as a criminal defense. *Fordham Urban Law Journal, 20*, 377–400.

DeNavas-Walt, C., Proctor, B. D., & Smith, J. C. (2008). *Income, poverty, and health insurance coverage in the U.S.: 2007*. Retrieved October 30, 2008, from *www.census.gov/prod/2005pubs/p60-229.pdf*.

Diamond, J. (Executive Producer). (1995, April 6). *America's war on drugs* [Television broadcast]. New York: ABC Broadcasting.

Drug Policy and Alliance Network. (2006). Reason, compassion, justice. New York: Author. Retrieved October 30, 2008, from *www.drugpolicy.org/communites/race*

Du Bois, W. E. B. (1899). *The Philadelphia Negro: A social study*. Millwood, NY: Kraus-Thomson Organization.

Du Bois, W. E. B. (Ed.). (1903). *Proceedings of the eighth conference for the study of Negro Problems*. Atlanta, GA: Atlanta University.

Dumont, M. P. (2000). Lead, mental health and social action: A view from the bridge. *Public Health Reports, 115*(6), 505–510.

Eitzen, D. S., & Baca Zinn, M. (2003). *Social problems* (9th ed.). Boston: Allyn & Bacon.

Fishbein, D. (2000). Neuropsychological function, drug abuse, and violence: A conceptual framework. *Criminal Justice and Behavior, 27*, 139–159.

Foucault, M. (1995). *Discipline & punish: The birth of the prison*. New York: Vintage Books.

Freeman, R. B. (1996). Why do so many young American men commit crimes and what might we do about it? *Journal of Economic Perspectives, 10*, 25–42.

Gilfus, M. (2002). *Women's experiences of abuse as a risk factor for incarceration*. Harrisburg, PA: National Resource Center on Domestic Violence. Retrieved January 1, 2010, from *new.vawnet.org/category/Main_Doc.php?docid=412*.

Glaze, L., & Boncazar, T. (2007). *Probation and parole in the United States, 2007*. Washington, DC: Bureau of Justice Statistics.

Greenberg, M., Dutta-Gupta, I., & Minoff, E. (2007). *From poverty to propensity: A national strategy to cut poverty*. Washington, DC: Center for American Progress.

Humphries, D. (1981). The dialectics of crime control. In D. Greenberg (Ed.), *Crime and capitalism* (pp. 209–255). Palo Alto, CA: Mayfield.

Hymowitz, K. S. (2005, Summer). The Black family: 40 years of lies. *City Journal*. Retrieved January 1, 2010, from *www.city-journal.org/html/15_3_Black_family.html*.

Irwin, J. J., & Austin, J. (1997). *It's about time: America's imprisonment binge* (2nd ed.). Belmont, CA: Wadsworth.

Jacobs, D. (1978). Inequality and the legal order: An ecological test of the conflict model. *Social Problems, 25*, 515–525.

Jacobs, D., & Helms, R. (1996). Toward a political model of incarceration: A time-series examination of multiple explanations for prison admission rates. *American Journal of Sociology, 102*(2), 323–357.

Johnson, T. D. (2008). *Census Bureau: Number of U.S. uninsured rises to 47 million: Almost 5% increase since 2005*. Retrieved October, 30, 2008, from *www.medscape.com/view-article/567737*.

Johnston, L. D., O'Malley, P., Bachman, J. G., & Schulenberg, J. E. (2006). *Monitoring the future. National results on adolescent drug use*. Bethesda, MD: National Institute of Drug Abuse.

Kozol, J. (1991). *Savage inequalities: Children in America's schools*. New York: Harper Perennial.

Lombroso, C. (2006). *Criminal man*. Durham, NC: Duke University Press. (Original work published 1876)

Lusane, C. (1991). *Pipe dream blues: Racism and the war on drugs*. Boston: South End Press.

Mann, C. R. (1993). *Unequal justice: A question of color*. Bloomington: Indiana University Press.

McCarthy, C., Laing, K., & Walker, J. (2004). *Offenders of the future?: Assessing the risk of children and young people becoming involved in criminal or antisocial behaviour.*

Newcastle, UK: Newcastle Centre for Family Studies, University of Newcastle upon Tyne.

McIntyre, C. L. (1992). *Criminalizing a race: Free Blacks during slavery.* Queens, NY: Kayode Publications.

McMillin, J. (2004). *The final victims: Foreign slave trade to north America, 1783–1810.* Columbia: University of South Carolina Press.

McVay, D. (Ed.). (2007). *Drug war facts* (6th ed.). Retrieved on October 30, 2008, from *www.drugwarfacts.org/cms.*

Muhammad, D., Davis, A., Lui, M., & Leondar-Wright, B. (2004). *The state of the dream: Enduring disparities in Black and White.* Boston: United for a Fair Economy.

Mumola, C. (2000). *Incarcerated parents and their children. Bureau of Justice Statistics Special Report.* Washington, DC: U.S. Department of Justice.

National Institute on Drug Abuse. (2005). *Principles of drug addiction treatment.* Washington, DC: National Institute on Drug Abuse and National Institute of Health.

National Organization for the Reform of Marijuana Laws. (2003). *European drug policy: 2002 Legislative update.* Washington, DC: Author. Retrieved January 1, 2010, from *norml.org/index.cfm?Group_ID=5446.*

Novas, H. (1994). *Don't look back.* New York: Muze Inc.

Ossorio, P., & Duster, T. (2005). Race and genetics: Controversies in biomedical, behavioral, and forensic sciences. *American Psychologist, 60*(1), 115–128.

Parenti, C. (1999). *Lockdown America: Police and prisons in the age of crisis.* New York: Verso.

Parrillo, V. N. (1997). *Stranger to these shores: Race and ethnic relations in the United States* (5th ed.). Boston: Allyn & Bacon.

Reiman, J. (2007). *The rich get richer and the poor get prison* (8th ed.). Boston: Allyn & Bacon.

Rusche, G., & Kircheimer, O. (1968). *Punishment and social structure.* New York: Russell and Russell. (Original work published 1939)

Russell, K. K. (1998). *The color of crime.* New York: New York University Press.

Schrantz, D., & McElroy, J. (2000). *Reducing racial disparity in the criminal justice system: A manual for practitioners and policymakers.* Retrieved October 30, 2008, from *www. sentencingproject.org/doc/publications/rd_reducingracialdisparity.pdf.*

Shaffer, J. N., & Ruback, R. B. (2002, December). Violent victimization as a risk factor for violent offending among juveniles. *Juvenile Justice Bulletin.* Retrieved January 1, 2010, from *www.ncjrs.gov/pdffiles1/ojjdp/195737.pdf.*

Siegel, L. (2008). *Criminology: The core.* Belmont, CA: Thomson Higher Education.

Spitzer, S. (1981). Notes toward a theory of punishment and social change. In S. Spitzer & R. Simon (Eds.), *Research in law and sociology* (Vol. 2, pp. 207–229). London: JAI Press.

Spohn, C., & Holleran, D. (2000). The imprisonment penalty paid by young, unemployed Black and Hispanic male offenders. *Criminology, 38*(1), 381–306.

Takaki, R. (1994). *From different shores: Perspectives on race and ethnicity in America* (2nd ed.). New York: Oxford University Press.

Tonry, M. (1995). *Maglign neglect: Race, crime and punishment.* New York: Oxford University Press.

U.S. Environmental Protection Agency, Office of Air and Radiation, Aerometric Information Retrieval System. (2004). Americas children and the Environment (ACE):

Measure E1: Excellances of air quality standards. U.S. EPA. Available at *www.epa.gov/economics/children/contaminants/e1-sources.html.*

Virkkunen, M. (1986). Reactive hypoglycemic tendency among habitually violent offenders. *Nutrition Reviews, 44*(Suppl.), 94–103.

Wacquant, L. (2003). Toward a dictatorship over the poor. *Punishment and Society, 5*(2) 197–205.

Walker, S., Sphon, C., & Delone, M. (2004). *The color of justice: Race, ethnicity, and crime in America.* Belmont, CA: Wadsworth.

Wallace, D., & Humphries, D. (1981). Urban crime and capitalist accumulation: 1950–1971. In D. Greenberg (Ed.), *Crime and capitalism* (pp. 140–157). Palo Alto, CA: Mayfield.

Weissman, M., Wolf, E., Sowards, K., Abate, C., Weinberg, P., & Marthia, C. (2005). *School yard or prison yard: Improving outcomes for marginalized youth.* Syracuse, NY: Center for Community Alternatives.

Willoughby, W. W. (1910). *The constitutional law of the United States* (Vol. II). New York: Baker, Voorhis.

Wilson, W. J. (1997). *When work disappears: The world of the new urban poor.* New York: Vintage Books.

Women's Prison Association. (1995). *Breaking the cycle of despair: Children of incarcerated mothers. New York: Author.*

Wright, L. E., & Seymour, C. B. (2000). *Working with children and families separated by incarceration: A handbook for child welfare agencies.* Washington, DC: CWLA Press.

Yaryura-Tobias, J. A., & Neziroglu, F. (1975). Violent behavior, brain dysrhythmia and glucose dysfunction: A new syndrome. *Journal of Orthopsychiatry, 4,* 182–188.

# Epilogue

ROBERT L. HAMPTON
THOMAS P. GULLOTTA

More than a quarter century ago, the landmark *Report of the Secretary's Task Force on Black and Minority Health* (U.S. Department of Health and Human Services, 1985) revealed large and persistent gaps in health status among Americans of different racial and ethnic backgrounds. This report not only served as an impetus for addressing health inequalities among racial and ethnic minorities in the United States but also led to the establishment of the Office of Minority Health within the Department of Health and Human Services, with a clear mandate to address these aforementioned disparities. Since the publication of the task force report, health-related issues and health reform have captured increased public and political attention. Discussions of racial disparities have become more prevalent in public media, and advocacy groups have become emboldened to speak out regarding inequities in the health care system. The societal dimensions of the problem are now better understood; many of these health disparities reflect inadequate access to care and other issues (e.g., where health care services are provided) that are associated with differentials in socioeconomic status (SES). It is clear to most, however, that SES is a central but incomplete explanation for health inequalities. Variance in SES does not account for all racial and ethnic disparities in health status, health care, and health-related outcomes.

In the preceding chapters, the reader has gained an understanding of the barriers that exist regarding African Americans' access to appropriate physical and mental health services and some specific issues of concern. Persistent economic and social adversity may afflict individuals over their life course and may have negative implications for both their own health and the health of their children. Consequently, efforts to eliminate the health disparity gap must address a more comprehensive set of factors than some early reformers had envisioned. The issue of health disparities is clearly more than a medical matter.

The economic downturn has been particularly acute for communities of color. Although the unemployment rate for African Americans has been consistently higher than for Whites, the growing number of jobless and uninsured people may exacerbate health disparities. When people lose their jobs, they often lose employer-sponsored health insurance. By mid-2009 one in four Blacks, one in five Hispanics, and about one in 10 Whites have lost health coverage as a result of the economic downturn (Berndt & James, 2009). Researchers have documented that uninsured Americans face significant barriers in accessing care. Compared with people with coverage, the uninsured are less likely to have regular health care providers and more likely to forgo needed care (Rowland, 2009). This tendency can lead to worse health outcomes and potentially more expensive treatments because patients' conditions may deteriorate when they postpone seeking assistance. For a host of diseases and conditions—stroke, cancer, congestive heart failure, diabetes, heart attacks, and hypertension, to name a few—people are likely to have worse outcomes if they lack insurance (Institute of Medicine, 2009).

With the election of Barack Obama to the presidency, there were some who presumed that this event would inaugurate a "postracial" America. In a postracial era, race and ethnicity would no longer significantly influence individual life chances whereby minorities are more disadvantaged than Whites. Race consciousness as we have come to know it would gradually diminish. Unfortunately, race still matters in most areas of American society. As activist Moya Bailey (2008) astutely noted, "It will take more than one man's rise to power to undo centuries old structured oppressions built along the axes of race, gender, sexuality, ability and age. The struggle continues." On the other hand, the new sense of optimism generated by the election could be the basis for positive self-perceptions and proactive health care actions among many who would not have considered either a few years ago.

Social factors are important drivers of health and well-being. Eliminating inequities in health status is clearly a matter that must be addressed by the entire health care industry in both policy and practice. We know, however, that African Americans' experiences outside of the health care practitioner's office, clinic, or department are likely to affect their perceptions and responses within health care settings. In this regard, the belief that we can move beyond race may be a positive sign that health care equity is not far behind.

Reducing the health disparity gap has been a national goal for nearly three decades, and significant work remains for federal, state, and local governments. A society is judged on the basis of how it treats its citizens, especially the most vulnerable. It is important for policymakers and those outside of government to understand that the continuation of inequality across racial and ethnic lines will have health, economic, social, and moral costs that we can no longer afford. Efforts to reduce the health disparity will ultimately benefit society as a whole. A true postracial society will exist when the total health of all of its citizens is realized.

## REFERENCES

Bailey, M. (2008). After the morning after, after the night before ... Retrieved September 16, 2009, from *theunapologeticmexican.org/elmachete/2008/11/10/after-the-morning-after-after-the-night-before-aap11*.

Berndt, J., & James, C. (2009). *The effects of the economic recession on communities of color.* Menlo Park, CA: Henry J. Kaiser Family Foundation. Retrieved September 30, 2009, from *www.kff.org/minorityhealth/upload/7953.pdf*.

Institute of Medicine. (2009). *America's uninsured crisis: Consequences for health and health care.* Washington, DC: National Academies Press.

Rowland, D. (2009). *Making health care work for American families: Medicaid and access to care.* Testimony before the U.S. House of Representatives Committee on Energy and Commerce Subcommittee on Health, March 24, 2009. Retrieved September 27, 2009, from *www.kff.org/healthreform/upload/7880.cfm*.

U.S. Department of Health and Human Services. (1985). *Report of the Secretary's Task Force on Black and Minority Health: Vol. I. Executive summary.* Washington, DC: U.S. Government Printing Office.

# Author Index

# Subject Index

Page numbers followed by *f* indicate figure; *n*, note; and *t*, table

584

# About the Editors

**Robert L. Hampton, PhD**, is Professor of Sociology and Social Work, and former Provost/ Executive Vice President, at Tennessee State University. He previously served York College of the City University of New York as President and Professor of Social Sciences. Prior to joining York College, he served as Associate Provost for Academic Affairs and Dean for Undergraduate Studies, Professor of Family Studies, and Professor of Sociology at the University of Maryland, College Park. In addition, Dr. Hampton has been a Research Associate at Children's Hospital in Boston and Dean of the College at Connecticut College, and held an academic appointment at Harvard Medical School. He has published extensively in the field of family violence, including several edited books, and is one of the founders of the Institute on Domestic Violence in the African American Community.

**Thomas P. Gullotta, MA, MSW**, is CEO of the Child and Family Agency of Southeastern Connecticut and a member of the Psychology and Education Departments at Eastern Connecticut State University. He has published extensively on adolescents and primary prevention, serving as senior author of the fourth edition of *The Adolescent Experience*, coeditor of *The Encyclopedia of Primary Prevention and Health Promotion*, senior book series editor for *Issues in Children's and Families' Lives*, and editor emeritus of the *Journal of Primary Prevention*. Mr. Gullotta also holds editorial appointments on the *Journal of Early Adolescence, Journal of Adolescent Research,* and *Journal of Educational and Psychological Consultation*. In 1999 he was honored by the Society for Community Research and Action, Division 27 of the American Psychological Association, with their Distinguished Contributions to Practice in Community Psychology Award.

**Raymond L. Crowel, PsyD**, is Vice President for Human Service Systems at ICF International, where he is responsible for the development and implementation of its National Technical Assistance and Evaluation Center, focused on strengthening the National Child Welfare system of care for children. Dr. Crowel also works on addressing issues of disaster/terrorism preparedness, response, and recovery, and has served as Director of Child and Adolescent Services for Baltimore Mental Health Systems, the local mental health authority for Baltimore City, where he developed and implemented mental health crisis and trauma response programs. While on the faculty at the School of Public Health at Johns Hopkins University, he served as director of an internationally recognized, federal- and state-funded initiative to develop integrated systems of care for children with serious emotional disturbance. Throughout his career in both public service and private practice, Dr. Crowel has focused on the role of mental health in the promotion of healthy development in children and families.

# Contributors

**Christon George Arthur, PhD,** is Associate Professor, Educational Administration, and Associate Dean, College of Education, Tennessee State University. His awards include Fellow, Organization of American States; Researcher of the Year, Department of Educational Administration; Faculty of the Year, Tennessee State University; and Marquis' Who's Who in America, 2006. His research agenda is catered around the psychosocial factors that explain/predict student learning. He has authored several publications and made many scholarly presentations on the topic.

**Rahn Kennedy Bailey, MD, FAPA,** is Chair of the Department of Psychiatry at Meharry Medical College, with clinical appointments at Tulane and Baylor Colleges of Medicine. He is dual-board-certified in general psychiatry and forensic psychiatry. Dr. Bailey has been featured live on MSNBC television as well as on CNN and on local TV/radio discussing psychiatric treatment, the insanity defense, and violent criminal behaviors. Dr. Bailey is currently the host of "Good Psychiatry Is Good Medicine," a weekly radio program on Voice America Internet Radio.

**Donna Holland Barnes, PhD,** is cofounder and President of the National Organization for People of Color against Suicide and a founding member of the National Council for Suicide Prevention. She has served on several national and local committees that pertain to suicidal behavior, sits on the board of the American Foundation for Suicide Prevention, and appears frequently on radio talk shows and in national magazines on the subject of suicide. Dr. Barnes is also Research Professor at Howard University's Psychiatry Department in Washington, DC, where she teaches suicide risk management to residents and third-year medical students and conducts research on families who have lost someone to suicide. She is the recipient of the Garrett Lee Smith Memorial Fund for Suicide Prevention on College Campuses through the Substance Abuse and Mental Health Services Administration for suicide prevention on Howard's campus.

**Bettina M. Beech** is Professor in the Division of Public Health Sciences and the Department of Pediatrics at Wake Forest University School of Medicine and Co-Director of the Maya Angelou Center for Health Equity. She has a unique interdisciplinary background that integrates public health, cancer prevention and control, health disparities, nutrition, and pediatric obesity prevention and treatment. Dr. Beech's research focuses on the role of nutritional factors in the primary and secondary prevention of chronic diseases, with a particular focus on childhood obesity and related problems such as diabetes, metabolic syndrome, and cancer. She is the lead editor of *Race and Research in Focus: Perspectives on Minority Participation in Health Studies*, published by the American Public Health Association.

**Derrick J. Beech, MD, FACS**, is Professor in the and Chair, Department of Surgery, Meharry Medical College. He has received numerous honors and awards, including membership in the Phi Kappa Phi Honor Society, Alpha Omega Alpha Honor Medical Society, and Who's Who in Medicine and Healthcare. A diplomat of the American Board of Surgery and a Fellow of the American College of Surgeons, Dr. Beech has been actively involved in medical education and the clinical practice of cancer surgery. He is a member of multiple national scientific organizations, including the American College of Surgeons, the American Association of Cancer Education, the Society of Black Academic Surgeons, and the Society of Surgical Oncology. He is a respected author in the field of surgery, with more than 170 publications; has delivered over 90 local and national presentations; and has served as visiting professor at many leading institutions.

**Rhonda BeLue, PhD**, is Assistant Professor of Health Policy and Administration at The Pennsylvania State University. She was formerly employed as a local public health worker responsible for the evaluation of community health programs for families in the Nashville, Tennessee, area. Dr. BeLue's research program involves the investigation of the complex interaction among risk factors for chronic diseases in African and African American populations. Her work examines the various contexts (individual, family, health care facility, and community) in which individuals must manage their illnesses. She is particularly interested in examining those conditions that have been most associated with stress-related inflammatory processes, such as cardiovascular disease, obesity, and diabetes.

**Holly L. Blackmon, BS**, is a senior research associate for Rahn Kennedy Bailey, as well as program administrator for several scientific sections (Psychiatry and the Behavioral Sciences, Anesthesiology, and Women's Health) for the National Medical Association (NMA). She oversees all grant-writing and research responsibilities along with other clinical projects for Dr. Bailey and the scientific sections of the NMA just listed. Ms. Blackmon is a member of the Alliance of Continuing Medical Education and has collaborated with Dr. Bailey on several projects, including a recent article in the *Journal of the National Medical Association*. She has assisted Dr. Bailey with forensic research for lectures on various topics, including confidentiality, the insanity defense, ethnic differences in psychopharmacology, competency, sexual violence, and medical student education.

**Richard Briscoe, PhD**, is Assistant Professor in the Department of Child and Family Studies at the University of South Florida. He has 30 years of experience in providing mental health and support services and in training mental health professionals. Dr. Briscoe specializes in training minorities in the mental health profession and in university–community partnerships. His interests are strengths of African American families, participatory community-based research with African American communities, and the development of strategies to improve service delivery systems within neighborhood-based programs.

**Deborah J. Burris-Kitchen, PhD**, is Associate Professor of Criminology at Tennessee State University. She is the author of *Female Gang Participation: The Role of African-American Women in the Informal Drug Economy and Gang Activities* and *Short Rage: An Autobiographical Look at Heightism in America*. She also coauthored an article on racism in higher education in the *College Student Journal*. Dr. Burris-Kitchen is an activist against violence, racism, exploitation, greed, and capitalism.

**Tamara M. Carter, MSW, LCSW**, is a lecturer in the Department of Social Work at Fayetteville State University. She has over 15 years of experience in social work practice, with a focus on family and children's services. Ms. Carter's research interests include social work and spirituality, foster care and adoptions, welfare reform, and adolescent pregnancy prevention.

**Ruth Chu-lien Chao, PhD**, is Assistant Professor at the University of Denver, where she teaches diversity, psychopathology, counseling theories, and practicum, among other subjects. Having taught at a marginally historically black university, Tennessee State University, she is strongly interested in African American psychology, specifically African Americans' distinctive well-being, support resources, and admirable resilience. Her recent book, *Multicultural Competencies in Counseling*, as well as her other publications, presentations, and book chapters, describe multicultural issues in counseling. Among her awards is the American Psychological Foundation Grant in Counseling Psychology for her research project "Multiculturally Sensitive Mental Health Checklist," which targets mental health among African Americans.

**Stacey Kevin Close, PhD**, is Professor of History at Eastern Connecticut State University, where he teaches such courses as African American History to 1877, History of the South, Black Nationalism, Churches and the Civil Rights Movement, and African American Religion. His publications can be found in the *Journal of Negro History*, *Connecticut Review*, *Connecticut History*, *The Griot*, *Illinois School Journal*, and *Edwin Mellen Press*. Dr. Close has presented papers at the Association for the Study of Afro-American Life and History, the Southern Conference on African American Studies, the Association for the Study of Connecticut History, and the Professional and Organizational Network.

**Michelle M. Cloutier, MD**, is Professor of Pediatrics at the University of Connecticut Health Center and Director of the Asthma Center at Connecticut Children's Medical Center. She has received numerous teaching awards from students and residents and has authored more than 100 journal articles and book chapters in the areas of airway epithelial transport and health services research in pediatric asthma.

**Donelda A. Cook, PhD**, a licensed psychologist and ordained clergy, is Assistant Vice President for Student Development, Director of the Counseling Center, and Affiliate Faculty of Pastoral Counseling at Loyola University in Maryland. Her scholarship and publications focus on multicultural psychology, with an emphasis on racial and cultural issues in clinical supervision, and the integration of spirituality and psychology in psychotherapy with African Americans. Dr. Cook serves on the editorial board of *Psychotherapy: Theory, Research, Practice, Training* and is an ad hoc reviewer for *Cultural Diversity and Ethnic Minority Psychology*. She has been a mental health consultant for African American churches since 1985.

**Lori E. Crosby, PsyD**, is Associate Professor of Pediatrics in the Division of Behavioral Medicine and Clinical Psychology at Cincinnati Children's Hospital Medical Center and the University of Cincinnati College of Medicine. Dr. Crosby has expertise in the assessment and treatment of anxiety disorders in children and adolescents. Her broad research interests are in community-based participatory research, health disparities, sickle cell disease, chronic pain, adolescent health, and anxiety and depression.

**Jacquelyn Duval-Harvey, PhD**, is Deputy Commissioner for Youth and Family Programs at the Baltimore City Health Department, where she is responsible for school health and adult services, maternal and child health programs, and the Office of Youth Violence Prevention. Dr. Duval-Harvey provides community education on attention-deficit/hyperactivity disorder through CHADD (Children and Adults with Attention Deficit/Hyperactivity Disorder) sponsorship.

**M. Kathleen Figaro, MD, MS**, is Endocrine Fellow at Vanderbilt University. She currently does research on the biological causes of insulin resistance. Dr. Figaro is especially interested in understanding and improving the inflammatory changes associated with diabetes to lessen its long-term physical impact on health.

**Shana Jeanelle Gage, MD**, is a second-year resident at Howard University Hospital. She has worked as an Upward Bound math and science mentor, creating and implementing curricula for underprivileged youth interested in the fields of science and medicine. Dr. Gage is a recent recipient of the Jeanne M. Spurlock Outstanding Resident Award given by the Black Psychiatrists of America and plans to pursue a rewarding career in the field of child and adolescent psychiatry.

**Tamika D. Gilreath, PhD**, is Assistant Professor of Social Work at the University of Southern California. Her research interests include tobacco-related health disparities, minority adolescent health, and adolescent tobacco consumption in sub-Saharan Africa. Dr. Gilreath has coauthored peer-reviewed articles and presented at national conferences on these topics.

**Thomas P. Gullotta, MA, MSW.** *See* "About the Editors."

**Robert L. Hampton, PhD.** *See* "About the Editors."

**Brenda Jones Harden, PhD, MSW**, Associate Professor in the Department of Human Development at the University of Maryland, College Park, is a developmental and clinical psychologist whose work has spanned the policy, practice, and research arenas. For over 30 years, she has focused on the developmental and mental health needs of young children at environmental risk, specifically those who have been maltreated, are in the foster care system, or are exposed to multiple family risks such as maternal depression, parental substance use, and poverty. She is the author of numerous publications, including the book *Infants in Child Welfare: A Developmental Perspective on Policy and Practice*.

**Aminifu R. Harvey, DSW, LICSW**, is Professor of Social Work at Fayetteville State University. He was the founder and executive director of the MAAT Center in Washington, DC, which provides culturally competent services to African American families and youth. Dr. Harvey is a pioneer in Africentric social work and the development of rites-of-passage programs and has also developed HIV/AIDS intervention programs. His area of interest is the development of culturally competent interventions for African Americans, especially males.

**David C. Henderson, MD**, is Associate Professor of Psychiatry at Harvard Medical School and Associate Psychiatrist at the Massachusetts General Hospital (MGH). He serves as Medical Director for the MGH Harvard Program in Refugee Trauma; Director of the MGH Chester M. Pierce, MD, Division of Global Psychiatry; Director of the MGH Schizophrenia, Diabetes, and Weight Reduction Research; Director of the MGH Clozapine Program; and Associate Director of the MGH Schizophrenia Program. Dr. Henderson is also editor of the *International Journal of Culture and Mental Health*. His main research interests focus on psychopharmacology, schizophrenia, glucose and lipid metabolism and cardiovascular disease, and the impact of ethnicity and culture on psychiatry. He also studies the impact of trauma in areas of mass violence and develops programs to assist vulnerable populations, including projects in Rwanda, Cambodia, East Timor, Bosnia, Peru, Liberia, New Orleans, and New York City.

**Charles H. Hennekens, MD, DrPH**, is currently the first Sir Richard Doll Research Professor in the Department of Clinical Science and Medical Education and Center of Excellence at Florida Atlantic University. He was the first John Snow Professor as well as the first Eugene Braunwald Professor of Medicine at Harvard Medical School. Dr. Hennekens's research includes investigations to reduce disparities in mortality between African Americans and Caucasians. From 1995 to 2005 he was the third most widely cited medical researcher in the world, and five of the top 20 were his former fellows and/or trainees.

**Oliver J. Johnson, PhD, LMSW, CAC-1**, is Assistant Professor of Social Work at Fayetteville State University. He has lectured and conducted workshops locally and nationally in a variety of forums on issues pivotal to the promotion of health and wellness among African American families.

**Gary King, PhD**, is a medical sociologist and Professor of Biobehavioral Health at The Pennsylvania State University. His primary interests are the smoking behavior of African Americans, international tobacco consumption in France and Africa, and uses of the race concept in health. Dr. King has been principal investigator of National Institutes of Health research and privately funded grants on tobacco control and was a contributing author to the 1998 *Surgeon General's Report on Tobacco Use among U.S. Racial/Ethnic Minority Groups*.

**Jaslean J. La Taillade, PhD**, is Assistant Professor in the Department of Family Science at the University of Maryland, College Park. Her research examines how culture-specific factors as well as factors common to all intimate relationships predict changes in satisfaction and stability for African American couples. She was awarded a National Institute of Child Health and Human Development Minority Supplement, in conjunction with Dr. Sandra Hofferth, to investigate how changes in relationship quality, residence, and stability affect fathering behaviors among African Americans. Dr. La Taillade's additional research focus is on couple therapy and domestic violence, and she is collaborating in an evaluation of a couple intervention program designed to prevent psychological and physical abuse.

**William B. Lawson, MD, PhD, FAPA**, is Professor and Chair of the Department of Psychiatry and Behavioral Sciences at Howard University College of Medicine; Distinguished Fellow of the American Psychiatric Association; a member of Alpha Omega Alpha, the medical honor society; past Chair of the Section of Psychiatry and Behavioral Sciences of the National Medical Association; and past President of Black Psychiatrists of America. Dr. Lawson is a recipient of the National Alliance on Mental Illness Exemplary Psychiatrist Award, the Black Psychiatrists of America Andrea Delgado Award, the American Psychiatric Association Jeanne Spurlock Award, and the E. Y. Williams Clinical Scholar of Distinction Award from the Psychiatry and Behavioral Sciences Section of the National Medical Association. He was also named one of "America's Leading Black Doctors" by *Black Enterprise* magazine. He has received state, federal, and foundation support for research in the cultural and biological aspects of the diagnosis and treatment of mental disorders and has authored over 100 publications.

**Robert S. Levine, MD**, is Professor of Family and Community Medicine at Meharry Medical College. He is certified as a specialist in preventive medicine, and his research focus is on elimination of racial disparities in health.

**Jessica Mazza, MSPH,** is a research assistant and a doctoral student at the University of Illinois at Chicago. She previously served as a research assistant at the Louis de la Parte Florida Mental Health Institute. Ms. Mazza is experienced in qualitative research and program implementation. Her research interests include mental health systems and community-based behavioral health services.

**Gwen McClain, MA,** is a social and behavioral researcher in the Department of Child and Family Studies, Louis de la Parte Florida Mental Health Institute, University of South Florida, where she is responsible for QA/CQI for the Florida's Center for the Advancement of Child Welfare Practice. She has 20 years of experience in quantitative and qualitative research methods. Her professional interests include strengths in African American families and communities, culturally competent research and development strategies that promote empowerment of individuals and communities, and social and economic justice.

**Annie McCullough-Chavis, MSW, EdD,** is Associate Professor of Social Work at Fayetteville State University. She has presented at national, regional, state, and local conferences concerning genograms and family assessment, assessment with African American families, and mentoring students in schools. Dr. McCullough-Chavis's research interests include genograms and assessment in family social work practice, assessment and intervention with African American families, cultural competency, and mentoring.

**April R. McDowell, MS,** is a family science doctoral student at the University of Maryland, College Park. As an undergraduate, she worked as a research assistant on a longitudinal study investigating continuity in parent–young adult relationships, published in the *Journal of Family Issues.* As a graduate student, she worked with Kevin Roy to code qualitative life history interviews from fatherhood data sets and presented the findings of her master's thesis, on men's perceptions of social support during incarceration and community reentry, at the annual meeting of the Association for Behavioral and Cognitive Therapies. Ms. McDowell is now working with Jaslean La Taillade on several research projects focused on Black and multiracial couples in the United States. Her primary research interests include chronic illness in families and couple relationships within Black and multiracial families.

**Peter Edmund Millet, PhD,** is an educator, administrator, and licensed clinical psychologist. Since 2004, he has served as Dean of the College of Education at Tennessee State University. Prior to becoming Dean, he served as Head of the Department of Psychology for 5 years. An avid researcher, for the last 8 years, Dr. Millet has served as Head of the University's Institutional Review Board for the Protection of Human Subjects. His scholarly interests focus on two primary areas: psychology and education.

**Angela Neal-Barnett, PhD,** Associate Professor of Psychology at Kent State University, is a national award-winning psychologist, author, and leading expert on anxiety disorders among African Americans. She is the recipient of grants from the National Institute of Mental Health, the National Institutes of Health, the National Science Foundation, the Ohio Children's Trust Fund, the Ohio Commission on Minority Health, the Ohio Board of Regents, the American Psychological Association, Pfizer, and the Health Priorities Trust Fund. Dr. Neal-Barnett is the author of *Soothe Your Nerves: The Black Woman's Guide to Understanding and Overcoming Anxiety, Panic, and Fear.*

**Teresa Nesman, PhD,** is Research Assistant Professor in the Department of Child and Family Studies at the Louis de la Parte Florida Mental Health Institute. Her work includes research on development of systems of care for children's mental health and evaluation of community-based programs focusing on Latino children and youth. Dr. Nesman has contributed to book chapters, monographs, articles, and reports on cultural competence in children's mental health, Latino student dropout, field-based experience in outcome evaluation, and interagency collaboration.

**Freida Hopkins Outlaw, PhD**, is Assistant Commissioner of the Tennessee Department of Mental Health and Developmental Disabilities. She has experience as a clinician, educator, and researcher in the delivery of psychiatric care in underserved areas. Dr. Outlaw has written extensively in the areas of cultural diversity, African American women and depression, management of aggression, seclusion and restraint, and the role of religion, spirituality, and prayer for persons with cancer.

**Marcus Pope, MEd**, is Associate Director of the Institute on Domestic Violence in the African American Community, a research and outreach institute housed at the University of Minnesota School of Social Work. He has a rich background in nonprofit management, project management, and direct services through community-based programs.

**Jessica M. Ramos, BA**, is a research assistant at the Child and Family Agency of Southeastern Connecticut. She has assisted in the editorial process of books on primary prevention, prevention and treatment of behavioral problems in childhood and adolescents, Asperger syndrome, promotion of prosocial behavior, and interpersonal violence in the African American community. She is involved in agency research and reviews cases for quality assurance.

**Kenneth M. Rogers, MD, MPH**, is a child and adolescent psychiatrist at the University of Maryland School of Medicine. His research and clinical interest is in the areas of aggression, violence, and juvenile justice.

**Bernadette Blount Salley, MM**, is a composer, performer, educator, and musical clinician with international experience. Her educational experience includes teaching music in public schools in Virginia and Ohio. In addition to teaching piano, Ms. Salley is Assistant Minister of Music and the principal accompanist at Arlington Church of God, Akron, Ohio.

**Wendy R. Schneider, RN, MSN, CCRC**, is Affiliate Clinical Instructor in the Department of Clinical Science and Medical Education and Center of Excellence at Florida Atlantic University. She also serves as Project Director at Florida Atlantic University of several multicenter investigator-initiated research trials and has served as Clinical Coordinator of individual clinical sites in multicenter randomized trials, especially for cardiovascular disease.

**Reginald D. Simmons, PhD**, is Assistant Professor in the Criminology and Criminal Justice Department of Central Connecticut State University, where he specializes in juvenile delinquency prevention, youth development, and culturally responsive intervention. He has provided direct clinical services to youth and families in school, community, and juvenile justice settings, as well as supervised programs and initiatives that provided behavioral health intervention to hundreds of youth and families of color in urban areas. Dr. Simmons, a licensed clinical psychologist, continues to see adolescents and families in private practice in the city of New Haven, Connecticut.

**Francis L. Stevens, MS**, is completing his doctorate in counseling psychology at Tennessee State University. His research looks at how aspects of identity such as race and gender affect an individual's psychological well-being. He has presented at numerous conferences, including the annual meeting of the American Psychological Association and the Annual Conference on Men and Masculinities. He recently defended his dissertation,

"Construction of an Authentic Gender Identity." Mr. Stevens has taught various courses in psychology as an adjunct instructor at Tennessee State University and Hudson Valley Community College and will be completing his clinical training as a psychology intern at the University of Rochester Counseling Center.

**Verla M. Vaughan, PhD, RN,** is Professor in the School of Nursing at Tennessee State University. She is a researcher in the field of diabetes. Her research focuses on interventions to improve health outcomes among elderly African Americans with diabetes.

**Gretchen Chase Vaughn, PhD,** has worked extensively on the health and mental health effects of behavioral interventions among ethnic-minority populations. She has devoted more than 20 years to national efforts in community-rooted prevention and mental health services for underserved populations. Dr. Vaughn, a licensed clinical psychologist, has designed and coordinated the evaluation of programs that address a range of public and behavioral health issues such as substance abuse, HIV/AIDS, parent skills training, and trauma. She has also worked extensively with academic institutions, state and federal agencies, and nonprofit organizations to provide consultation, supervision, training, technical assistance, evaluation support, and policy analysis.

**Guy-Lucien Whembolua, PhD,** a Congolese (DRC) citizen, is a postdoctoral research associate in the Program in Health Disparities Research in the Department of Family Medicine and Community Health at the University of Minnesota. His primary research interests include using biomarkers to understand the etiology of drugs of abuse and drug abuse–related health disparities. The primary aim of his research is to elucidate biobehavioral factors to be targeted through preventive interventions within minority communities in the United States and abroad.

**Jamell White, MSW, LCSW-C, MS,** is a doctoral student at the University of Maryland, College Park, Department of Human Development. She is a therapist and case manager specializing in children with autism spectrum disorders and other developmental disabilities. Her research area of interest is the social and emotional development of young children.

**Kristin N. Williams-Washington, MA,** is an American Psychological Association Minority Fellow and doctoral candidate in clinical psychology with a concentration in diversity and multiculturalism at Argosy University in Washington, DC. Her areas of interest include underserved populations, cultural and linguistic competence, cultural disparities, and the biopsychosocial effects of trauma.

**Maxine Woodside, EdD,** is a community leader and chair of Tampa Bay Community and Family Development Corporation, a collaborative of community residents, representatives from community agencies, schools, and partners from the university to enhance the health, educational, and social services and the quality of life of neighborhood residents. Dr. Woodside is a pastor of community involvement for a faith-based community and family development corporation and is an ordained minister. She has served various positions with the public school system in the area of youth services.